DRUGS IN VETERINARY PRACTICE

DRUGS IN
VETERINARY PRACTICE

Joseph S. Spinelli, D.V.M.

Associate Clinical Professor of Veterinary Medicine,
School of Pharmacy; Director, Animal Care Facility,
University of California, San Francisco, California

L. Reed Enos, Pharm.D.

Chief Pharmacist, Veterinary Medicine Teaching Hospital;
Lecturer, Department of Medicine, School of Veterinary Medicine,
University of California, Davis, California;
Clinical Instructor, Division of Clinical Pharmacy,
School of Pharmacy, University of California,
San Francisco, California

with 92 illustrations

The C. V. Mosby Company

Saint Louis 1978

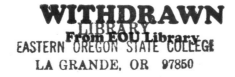

The C. V. Mosby Company
11830 Westline Industrial Drive, St. Louis, Missouri 63141

Library of Congress Cataloging in Publication Data

Spinelli, Joseph S   1937-
    Drugs in veterinary practice.

    Bibliography: p.
    Includes index.
    1. Veterinary drugs. 2. Veterinary medicine—
Practice. I. Enos, Laurence Reed, 1942-   joint
author. II. Title. [DNLM: 1. Animal diseases—
Drug therapy. 2. Veterinary medicine. SF915 S757d]
SF917.S73   636.089′5′1   78-7046
ISBN 0-8016-4749-5

GW/CB/CB   9 8 7 6 5 4 3 2 1

Preface

The delivery of quality health care for animals is becoming more dependent on the combined efforts of various professional groups. Examples of this interdependence include the practice of clinical pharmacy in numerous veterinary medical teaching hospitals, the growing professionalism of animal health technicians, and the teaching of courses of veterinary drugs in numerous schools of pharmacy.

The purpose of this text is to discuss the use of drugs and biologicals in the prevention and treatment of animal diseases. The material is directed primarily to students and practitioners of pharmacy and animal health technology. It is our belief that there is a largely unexploited need for pharmacists to participate in veterinary therapeutics at the clinical level. It is our hope that this text will spark pharmacists' interest in veterinary therapeutics and will encourage them to modify their skills in an appropriate manner to enable them to make a contribution to the drug therapy of animal diseases.

Because animal health technicians will administer drugs discussed in this text, it is important for them to have an understanding of why the drugs are used, how they work, and their effects, toxicity, doses, and administration.

Although many animal diseases are discussed in this text, it is not a book about animal diseases. Rather it is a book about drugs. Diseases are only discussed to put the use of drugs in a clinical rather than abstract framework. Because diseases are used to illustrate drug use, the only diseases discussed in this text are those which best illustrate the proper use of veterinary drugs. Many important animal diseases are therefore not discussed here.

Throughout the text, drugs are referred to by their generic names. For the most part, the generic names of drugs are the same as used by I. S. Rossoff in *Handbook of Veterinary Drugs.** In Appendices H and I, examples of veterinary brand names are listed for the biologicals and generic drugs discussed in the text. The inclusion of brand names does not constitute our endorsement of the products, neither does failure to include brand names constitute our nonendorsement of those brands.

All dosage forms discussed in the text are expressed in milligrams per kilogram. For those who prefer the more traditional grains, ounces, and pounds, conversion tables in Appendix D can be used. To clarify words and phrases that appear in the text, definitions are provided in the Glossary (Appendix J).

---

*Rossoff, I. S.: Handbook of veterinary drugs, New York, 1974, Springer Publishing Co.

Doses for drugs are recommended throughout the text. The doses were obtained from the latest clinical and research information in the literature. Although we have done everything possible to check the accuracy of recommended doses, we cannot be responsible for ineffectiveness or toxic reactions resulting from the use of drugs as recommended in the text. Before any drug discussed here is used, the most recent recommendations of the manufacturer should be consulted. When that information is compared to the information in this text, a judgment regarding the most appropriate dose can be made.

One important group of drugs, veterinary anesthetics, is not discussed in the text. Our intent is to discuss drugs used in the prevention and treatment of animal diseases. Anesthetics are not generally used in the therapy of animal diseases but rather as tools to facilitate diagnostic, surgical, and therapeutic procedures. The proper application of anesthetics is a complex and exacting science: anesthesiology. Anyone who would use these drugs should have a thorough training in veterinary anesthesiology. Because a full discussion of anesthesiology and anesthetics would necessarily go far beyond the scope of this text, and since excellent textbooks on veterinary anesthesiology exist,* we decided not to attempt to cover this subject in these pages.

We would like to thank all those whose efforts during the past three years have resulted in this text. Yvonne Drisdell coordinated the literature search and all phases of the manuscript preparation. When we bogged down, her optimism often gave us the will to keep going. We particularly thank her for her patience and for never suggesting

that we drop this project and direct our energies elsewhere. For the sake of brevity, the names of those who made such suggestions will not be listed here. Many others have been involved with the typing of various stages of the manuscript. We thank them and particularly thank Rae Weinstein, who coordinated that effort during the "home stretch." We appreciate the long hours and hard work of Kathleen Schmidt to produce all the original drawings for the text. We believe that her drawings clearly illustrate many principles of anatomy and physiology necessary for the understanding of the use of veterinary drugs. We are also grateful to Debbie Hecht, a fourth-year pharmacy student at the University of California, for her preparation of the generic–brand name list (Appendices H and I). Ms. Schmidt is an aspiring medical illustrator, and Ms. Hecht is aspiring to a career in veterinary pharmacy. We believe that the quality of the work they performed in the preparation of this text indicates that both can look forward to promising careers. We are also indebted to the many students and colleagues at both the Davis and San Francisco campuses of the University of California who reviewed and commented on portions of the manuscript.

Jerome Fried, who worked as an editorial consultant on the book, was killed in an automobile accident after editing half the chapters. In those chapters he converted our material from what we said to what we meant to say. Whereas we were primarily concerned with the technical accuracy of the manuscript, his concern was with both the technical aspect and also that the reader understand what we were saying. We have attempted to style all the chapters after the model that he provided us. His tragic and untimely death reminded us that in addition to various noninfectious and infectious diseases, the automobile is a major cause of death and injury to both people and animals.

Joseph S. Spinelli
L. Reed Enos

---

*Lumb, W. V., and Jones, E. W.: Veterinary anesthesia, Philadelphia, 1973, Lea & Febiger; Short, C. E.: Clinical veterinary anesthesia: a guide for the practitioner, St. Louis, 1974, The C. V. Mosby Co.; Soma, L. R.: Textbook of veterinary anesthesia, Baltimore, 1971, The Williams & Wilkins Co.

Contents

Appendices

DRUGS IN VETERINARY PRACTICE

1

INTRODUCTION TO THE USE OF
Veterinary drugs

THE USE OF VETERINARY DRUGS

A drug in veterinary practice is broadly defined as any chemical used to prevent, diagnose, or treat diseases in domestic animals. A distinction is usually made between drugs and biologicals.

A biological is a product such as a vaccine, toxoid, serum, antigen, or antitoxin. Biologicals tend to be identified by the source and/or purpose for which they are used, for example, feline panleukopenia vaccine, tetanus toxoid, canine distemper antiserum, flea antigen, and tetanus antitoxin.

A drug is described by a generic name, which refers to the active components of the preparation. When the chemical formula of a drug is known, the drug may also have a chemical name. For example, the generic name of a commonly used veterinary pesticide is dichlorvos. The chemical name is 0,0 dimethyl-2,2-dichlorovinyl dimethyl phosphate. For some drugs the generic and chemical names are the same, for example, 20% calcium gluconate.

The use of drugs affects the course of a disease in one of three ways: it may have no influence on the outcome of the disease, it may speed the recovery of the animal, or it may make the animal worse.

Because the use of drugs and biologicals is so common in the twentieth century, one can easily get the impression that drugs and biologicals are as necessary for the survival of animal life as food, water, and air. One often forgets that the development and use of safe and effective drugs and biologicals in veterinary medicine are relatively recent occurrences. Although there is little question that the proper use of drugs and biologicals can improve the health and well-being of both humans and animals and can be extremely important to individual members of any species, they are not necessary for the survival of the human or animal species discussed in this book. Both animals and humans evolved in an environment in which biologicals and drugs were not used.

Emphasis on technology in discussing improvements in human and animal health over the past century may lead one to the conclusion that these advances have stemmed primarily from the availability of biologicals,

1

drugs, and surgical skills. Although these factors are important, many improvements in the quality of human and animal life have resulted from technologies not generally associated with either human or veterinary medicine. For example, probably the greatest contribution to the health of man has been the utilization of a closed sewer system that prevents the spread of a wide variety of viral, bacterial, and parasitic diseases. In addition, improved nutrition for the masses has resulted in maximizing the genetic potential for disease resistance. Like humans, animals have the best chance of remaining healthy when they are kept in environments which allow them to maximize the potential resistance to disease that has developed through millions of years of evolution and survival of the fittest. However, domesticated animals are captive, and their environment is totally at the control of their captors, man. In the wild, animals are able to select nutritious diets and to range over an area sufficiently wide to be relatively free of fecal contamination. However, humans control the level of nutrition and the amount of feces in the domesticated animal's environment.

Generally, animals living in a good environment without drugs and biologicals will be healthier than animals living in a bad environment but supported by biologicals and drugs. Therefore those involved with animal health must evaluate animal diseases in light of the environment in which animals live. Frequently, improving that environment is more important than falling back on drug therapy.

Most sick animals would survive without the intervention of drugs. Thus the first decision that must be made by a veterinarian faced with a sick animal is whether to attempt to shorten the course of the disease by using drugs. If the decision is made to use drugs, then many factors are involved in the choice of those drugs. The factors that influence the choice of a veterinary drug to treat a particular disease are discussed in Chapter 2. The most important of these factors are the safety and the efficacy (effectiveness) of the drug.

One must weigh the benefit that will be derived from the drug against the damage that it may do. If the chances are high that the animal will succumb to a disease, a relatively toxic drug may be chosen. On the other hand, if the chances are high that the animal will recover without drug intervention, it would be unwise to select a drug with a high toxic potential.

Drugs must be continually investigated both experimentally and clinically to determine whether they are truly effective. That a drug has been traditionally used to treat a specific condition is not necessarily an indication that the drug is effective. If animals are ill and are given a drug and they recover, the conclusion can be that the drug caused the cure. However, a look at a population of animals with the same disease that received no drug might reveal that just as many animals recovered; one might therefore conclude that the recovery was due to nature and not the drug.

Our basic approach in this book will be a brief examination of conditions in animals for which drugs and biologicals are used, a brief discussion of the actions of the drugs and biologicals, an evaluation of them in terms of their safety and effectiveness, and presentation of information on dosage and administration.

INTERDEPENDENCE OF HUMAN AND ANIMAL HEALTH

The domestic animal population of the United States far exceeds the human population. According to the Animal Health Institute, the livestock population of the United States in 1972 was 3 billion broiler chickens, 3 hundred million laying hens, 94 million hogs, 43 million beef cattle, and 12 million dairy cattle. In addition, the Unites States dog population has been estimated at 25 to 35 million and the cat population at 30 million.[3]

Human and animal health are related in the following ways:

1. *Some infections are transmitted from animals to humans.* These infections are

called "zoonotic infections." Perhaps the most feared zoonotic infection is rabies, since once the symptoms are evident in humans, the disease is almost universally fatal. The most common source of infection in humans is dog bites. The incidence of rabies in humans has been reduced through massive immunization programs against rabies in dogs. In the United States the number of cases in humans have decreased from an average of 22 per year in the years 1946 to 1950 to only one or two per year since 1963. A similar decrease of the disease has occurred in the canine population. In 1946 there were more than 8000 cases of rabies in dogs compared with 129 in 1975.

In the early 1900s in the United States tuberculosis was the leading killer of people. The type that was responsible for almost all tuberculosis of the bones and joints, the digestive system, and all other organs except the lungs was contracted by humans from cattle. In addition, as much as 10% of pulmonary tuberculosis in humans was contracted from cattle. The high incidence of tuberculosis in cattle not only resulted in human infections but lowered the value of the cattle as food-producing animals. Today in the United States tuberculosis is not as serious a human killer as it once was; nonpulmonary tuberculosis has almost entirely disappeared. A major reason for this has been the direct and indirect effects of a successful nationwide campaign that has nearly eliminated tuberculosis from American cattle.[10]

In 1947 when a program to eliminate brucellosis from cattle commenced, the incidence of the disease in humans was 4.4 cases per 100,000 people. With the progress in the control of the disease in the livestock population, the level was reduced to 0.13 cases per 100,000 people in 1965.[10]

2. *Animals produce protein for human nutrition.* Products from domestic animals—meat, dairy products, and eggs—provide a major source of dietary protein of high biological value. The health of livestock influences the average rate of productivity for the species (for example, pounds of meat gained or pounds of milk produced during a period of time) and the efficiency of feed conversion (that is, the rate of gain compared with pounds of feed consumed). In an attempt to meet the world's expanding protein needs, the livestock industry has had to increase its efficiency substantially. Animal health has been a major factor in the dramatic increases that have occurred in livestock production over the past thirty years. For example, according to the Animal Health Institute, in 1947 in the United States 500 million broilers were raised yearly, and 30% of these were lost to disease. In 1972, 3 billion broilers were raised, with less than a 3% loss.

3. *Animals contribute to the psychological well-being of man.* Both children and adults develop strong emotional ties with their animal companions. A wide variety of animals have been domesticated as pets. Young children often make pets of small rodent species. They have the opportunity to see within a couple of years the complete life cycle of the species and from that learn the meaning of birth, life, and finally death. Having to care for a pet can instill some sense of responsibility in a child. In a similar way, being involved with domesticated farm animals in a 4-H or Future Farmers of America project teaches those living in rural environments the responsibility of attending to the needs of domesticated livestock. Horses provide companionship and a form of recreation for many people, and companion pets provide comfort for the elderly, who frequently live alone.

For many years, it was thought that keeping pets was a luxury. However, who is to say that it is a luxury for a child to have the companionship and responsibility of caring for a pet? Who is to say that it is an extravagance for an elderly person living alone to have a pet bird, cat, or dog?

The demand by pet owners for high-quality veterinary care has resulted in veterinarians developing clinics and modes of treatment that rival those provided for human patients. In addition, the use of high-quality animal health products to prevent and treat diseases in companion animals helps to assure pets a maximum life span relatively free from disease.

4. *The human environment can become contaminated with veterinary drugs.* Because a wide variety of animal health products are used in the livestock population, there is always a danger that meat, dairy products, and eggs will be contaminated by those drugs. The amount and type of contamination will determine the seriousness of the problem for the humans who eat such products. There is concern that resistant forms of bacteria that cause diseases in humans may result from the widespread use of antibiotics in livestock.

Another potential problem with veterinary drugs is their misuse by individuals for the prevention or treatment of diseases in themselves or others. Many drugs that require a prescription for human use are sold over the counter (OTC) for use in animals.

VETERINARIAN'S ROLE ON THE ANIMAL HEALTH TEAM

To obtain a doctor of veterinary medicine degree (D.V.M.), the student must pursue an intensive preprofessional and professional curriculum. The preprofessional curriculum, normally requiring two years, is aimed at providing information that will enable the student to successfully complete courses in veterinary school. In addition, grades earned during the preveterinary phase are used as one criteria for evaluating students for admission to colleges of veterinary medicine.

Professional study in veterinary school lasts four years. Because of limited space within the eighteen veterinary schools in the United States, a large number of those enrolled in preveterinary curriculum are never admitted to professional schools.

Generally, the first two years of veterinary school are spent in the study of the basic sciences: anatomy, physiology, biochemistry, microbiology, parasitology, pathology, and pharmacology. The last two years are generally spent in such clinically oriented courses as medicine, public health, radiology, and surgery. A large percentage of time in these last two years is spent working in university veterinary clinics under the direction of veterinarians. The necessity for universities to operate large- and small-animal clinics causes the veterinarian to be one of the most expensive students to educate.

To practice within a state, the veterinarian must become licensed. Licensing usually requires passing a written and a practical examination.

Veterinarians fill a large number of roles. Practitioners may care for a wide variety of companion and food-producing animals (mixed practitioners) or limit their practice to one or two species. Large-animal practitioners generally care for farm animals and horses. However, they may limit their practice to an individual species (such as an equine practitioner) or to a type of activity (such as dairy practitioner).

Since dairy and beef cattle are managed in entirely different ways, they are subject to different disease problems. Therefore some large-animal practitioners limit their practice to only dairy cattle or only beef cattle.

Small-animal practitioners generally care for household pets. The National Academy of Sciences estimates that approximately 42.2% of veterinarians engage primarily in small-animal practice.[11] Some small-animal practitioners specialize in disciplines paralleling those in human medicine, such as veterinary ophthalmology, veterinary radiology, and veterinary surgery. The following list contains the specialty boards recognized by the American Veterinary Medical Association[1]:

American Board of Veterinary Public Health
American Board of Veterinary Toxicology
American College of Laboratory Animal Medicine
American College of Theriogenologists
American College of Veterinary Internal Medicine
American College of Veterinary Microbiologists
American College of Veterinary Ophthalmologists
American College of Veterinary Pathologists
American College of Veterinary Radiology
American College of Veterinary Surgeons

In addition to private practice, veterinarians engage in laboratory animal medicine (caring for laboratory animals in research and drug testing centers), public health, military service, regulatory veterinary medicine, meat inspection, industrial veterinary medicine, and teaching and research.

DISPENSING OF ANIMAL HEALTH PRODUCTS BY VETERINARIANS

An important difference between human and veterinary medicine, aside from the fact that they provide care to different species, is that veterinarians generally dispense drugs, whereas physicians prescribe them. In addition, many products that require prescriptions for humans are sold OTC for use in animals.

A major reason veterinarians dispense drugs is that it represents a significant portion of their total income.[8] Some large-animal practitioners in particular believe that they cannot adequately charge for their time and therefore must supplement their income by the sale of veterinary drugs. They must also have on hand a wide variety of animal health products to administer to animals when making visits to a ranch or farm. For example, it is not practical to restrain a range cow in a location twenty miles from the nearest town, have the veterinarian examine her, and then write a prescription for the appropriate drug to treat her. The general practice is for the veterinarian to administer the drug at the time he sees the animal and then dispense medication for follow-up treatment.

If large-animal practitioners were to prescribe drugs, pharmacies would be required to stock specific veterinary items. Many times the drugs used in large farm animals are different from those used for humans. Drugs that are used in both humans and farm animals are often dispensed in a unique form and concentration for farm animals.

Even though some small-animal practitioners are beginning to write more prescriptions, the majority of them still dispense drugs. When the environments in which physicians and veterinarians practice are compared, the reason that veterinarians dispense more drugs than physicians becomes apparent. Physicians generally practice in offices removed from a hospital. However, small-animal practices are conducted in veterinary hospitals operated by the veterinarians who own the practice. Because there is a necessity to treat hospitalized patients, veterinarians stock a wide variety of small-animal health products. Therefore they find it convenient and profitable to dispense drugs for their outpatients as well.

As with large-animal practitioners, before establishing a policy of writing prescriptions, small-animal practitioners must be assured that the appropriate veterinary drugs are available in local pharmacies. In an attempt to assist veterinarians and pharmacists to determine which human pharmaceuticals are similar to veterinary products, the American Pharmaceutical Association Academy of General Practice of Pharmacy has published a comparative guide to veterinary and human pharmaceuticals.[4]

ANIMAL TECHNICIAN'S ROLE ON THE ANIMAL HEALTH TEAM

Like other health professionals, veterinarians need highly trained assistants. These assistants are called by various names, such as "veterinary assistants," "veterinary nurses," "animal health technicians," or "veterinary paramedics."

Originally in small-animal practices the kennel help would occasionally be asked to assist the veterinarian. Eventually many veterinarians realized that they had a need for more intensively trained aides. Therefore they trained their employees to assist at various procedures. The degree of involvement by these assistants varied from practice to practice. In some practices, assistance was limited to merely restraining animals during treatment. In others the assistant administered gaseous anesthetics or assisted at surgery. In other practices the assistant worked semiindependently by administering medications that the veterinarian had prescribed for animals, administering routine immunizations, and performing minor procedures such as cleaning the animal's teeth. Although a legal precedent was established for paramedical staff members performing similar procedures in the practice of human medicine and dentistry, the legal status of animal health technicians until recently was cloudy. State veterinary licensing acts did not make provisions for "veterinary nurses" or for "veterinary dental assistants."

Recently there has been a move to clarify the status of veterinary assistants. The type of training they should receive and the conditions under which they should be licensed are being defined in various states. This has come about because of a shortage of veterinarians in the United States. It has been recognized that not all the procedures performed by veterinarians require the intensive education that veterinarians receive. Therefore it becomes more economical to train animal health technicians so that they can perform routine procedures in veterinary practice, which allows veterinarians to spend their time diagnosing diseases and performing surgical procedures.

Recently in California a law was passed establishing certification for animal health technicians. Various two- and four-year programs are available throughout the United States for this new specialty. The American Veterinary Medical Association has an accreditation program for college level courses for animal health technicians.

One duty of the animal health technician is to administer drugs to animals on the order of a veterinarian. Therefore animal health technicians should have some background regarding the types and actions of drugs used in veterinary medicine. They must also be alert to the toxic reactions of drugs.

PHARMACIST'S ROLE ON THE ANIMAL HEALTH TEAM

Pharmacists can be valuable members of the animal health team. Probably the most valuable role pharmacists can fill for veterinarians is that of drug consultant. Their education and training make them ideally suited to be a source of drug information. With some effort on the part of pharmacists, they can gain the knowledge necessary to apply their expertise in drugs and therapeutics effectively in the veterinary setting. By using their professional expertise in advising veterinarians, by stocking and dispensing appropriate animal health products, and by participating in certain community programs, pharmacists can help to improve both animal and human health in their areas. The following are a few examples of ways that pharmacists can participate as a member of the animal health team in their communities:

- Educating their clients regarding such animal health matters as rabies vaccination clinics, spay clinics, and prevention of various zoonotic infections such as visceral larval migrans (Chapter 11)
- Encouraging ranchers to initiate measures that will prevent disease in their livestock
- Stocking appropriate animal health products and providing those who purchase them with appropriate information regarding their use
- Advising their clients to seek veterinary medical attention for their animals when appropriate
- Remaining informed about and providing drug information to veterinarians
- Advising public regulatory bodies regarding the appropriate use of animal health products

Currently the livestock producer can purchase animal products from a veterinarian, a pharmacist, or various persons with no professional training in the use of biologicals and pharmaceuticals in animals. Since there is an acute shortage of livestock veterinarians (large-animal practitioners), it would seem highly desirable to have pharmacists more actively involved in dispensing animal health care products. Unfortunately, however, many pharmacists have dispensed such products with no more knowledge about the proper use of veterinary drugs than their lay competitors. It is reasonable for a rancher to expect little, if any, information on the use of veterinary drugs from a lay distributor, but he would expect a pharmacist to be knowledgeable about veterinary drugs that he dispenses. It is hoped that through this text, courses in schools of pharmacy, and continuing education programs, pharmacists will become thoroughly familiar with animal health products and join veterinarians in providing for the animal health needs of their community.

DISPENSING OF ANIMAL HEALTH PRODUCTS BY PHARMACISTS

The decision whether to sell veterinary drugs in a pharmacy will depend on the following:

1. *The type and size of store.* A small store in a multistory medical building with a small percentage of its trade in OTC products is less likely to carry veterinary products than a large store with a high percentage of OTC sales.

2. *Location.* The animal population is determined by the local environment. It varies markedly from an urban to a rural location. The surrounding animal population will dictate the type of veterinary products that could be reasonably handled by a retail outlet.

3. *The pharmacist's relationship with local veterinarians.* An increasing number of veterinarians desire to write prescriptions rather than dispense to their clients. This technique is likely to be adopted by veterinarians who have a busy small-animal (dog and cat) practice and find that they can serve their clients better by rendering professional skill through diagnosis and prescribing rather than merchandising drugs.[5]

4. *The relative profit that can be made on animal health products as opposed to other items the pharmacist may stock for OTC sale.* The sale of animal health products constitutes a sizable industry within the United States. In 1973 at the distributor's price level, 691 million dollars of animal health products were sold in the United States.[7] These are broken down as follows*:

Drugs placed in feed to increase agricultural production	54%
Pharmaceuticals	35%
Biologicals	11%

---

*From Animal Health Institute Domestic Net Sales Report, 1973.

Even though veterinarians dispense substantial amounts of animal health products, virtually all feed additives, about 63% of veterinary pharmaceuticals, and about 41% of biologicals are sold through nonveterinary channels.

5. *The desire of the pharmacist to provide community service.* The willingness of the pharmacist to stock veterinary pharmaceuticals and biologicals can provide an important resource that helps to protect the health of both animals and humans.[9] In addition, pharmacists dispensing animal health products can significantly contribute to the economic well-being of a livestock-producing area.

INTERPROFESSIONAL RELATIONSHIPS

Because veterinarians dispense a large amount of drugs and because pharmacists can dispense a wide variety of veterinary products OTC, poor relationships between pharmacists and veterinarians can result. In an attempt to develop an ethical relationship between the two professions, the American Pharmaceutical Association and the American Veterinary Medical Association have developed a code of interprofessional relations, which is shown on p. 8.

In addition to ethical relationships, both veterinarians and pharmacists must comply with the laws and regulations governing the dispensing and prescription of veterinary products. One factor that can add confusion and impede cooperation between pharmacists and veterinarians is the policy of some drug companies to restrict the sale of their products to veterinarians only. The purpose for doing this is apparently to develop good relations with veterinarians by refusing to sell to their "competitors." Many of these companies, however, sell the same generic compounds under different brand names through their subsidiaries to nonveterinary distributors. Companies that restrict the sale of their products to veterinarians will generally place "sold to veterinarians only" on the label. That statement in no way relates to legal control of drugs but rather to a sales policy of the company.

PHARMACIST-VETERINARIAN CODE OF INTERPROFESSIONAL RELATIONS*

The purpose of this Code of Interprofessional Relations is to improve relations between doctors of veterinary medicine and pharmacists. Its provisions are intended as guides for veterinarians and pharmacists in their interrelated practices. It is the hope of the parties who have participated in the development of this Code of Interprofessional Relations that by an improved and closer relationship between the two professions the public will be better served.

The Code of Interprofessional Relations is not a pronouncement of law. It recommends rules of conduct for the members of these two professions subject to the principles of ethics and practice governing the members of the respective organizations.

This code recognizes that doctors of veterinary medicine and pharmacists are interdependent upon one another in serving the farm and city communities.

The pharmacists shall not diagnose, treat, administer to, or operate on animals, and shall use professional discretion in commenting upon the prescribed medication or treatment. The pharmacist should refer persons requesting such assistance to a doctor of veterinary medicine.

The sale of a veterinary proprietary product that has been approved by the Federal Food and Drug Administration for over-the-counter sale, requested as a result of diagnosis made by the individual requesting the product, shall not be considered counter prescribing by the pharmacist. Nor shall it be construed as violating the practice of veterinary medicine when the pharmacist advises the purchaser of a veterinary proprietary product with regard to contraindications, cautions, dosage and instructions for administration, insofar as this information is contained on the product label or the package insert.

The pharmacist shall provide an adequate supply of veterinary products, including biologicals, which the doctor of veterinary medicine may obtain, through direct purchase or which an animal owner may obtain by prescription. He shall serve as a source of information on new drugs in order that the veterinarian may have advantage of the latest pharmaceutical developments.

The veterinarian should recognize the specialized training of the pharmacist, and utilize his professional services whenever they serve the best interest of the farm and city community.

In the AVMA Principles of Veterinary Medical Ethics, it is stated that dispensing by the veterinarian is interpreted to mean providing veterinary products for lay use, only on the supposition that the veterinarian has previous knowledge of the particular case or general conditions which apply to the specific farm or kennel (or other place of confinement). Distribution of biologicals and pharmaceuticals solely for profit by veterinarians or pharmacists without due consideration for the patient or patients receiving such product should not occur.

The veterinarian and the pharmacist should have a mutual respect for each other's profession, and through cooperative efforts cultivate this respect. By so doing, each will better serve the public health and animal health and add to the stature of his own profession.

*Jointly prepared by American Pharmaceutical Association and American Veterinary Medical Association, 1966.

LAWS REGULATING ANIMAL HEALTH PRODUCTS
OTC and legend veterinary drugs

Veterinary drugs that are prescription items, known as "legend drugs," carry the following statement on the label of the container in which they are dispensed: "Caution: Federal law restricts this drug to use by or on the order of a licensed veterinarian." By comparison, OTC drugs require no prescription and may be bought by anyone.

Since 1975 OTC anthelmintic drugs (those that are used to treat internal parasitic infections in animals) and animal feeds containing anthelmintics have had to carry the following label instruction: "Consult your veterinarian for assistance in the diagnosis, treatment, and control of parasitism."

Among the various factors that determine whether a veterinary drug is a prescription item are the following:

1. *An inability to develop adequate directions by which clients can use a drug or device safely for the purpose for which it is intended.* Adequate directions include dose, frequency, time, and route of administration; directions for use include statements of purposes for which it is prescribed and recommended or suggested.

Some drugs can be dispensed OTC when used in one way but require a prescription for another use.[6] If the drugs are safe and efficacious and adequate directions can be developed for one method of administration, they can be dispensed OTC. For another use, writing adequate directions may be virtually impossible; thus a prescription would be required for that use. For example, the use of injectable iron preparations to treat anemia in baby pigs is common. Writing adequate directions for such a use is feasible. Therefore injectable iron for the prevention or treatment of iron deficiency anemia in baby pigs is an OTC product. Diagnosing this condition in adult animals, however, is difficult, and special skills are required. Simple and adequate directions for the use of injectable iron preparations cannot be developed. Therefore injectable iron for use in adult animals requires a prescription.

2. *Drugs potentially harmful for animals or humans or subject to human drug abuse.* Examples of drugs falling in this category are tranquilizers, narcotics, and barbiturates. This is the reason that so many veterinary drugs are legend drugs.[2] Regulations concerning the veterinary use of such controlled substances are discussed in Appendix G.

3. *Drugs requiring long withdrawal periods between the time of administration and the time that the animal is either slaughtered or its milk or eggs could be used for human consumption.* Withdrawal times are established for various animal health products to prevent residues of drugs in meat, milk, or eggs. For those drugs requiring a long withdrawal time the U.S. Food and Drug Administration (FDA) believes that use of the drug should be under the supervision of a veterinarian.

4. *Those antibiotics highly effective against organisms resistant to common anti-infective drugs.* Because of the danger of allowing further development of strains of organisms that are resistant to highly effective antibiotics, such products are required to be prescription drugs.

One confusion arises regarding dispensing drugs that require prescriptions for humans but can be dispensed OTC for veterinary use. It is said that the product can be dispensed if a statement to the effect that the drug is a hazardous livestock remedy and not for human use is added to the label. This is not true. It is legal for a pharmacist to take a product that was intended by its manufacturer for human use and label that product for veterinary use and sell it without a prescription, provided that this drug is one which may be legally sold for veterinary use without a prescription. The pharmacist, however, must supply complete labeling for the product that is sold. A special knowledge of veterinary medicine is required to supply adequate directions for use and the appropriate warnings that should be on the package. Therefore it is recommended that the pharmacist purchase drugs labeled by the manufacturer for veterinary use with complete directions for such use.

A licensed veterinarian may purchase human prescription drugs for use in animals. A licensed veterinarian is also entitled to write prescriptions for human prescription items for use in animals. The FDA, however, does not encourage such practices because of the lack of specific directions for the use in animal species. Since it is unlikely that tolerances for such products have been established in food-producing animals, the use of such products could cause serious drug residue problems if used in these animals. The veterinarian can be held legally responsible for such residues and losses incurred as a result of the residues.

Drug residues

On a practical basis the problem of drug residues in food-producing animals is probably the greatest legal problem encountered in the dispensing of animal health products. The types of drugs that can be used in food-producing animals differ from those for other species. Even a drug that has been cleared for use in horses often carries the statement that the drug shall not be used if the horse is to be used for human consumption.

Generally, drugs in livestock are used in two ways. One is at therapeutic levels to treat a disease. Another is at subtherapeutic levels either to prevent disease or to increase the rate of gain and feed conversion.

Drug residues in animal products are likely to occur when either an improper dose is used or the time between administration of the drug and slaughter of or the taking of milk or eggs from the animal (withdrawal time) is not as long as it should be. To prevent problems of residues in animals, those dispensing animal health products should check the label and become familiar with appropriate dose and withdrawal times. These should be pointed out to drug purchasers.[5]

Preslaughter withdrawal times are expressed in days. In establishing withdrawal times, the FDA considers 1 day as equal to 24 hours. Therefore a withdrawal time of 5 days means that a minimum of 120 hours must elapse between the time a drug is given and the animal is slaughtered. If the time between administration of the drug and slaughter is less than the established withdrawal time, illegal drug residues could result.

When drugs are administered to dairy cattle, milk may often not be used for human consumption for a specified time after the last drug administration. For each day of withdrawal time, 24 hours must elapse from the last administration, and two milkings per day must be discarded. Therefore if a drug requires a 3-day milk withdrawal time, a minimum of 72 hours must pass and the milk from at least six milkings must be discarded before the milk from these cows may be used for human consumption.

When animals receive medicated feed or water, the withdrawal time does not start until the animals no longer have access to the medicated feed or water.

The government essentially recognizes two types of tolerance of drugs in meat, eggs, and milk. One allows a certain detectable level of a drug, and the other states that no detectable level of a drug may exist in these products. The FDA sets the tolerance for each drug.

The FDA is concerned about three kinds of drug residues[12]:

1. *Residues that induce cancer.* Under the Delaney clause, if it can be shown that a chemical induces cancer in any animal species, this substance cannot be permitted in any amount in a food product. *It does not have to be shown that the product is capable of causing cancer in humans.*

2. *Residues that may cause allergic reactions in human consumers.*

3. *Antibiotics that may result in the development of resistant organisms in animals.* Even a low level of feeding antibacterials to cattle allows proliferation of intestinal bacteria resistant to antibiotics. In recent years it has been found that these resistances are transferable from one species of bacteria to another. The concern is that such resistance might be transferred to organisms that infect humans.

References

1. American Veterinary Medical Association Directory, Chicago, 1974, American Veterinary Medical Association.
2. Cazier, P. D.: The FDA viewpoint, Vet. Econ. **17**:26, March 1976.
3. Feldmann, B. M., and Carding, T. H.: Free roaming urban pets, Health Serv. Rep. **88**:956, 1973.
4. Hansell, D. N., and Scheu, J. D.: Comparative guide of veterinary and human pharmaceuticals, Washington, D.C., 1973, American Pharmaceutical Association.
5. Jones, L. M.: Professional interrelations of pharmacy and veterinary medicine, J. Am. Vet. Med. Assoc. **151**:1772, 1967.
6. Kingma, F. J.: Distribution of human prescription drugs to veterinarians, J. Am. Vet. Med. Assoc. **151**:1056, 1967.
7. Linney, J. J.: Don't count out large animal drugs just yet, Vet. Econ. **15**:44, Oct. 1974.
8. Reed, G. B., and Norris, G. D.: Why we dispense, Vet Econ. **8**:23, Aug. 1967.
9. Schwabe, C. W.: Veterinary medicine and human health, Baltimore, 1964, The Williams & Wilkins Co.
10. Schwabe, C. W., and Ruppanner, R.: Animals diseases as contributors to human hunger problems of control, World Rev. Nutr. Diet. **15**:185, 1972.
11. Terry, L. L., and others: New horizons for veterinary medicine, Washington, D.C., 1972, National Academy of Sciences.
12. Van Houweling, C. D.: The FDA and the practicing veterinarian, Vet. Econ. **14**:40, Aug. 1973.

Additional readings

A survey of the veterinary dispensing problem, Vet. Med. **58**:29, Jan. 1963.

Azelton, R. P.: Professional responsibility in prescribing and dispensing animal health products, Vet. Med. Small Anim. Clin. **61**:418, 1966.

Black, and others: Drugs and the veterinary profession, Can. Vet. J. **14**:175, Aug. 1973.

Cockerill, V. L.: The "legally-available" drug controversy, Vet. Econ. **16**:26, June 1975.

Jolly, D. W.: This residue business, Mod. Vet. Pract. **41**:30, April 1960.

Kingma, F. J.: Multiple use drugs require adequate restrictions, J. Am. Vet. Med. Assoc. **151**:746, 1973.

Lindley, W. H.: No visible action has resulted, Vet. Econ. **17**:23, June 1976.

Pals, C. H.: Biological residues; a challenge to veterinarians, J. Am. Vet. Med. Assoc. **146**:1427, 1965.

Pierson, R. E.: Herd health for a large feedlot operation, J. Am. Vet. Med. Assoc. **157**:1504, 1970.

Pritchard, W. R.: Animal disease constraints to world food production, Theriogenology **6**:305, 1976.

Schwabe, C. W.: Diseases in animals and man's well-being, University Lectures, No. 24, University of Saskatchewan.

Spencer, R. H.: Disease problems in feedlot practice, J. Am. Vet. Med. Assoc. **155**:1904, 1969.

Turpin, J. T.: Time to strike back, Vet. Econ. **17**:20, June 1976.

Wenning, G. B., Schmiesing, D. E., and Coe, P. H.: Why not dispense drugs competitively? Vet. Econ. **15**:32, Nov. 1974.

2

INTRODUCTION TO
Veterinary therapeutics

VETERINARY THERAPEUTICS
Definition

As used in this text, veterinary therapeutics is the use of drugs in the treatment and prevention of disease. The process of selecting the best possible regimen of drug therapy for a particular animal at a particular time is extremely complex. Veterinarians must consider many factors in their drug selection to be sure that their choice of therapy is both scientifically and practically sound. Like physicians, veterinarians must first concern themselves with the safety and efficacy (effectiveness) of the therapeutic regimen.

The selection of a treatment regimen requires a careful and deliberate assessment of a drug's inherent liabilities with regard to toxicity and side effects and the expected beneficial effects to be gained from its use.

Physicians are concerned primarily with safety and efficacy. They may be concerned secondarily with other factors like convenience, price, and patient acceptance but only after making sure that safety and efficacy are not compromised. Veterinarians, on the other hand, must consider many factors in addition to safety and efficacy, and frequently they must give these factors equal or nearly equal weight in the decision-making process. To indicate how sound judgments are made in the application of drug therapy to animal patients, we will briefly discuss these other decision-making factors. One should keep in mind that this is not a comprehensive review of veterinary therapeutics and that examples used here have been selected to illustrate how drug therapy for animals may differ in principle, method, or goal from drug therapy in humans. These examples are offered only to give an appreciation of the problems encountered in the veterinary therapeutic situation.

Economic considerations

The veterinarian's relationship with the patient is somewhat different from that of the physician. The physician's services are generally enlisted by the patient. There are, of course, exceptions to this in the treatment of children or of patients who are too sick or not competent to communicate with the physician. The veterinarian's services, on the other hand, are always enlisted by the patient's owner, the veterinarian's client. This arrangement results in a delicately balanced relationship indeed. The veterinarian must satisfy the needs of the patient and also those of the client. It is both legally and morally recognized that the owner of an animal has ultimate authority over the disposition of that animal. Therefore the veterinarian must include the wishes of the client in the treatment plans.

The economics of a therapeutic regimen must always be taken into consideration. The veterinarian must determine an optimum therapeutic regimen within the economic limitations agreed on by himself and the client.

Veterinary practice can be divided into two categories: pet and companion animal practice and agricultural or commercial animal practice. Pet and companion animal practice provides health care primarily for dogs and cats but also extends to other animals, such as horses, that are kept for companionship, protection, or enjoyment. These animals are of varying value to their owners; a value is established subjectively by the owner. Indeed some of these animals are considered family members and enjoy all the privileges, economic and otherwise, such status implies. The economic limitations on treatment of pet and companion animals then are generally less limiting than might be the case for animals kept for other reasons. It is not uncommon, for instance, for the veterinarian to treat malignancies or metabolic diseases with drugs costing more per treatment than the original purchase price of the animal. Even though economic limitations in the treatment of companion animals are based on the client's subjective evaluation of the animal, they are nonetheless real limitations, which must be included in the consideration of any treatment regimen. The well-intentioned therapeutic plan based on the most scientifically sound medical data is of little value if the owner of the animal will not accept the costs of that treatment.

The other major category of veterinary practice, agricultural or commercial animal practice, deals with the health care of animals raised for their commercial value. Dairy cattle, beef cattle, sheep, poultry, and breeding stock comprise the bulk of these animals. Unlike the owner of the companion animal, the owner of commercial animals does not establish the value of his animals subjectively. Each animal in his herd or flock has an absolute dollar value as a part of the owner's business operation. Thus economic considerations are of prime concern in providing health care for these animals. Any expenditure for drugs or treatment must fit within the profit-loss structure of the specific business. The cost of a therapy must be considered an investment, and, as with any business investment, there must be a promise of sufficient return on money so invested. For example, if a veterinarian were treating a cow infected with a penicillinase-producing staphylococcus, economic considerations would influence his choice of the appropriate antibiotic. If the veterinarian were to consider only the most rational drug use, the choice would be one of the penicillinase-resistant penicillins. However, the use of such a drug would cost about $100 a day. Such cost would not be economically justified in treating an ordinary cow. The veterinarian would likely decide to use tetracyclines or sulfonamides, with a treatment cost of approximately 50¢ per day. Even though these drugs are not as likely to be as effective as the more expensive antibiotics, their use is rational when economic factors are considered.

In summary, economic considerations are always present, albeit to differing degrees, in the therapy of animal patients. It is imperative that anyone who becomes involved in the process of designing rational drug therapy for animals, especially for commercial animal patients, have a complete understanding of the economic realities within which the veterinarian's client is obliged to function.

Physical factors

Many physical factors can and do influence the selection of a drug and dose schedule in the animal patient. Frequently, particularly with large, wild, or aggressive animals, physical restraint of the animal becomes necessary to permit administration of a drug. The problems involved in such restraint must be considered when deciding what drug and dose schedule to employ. In the horse, for example, any oral medication that is not voluntarily consumed by the animal is usually administered by means of a stomach tube. This tubing procedure, although not uncommon, often prohibits the use of an oral drug on a continuing basis. Tubing is a fairly safe and simple procedure for administering one dose, but in most cases it is too troublesome and dangerous to perform three or four times a day for several days.

Many animals not used to being handled are difficult to catch and restrain. Few owners will administer a drug on a continuing schedule if catching and restraining the animal becomes too great a task. In addition to the problems encountered by the individuals applying restraint, many animals, especially exotic and wild animals, are severely stressed by restraint and handling. The therapeutician, the one who recommends a course of drug therapy, must always be satisfied that the recommended regimen does not produce more harm to the animal by stress than benefits by pharmacological action.

Another factor that must always be considered in the restraint of any animal is the safety of the persons applying the restraint. Asking a client with limited experience, equipment, and facilities to restrain a thousand pounds of intractable horse several times a day is certainly not in the best interests of veterinarian-client relations or of public safety. The veterinarian as animal health expert must accept responsibility for judgment as to the safety and practicality of a prescribed method of treatment, taking into account the client's inexperience and limitations when they exist.

Behavioral variations

The veterinarian is commonly called on to treat at least ten species of domestic animals and sometimes many more species of wild and domestic animals.[9] Each of these species is the product of a long process of evolutionary adaptation and often generations of selective breeding by man. As a result, the veterinarian is faced with creatures of widely varying behavioral characteristics. An understanding of these behavioral characteristics is essential to the rational application of drug therapy.

The domestic cat, for example, is a constant groomer. Any drug substance applied to cats topically, that is, directly to a surface such as the skin, is likely to be ingested by the animals during their licking and grooming behavior. Disinfectants and chemicals applied to environmental surfaces like floors, cat boxes, and cages are picked up on the cat's feet and eventually ingested. Therefore care must be exercised in the selection of drugs and chemicals to be used on or around cats. A disinfectant perfectly safe for use around canines may indeed prove troublesome or even fatal in the cattery.

Behavioral patterns of a breed within a species may also present problems in drug selection. The modern flea collar, which consists of an organic phosphate pesticide incorporated into a plastic resin (so that the volatile pesticide is slowly released from the collar), has proved to be a great aid in the control of fleas and the problems that they cause in dogs. However, care must be exercised not to allow such a collar to become wet while on the dog. When the collar does become wet, a severe reaction can occur where the collar is in contact with the animal's skin. Although this problem may occur in any dog, it is much more likely to occur in the Labrador retriever and other water-loving breeds.

Anatomical variations

The selective processes at work in the development of the various animal species have produced wide anatomical variations. Anatomical considerations play an important role in the veterinarian's selection of drug therapy for the animal patient. For example, the bovine and several other species have a complex stomach (pp. 172 and 173) that enables them to use fibrous plant celluloses. The rumen, the largest part of the ruminant stomach, provides a large chamber (40-gallon capacity in cattle) for storage and fermentation by microorganisms of foodstuffs to render them absorbable and allow their utilization by the animal. Ingested material is retained in the rumen for 1 to 3 days. During this time the foodstuffs are acted on by ruminal microorganisms. The rumen contents are mixed with rumen liquor by contractions. These contractions are also involved in the eructation of the large amounts of gases produced by the fermentation process. This delicately balanced fermentation system presents certain problems in the application of drug therapy to ruminant animals. For example, the oral administration of antibiotics to ruminants can upset the population balance of rumen microorganisms and cause severe digestive problems.

The rumen may also have an effect on the absorption and distribution of many drugs. Digitalis has little effect in ruminants. This is thought to be a result of the drug's being destroyed in the rumen.[9] Orally administered chloramphenicol has been shown not to be absorbed in the goat, a ruminant; however, the levels found in the blood after parenteral administration, that is, by routes other than oral, are adequate.[3]

Another example of the effect of anatomy on drug response can be found in the racing breeds of dogs—greyhounds, whippets, and the like. These animals exhibit abnormally long sleeping times in response to the barbiturate anesthetics. The distribution of these lipid-soluble (soluble in fats) barbiturates into body fat is responsible for a rapid decline of their concentration in the plasma and the central nervous system. Thus the presence of body fat tends to shorten the action of barbiturate anesthetics. The greyhound and whippet breeds are extremely lean and do not have sufficient body fat to accept a standard dose of these barbiturates, calculated on a body weight basis.

The great variation in anatomical mass may also influence the response to drug therapy. The veterinarian's patients may vary from a few ounces to several tons. Extremely large animals present problems in the use of anesthetics and depressant drugs. The great weight of the elephant, for instance, can interfere with its respiration when it is unconscious. The weight of the body wall in a laterally recumbent elephant results in such enormous gravitational force on the chest cavity and lungs that mechanical ventilation becomes difficult and in fact impossible without specialized equipment. Similarly, the horse, whose respiratory system moves extremely large volumes of gases, must be adequately ventilated when anesthetized. Specially designed anesthesia machines currently available can move large volumes of gases and safely anesthetize these animals.

Metabolic factors

The phylogenetic differentiation of animal species has resulted in many other differences, less obvious than the behavioral and anatomical variations mentioned previously. The ability to metabolize drugs, that is, to change them chemically, varies greatly between species. Organic compounds that are soluble in tissue fluids are generally easily and rapidly eliminated by the mammalian kidney (Fig. 2-1). These compounds pass well into the urine, and their relative insolubility in fat does not favor reabsorption through the fatty membranes of the kidney tubules. The kidney's inability to excrete substances that are soluble in fat (lipid) is of such magnitude that highly lipid-soluble drugs such as thiopental would have a biological half-life (the period of time for the animal to eliminate one half the total dose of a drug) of up to 100 years if they were not changed to water-soluble compounds (Fig. 2-2).[2]

The enzymes responsible for the metabolism of drugs to more easily excreted compounds were developed by selective adaptation to enable the species to dispose of foreign substances to which they were exposed.

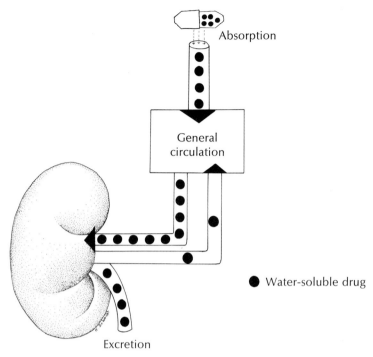

Fig. 2-1. Excretion of water-soluble drugs. Drugs that are water soluble are easily and rapidly excreted by the kidneys.

The levels of these various enzymes, then, vary among the species. Thus various species differ in their ability to metabolize lipid-soluble drugs as well as in the rate at which this is accomplished. The domestic cat, for example, has been shown to be relatively deficient in the ability to form glucuronides.[10] The cat's sensitivity to phenolic compounds can be explained by this relative inability to form glucuronides. Conjugation with glucuronic acid to form water-soluble glucuronides is one of the major pathways in the metabolism of phenolic compounds.[13] The unusually slow metabolism of these compounds in the cat results in accumulation of phenolics in the tissues and leads to increased susceptibility and central nervous system toxicity.

It is becoming increasingly common for drug manufacturers to market their new drugs only in the field of human medicine or at best to release them in the veterinary market with recommendations and data support-ing use in only one or two species. Information regarding species variation in drug response is scarce, and what is available is scattered widely in the medical, biochemical, and physiological literature. These species variations in drug response become a problem that veterinary therapeuticians must handle. It would certainly be unsatisfactory for the therapeutician to avoid using the multitude of available drugs about which questions of species variation are unanswered. Assuming then that the decision has been made to use a drug in an animal when the species variability in response is not known, what can be done to minimize the risks inherent in such a decision? The variation in response between species is generally in degree rather than in the mechanism of the drug's action. The availability of the drug to its site of action or receptor site is determined by the concentration of the drug in the plasma and tissue fluids. When a species exhibits a slow-er rate of excretion of a given drug, the bio-

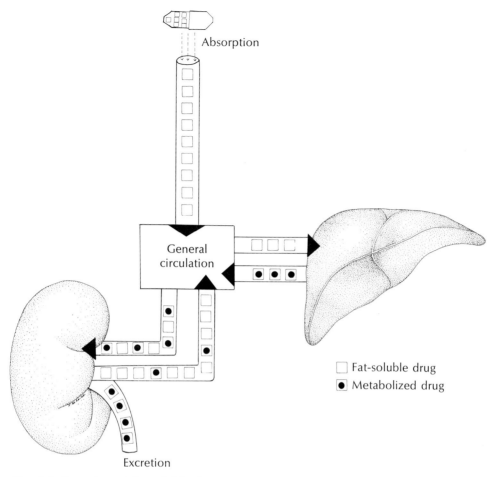

Absorption

General
circulation

☐ Fat-soluble drug
● Metabolized drug

Excretion

Fig. 2-2. Excretion of fat-soluble drugs. Fat-soluble drugs must be metabolized prior to being excreted. Rate of metabolism will vary significantly among different species.

logical half-life of the drug is prolonged, that is, the period in which the body excretes or changes half the administered drug is longer. Equivalent doses at equivalent intervals result in much higher concentrations of the drug in tissues; the drug will accumulate more than it will in species exhibiting more rapid excretion or metabolism of the compound, that is, a shorter half-life. This phenomenon has been observed with many drugs. For example, the half-life of phenylbutazone in humans is 45 to 72 hours, and in the rat it is 6 hours.[4] The dose of phenylbutazone required to produce sodium retention in humans and the rat is 5 to 10 mg/kg and 400 mg/kg, respectively. However, the plasma levels attained with these doses are essentially identical. Barbiturates exhibit a wide variation in rates of metabolism, distribution, and duration of action among species. Careful measurement of plasma levels, however, indicates that at the time of recovery from barbiturate-induced sleep, the plasma levels are the same.[2]

Although information about the rate of excretion or metabolism of a new drug in a particular species is often nonexistent or at least difficult to obtain, the veterinary therapeutician is not without recourse. Generally, information is available describing the metabolism and excretion of the drug in one animal species or at least in humans. From this information the alert therapeutician may make certain assumptions.

First, if available data indicate that the drug is excreted primarily by the kidney in unchanged form, the variation in half-life between species will be slight. The water-soluble antibiotics are an example of this type of drug. The half-lives of penicillin G, gentamycin, and many other antibiotics differ little among species (Table 2-1). Certainly when the biologic half-life of a compound is essentially invariable, dosage calculations may be made with a reasonable degree of confidence. On the other hand, the half-life of drugs that depend on the action of drug-metabolizing enzymes to facilitate their excretion is subject to the variability found among the spe-

cies with respect to these enzymes. The rate of excretion of these drugs will naturally vary from species to species so that dosage calculations often cannot be made safely with available data. This is illustrated clearly in the case of the drug meperidine. The half-life of meperidine in man and dog differs by a factor of six (Table 2-1). It is obvious that if the dose of this drug for humans was simply extrapolated to the dog, the drug would not reach sufficient plasma concentration in the animal to produce the desired effect.

Second, the veterinarian should be aware of the intrinsic toxicity of the drug. Drugs that have a wide margin of safety and a low degree of toxicity can of course be employed with less trepidation than those which are in-

Table 2-1. Excretion characteristics and comparison of biological half-life (T½) of some drugs in different species

Drug	Excretion characteristics[5]	Species	T½ (hr)
Acetazolamide	Primarily in urine unchanged (tubular secretion)*	Man	1.58[6]
		Dog	1.8[6]
Antipyrine	5% in urine unchanged, 40% in urine after oxidation, 55% undetermined	Man	12.0[6]
		Dog	1.7[6]
Cephaloridine	Primarily in urine unchanged (glomerular filtration)*	Man	0.83[6]
		Dog	0.5[12]
Chloramphenicol	5% to 10% in urine unchanged, remainder in urine after conjugation or hydrolysis	Man	1.5-3.5[5]
		Dog	4.2[3]
		Cat	5.1[3]
		Pony	0.9[3]
		Goat	2.0[3]
		Swine	1.3[3]
Dexamethasone	20% in bile, remainder in urine after glucuronide or sulfate conjugation in liver	Man	3.34[6]
		Dog	1.0[6]
Diphenylhydantoin	Dog and man: 2% in bile, remainder primarily in urine after parahydroxylation in liver	Man	23.5-11[6]
		Dog	7.3-1.2[6]
Gentamycin	In urine unchanged (glomerular filtration)	Man	1-1.5[6]
		Dog	1.5[4]
Kanamycin	In urine unchanged (glomerular filtration)	Man	4.0[6]
		Dog/cat	4.0[6]
Meperidine	In urine after N-demethylation hydrolysis or conjugation	Man	5.5[6]
		Dog	0.9[6]
		Monkey	1.2[6]
Penicillin	Primarily in urine unchanged (tubular secretion)	Man	0.5-1[6]
		Dog ⎫ Horse ⎭	0.4-1

*For a discussion of tubular secretion and glomerular filtration see Chapter 17.

herently toxic and which have a narrow margin between therapeutic and toxic levels in the tissues.

In summary, species variations in rates of metabolism of drugs present real problems in therapy of diverse animal species. The enterprising therapeutician can, however, considerably reduce the risk involved by careful consideration of the metabolic and excretion characteristics of the drug.

Administration of drugs

When a drug is administered to an animal the dose must be adequate and the drug must be administered in such a way that it will be delivered to the site of action in an effective concentration. For example, if follicle-stimulating hormone is given intramuscularly to stimulate the ovaries, it must be absorbed into the blood from the injection site, and then only the relatively small portion taken up from the blood by the ovaries will bring about increased ovarian activity.

Generally, an equilibrium is established between the site of action and the concentration in the blood.

Various factors affect the level of drug concentration available at the site of action, including the following:

- The dose administered
- The rate of absorption from the site of administration
- The tendency of the drug to bind to substances such as fat or proteins, which reduces the amount of free drug available at the site of action
- The rate of excretion of the drug from the body
- The rate at which the drug is metabolized by the body
- The frequency of administration

One factor that determines how quickly a drug will be absorbed from the site of administration is the route by which it is administered. As in human medicine, veterinary drugs are administered by a variety of routes.

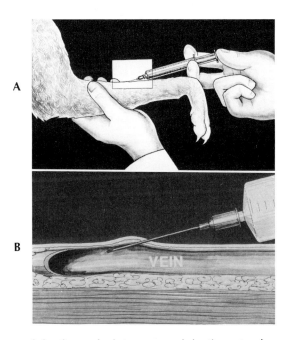

Fig. 2-3. Intravenous injections. **A,** Intravenous injections to dogs are given in the cephalic vein, **B,** which runs along anterior surface of front legs. (From Spinelli, J. S., Evans, J. L., and Merrill, I. R.: Laboratory animal care, Pub. 74-1B, 1973, Joliet, Ill., American Association for Laboratory Animal Science.)

Drugs may be applied topically. When thus applied, drugs may affect only the area to which they are applied. If a drug is not absorbed by the tissue on which it is placed, the drug may be given systemically so that it will get into the blood and be carried to the cells.

As with topical administration of drugs to the skin, the administration of a nonabsorbable drug orally affects only the surface cells of the gastrointestinal tract. If deeper tissues must be affected by the drug, then systemic administration is necessary. The systemic administration of drugs results in their being absorbed into the blood and distributed throughout the body.

When drugs that are absorbed by the intestinal tract are given by the oral route, they are carried by the circulatory system to target tissues. Under ideal circumstances the oral route is preferred because it is less hazardous to the animal. However, some drugs are destroyed by gastrointestinal secretions or are not adequately absorbed from the gastrointestinal tract. Such drugs have to be administered parenterally, that is, by injection. Drugs for parenteral administration must be sterile and given in such a way that their sterility is maintained.

Intravenous administration (Fig. 2-3) is made to get a drug into the bloodstream rapidly. In addition, some drugs are given by the intravenous route because they are highly irritating. Because they are diluted immediately by the blood, their irritating effect is mediated. However, if they are injected into surrounding tissues instead of into the blood vessel, their irritating effects may be concentrated to the extent that they cause tissue death in the surrounding area. Therefore when making intravenous injections, one must be absolutely sure to get the entire dose in the vein. If the drug is accidentally injected outside the vein, then either it must be diluted with sterile saline or other drugs must be injected into the area to neutralize the irritating effect of the compound.

When drugs are administered intramuscularly (Fig. 2-4), they are absorbed into the

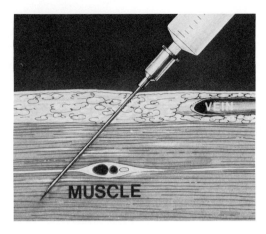

Fig. 2-4. Intramuscular injection. (From Spinelli, J. S., Evans, J. L., and Merrill, I. R.: Laboratory animal care, Pub. 74-1B, 1973, Joliet, Ill., American Association for Laboratory Animal Science.)

blood quickly unless they have been placed in material (the vehicle) that causes them to be retained in the tissues. When drugs are given intramuscularly, the volume that can be placed at any one site is limited. Usually no more than 2 ml are given per site for small animals such as dogs and cats and 10 ml per site for large animals such as horses and cattle.

The subcutaneous route (Fig. 2-5) generally results in slower absorption of drugs into the blood than the intramuscular route.

In addition to the route of administration, the other major factor that determines the rate at which a drug is absorbed from the site of injection is the nature of the drug or the material in which the drug is dissolved or suspended. This material is referred to as the "vehicle" because the drug is carried in it to the injection site. Generally, drugs that are dissolved in water or saline are quickly absorbed from the injection site. Drugs that are suspended in water or saline or in an oily vehicle are more slowly absorbed. In addition, certain oral preparations can be produced so that drugs are slowly absorbed into the circulatory system from the digestive tract.

When a drug is absorbed, an equilibrium

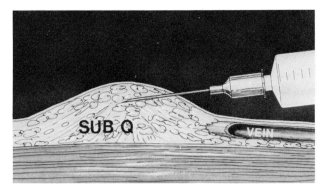

Fig. 2-5. Subcutaneous injection. (From Spinelli, J. S., Evans, J. L., and Merrill, I. R.: Laboratory animal care, Pub. 74-1B, 1973, Joliet, Ill., American Association for Laboratory Animal Science.)

is established between the concentration of the drug in the blood and that in the body tissues.

Some drugs have a great affinity for certain tissues, for example, fat, and tend to become highly concentrated in those tissues. Others combine with certain chemicals in the body, such as proteins. Such events have been described as the drugs moving into a tissue reservoir. The movement of drugs into tissue reservoirs is highly significant and will result in one or more of the following:

1. When a drug is first given, the blood concentration of free drug tends to rise and then drop as the drug moves to the tissue reservoir.

2. Once the tissue reservoir is saturated, further administration of the drug will increase the blood concentration of free or active drug.

3. When a significant amount of the drug is present in a tissue reservoir and administration of the drug is discontinued as the blood level drops, the drug moves from the tissue reservoir to the blood, thus prolonging the presence of the active drug in the blood.

The barbiturate anesthetics, which are given intravenously, are a good example of the three principles just given. Barbiturate anesthetics cause generalized anesthesia by their activity in certain tissues of the brain.

The brain has a high fat content. However, in addition to the brain, barbiturates have an affinity for all fatty tissue. Therefore when one of these drugs is administered intravenously, there is an initial rise in the blood levels. Almost immediately, however, the barbiturate starts to move from the blood into fat. This reduces both the blood levels and concentrations of this drug in the brain. (It is their high affinity for fat that causes the short anesthetic time after initial administration of the ultrashort-acting barbiturates.) As additional amounts of the drug are given, the fat eventually becomes saturated and blood levels rise. Prior to the metabolism and excretion of the drug, it must be reabsorbed from the fat. Therefore, with barbiturate anesthetics, even the ultrashort ones, once fat reservoirs are saturated, blood levels achieved with subsequent doses will remain high, and recovery from the anesthetic is prolonged.

Whereas some drugs have an affinity for fat, others have a tendency to be bound to blood or tissue proteins. Generally, the bound portion is inactive and does not cause toxicity. If doses are calculated on the assumption that a certain percentage of the administered dose will be bound to protein, anything that interferes with that binding will effectively increase the concentration of available (nonbound) drug. If the drug is relatively toxic, the release of a substantial portion of normally bound drug by simultaneously administered compounds that have a greater affinity for binding to proteins can result in toxic and even fatal levels.

The speed at which a drug is excreted from the body will have a profound effect on the concentration of the drug in the blood. In the most simple system, drugs are excreted from the blood in an unchanged form, usually by the kidneys. Other drugs must be metabolized, often by the liver, before they are excreted. When the blood concentration to maintain effective tissue concentrations at the site of action is known, the drug can be administered at set frequencies so that the drug lost by excretion is equal to that replaced by maintenance doses. However, if there is damage to the organ responsible for the metabolism of the drug or to the organ that excretes the drug, usually the liver and kidney, respectively, then average recommended doses will be excessive or the normal interval at which the drug is given will be too short.

DRUG INTERACTIONS

A drug interaction occurs when the effects of one drug are modified by the prior or concurrent administration of another drug. In recent years the clinical significance of drug interactions has been realized and much of the human medical literature has been devoted to discussion of interactions. More recently, attention has begun to be given to drug interactions in veterinary medicine. The study of drug interactions is a complex one, and a comprehensive review is beyond the scope of this chapter. It is our intention to explore the ways in which drugs might interact and to list some possible interactions that may be of importance in veterinary medicine (Table 2-2).

The classification of drug interactions is somewhat arbitrary, and frequently in the clinical setting a combination of factors comes into play. A number of sources dealing with drug interactions are now available.[1,7,8,11] In practice, an understanding of some of the ways in which drugs interact will perhaps

facilitate prediction, detection, and handling of such interactions. Such an understanding is of particular value in instances in which the two drugs involved are not listed in drug interaction tables and other literature.

Table 2-2 is a compilation of some drug interactions with which the veterinary practitioner might be confronted. It should be emphasized that this list is not complete but includes interactions that we think are particularly important or unique to veterinary medicine.

Drugs interact in a variety of ways. These are briefly discussed here.

Physical or chemical reaction

Physical or chemical drug interactions include those in which activity of one drug is prevented by its chemical reaction with another drug. The chelation (the binding of metals in soluble chemical complexes) of lead with EDTA solutions is an example.

Alteration of gastrointestinal absorption

If drugs are to be absorbed from the gastrointestinal tract, they must pass through cell membranes. Most drugs are weak acids or weak bases and exist in solution in an equilibrium between the ionized and nonionized forms. Generally, it is the nonionized species in solution that is able to pass through a membrane and thus be absorbed. Drugs that change intestinal pH may then affect the rate of absorption of other drugs by shifting the equilibrium in the direction of either the ionized unabsorbable species or the nonionized absorbable species. In the case of a weak base, for example, an increase in pH in the gut will result in a higher concentration of nonionized drug and increase absorption. With drugs that are weak acids, the reverse is true.

Other alterations in gastrointestinal absorption can be found with drugs that alter blood supply to the area of absorption and substances that chelate, precipitate, hydrolyze, or otherwise render a drug inactive or unabsorbable. An example of the latter is the interference with gastrointestinal absorption of tetracyclines by divalent ions like calcium.

Table 2-2. Drug interactions of commonly used veterinary drugs

Drug	May react with (agent)	Comment
Adrenocortical steroids	Salicylates	Risk of gut ulceration is increased
	Diuretics	Potentiation of potassium wasting effects may occur when these are used together
	Diphenylhydantoin	Metabolism of hydrocortisone is stimulated by enzyme induction
Analgesics		
Dipyrone	Chlorpromazine	Fever-reducing (antipyretic) effect of dipyrone may be increased, resulting in a severe drop in body temperature (hypothermia)
Salicylates	Corticosteroids	Risk of gut ulceration is increased
	Phenobarbital	Effect of salicylates is decreased due to enzyme induction
Anesthetics		
Barbiturate anesthetics	Chloramphenicol	Duration of anesthesia may be increased
General anesthetics	Hypotensive drugs and drugs that can lower blood pressure (e.g., phenothiazines)	Hypotensive effect may be enhanced
	Kanamycin Neomycin Streptomycin	Muscular paralysis with respiratory arrest may result when these drugs are given in high doses to animals receiving general anesthetics
Cyclopropane and halothane	Doxapram	Increase in epinephrine release may result, to which heart is more responsive in presence of cyclopropane and halothane
	Epinephrine Norepinephrine	These anesthetics sensitize myocardium to these agents, thus increasing chances of fibrillation or tachycardia
	Tubocurarine	Enhanced neuromuscular blocking effect dosage of tubocurarine should be reduced
Anticancer drugs		
Methotrexate	Sulfonamides	Methotrexate may be displaced from binding sites, and toxic reaction to methotrexate may result
Anticholinergics	Antihistamines Phenothiazines Tricyclic antidepressants	These drugs exhibit some anticholinergic activity and may be additive
Anticonvulsants	Diazepam (Valium)	When diazepam is used as adjunct to anticonvulsant therapy, increase in the dose of standard anticonvulsant may be necessary
	Phenothiazines	Convulsive threshold can be lowered
Barbiturate anticonvulsants	Phenothiazines	Although these agents will potentiate depressant effects of barbiturates, they do not potentiate anticonvulsant effects

Continued.

Table 2-2. Drug interactions of commonly used veterinary drugs—cont'd

Drug	May react with (agent)	Comment
Diphenylhydantoin	Corticosteroids	Metabolism of hydrocortisone is increased by enzyme induction
	Phenobarbital	Effect of diphenylhydantoin can be decreased by stimulating its metabolism
	Phenylbutazone	Depressive effect of diphenylhydantoin on central nervous system is enhanced by inhibition of its metabolism
	Salicylates	Large doses of aspirin have been reported to enhance effect
Anti-infectives		
Chloramphenicol	Other drugs that may cause bone marrow depression	Concurrent use should be avoided
	Phenobarbital	Some studies show that pretreatment with phenobarbital may decrease plasma levels and effectiveness of chloramphenicol
Colistin and polymyxin	Muscle relaxants or antibiotics kanamycin, neomycin, or streptomycin	These drugs interfere with nerve transmission at the neuromuscular junction; concomitant use should be undertaken with caution
Erythromycin Gentamycin Kanamycin	Urinary alkalinizers	Antibacterial activity is enhanced in alkaline urine
Griseofulvin	Phenobarbital	Concurrent administration results in lower blood concentration of griseofulvin
Streptosidine antibiotics	Anesthetics Muscle relaxants	Neuromuscular blockade potentiated
	Antihistamines Antinausea drugs	Ototoxic effects of antibiotics may be masked
Lincomycin	Kaopectate	Absorption of lincomycin is severely inhibited
Penicillins	Bacteriostatic antibiotics	Activity of penicillins is inhibited
	Dactinomycin	Action of penicillins can be antagonized
	Probenecid	This can enhance activity of penicillins by inhibiting their tubular excretion
Tetracyclines	Divalent and trivalent cations Antacids Milk	These combine with tetracyclines in gastrointestinal tract to form compounds that are not readily absorbed
	Methoxyflurane	Oxlate crystals are formed, causing glomerular necrosis
Idoxuridine	Boric acid	Boric acid is irritant in presence of idoxuridine
	Corticosteroids	Spread of viral infection may be accelerated

Table 2-2. Drug interactions of commonly used veterinary drugs—cont'd

Drug	May react with (agent)	Comment
Sulfonamides	Urinary alkalinizers	Excretion of sulfonamides is increased
	Antacids	Absorption of sulfonamides from gut may be compromised
	Phenylbutazone	Sulfonamide activity may be increased by displacement from binding sites
Central nervous system drugs		
Sympathomimetics	Doxapram	Pressor effect of sympathomimetics enhanced
	Halothane Cyclopropane	Myocardium is sensitized to sympathomimetics
Phenothiazines	Piperazine	Phenothiazines sometimes cause tremors or shaking; this effect can be potentiated by piperazine
Norepinephrine	Diuretics	Arterial responsiveness to norepinephrine may be decreased
Digitalis glycosides	Diuretics	Diuretics cause potassium loss; if hypokalemia is not corrected, heart becomes more sensitive to digitalis
Diuretics	Corticosteroids ACTH	Additive potassium loss occurs when these are given together
	Digitalis	See above
Gastrointestinal agents		
Lomotil	Barbiturates	Barbiturates may be potentiated
Mineral oil	Dioctyl sodium sulfosuccinate (DSS)	Absorption of mineral oil is increased; these should not be given together for prolonged periods of time
Muscle relaxants	Anticholinesterases Neostigmine Edrophonium Organophosphates*	Effects of succinylcholine and decamethonium are potentiated

*The potential for interactions due to organophosphates is of particular and increasing importance in veterinary medicine. The use of these agents as anthelmintics and pesticides and in flea collars and medallions is extensive. The nature of these products is such that they are often employed by the owner at home or on the farm. For this reason a carefully taken history is essential to prevent drug interactions with the organophosphates.

Alteration of renal excretion

There are three basic mechanisms by which one drug might alter the renal excretion of another:

1. Some drugs have a direct effect on the kidney and produce changes in glomerular filtration rate, thereby altering the rate of excretion of drugs whose excretion is by this mechanism. Examples of drugs affecting glomerular filtration are some diuretics and the adrenocortical steroids.

2. Active tubular secretion is a process by which some drugs are secreted into the urine against a concentration gradient. This process is thought to be dependent on a carrier molecule to which the drug attaches for transport across the tubular membrane. Other drugs may interfere with this process. p-Aminohippurate, for example, competes with penicillin for a common carrier, thus reducing the rate of excretion of penicillin. Probenecid disables the carrier for penicillin. This phe-

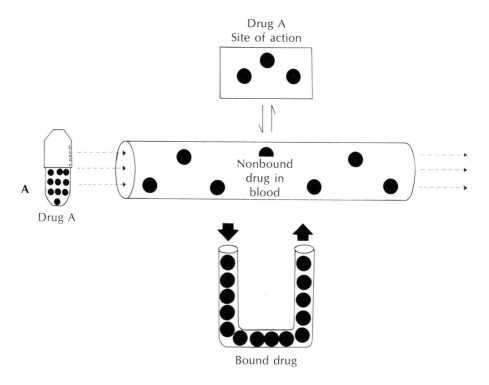

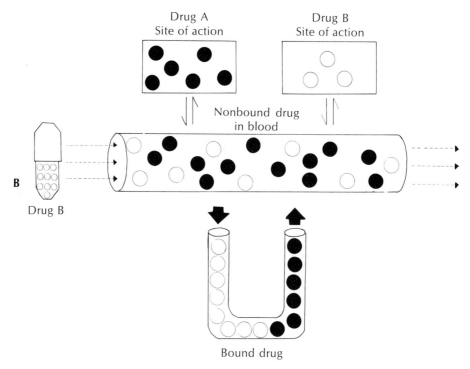

Fig. 2-6. Replacement of one bound drug with another. **A,** When a drug *(drug A)* is bound to tissue-binding sites, equilibrium is established with nonbound (active) drug in blood and at site of action. **B,** When bound drug is replaced by another *(drug B)*, concentration of active drug in blood and at site of action rises dramatically.

nomenon has been used to therapeutic advantage to increase and prolong circulating penicillin levels.

3. Many drugs pass into or out of the urine by passive tubular diffusion. pH changes in the urine can effect the ratio of diffusion in much the same manner as those discussed in gastrointestinal absorption. An increase in urine pH will favor excretion of acidic drugs like the barbiturates, salicylates, and nitrofurans. A decrease in urine pH will favor the excretion of basic drugs like meperidine, quinidine, and procaine.[8] Alterations in renal excretion by this mechanism are of sufficient magnitude, for example, to be of some value in increasing the rate of excretion of salicylates in salicylate intoxication.

Alteration of drug metabolism

The elimination of many drugs is dependent on their being metabolized to more easily eliminated substances. Prior exposure to many drugs can alter significantly the rate at which other drugs are metabolized.

Enzyme induction. Many drugs stimulate the production of enzymes responsible for the metabolism of other drugs. For example, prior exposure to phenobarbital greatly accelerates the metabolism of diphenylhydantoin, hexobarbital, warfarin, griseofulvin, and others. Obviously in this situation the prior exposure to one drug results in a shorter biological half-life and therefore lower concentrations and diminished effects of the other.

Metabolic inhibition. Just as the metabolism of a drug can be stimulated by prior administration of another drug, there are also instances in which the reverse is true. For example, oxyphenbutazone has been shown to inhibit metabolism of warfarin and thereby increase its anticoagulant action.

Alteration of drug distribution

The effect a drug produces is proportional to the concentration of that drug at the receptor sites. The distribution of many drugs includes, in part, the binding of part of the drug to tissue storage sites. Tissue storage sites include plasma proteins, connective tissue binding sites, fat, and even intracellular binding sites. The dose of a drug, determined by in vivo testing, often empirically allows for an amount of drug bound to tissue binding sites. Should the ratio of free to bound drug be altered by the intervention of another drug, the effects of the drug may vary considerably from what is expected (Fig. 2-6). Phenylbutazone or aspirin, for example, will displace anticoagulant drugs from albumin-binding sites, increasing the concentration of unbound drug at the receptor site and significantly increasing the anticoagulant effect of a given dose of these drugs.

Pharmacological interaction

One final mechanism by which drugs might interact can be classified as pharmacological interaction. This classification includes what have long been known as therapeutic incompatabilities. Although these interactions are often the most easily predictable, they do occur frequently. They include the administration of drugs of similar pharmacological action, resulting in additive or even synergistic action and the employment of drugs of opposing pharmacological action. In the latter, one often risks the side effects of both drugs and gains little or no beneficial effect, since the response to one drug is essentially reversed by the other.

References

1. American Pharmaceutical Association, Evaluation of drug interactions, ed. 1, Washington D.C., 1973, American Pharmaceutical Association.
2. Brodie, B. B., and Watson, R. D.: Some pharmacological consequences of species variation in rates of metabolism, Symposium on Comparative Pharmacology, Fed. Proc. **26:**1062, 1967.
3. Davis, L. E., and others: Pharmacokinetics of chloramphenicol in domesticated animals, J. Vet. Res. **33:**2259, 1972.
4. Enos, L. R.: Unpublished data.
5. Goodman, L. S., and Gilman, A.: The pharmacological basis of therapeutics, ed. 4, New York, 1970, Macmillan Co.
6. Franke, D. E., and Whitney, H. A.: Perspectives in clinical pharmacy, ed. 1, Hamilton, Ill., 1972, Drug Intelligence Publications.

7. Hansten, P.: Drug interactions, Philadelphia, 1971, Lea & Febiger.
8. Hartshorn, E. A.: Handbook of drug interactions, Cincinnati, 1970, Donald E. Francke.
9. Jones, L. M.: Veterinary pharmacology and therapeutics, ed. 3, Ames, Iowa, 1965, Iowa State University Press.
10. Robinson, D., and William, R. T.: Do cats form glucuronides? Biochem. J. **68:**23, 1958.
11. Szabuniewcz, M., Bailey, E. M., and Wiersig, D. O.: Clinical aspects of drug actions and interactions in veterinary practice, Vet. Med. Small Anim. Clin. **68:**1048, 1973.
12. Wells, J. S., and others: Toxicity, distribution and excretion of cephaloridine in laboratory animals, Antimicrob. Agents Chemother., p. 863, 1965.
13. Wilson, C. O., and Gisvold, O.: Textbook of organic medicinal and pharmaceutical chemistry, ed. 4, Philadelphia, 1962, J. B. Lippincott Co.

3

INTRODUCTION TO PREVENTION AND TREATMENT OF

Infectious diseases

MICROORGANISMS

Disease in animals may come from any of a great number of causes. Among the most common causes are microorganisms, and this chapter will be concerned with diseases caused by microorganisms, their prevention, and treatment.

Not all microorganisms produce disease. Some are essential to life. For example, the bacteria, fungi, and protozoa that make up the normal flora of the rumen of cattle and sheep are aids to the digestion of the food these animals ingest and are essential to the well-being of these species. Numerous microorganisms live on or in animals and cause no problems for the host. However, other microorganisms cause diseases in animals, and these are referred to as "pathogenic microorganisms."

Pathogenic microorganisms that will be discussed in this chapter include viruses, bacteria, fungi, and protozoa.

MANAGING INFECTIOUS DISEASES

Generally, there are two approaches to managing infectious diseases: prevention and treatment. In the following sections we will discuss various aspects of prevention and treatment of infectious disease.

PREVENTING INFECTIOUS DISEASES

Animals are continually exposed to pathogenic microorganisms. Whether those exposures will result in disease is a function of three factors: the microorganism, the environment, and the physiological state of the animal. In endeavoring to prevent diseases in animals an attempt must be made to manipulate one or more of these interrelating factors. Let us examine each of these factors and discuss how they can be manipulated to prevent diseases in animals.

The organism

For our purposes, the most important characteristic of a microorganism is its ability to produce disease. This is called the "virulence" of the organism. Certain strains of microorganisms that can produce disease have a greater virulence than other strains.

The virulence of an organism stems from its ability to propagate in tissues or on the surface of the host. Virulence is also determined by the ability of the organism to produce chemicals that kill or injure cells. These chemicals that poison tissues or cells are called "toxins."

There are two types of toxins. *Endotoxins* are present in the cell wall of bacteria and affect the tissues inhabited by the bacteria. The toxic effects they usually produce are fever and increased capillary permeability, which results in inflammation, hemorrhage, and shock. Such toxins do not tend to stimulate the production of protective antibodies in the host.

Exotoxins are excreted by bacteria. The effect of exotoxins is frequently seen in organs distant from the actual site of infection. For example, when an animal contracts tetanus, the point of infection is usually in an extremity. However, the exotoxins produced by the bacteria act on the central nervous system to produce the typical rigid muscular contractions associated with the disease.

Specific exotoxins affect specific systems in the body. Examples are neurotoxins, which affect the nervous system; hemolytic toxins, which destroy the red blood cells; and leukotoxins, which destroy white blood cells. Exotoxins stimulate formation of protective antibodies by the host.

In addition to their virulence, another primary characteristic of infectious organisms that determines whether disease will be produced in the host is the number of organisms to which the host is exposed. The combination of these two factors, number of organisms and virulence, can determine whether disease will be produced and, if it is, the severity of the disease. A large number of organisms with relatively low virulence is necessary to produce disease, whereas a relatively small number of highly virulent organisms could possibly produce serious disease. Reducing the number of organisms to which an animal is exposed can substantially reduce the probability of that animal developing an infectious disease.

Environmental factors

The environment can play an important role in determining whether an animal will contract an infectious disease. The environment influences the general health status of the animal, and this health status is a determining factor of the animal's resistance to infection by microorganisms. Factors such as whether animals are overcrowded, environmental humidity, exposure to noxious substances, and the type of feed available play a major role in the animals' ability to combat infection successfully.

Characteristics of the host

One of the most important characteristics of the host is partial or complete genetic resistance to infection by certain microorganisms. An example of complete genetic resistance is the inability of cats to become infected with canine distemper virus.

Even within a given species, genetic differences exist in the susceptibility of infection by given microorganisms. For example, Brahman cattle are more resistant than other kinds of cattle to natural infection from the protozoans of *Babesia* species, which cause destruction of red blood cells. The resistance is in part due to resistance to infestation by an intermediate host, ticks.

When an animal is capable of being infected by microorganisms and is exposed to a suitable number of microorganisms with adequate virulence to cause disease, its overall state of health will likely determine whether disease results. Animals in a good state of health have numerous primary and secondary defense mechanisms to combat invading microorganisms. However, when animals are in poor health, their defense mechanisms are seriously compromised.

The primary defenses consist of the skin and mucous membranes, which must be penetrated if an invading organism is to establish an infection. These surfaces have numerous mechanisms by which they can prevent invasion by microorganisms. For example, tears wash organisms away from the epithelium of the eye, and various mucous membranes and the skin secrete substances that destroy microorganisms. When organisms are swallowed, they pass into a highly acidic environment in the stomach that destroys many organisms.

Secondary defenses include the body's various biochemical systems of defense, antitoxic immunity, and antibodies formed against the organisms. Most animal tissues and fluids contain an enzyme, lysozyme, which has the ability to destroy bacteria. Various tissues in the body contain other chemical substances that can destroy invading microorganisms. The body also produces antibodies that render invading microorganisms harmless. These antibodies are the basis of the use of biologicals in medicine. The ability of an animal to produce antibodies is directly related to its state of general health and nutrition. For these reasons veterinarians often recommend a thorough examination and deworming program before beginning vaccination routines in small animals. The general health and state of nutrition should also be considered before immunization procedures are initiated in large farm-type animals.

Controlling organisms, environments, and hosts

An enormous amount of control can be exercised over the numbers of organisms to which animals are exposed, the type of environment in which animals live, and the health and immune status of animals. About the only factor that cannot be controlled is the virulence of the organisms to which the animal is exposed. However, this is just one of a multitude of factors that determine whether an animal will develop an infectious disease.

Through management one can do most to prevent infectious diseases in animals. Choosing animals from a genetic stock less susceptible to a particular disease is one available management process. However, the most important and practical processes relate to good husbandry practices. Animals should receive balanced diets, they should be kept in clean surroundings, and they should be housed under conditions that minimize the environmental stresses of extreme heat and cold.

By means of intense and expensive processes, infectious organisms that are responsible for a particular disease can be eliminated or substantially reduced in a given area. Through a method of testing all animals and slaughtering those infected, foot and mouth disease has been eradicated from the United States. As a result of vigorous vaccination programs and quarantine procedures, rabies has been eliminated from England. When it is not practicable to eliminate diseases totally from an area, animals can sometimes be protected by artificially inducing immunity in them.

Acquired immunity

Immunity is that process through which animals can, by developing appropriate antibodies, become partially or totally resistant to a given microorganism. The antibodies react with either microorganisms or toxins to render them harmless to the animal. Antibodies work by one of the following mechanisms: neutralizing a toxic product of the infecting organisms, killing the infecting organism, promoting their ingestion by phagocytic cells, or preventing entry of the organism into host cells in which the organism may reproduce.[2]

Antigens are substances that stimulate the production of antibodies. In response to an antigen, various types of antibodies will be formed by the body. Some of these antibodies will confer immunity to the host; others may not. Unfortunately many serological tests for the presence of antibodies measure antibodies that do not confer immunity. Therefore many such tests are not reliable in determining the immune status of animals.

If antibodies are to be effective in preventing disease, they must be present in significant concentration in tissues that will be invaded by either microorganisms or the toxin they produce. For some diseases the level of antibodies in the serum is a good measure of the available antibodies to prevent infection. For others it is not. The measure of antibodies in the respiratory or gastrointestinal tracts may be far more important for diseases affecting the respiratory or digestive system than serum antibodies.

Independent of the development of immunity to particular diseases, the antigen-antibody relationship has a strong influence on the health of animals, in many cases negative. The formation of antibodies is the basis for the development of allergies and autoimmune diseases (in which an animal destroys its own tissues). Defects in the immunologi-

cal system very likely play an important role in the development of cancer. Discussions of these phenomena are for the most part beyond the scope of this text. For an understanding of basic immunological phenomena the student is referred to Roitt.[11]

One should be careful not to confuse the term "antibodies" with "antibiotics." Antibodies are large complex proteins manufactured by the body as a response to the stimulus of an antigen. The antibody reacts with that antigen in some demonstrable way. Antibiotics, on the other hand, are produced by microorganisms and are chemicals that have inhibiting or lethal effects on other microorganisms. They are developed commercially for use in animals to combat certain microorganisms, usually bacteria.

Active immunity. There are two types of

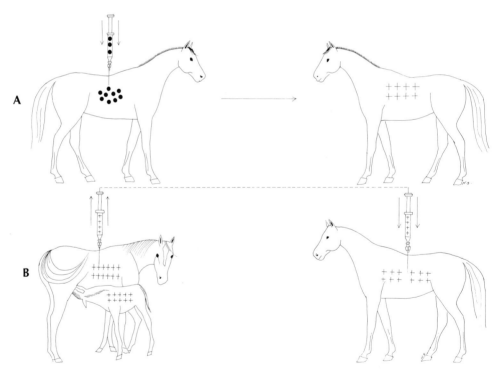

Fig. 3-1. A, Active immunity. Animal takes in antigen (●) either by natural exposure or by inoculation *(top left)* and responds by producing antibodies (+) *(top right).* **B,** Passive immunity. Immune animal can transfer antibodies (+) to offspring either through placental transfer or in colostrum *(lower left),* or serum containing antibodies can be taken from immune animal and transferred to another animal *(lower right).*

immunity: active and passive (Fig. 3-1). Active immunity results when an animal produces antibodies and develops an immune status as a result of being exposed to an antigen. Exposure to the antigen can be natural, such as occurs when an animal is naturally infected. The natural infection may produce a disease state, or the infection may be subclinical. Active immunity also results from artificial introduction of antigens to the animal. This occurs during immunizing procedures. In either case the immunity that develops may be short lasting or result in lifetime protection. Even when the antibody level drops, animals once immunized often have the ability to rapidly develop high levels of antibodies when they are once again exposed to the antigens, which is known as the "anamnestic response."

The active production of antibodies can be reduced by the concurrent administration of corticosteroids. This is one mechanism by which corticosteroids increase an animal's susceptibility to infections. The significance of this effect at clinical doses is in question.

Passive immunity. Passive immunity develops by transferring antibodies from one animal to another. The animal itself does not actively produce the antibodies. Such transfer occurs in nature by the placental transfer of antibodies from mother to fetus or by the animal receiving antibodies in the colostrum (the milk that the animal receives during the first few days of life). In humans the natural transfer of antibodies from mother to child occurs primarily in utero through the placenta. In the animals considered in this text the transfer is largely or wholly by way of the colostrum.

Generally, an animal cannot absorb antibodies through its intestine. However, in many species, newborn animals have the ability to ingest antibodies and absorb them from the intestinal tract intact.

Passive immunity may develop in another way. In animals, antibodies can be artificially transferred by administering serum, antitoxins, or gamma globulins, usually by subcutaneous inoculation.

All antibodies obtained by the passive route are short-lived. They do not give the animal an increased ability to produce its own antibodies when it is exposed to the antigens. In fact, in some instances the presence of passive antibodies severely limits the ability of the animal to respond immunologically to the antigen.

The relationship between passive antibodies and the ability of the animal to produce its own antibodies is complex. In some species, newborn animals are incapable of immunologically responding to an antigen, since the tissues responsible for the production of antibodies are not fully developed. In other species, such as the dog, animals are potentially able to produce antibodies shortly after birth, but the presence of passive antibodies actually prevents the animal from responding immunologically to an antigen. For example, 2-week-old puppies that have received no anti–canine distemper antibodies in the colostrum or artificially can respond to distemper vaccine, but puppies that have received anti–canine distemper antibodies in the colostrum or artificially may be unable to respond for as long as 12 weeks. In other species an immune state can be developed by the simultaneous inoculation in different sites with antisera (sera containing antibodies) and appropriate antigens. For example, hogs can be inoculated with virulent hog cholera virus in one leg and hog cholera antiserum in the other. If the doses given are correct, the animals not only fail to develop hog cholera but also develop immunity to the disease. This would not happen if dogs were inoculated with canine distemper antiserum and virulent distemper virus. The reasons for these differences are beyond the scope of this text. However, it is important to be aware that these differences exist. The proper techniques for immunizing both young and mature animals against various diseases will be discussed in subsequent chapters.

BIOLOGICALS

Those products used in animals that confer active or passive immunity against either the organism responsible for infectious disease or the toxins it produces are called "biologicals." Potency of biologicals is often described in terms of units rather than milligrams as used for drugs. A unit is a measure of biological activity defined for the specific biological. For example, doses of tetanus antitoxin are measured in units. A dose recommended for prevention of tetanus in the horse is 1500 units.

Biologicals that produce active immunity (vaccines and toxoids)

Vaccines and toxoids are used to produce active immunity. Vaccines contain living or dead microorganisms. Toxoids contain nonpathogenic chemicals closely related to exotoxins. Adjuvants are often added to vaccines. Adjuvants are substances that, when added to an antigen, increase the immune response. Generally, adjuvants delay the absorption of biologicals from the site of administration, which results in a higher level of antibody response. For example, aluminum hydroxide is frequently used as an adjuvant in veterinary vaccines.

Vaccines and toxoids are classified according to the type of antigen they contain.

Vaccines containing living organisms. There are three possible means by which living organisms may be used to produce immunity without causing disease. Virulent organisms may be either administered in a dose that will produce subclinical infection or inoculated in an abnormal site. For example, to immunize chickens against laryngotracheitis (a disease infecting the upper respiratory system) the virulent virus is brushed into the mucous membranes of the cloaca, which is the genital area of the chicken. Another example is inoculation against ovine ecthyma, a virus disease of sheep that causes blisterlike lesions on the skin of the lips and sometimes around the nostrils and the eyes. The virulent virus is scarified into the skin on the inner aspect of the thigh.

The most common biologicals containing living organisms are made up of attenuated organisms, which by manipulation have been reduced in virulence. These organisms still contain suitable antigens to produce an active immunity against virulent organisms, but they are not likely to cause disease states in the animals to which they are administered. Various methods are employed for attenuating virulent organisms. These include drying, growing at unfavorable temperatures, growing in a less susceptible host, growing in an artificial medium, selecting a relatively avirulent colony, adding chemicals or heat to living colonies, or serial passage of the organisms into animals or animal tissue. Serial passage involves injecting the organism into an animal or animal tissue, permitting its multiplication in the host for a time, then passing it to a second animal or animal tissue, then to a third, and so on until the desired level of attenuation is reached. In general, the more times it is passed the greater the attenuation.

Biologicals often are named by the method used to attenuate the organisms they contain. For example, one class of biologicals contains modified live viruses. The term "modified live virus" is another way of saying that the virus is attenuated. Commonly the virus is attenuated by serial passage of the virus in eggs. Thus some biologicals are referred to as "modified live virus duck embryo origin." Another common way of modifying viruses is by producing them in tissue culture. These vaccines are referred to as "tissue culture origin modified live virus" products.

Tissue cultures are produced by harvesting living cells and growing those cells in artificial media. Kidney cells are used commonly. Because the tissue culture environment is substantially different from that of the cells within the body, viruses often become attenuated, even when grown in tissue culture in cells from a host that the virus normally would affect. For example, the canine distemper virus can be attenuated in canine kidney cell culture.

Cells used to produce tissue culture vaccines may be primary cells (recently harvested from animals and transferred from one cell culture to another less than ten times) or established cell lines that have been thus transferred ten times or more. When placed in cell culture, cells tend to develop new characteristics and in many cases new chromosome numbers. Usually only established cell lines that have stabilized (developed certain defined characteristics from generation to generation) are used.

Because living organisms, including those that are attenuated, actually invade tissues of the animal and in many cases reproduce in the animal, it is generally assumed that they produce better immunity than killed products. With living vaccines, one has the best chance of obtaining antibodies in the tissues that are likely to be infected.

Vaccines containing killed organisms. Viral and bacterial vaccines can be prepared by killing the infective organism. This is usually done by adding chemicals such as phenol to the organisms or by heating them to a temperature at which they are destroyed. The dead organisms are incapable of producing a disease state within animals. However, they still contain antigens necessary to bring about an antibody response.

Bacterins are vaccines containing killed bacteria. Commercially available bacterins are prepared from well-characterized cultures of bacteria. In addition, autogenous bacterins are prepared from pathogenic bacteria isolated from diseased animals. They are intended for use in animals in the herd from which the organism was originally isolated.

Bacterins can be prepared by chemically killing bacteria in whole liquid culture or from bacteria washed from solid cultures. When whole liquid cultures are used, the bacterin contains the antigens associated with the bacteria cell as well as metabolic products of bacterial growth. When prepared from solid cultures, the bacterin is more limited in the amount of antigenic metabolites present.

Toxoids. In some instances, the exotoxins excreted by infectious organisms cause disease. In such infections it may be more important to develop antibodies in the animal against the toxins rather than against the offending organisms. For this purpose, toxoids are used, chemicals that have a similar structure to the toxin and are therefore capable of eliciting an antibody (antitoxin) response in the animal without causing toxic effects. Toxoids can be produced by allowing toxins to age, which causes them to lose their toxic properties. Toxins can also be converted to toxoids chemically by adding chemicals such as formalin to fresh preparations of toxins. Toxins are harvested from cultures of the organisms that produce them.

Biologicals that confer passive immunity

Biologicals that transfer passive immunity to an animal are not nearly as effective in preventing disease as those that produce active immunity. In some instances they are even counterproductive. For example, the use of canine distemper antiserum does not provide adequate protection against the disease. However, it prevents the animal from responding immunologically when distemper vaccine is administered.

Antisera and gamma globulins. Antibodies are passively transferred to animals by injecting them, generally subcutaneously, with serum containing antibodies that have been actively produced in another animal. This serum is usually standardized so that equivalent commercial products have equivalent levels of antibodies. In some cases, instead of using the serum, the gamma globulins from the serum are isolated. Gamma globulins contain the various immunoglobulins that contain the antibodies. Administration of gamma globulins requires a less massive injection than administration of antiserum.

Antitoxins. Antitoxins are preparations containing antibodies that act against bacterial toxins rather than against the bacteria. Preparations of antitoxins are standardized against known quantities of bacterial toxins. Like antisera, antitoxins are not as effective in protecting animals as the development of active immunity by administering a toxoid.

Factors determining effectiveness of biologicals

A primary factor determining the effectiveness of an active response to the administration of biologicals is the route of administration. The level of antibodies in tissues likely to be invaded by the organism will determine whether the animal is truly immune to infection. The route of administration can substantially affect the area in which antibodies are primarily developed. For example, in the management of respiratory disease it may be more suitable to administer vaccines by the intranasal route so that high levels of antibodies are reached in the membranes of the upper respiratory tract.

Although most vaccines are currently given subcutaneously or intramuscularly, there are indications that the development of new products will result in new routes of administration to make vaccines more effective.

There is one important difference between the use of biologicals and the use of most pharmaceuticals. Doses are usually established for biologicals on a per animal basis rather than on a weight basis. Therefore a chihuahua receives as much rabies vaccine as a great dane. The reason is that it requires a certain amount of antigen (antigenic mass) to elicit the antibody response within the animal. Great risk of compromising the future immune status of an animal is taken if a smaller dose is given because the animal is smaller than most members of its species. *The recommendations of the manufacturers of a particular biological should always be followed for both the amount of the product administered to an animal and the route of administration.*

How biologicals are handled will also determine whether they will be effective when administered to animals. It is important that, when administering vaccines with living organisms, no disinfectants be used to sterilize syringes unless they are thoroughly rinsed prior to administering the product. If residues of disinfectant linger in the syringes, they may kill the living organism and render the product useless. (Although many biologicals contain dead organisms and are effective, it is a safe generalization that those biologicals containing living organisms will not be effective when administered if the organisms have been inadvertently killed.)

Many biologicals are destroyed by heat and sunlight. It is essential to keep biologicals adequately refrigerated until they are ready to be used. Many livestock owners and veterinarians use picnic ice chests to protect biologicals when immunizing large herds of animals. The users of biologicals must also be assured when receiving biologicals from the manufacturer that they have not been exposed to extreme light or heat.

As already mentioned, for some species of animals the presence of passive antibodies prevents active response against an antigen. An adequate period of time must therefore have elapsed before an animal is inoculated with a biological after it has been given antisera. This will be discussed in specific detail in subsequent chapters.

The production of antibodies by animals can also be impaired if certain combinations are administered. There is no rule of thumb in this regard; it is suitable to administer certain combinations, whereas others prevent the active production of antibodies. This subject too will be discussed in greater detail in later chapters.

Hypersensitivity

Ideally, when biologicals are administered to an animal to produce an active antibody response, the antibodies so produced are the type that prevent subsequent infection by the specific virulent organisms. However, administration of any biological, including antiserum, can result in the development of a hyperimmune status. With hyperimmunity, subsequent administration of antigens will result in undesirable reactions. These reactions, which can also occur from administration of pharmaceuticals such as penicillin, may result in anything from relatively mild signs such as a generalized rash to a major reaction such as anaphylaxis, which if untreated kills the animal. In anaphylaxis, smooth muscles surrounding the bronchi and upper respiratory tract constrict the air passages, preventing the animal from breathing. In addition, general circulatory collapse may occur. Unless epinephrine is administered immediately, the animal will die. For this reason one should always have epinephrine immediately available when administering biologicals.

Other undesired hypersensitivity reactions that may occur after administering biologicals include fever, joint pain, and diarrhea. Animals exhibiting such signs after receiving biologicals should be closely observed by a veterinarian.

Summary

Many infectious diseases of animals are prevented by the use of biologicals. To use biologicals to advantage, one must know the organism responsible for the disease. Familiarity with the factors governing administration of biologicals is also essential. These factors include the age of the animals, the time of year at which the biological is administered, and the method and route of administration. For various diseases these factors will be discussed in detail in subsequent chapters.

TREATING INFECTIOUS DISEASES
Chemotherapy

Chemotherapy is the use of chemicals (drugs) for the treatment of disease. The term was first used to describe the use of chemicals to treat infectious diseases. More recently chemotherapy has included the use of chemicals in the treatment of cancer.

Three principal classes of drugs are used to combat infectious diseases: sulfonamides, antibiotics, and nitrofurans. These anti-infective drugs function in one of two ways. They either kill the microorganisms (those that kill bacteria, for instance, are referred to as "bactericidal"), or they prevent the microorganisms from multiplying (those that prevent bacteria from multiplying are referred to as "bacteriostatic"). Bacteriostatic drugs act by preventing multiplication of the pathogens, thereby containing the infection and allowing the natural defenses of the body to resolve the infection.

The various genera, species, and strains of microorganisms have varying susceptibilities to the anti-infective drugs. Since the introduction of anti-infective drugs, microor-

ganisms have tended to become more resistant to their effects. Microorganisms genetically more resistant to the effects of the anti-infective drugs have possibly been selected for survival by the widespread use of such drugs. Therefore the population of microorganisms among animals over the years has changed from those microorganisms that were highly sensitive to anti-infective drugs to those that are more resistant.

A genetic component of some bacteria causes them to be resistant to certain types of antibiotics and is called the "resistance factor." This resistance factor may contain genetic information capable of producing resistance to one or several antibiotics. Unfortunately it is possible for bacteria containing the resistance factor to transfer that factor to other bacteria, even those of different species. This has contributed to the increasing resistance of bacteria to antibiotics.

Principles of use

Numerous factors will determine whether an antibacterial is effective in clinical use.

Appropriateness of the anti-infective for the organism. For an anti-infective drug to be of benefit, the disease that it is being used to treat must be caused by an infective organism susceptible to the particular anti-infective. If veterinarians prescribe anti-infective drugs for diseases not caused by infective organisms or if they are used against a resistant organism, the drugs and treatment will be of no value.

To select a rational therapeutic regimen for treating an infectious disease, one must know something about the offending organism. Ideally a culture and sensitivity test will be run; that is, the offending bacteria is grown on a culture medium and identified, and its susceptibility to various antimicrobial drugs is determined. In practice a culture and sensitivity test are not always possible or practical. When this is the case, the practitioner selects an anti-infective drug on the bases of which one of several organisms are most likely to be involved and his experience with anti-infective drugs.

The surest determination of the effectiveness of an antibacterial is the clinical response. Generally, if marked improvement is not seen within 24 to 48 hours, the diagnosis should be reevaluated and if an infectious process is still suspected, then a reevaluation of therapy should be considered.

Dose. For an anti-infective drug to be effective, it must reach the site of infection at a suitable concentration. Reaching an effective concentration may require administering an initial dose to raise the concentration of the drug in the blood and then periodically giving maintenance doses to maintain the concentration as the body destroys or excretes the anti-infective drug. Although administering proper dose levels is rarely a problem in small-animal practice, it is often a problem in treating large domestic animals. Horses and cattle are frequently given ineffective doses of anti-infective drugs. However, it has been reported that lethal doses of tetracycline would have to be given to adult cattle and horses to treat them effectively for infections with organisms semiresistant to that antibiotic.[1] In small-animal practice, animals are often administered streptomycin at long intervals, so that the blood level drops below therapeutically effective concentrations (p. 52).

Even when adequate doses are administered, physical barriers may prevent effective concentration at the infected site. The thick walls of abscesses may prevent the diffusion of anti-infectives into the lesion, thus preventing their effectiveness. Even when antibiotics are able to penetrate abscesses, their effectiveness may be reduced by the chemical or physical nature of the area.

The effectiveness of anti-infective drugs can be reduced in the urinary tract, depending on the pH of the urine. Generally, antibacterials are highly effective in treating urinary infections because many are excreted unchanged into the urine. Novobiocin and the tetracyclines are examples of drugs whose effectiveness is increased in acidic urine. On the other hand, the effectiveness of erythromycin and the aminoglycosides (streptomycin, neomycin, kanamycin, and

gentamicin) is increased in alkaline urine. Therefore one should monitor the pH of urine during treatment of urinary infections and either adjust the pH to meet the needs of the selected antibacterial or select an antibacterial drug effective in the existing pH.

To obtain effective levels of anti-infective drugs at the site of the infection, the route of administration is important. For example, for most infections procaine penicillin G must be administered parenterally for it to be effective. Many anti-infective drugs, although useful in the intestinal tract, are not absorbed systemically and therefore have no value in the oral treatment of systemic infections.

Duration of treatment. Infections are likely to recur if anti-infective drugs are discontinued too soon after apparent clinical recovery. Infective organisms can multiply rapidly within the body and may do so if anti-infective drugs are removed from their environment. Bacterial urinary tract infection in dogs and cats should be treated for a minimum of 3 weeks and often for 6 to 8 weeks. Other infections requiring prolonged treatment include bacterial endocarditis (4 to 6 weeks) and pneumonia (2 to 4 weeks),[16] even though the animal has stopped showing signs of the disease early in treatment.

Combinations of anti-infective drugs. Generally, only one anti-infective drug is indicated to treat a particular infection. However, sometimes combinations are advantageous. For example, gentamycin and ampicillin are often synergistic. Ampicillin probably allows gentamycin better access to the bacterial cell. Problems from combinations can result, however. In some instances, combinations are pharmacologically incompatible. For example, penicillin is effective only against metabolically active bacteria. The tetracyclines, being bacteriostatic, slow down the metabolic rate. If these drugs are given in combination, the tetracycline may still be effective but it will inhibit the activity of penicillin.

Even if combinations of anti-infective drugs are pharmacologically compatible, physically or chemically they may be incompatible. Preparations prepared by commercial pharmaceutical companies are physically and chemically compatible of course. However, attempts to mix anti-infectives in syringes involve the risk of encountering a physical or chemical incompatibility that would render one or more of the active ingredients useless.[1] For example, the simultaneous administration of calcium solutions and sulfonamide in the jugular vein of cattle has resulted in death. This happens because calcium forms gels at the high pH characteristic of many sulfonamide solutions. If combinations are used or if antibacterials are administered with other drugs, they should be put in different syringes and injected in different sites.

Tetracyclines should not be administered orally with any calcium, aluminum, manganese, or iron salt because unabsorbable complexes are formed. When given orally, tetracycline should not be given within 2 hours of the ingestion of feed that has high levels of calcium.

Toxic effects. Many anti-infective drugs possess toxicity. Anyone administering them should be familiar with these toxic effects. For example, use of some antibiotics can result in a curare-like flaccid paralysis of the skeletal muscles. The aminoglycosides (neomycin, streptomycin, dihydrostreptomycin, kanamycin, and gentamycin), tetracycline, lincomycin, and polymyxins have been implicated. The same compounds plus chloramphenicol have been reported to cause cardiovascular depressant effects. Chloramphenicol and chlortetracycline have been indicated in inhibiting detoxification of drugs by the liver. Chloramphenicol has been shown to increase the amount of time necessary for a cat to recover from barbiturate anesthetics. Various antibiotics may suppress the immune response in animals.[14] If they are effective, this may not be too important. However, if antibiotics are given to an animal with an infection and they are not effective, suppressing the immune response opens the animal to greater danger.

Specific toxicity effects of various anti-infectives will be discussed later in this chapter.

Prophylactic use. The prophylactic use of anti-infective drugs involves their use to prevent infection by microorganisms against which the drugs are effective, even when such an infection does not already exist in the animal. Anti-infectives are used prophylactically far too often in animal patients. The dangers of prophylactic use include the following:

1. Increased chance that organisms develop resistance
2. Exposure of potentially debilitated animals to the toxic effects of drugs
3. Possible reduction of the animal's immune response
4. Increased risk of infections by viruses or other resistant organisms

Prophylactic use of anti-infective drugs may be indicated when the body's defenses are being reduced as a result of the use of certain drugs, when it is known that surgical intervention will cause contamination, and in certain well-defined conditions, for example, in the prevention of certain streptococcal infections. It should be noted that in surgical procedures the use of prophylactic antibiotics should not replace general aseptic procedures or the establishment of appropriate surgical drains and removal of debilitated tissue.

Anti-infective drugs
Sulfonamides

The sulfonamides were the first clinically useful antibacterial drugs. They are bacteriostatic in action, that is, they do not kill organisms but limit their reproduction and growth. Therefore successful treatment is dependent on the defense mechanisms of the host. Over 3300 sulfonamides have been prepared, but only a few are clinically useful.

The spectrum of activity of the sulfonamides is potentially broad, including many gram-positive and gram-negative organisms. The many sulfonamides available are essentially identical in spectrum and differ pri-

Table 3-1. Sulfonamides commonly used in veterinary medicine

Sulfonamide	Group*	Duration of blood levels†	Dose	Comment
Salicylazosulfapyridine	SA	S	Oral: 44-55 mg/kg three times daily, no more than total dose of 6 gm/24 hr	For ulcerative colitis in dogs; prolonged use associated with keratoconjuctivitis sica
Sulfabromomethazine	A	L	Oral: 220 mg/kg every 48 hours; IV‡: 30-70 mg/kg	May cause abortions in cattle
Sulfacetamide	SA	S	Topical in eye as 5%-20% solution	May not penetrate cornea of dog
Sulfadiazine	A	L	Oral or IV: 220 mg/kg, then 100 mg/kg twice daily	Seldom used; other sulfas generally preferred
Sulfadiazine and trimethoprin	A	L	30 mg/kg/24 hr of sulfadiazine	Trimethoprin is reported to increase effectiveness of sulfadiazine[6]
Sulfadimethoxine	A	L	Oral or parenteral: 55 mg/kg, then 25 mg/kg/24 hr	Enjoys considerable veterinary use; some think dosage recommended is inadequate
Sulfadimethoxine—sustained release	A	PR	Oral: 137.5 mg/kg/24 hr	Provides effective blood levels for 4 days
Sulfaguanidine	E	NA	Oral: calves, 2.5 gm twice daily; poultry, 0.5%-1.5% in feed	Not absorbed from gut
Sulfamerazine	A	S	Oral or parenteral: 130 mg/kg, then 45 mg/kg three times daily	
Sulfamethazine	A	L	Oral or parenteral: 130 mg/kg, then 65 mg/kg twice daily	Blood concentration of sufficient duration to allow dosage two times a day
Sulfamethazine—prolonged release (Hava Span)	A	PR	Oral: cattle, 495 mg/kg every 4 days[4]	In cattle, will provide effective blood levels about 18 hours after administration; to obtain rapid blood levels, concurrent parenteral administration of sulfonamide is recommended[4]
Sulfamethizole	A	S	130 mg/kg, then 45 mg/kg three times daily	

*Group: SA = sulfonamides with special application; A = absorbable sulfonamides, E = poorly absorbed, enteric sulfonamides.
†Duration of blood levels: S = short-acting (must be given more than two times a day); L = long-acting (given once or twice a day); PR = prolonged release (can be given less than once a day); NA = not applicable.
‡IV = Intravenous.

Table 3-1. Sulfonamides commonly used in veterinary medicine—cont'd

Sulfonamide	Group	Duration of blood levels	Dose	Comment
Sulfaquinoxaline	E	NA	Poultry, lambs, pigs: 0.0125%-0.025% in drinking water	Primary use in coccidial infestations and swine diarrhea
Sulfathiazole	A	S	130 mg/kg, then 45 mg/kg three times daily	
Sulfisoxazole	A	S	130 mg/kg, then 45 mg/kg three times daily	Primarily used in urinary tract infections

marily in their absorption, distribution, solubility, and duration of action.

Sulfonamides are used to treat various infectious diseases of animals. They find some use in infections of the respiratory system and the urinary tract, bacterial diarrheas, foot rot, coccidial infestations, uterine infections, mastitis, and various other infectious conditions.

For purposes of this discussion the sulfonamides will be categorized into three groups: the poorly absorbed sulfonamides, the absorbable sulfonamides, and the sulfonamides for special application. No attempt will be made to discuss every available sulfonamide, but those most commonly encountered in each group are listed in Table 3-1.

Poorly absorbed sulfonamides. The poorly absorbed sulfonamides are those that are not absorbed from the gastrointestinal tract in sufficient quantity to produce adequate systemic concentrations. The use of these drugs is limited to infections confined to the lumen of the gastrointestinal tract.

Absorbable sulfonamides. The sulfonamides in this group are absorbed from the gut in sufficient quantity to be of value in the treatment of systemic infections. These sulfonamides find use in various infectious diseases. They are employed most commonly in large animals in the treatment of pneumonia, foot rot, infections of the nervous system, and various other infections. Absorbable sulfonamides are available in many dif-

ferent dosage forms: tablets, boluses, oral suspensions, injectable solutions, and solutions or soluble powders for use as feed or water additives. The absorbable group of sulfonamides can be further divided on the basis of duration of action.

Short-acting sulfonamides. Short-acting sulfonamides must be given three or more times a day. The usual dosage of these drugs is given in Table 3-1. Short-acting sulfonamides are used in both large and small animals. In small animals they find particular use in urinary tract infections.

Long-acting sulfonamides. These sulfonamides are either absorbed slowly or excreted slowly so that the duration of blood levels is extended. As a result they are administered only once or twice a day. The primary advantage lies in the fact that these drugs need not be given as often as those of the short-acting group. This is of value in the treatment of large animals or animals that are difficult to restrain.

Prolonged-release sulfonamides. These drugs are absorbed extremely slowly and are administered less than once a day. Because it may take 12 to 18 hours for prolonged-released sulfonamides to reach therapeutic blood levels, it is wise to administer a short-acting sulfonamide concurrently with the first dose.[4]

Sulfonamides for special application

Sulfacetamide. This sulfonamide is soluble in water (1:140). Its primary use is in the topical treatment of ophthalmic infections. The sodium salt in a 10% to 30% solution can be employed and is nonirritating to the sensitive tissues of the eye. Some question of the drug's usefulness is raised by the fact that it apparently does not penetrate the cornea of the dog's eye (Chapter 15).

Salicylazosulfapyridine (Azulfidine). This sulfonamide is used in the treatment of ulcerative colitis in dogs. The mechanism of action is unknown, but it is thought not to be related to the antimicrobial activity of the drug. Salicylazosulfapyridine is broken down in the gut to sulfapyridine and 5-aminosalicylate. It is the experience of one of us (L. R. E.) that this drug is contraindicated in cats and has been associated with keratoconjunctivitis sicca (inflammation and drying of the cornea and conjunctiva) in dogs.

Toxicity and liabilities of sulfonamides. As is the case with any large group of drugs that has enjoyed widespread use over many years, the number and kinds of toxicities and side effects that have been associated with the sulfonamides are overwhelming. The most commonly encountered acute toxicity to sulfonamides is primarily seen after the intravenous injection of these drugs, particularly following a large dose or rapid injection. Acute toxicity is usually exhibited as central nervous system stimulation. Cattle become uncoordinated, exhibit mydriasis (pupils dilate), are unable to focus, and display muscular weakness. They may collapse, and death is not rare. A related, if not identical, toxicity has been seen in dogs after large oral or intravenous doses. Affected dogs exhibit nystagmus (horizontal oscillation of the eyes), involuntary running movements, nausea, and vomiting. In severe cases, convulsions may result; these can be controlled with pentobarbital.

Skin rashes and other hypersensitive (allergic) manifestations have also been seen in animals treated with sulfonamides.

Sulfonamides have limited solubility in urine. As a result, precipitation can occur, resulting in a condition called "crystalluria," in which the insoluble crystals formed in the urine can result in renal obstruction. The signs of crystalluria include those of renal failure: loss of appetite, rough hair coat, depression, blood in urine, colic, lack of urine flow, and accumulation of whitish precipitate on preputial or vulvar hairs. The occurrence of this condition is dependent on several factors: water intake, urine pH, individual and species susceptibility, and the solubility of individual sulfonamides, which varies. The triple sulfa tablet (trisulfapyrimidines, USP) is a combination designed to minimize crystalluria. The three sulfonamides contribute to bacteriostatic activity, although the solubility of each remains independent.

Prolonged application of sulfonamides has also been associated with decrease in tear production, decreased milk production, decrease in rumen motility, and vitamin K deficiencies.

Solutions of sulfonamides for injection are extremely alkaline. These solutions are irritating to tissues, and their use by other than intravenous routes is to be discouraged. For example, for intramammary infusion, suspensions of free sulfonamides and not solutions of their sodium salts are to be used. The pH of the solutions will cause irritation and destruction of the udder.

Evaluation of sulfonamides. The use of sulfonamides in veterinary medicine has declined with the introduction of the many antibiotics now available. Specific indications in small animals and the economy of their use in large animals, however, ensure a continuing place for sulfonamides on the veterinary drug shelf.

Miscellaneous anti-infectives

Nitrofurans. Of the several compounds belonging to the nitrofuran group, three find extensive use in veterinary medicine: furazolidone, nitrofurantoin, and nitrofurazone. The exact mechanism of action of the nitrofurans is unknown. It is presumed, however, that they exert their effect by interfering with enzymatic reactions essential to bacterial cells. Nitrofurans possess a broad spectrum of action, that is, they are effective against a wide variety of bacteria. Their activity may be bactericidal or bacteriostatic, depending on both the concentration of the drug and the bacteria in question. Bacteria have not readily developed resistance to the nitrofurans.

Furazolidone

Use. Furazolidone is used primarily for infections of the gastrointestinal tract. It is effective against a wide range of enteric (intestinal) bacterial organisms and some protozoa, particularly in poultry.

Furazolidone is not water soluble so it is used in powder or granular form as a feed mix. In the United States, furazolidone is recommended only for use in chickens, turkeys, and swine.

Toxicity. The toxic manifestations of this drug appear in the central nervous system, and it is our opinion that nearly all instances of toxicity are a result of incorrect dosage.

Dose and administration. The dosage of furazolidone varies, depending on the condition and species being treated (Table 3-2). The labeling includes dosage information and should be followed accurately.

Nitrofurantoin

Use. Nitrofurantoin is used primarily in the treatment of urinary tract infections. This drug is rapidly absorbed from the intestinal tract and rapidly excreted in the urine; it is excreted so quickly that it probably does not reach therapeutic levels in tissues when used systemically. Even though nitrofurantoin is recommended for systemic infections, because of the rapid urinary excretion and lack of adequate tissue levels, it is probably ineffective.

Nitrofurantoin is available as tablets, oral suspension, and injectable solution. There are two types of nitrofurantoin tablets, those made with microcrystalline powder and those made with macrocrystalline powder. The former are absorbed much faster, but the latter cause less nausea and vomiting, a commonly encountered problem in oral administration of nitrofurantoin.

Toxicity. Toxicity of nitrofurantoin is rarely encountered at normal doses (Table 3-2). At elevated doses, damage has been done to peripheral nerves. Nitrofurantoin is metabolized to various compounds, which impart a brownish color to the urine. Mentioning this to the animal owner often will prevent later anxiety when this color is noticed in the animal's urine.

Dose and administration. The dose for nitrofurantoin is shown in Table 3-2.

Nitrofurazone

Use. Nitrofurazone is used both topically and systemically in veterinary medicine. Topically the drug is available in many dose forms: ointment, solution, powder, and aerosol powder. For systemic use it is supplied as a soluble powder for mixing in drinking water. The topical forms of nitrofurazone are used as antimicrobial dressings for abrasions, burns, cuts, and ulcers. The preparations are nonirritating.

Systemically, nitrofurazone is used primarily for bacterial infections in swine and poultry.

Toxicity. The drug exhibits central nervous system toxicity at high dosages, particularly in young cattle.

Dose and administration. The dosage recommendations on the label should be carefully complied with (Table 3-2). Since it is

Table 3-2. Dosages of nitrofurans*

Drug	Species	Dose
Furazolidone	Calf	0.25-1.0 gm twice daily orally
	Foal	15-25 mg/kg/24 hr for 4 days
	Swine	150 gm/ton of feed
Nitrofurantoin	Horse	250 mg/kg three times daily orally
	Dog	4.4 mg/kg three times daily orally
Nitrofurazone	All	0.2% topically
	Dog	4-8 mg/kg three times daily orally

*Based on data from Rossoff, I. S.: Handbook of veterinary drugs, New York, 1974, Springer Publishing Co.

used extensively in the water of large herds of animals, special attention should be given to the fact that the drug is unstable in galvanized water containers.

Methenamine. Methenamine is a urinary antiseptic found in many common veterinary preparations for urinary tract infections of dogs and cats. Its mechanism of action depends on the slow release of formaldehyde in acidic solution. Methenamine is frequently found as the salt of an organic acid such as hippuric or mandelic acid. These acids are slightly antiseptic in their own right and also help to acidify the urine to ensure the activity of the methenamine. Methenamine and its salts have largely been replaced by other drugs, primarily sulfas and antibiotics.

Results of therapy with methenamine have been marginal at best. However, when used, it can only be effective in acidic urine of pH 6 or less. Methenamine is given orally to cats at a dose of 100 to 500 mg twice a day. It is given orally to dogs at a rate of 0.1 to 2 gm twice to four times a day.[12]

Antibiotics

The largest and most commonly used group of anti-infective drugs is the antibiotics. An antibiotic is a substance produced by microorganisms, which has the ability to kill or inhibit other microorganisms. That they are produced by microorganisms is what separates this group of anti-infectives from the sulfonamides or nitrofurans. Many antibiotics are currently being produced for the veterinary market, and it is not uncommon for antibiotics produced only for the human market to be employed by veterinarians. Because of their ability to cure disease, antibiotics are perhaps the most important and

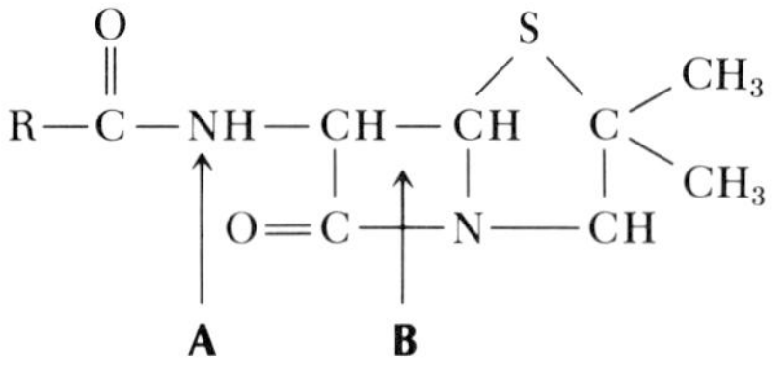

useful group of drugs available to the veterinarian. Their rational and judicious use can relieve animal suffering, increase food production, and protect the public health. Their injudicious use can and unfortunately often does produce serious and far-reaching deleterious effects on animal, man, and the environment.

Penicillins. One of the most significant developments in medical science has been the discovery and clinical application of the penicillins. Penicillin G, or benzylpenicillin, was the first of the penicillins to be used clinically. Penicillin G remains one of the most effective and safe of the antibiotics and the prototype of the penicillin group of drugs.

All the penicillins share a common β-lactam fused ring structure that is essential to their antibiotic activity. Substitution of different groups at the 6-amino position has resulted in variations in activity or stability to enzymatic or acid hydrolysis (Fig. 3-2). Such substitutions have produced the various penicillins currently available. The penicillins also share a common mechanism of action. They exert their bactericidal effect by interfering with cell wall synthesis by the bacteria.

The characteristics and commonly used doses of the penicillins are listed in Table 3-3.

Penicillin G (benzylpenicillin). Penicillin G is the most commonly used penicillin in veterinary medicine. The spectrum of action of penicillin G is primarily gram-positive. Gram-positive bacteria are those that take up the Gram stain; gram-negative bacteria do not. This staining characteristic of bacteria is a convenient means of general classification (Table 3-4).

Penicillin G is effective against most streptococcal and many staphylococcal species. Some strains of staphylococci elaborate an enzyme, penicillinase, which hydrolyzes penicillin G. The products of such hydrolysis have no antibiotic activity. Penicillin G is also effective against many strains of *Corynebacterium*, *Clostridia*, and *Leptospira*, *Bacillus anthracis*, *Actinomyces bovis*, and others.

Penicillin G is marketed in various preparations for veterinary use. Oral tablets of

Fig. 3-2. Structure of penicillin. A = 6-Amino position; B = β-lactum–fused ring.

Table 3-3. The penicillins

	Route of administration*	Acid stable	Penicillinase resistant	Altered spectrum	Dose†
Penicillin G‡	Oral, IV, IM, SC	No	Not resistant	No	Oral: 22,000-44,000 units/kg three or four times daily
				-	Injection: 22,000-44,000 units/kg for domestic species§
Procaine penicillin G‖	IM, SC	No	Not resistant	No	22,000-44,000 units/kg one or two times daily for domestic species
Benzathine penicillin G‖	IM	No	Not resistant	No	22,000-88,000 units/kg every 2-10 days for domestic species
Phenicillin V	Oral	Yes	Not resistant	No	5-25 mg/kg three or four times daily for dogs and cats
Phenethicillin	Oral	Yes	Not resistant	No	5-25 mg/kg three or four times daily for dogs and cats
Methicillin¶	SC, IV, IM	No	Resistant	No	10-40 mg/kg every four to six hours for dogs and cats
Nafcillin	Injection, IV, IM	Yes	Resistant	No	10-40 mg/kg every four to six hours for domestic species
Oxacillin	Oral, IV, IM, SC	Yes	Resistant	No	10-40 mg/kg three or four times daily for domestic species
Cloxacillin	Oral	Yes	Resistant	No	10-40 mg/kg three or four times daily for dogs, cats, and horses
Dicloxacillin	Oral	Yes	Resistant	No	10-40 mg/kg three or four times daily for dogs, cats, and horses
Ampicillin	Oral, IM, IV, SC	Yes	Not resistant	Yes	10-40 mg/kg three or four times daily for domestic species
Amoxacillin#	Oral	Yes	Not resistant	Yes	5-40 mg/kg three or four times daily for dogs and cats
Hetacillin#	Oral	Yes	Not resistant	Yes	10-40 mg/kg three times daily for dogs and cats
Carbenicillin**	IV, IM	No	Not resistant	Yes	10-20 mg/kg three times daily for dogs and cats

*Route of administration: IV = intravenously; IM = intramuscularly; SC = subcutaneously.
†Doses of all antibiotics and especially the penicillins are variable, depending on clinical picture and experience. These doses represent usual ranges. Doses exceeding these are often used and may well be indicated. Before using any of these in food-producing animals, check the package insert to be sure that use has been cleared by the FDA.
‡Although not acid stable, penicillin G has been found to be effective after oral administration to dogs.
§Domestic species are those species discussed in this text: dogs, cats, cattle, horses, sheep, and swine.
‖Active species is penicillin G. Salt form slows absorption.
¶This penicillin is exceptionally unstable. In our opinion, its usefulness has been replaced by other members of this group.
#Derivative of ampicillin.
**Only penicillin active against *Pseudomonas* species.

Table 3-4. Gram-staining characteristics of bacteria that commonly infect domestic animals

Gram-positive bacteria	Gram-negative bacteria
Bacillus anthracis	Brucella abortus
Actinomyces bovis	Enterobacter aerogenes
Clostridium species*	Escherichia coli
Corynebacterium species	Fusobacterium necrophorum
Erysipelothrix rhusiopathiae	Haemophilus species
	Pasteurella species
Staphylococcus species	Proteus species
	Pseudomonas species
Streptococcus species	Salmonella species
	Vibrio fetus

*Mostly gram-positive, but some gram-variable organisms do occur.

potassium penicillin G are available. Although the stability of orally administered penicillin G in gastric acid results in erratic and incomplete absorption from the gastrointestinal tract, appropriate doses will generally produce adequate blood levels in the dog. Care should be taken that penicillin is not given orally after a meal when the acid content of the stomach is especially high. Oral penicillins are not practical for use in large animals such as horses and cattle.

The sodium and potassium salts of penicillin G are available for reconstitution with sterile water or saline to provide aqueous solutions of penicillin G. These solutions can be injected intravenously, subcutaneously, or intramuscularly. Such injections result in rapid high blood levels. The excretion rate of penicillin G is rapid. To maintain adequate blood levels of penicillin G, therefore, frequent administration of these solutions is necessary. Some preparations, however, are absorbed more slowly when given intramuscularly or subcutaneously, so that injections can be given at longer, more practical intervals. These preparations are suspensions of insoluble salts of penicillin G, which are slowly absorbed from the injection site. The two most commonly encountered prepara-

tions are procaine penicillin G and benzathine penicillin G.

Penicillin G and procaine penicillin G are also commonly employed in the local treatment of mastitis. The drugs are usually suspended in a nonirritating viscous base and packaged in plastic syringes for intramammary infusion.

Acid-resistant penicillins. The acid-resistant penicillins, phenoxymethyl (penicillin V) and phenoxyethyl (phenethicillin), are derivatives of penicillin with various substituents at the α-carbon, which increase their resistance to attack by gastric acid. For this reason these derivatives enjoy more complete and predictable absorption after oral dosage. The spectrum of activity and side effects are generally like penicillin G. Penicillin V, however, is several times less active against some bacterial strains than is penicillin G.

Penicillinase-resistant penicillins. The penicillinase-resistant penicillins include methicillin, nafcillin, oxacillin, cloxacillin, and dicloxacillin. These penicillins are substituted in such a way as to prevent hydrolysis by the enzyme penicillinase. The exact mechanism of this resistance is unknown, but it is thought to be due to stearic hindrance; that is, the substitution groups prevent the enzyme from obtaining appropriate proximity to the molecule to effect hydrolysis. These penicillins may be acid labile (methicillin) or acid stable (nafcillin, oxacillin, cloxacillin, dicloxacillin). Acid-stable penicillins may be used orally. These penicillins tend to exhibit the same spectrum of activity as penicillin G and V but are also effective against penicillinase-producing staphylococci.

Resistance to penicillinase by this group of penicillins allows the veterinarian to employ potent, safe drugs with the attributes of penicillin G in the treatment of infections caused by penicillinase-producing staphylococci. Penicillinase-resistant penicillins are less effective by weight than penicillin G against streptococci and other gram-positive organisms. It can require a ten to fifty times greater concentration of these penicillins to have the same effect on organisms as penicillin G.[5]

Altered-spectrum penicillins. The newest group of penicillins are those in which substitutions in the side chain increase the activity of the drug against certain gram-negative bacilli. These penicillins are not resistant to penicillinase. The first of the altered-spectrum penicillins to be developed was ampicillin. Ampicillin has the same gram-positive spectrum of action as penicillin G but is also active against many gram-negative organisms. Many strains of *Haemophilus, Salmonella, Shigella, Escherichia coli*, and *Proetus mirabilis* are sensitive to ampicillin. Although the gram-positive spectrum of ampicillin parallels that of penicillin G, ampicillin is often slightly less active than penicillin G against many of these organisms.

Hetacillin, which is widely promoted and used in the veterinary market, is hydrolyzed in vivo to acetone and ampicillin. This drug possesses no apparent advantage over ampicillin.

A third member of this group of penicillins is carbenicillin. Carbenicillin is active against many gram-negative organisms, but most important clinically is its activity against many strains of *Pseudomonas aeruginosa.* Although this antibiotic is finding some use in veterinary medicine, it is expensive, and economics limit its use.

The most recently developed antibiotic in this group is amoxicillin, a hydroxylated derivative of ampicillin. Its spectrum of activity is similar to that of ampicillin. The levels reached in the serum after oral administration are approximately double those achieved with ampicillin. The concentration required to inhibit the growth of many organisms in vitro, however, is often higher.[9]

Clinical experience with amoxicillin is limited at this time, so it remains to be seen whether the drug will prove to possess any advantage over ampicillin.

Toxicity and side effects of penicillins. The penicillins possess a low order of toxicity to mammalian cells. They are all capable of producing central nervous system toxicity in high doses. Although uncommon, this toxicity can be serious; convulsions and death may result. The most common adverse reactions to the penicillins are hypersensitive in nature. Hypersensitivity to penicillins is occasionally seen in all species. These reactions may be manifested as hives, fever, joint pain, or even anaphylactoid reactions. There seems to be complete cross sensitivity between the penicillins, so a serious reaction to one penicillin should preclude the use of any other penicillin.

Use of penicillin in horses. It is difficult to obtain adequate blood levels of antibiotics in large animals such as horses. The administration of sodium penicillin at the rate of 6600 units/kg (approximately 3,000,000 units per animal) has been reported to produce blood levels in horses that reach approximately 3 μg/ml. Blood levels of 3 μg/ml would be adequate to treat most gram-positive infections sensitive to penicillin. The more commonly used procaine penicillin, when administered at rates as high as 13,200 units/kg (approximately 6,000,000 units per animal), will result in blood levels of approximately 0.1 μg/ml. This level would be effective against some gram-positive organisms and not high enough for others.[5] Large volumes of procaine penicillin G would have to be administered to reach this relatively low blood level. The standard preparation of procaine penicillin G consists of 300,000 units/ml. Twenty milliliters (usually 10 ml in each site) would have to be administered daily to an adult 450 kg horse to obtain these values. For routine treatments we recommend much higher doses, ranging from 10 to 20 million units/ 450 kg horse. This is equivalent to about 33 to 66 ml of the standard procaine penicillin. This should be divided into 10 ml volumes per injection site.

Increasing the dosage of benzathine penicillin for horses does not greatly increase the blood level. Primarily, increases in dose prolong the duration of action. It is therefore difficult to obtain high enough blood levels with the benzathine penicillins in the horse.

Use of penicillin in cattle and sheep. If

procaine penicillin is given at the rate of approximately 6600 units/kg in cattle, blood levels will reach a maximum of 1.25 μg/ml in about an hour. At the end of 24 hours, blood levels will drop to approximately 0.2 to 0.3 μg/ml. Massive doses such as 33,000 units/kg will result in blood levels of approximately 4.3 μg/ml.[5]

When a dose of 12,100 units/kg of procaine penicillin is administered to sheep, blood levels of approximately 1.1 μg/ml are obtained. Such levels decrease to about 0.01 μg/ml in 24 hours.[5]

Summary. The penicillins represent the safest and most effective group of antibiotics available. Their attributes and relative lack of liabilities make the penicillins the most used antibiotics. In infections that are susceptible to one or more of the penicillins, there is probably no better choice of drugs to be employed.

Cephalosporins. Eight antibiotics in the cephalosporin group are in use in medicine. Only four are of sufficient interest to veterinary medicine at this time to warrant discussion in this chapter. All the cephalosporins are derivatives of 7-aminocephalosporanic acid. All share a similar spectrum of activity and mechanism of action. They are bactericidal and act by interfering with cell wall synthesis, much like the penicillins. Cephalosporins exhibit cross antigenicity with one another and sometimes with the penicillins. Their spectrum includes penicillinase-producing staphylococci, other gram-positive cocci, and some gram-negative organisms. They are effective against most *Salmonella* species, most *Shigella* species, most *Proteus mirabilis*, many *Escherichia coli*, and many strains of *Klebsiella*.

Individual cephalosporins of interest in veterinary medicine include the following.

Cephalothin. Cephalothin is not absorbed well from the gastrointestinal tract. It is administered either intravenously or intramuscularly. Levels are obtainable in serum and tissues that are adequate for treatment of systemic infections. Urine levels are also adequate. The drug produces considerable pain on injection and may cause damage to the vein. Cephalothin is not available under veterinary label.

Cephaloridine. Cephaloridine also must be given by injection. The veterinary brand, Loridine, is available as a suspension in oil for intramuscular administration. The manufacturer recommends a dose of 11 mg/kg twice daily. Rossoff[12] recommends 25 mg/kg twice daily for infections other than of the urinary tract. In our opinion, the dose recommended by the manufacturer frequently may be insufficient.

Cephaloridine has been shown to cause kidney pathology in humans, rats, mice and rabbits at high doses. There is no reason to believe these adverse effects are limited to those species.

Cephaloglycin. Cephaloglycin is absorbed orally and is available in capsule form. Excretion of cephaloglycin is rapid. High levels of this drug are found in the urine, but levels attained in the plasma are generally inadequate. Its use therefore is recommended only for infections of the urinary tract. The dosage of cephaloglycin in animals has not been established. We think that doses in the range of 5 to 15 mg/kg three to four times a day are adequate.

Cephalexin. This compound is well absorbed from the gastrointestinal tract. Adequate levels are attained in both serum and urine. In humans more than 90% of the dose is excreted in the urine unchanged, which suggests that the half-life of the drug is probably similar in most species. For this reason, to maintain adequate serum levels for treatment of systemic infections, we prefer a dosage interval of 6 to 8 hours over twice daily administration. The dosage of cephalexin has not been established in animals. Again, in our opinion, 5 to 15 mg/kg three to four times daily will prove adequate.

Summary. The cephalosporins are relatively safe and effective antibiotics. The cost of these drugs and the risk of increasing the number of resistant strains of bacteria suggest that they should be employed only when definitely indicated; that is, when the infection is only sensitive to cephalosporins. The inappropriate use of cephalosporins in human medicine has been documented,[10] and we hope that their use in veterinary medicine will not follow a similar pattern.

Tetracyclines

Use. The tetracyclines are closely related chemically. They share essentially the same spectrum of activity. All the tetracyclines are absorbed incompletely but adequately from the gastrointestinal tract. Tetracyclines exert their effect on the organism by interfering with protein synthesis. They exert their action within the bacterial cell and are bacteriostatic rather than bactericidal. The spectrum of activity of the tetracyclines includes a wide range of both gram-positive and gram-negative bacteria; species of *Rickettsia*, *Mycoplasma*, and *Chlamydia*; and some protozoa. Many bacterial organisms for which tetracyclines have been indicated in the past are now better treated by newer, less toxic, and more effective antibiotics.

Oxytetracycline, chlortetracycline, and tetracycline are excreted primarily in the urine in active form, so that levels in the urinary tract are high. Urinary excretion is by means of glomerular filtration and thus is significantly affected by diseases that compromise renal function.

Doxycycline and minocycline are newer derivatives of tetracycline. These compounds have longer half-lives in the plasma and therefore can be given in smaller doses and less often. These compounds are not found in the urine in high concentrations. Their half-lives then are not dependent on renal function.

Toxicity. The use of the tetracyclines is not without liability. Hypersensitivities to the tetracyclines do occur. Anaphylaxis, skin rashes, fever, and angioedema (painful swelling) may be seen. It is important to note that tetracyclines exhibit an essentially complete crossover in hypersensitivity; sensitivity to any one indicates sensitivity to all. This group of antibiotics is irritating, and nausea and/or vomiting or diarrhea often occur after oral doses. Tetracyclines are also irritating when injected, and thrombophlebitis frequently follows repeated intravenous injections. The tetracyclines are also toxic to the liver. This hepatotoxicity occurs especially after large parenteral doses and during pregnancy. In growing animals, tetracyclines bond with calcium in the bone and can interfere with the development of bones and teeth in young animals or the fetus. Suprainfections, that is, infections by resistant bacteria, yeast, or fungi, sometimes occur during tetracycline therapy. The clinician must be prepared to differentiate between irritative diarrheas and bacterial suprainfections in the gut of animals being treated with a tetracycline.

Distribution of chlortetracycline is much like that of oxytetracycline and tetracycline. A far greater amount of chlortetracycline is

Table 3-5. Dosage of tetracyclines

	Route	Large animals	Small animals
Tetracycline	Oral	Not used by this route	20 mg/kg three times daily
Oxytetracycline	IM, IV	2.5-10 mg/kg/ 24 hr	6 mg/kg daily; use one-half dose for very small dogs and double dose for large dogs; 10-20 mg/kg three times daily
Chlortetracycline	Oral	10 mg/kg/24 hr in feed	
	Intrauterine	0.5-1 gm	
Doxycycline	Oral	Not used	5 mg/kg twice daily
Minocycline	Oral	Not used	2-4 mg/kg twice daily

excreted in the bile, however, and the risks of upsetting the bacterial balance in the gut and suprainfection may be greater.

Dose and administration. Tetracycline, oxytetracycline, and their salts are available for injection or oral administration. Adequate levels of the drug are produced in most tissues, including the liver, spleen, kidney, and lung. Only minimal levels are obtained in the cerebrospinal fluid.

Chlortetracycline is not suitable for intramuscular injection because it is irritating. Chlortetracycline is available for oral administration in many forms: capsules, water-soluble power, and feed mixes. Doses and routes of administration for the tetracyclines are shown in Table 3-5.

Chloramphenicol

Use. Chloramphenicol is primarily a bacteriostatic antibiotic. The spectrum of activity of chloramphenicol is wide, including many gram-negative and gram-positive organisms, *Rickettsia* species, and *Mycoplasma* species. Chloramphenicol exerts its action on bacteria by inhibiting protein synthesis. It is absorbed well orally. The drug is excreted in the urine both as active chloramphenicol and inactive metabolites. Good liver function is essential for normal excretion of chloramphenicol; plasma levels will accumulate after normal doses in animals with less than normal liver function. Thus its use in young animals, old animals, or animals with liver disease must be avoided or approached with extreme caution. Chloramphenicol should not be used in food-producing animals.

Toxicity. The hypersensitivity resulting in pancytopenia (a decrease in all blood cellular components) and aplastic anemia, which has been seen in humans treated with chloramphenicol, has not been reported in animals. A dose-related and reversible bone marrow depression occasionally occurs, especially with high doses over prolonged periods of time. Chloramphenicol can cause prolonged sleeping times in dogs to which pentobarbital anesthesia has been administered.[3] Hypersensitivities that are manifested as skin rashes and/or angioedema of the face and head occur rarely. Gastrointestinal irritation, nausea, and vomiting are the most frequently encountered side effects.

Dose and administration. Chloramphenicol is available in oral form as capsules and the palmitate ester oral suspension. Injectable forms are also available, as are several otic, ophthalmic, and topical preparations. Chloramphenicol sodium succinate for intravenous use is inactive until hydrolyzed by enzymes in the plasma. This should be kept in mind, since it is ineffective topically. The flushing of surgical sites or joints with this form is probably also ineffective, since the necessary esterases usually are not present.

Because of the complete absorption of orally administered chloramphenicol in nonruminants, parenteral and oral dosages are the same. Recent studies on the plasma levels attained with chloramphenicol indicate that the following doses are necessary to achieve and maintain plasma concentrations above 5 μg/ml[7]:

Horse	25 to 50 mg/kg every 6 to 8 hours
Dog	25 to 50 mg/kg every 6 to 8 hours
Cat	20 to 50 mg/kg every 8 to 12 hours

Macrolide antibiotics. The antibiotics in this group include erythromycin, oleandomycin, and tylosin. The spectrum of the macrolide antibiotics include *Mycoplasma* species and most gram-positive and occasionally gram-negative organisms. These antibiotics are unaffected by penicillinase and are effective against penicillinase-producing staphylococci. Their use against these organisms, however, has largely been replaced by the penicillinase-resistant penicillins. The macrolides are bacteriostatic in action. Suprainfection in the gut is the most commonly encountered adverse effect of the macrolides. Hypersensitivity to these drugs seems to be rare, and other toxic reactions are seldom seen clinically.

Of the macrolides, erythromycin and tylosin are most commonly used. Because it is expensive and has an antibacterial activity similar to the penicillins, oleandomycin is

Table 3-6. Doses of macrolide antibiotics*

	Erythromycin base	Erythromycin ethylsuccinate	Erythromycin stearate	Tylosin
Dogs	IM: 4.4 mg/kg/24 hr or every other day	IM: 4.4 mg/kg/24 hr or every other day	Oral: 11 mg/kg once or twice daily	IM: 6.6-11 mg/kg/24 hr Oral: 7-15 mg/kg three times daily
Cats	IM: 4.4 mg/kg/24 hr or every other day	IM: 4.4 mg/kg/24 hr or every other day	Oral: 11-22 mg/kg once or twice daily	IM: 6.6-11 mg/kg/24 hr Oral: 7-15 mg/kg three times daily
Cattle	IM: 2.2-4.4 mg/kg/ 24 hr	IM: 2.2-4.4 mg/kg/ 24 hr	Not used	IM: 2.2-4.4 mg/kg/ 24 hr (as base)
Horses	IM: 2.2-4.4 mg/kg/ 24 hr	IM: 2.2-4.4 mg/kg/ 24 hr	Not used	Not used
Sheep	IM: 2.2 mg/kg/24 hr	IM: 2.2 mg/kg/24 hr	Not used	Not used
Swine	IM: 2.2-6.6 mg/kg/ 24 hr	IM: 2.2-6.6 mg/kg/ 24 hr	Not used	IM: 2.2-4.4 mg/kg/ 24 hr, not over three injections

*Based on data from Rossoff, I. S.: Handbook of veterinary drugs, New York, 1974, Springer Publishing Co.

not commonly used in veterinary medicine to treat species discussed in this text.

Dose and administration. The dose and route of administration for erythromycin and tylosin are shown in Table 3-6.

Lincomycin

Use. Lincomycin is a bacteriostatic antibiotic. Its spectrum of activity is primarily against gram-positive organisms but does not include most strains of enterococci. The structure of lincomycin is not related to any of the other antibiotics discussed here; thus there is no crossover in hypersensitivities. Lincomycin has been vigorously promoted in the veterinary market. In our opinion, such promotion has resulted in overuse of the drug.

Lincomycin is certainly not without value. Because it is structurally unrelated to other antibiotics, lincomycin is of value as an alternate choice for treating infections caused by sensitive organisms in animals that exhibit hypersensitivity or other untoward effects to other antibiotics.

Toxicity. The use of lincomycin in animals is not without risk. Although hypersensitivities are rare with this drug, other untoward effects are associated with its use. Gastrointestinal upset and floral disturbance are not infrequent. Vomiting is not uncommon in cats; and diarrhea has been seen in cats, dogs, and frequently in swine. Lincomycin at a dose rate of 10 mg/kg has been fatal in hamsters. Its use in horses is to be avoided, since severe intestinal floral disturbances and serious diarrheal conditions are common. A sometimes fatal pseudomembranous colitis associated with lincomycin has been reported in humans.[13] The intramuscular injection of lincomycin in dogs has resulted in necrosis and scarring of nerves in the area of the injection site.

Dose and administration. Rossoff[12] recommends the following dosages of lincomycin in cats and dogs:

Oral	22 mg/kg twice a day
	15 mg/kg three times a day
Intramuscular	22 mg/kg/24 hr
	11 mg/kg twice a day

Aminoglycoside antibiotics. The aminoglycosides include streptomycin, dihydrostreptomycin, gentamycin, kanamycin, and neomycin. The chemical structures of aminoglycosides are similar. They exert their effect on the microorganism by interfering with protein synthesis. These antibiotics may be bactericidal or bacteriostatic, depending on the organism involved and the concentration of the drug.

All the aminoglycosides are neurotoxic and nephrotoxic; they exhibit these toxicities to varying degrees (see individual drugs). High doses of aminoglycosides can potentiate neuromuscular blocking drugs. The neuromuscular blockade produced by the aminoglycosides can be reversed with neostigmine and calcium gluconate.

The aminoglycosides are poorly absorbed from the gastrointestinal tract and must be given parenterally to achieve adequate therapeutic levels in the plasma. These antibiotics are all excreted primarily by means of glomerular filtration. Because of this, the levels of antibiotic in the urine are high. Aminoglycosides tend to accumulate in animals with compromised renal function, and the kinetics and half-life vary little between species.

Streptomycin and dihydrostreptomycin

Use. Because it is stable in solution, dihydrostreptomycin is most commonly available under veterinary label. The spectrum of activity of streptomycin and dihydrostreptomycin, although potentially broad, has been severely limited by the development of resistance by many organisms.

Toxicity. Neurotoxicity, specifically ototoxicity (damage to the eighth cranial nerve with resultant loss of hearing and loss of balance), is more likely to be seen clinically than is kidney damage with these drugs.

Dose and administration. Dosage recommendations for dihydrostreptomycin range from 5 to 20 mg/kg to be repeated every 12 to 24 hours. The half-life of streptomycin is short in animals with normal renal function (approximately 1.5 hours in the dog). Therefore in our opinion the dosage regimen of this drug should be 5 to 10 mg/kg given at 6- to 8-hour intervals.

Kanamycin. The spectrum of activity of kanamycin is broad. It includes many *Pro-*

teus, Escherichia coli, and other gram-negative organisms and many *Staphylococcus* but not *Pseudomonas* species. The resistance limitations are not as great as they are with streptomycin, but with continued use of the drug they are increasing. There is generally a one-way crossover in resistance with streptomycin: a positive sensitivity to streptomycin also indicates sensitivity to kanamycin, whereas the reverse is not necessarily true. The dosage recommended by the manufacturer is 5.5 mg/kg twice daily. The half-life of kanamycin in most species is probably short enough to warrant dosing at 6- to 8-hour intervals.

Gentamicin. The clinician may see kidney toxicity, neurotoxicity, or both with this antibiotic. The spectrum of gentamicin is broad, including many gram-negative and gram-positive organisms. Most strains of *Pseudomonas* are sensitive to this drug. However, because of the potential renal toxicity of gentamycin, the renal function of all animals receiving this drug should be assessed at the beginning of therapy and periodically during treatment. The manufacturer recommends a dosage of 4.4 mg/kg twice for the first day, then 4.4 mg/kg once daily. The half-life of gentamicin is not long (1.5 hours in the dog).[8] The adequacy of 24-hour dosage intervals with a drug that is excreted at such a rate might be questioned. We think a dose of 2 to 3 mg/kg four times daily is a more adequate therapeutic regimen.

Neomycin. The spectrum of neomycin is essentially like that of kanamycin. Neomycin is the most nephrotoxic of the aminoglycosides. For this reason, it is used primarily for topical application. However, hypersensitivity or allergy to topically applied neomycin also occurs. Because it is not absorbed from the intestine to a significant degree, it is given orally for its effect on organisms within the lumen of the gut. It is often employed in 0.5% to 1% concentrations in ointment or solution form to control bacteria in wounds or on the surface of the skin.

Polymyxins. The members of this group of antibiotics are polymyxin B and polymyxin

E (colistin). These drugs are both nephro-toxic and neurotoxic. They are not adequately absorbed orally. Polymyxin B is excreted rapidly in the urine, and considerable doubt exists that adequate tissue levels can be obtained even with parenteral administration. Polymyxins, like the aminoglycosides, can produce a neuromuscular blockade and will potentiate other neuromuscular blocking agents. Their neuromuscular blocking effects, however, are not reversed by neostigmine or calcium gluconate. The polymyxins are active against many gram-negative organisms, including many strains of *Pseudomonas*.

Because of their systemic toxicity, the polymyxins find use primarily in topical preparations, in eye and ear ointments and drops, and as pseudomonocidal preservatives for various preparations.

Amphotericin B. Amphotericin B is an antibiotic used to treat certain fungal infections, such as coccidiomycosis, blastomycosis, histoplasmosis, and cryptococcosis. Amphotericin B acts by binding sterols in the fungal cell membrane, with resultant changes in membrane permeability. This change in membrane permeability allows intracellular components to be lost. Mammalian cell walls also contain sterols; thus damage to body cells and damage to fungal cells may share a common mechanism. The major factor limiting the use of amphotericin B is its severe toxic effects on the kidneys. This toxicity can be monitored by determining the blood urea nitrogen (BUN) levels and blood creatinine levels. In dogs and cats the BUN should be kept below 70 mg/100 ml and the creatinine, below 3.5/100 ml. If the BUN or blood creatinine rises above these levels, administration should be temporarily discontinued to prevent permanent kidney damage.

In dogs the dose normally ranges from 0.25 to 0.50 mg/kg administered intravenously daily or three times a week over a 2- to 3-month period.[12] The total dosage is normally 10 to 25 mg/kg.

For cats it appears that the dose should be smaller than that used in dogs.[15] The dose ranges between 0.07 to 0.42 mg/kg diluted to a volume of 10 ml with 5% glucose and given by intravenous injection three times a week for 3 months. This provides a total dose of approximately 5 mg/kg. However, since little information is available on the use of amphotericin in cats, the clinician must proceed with extreme caution.[15]

References

1. Aronson, A. L.: The use, misuse, and abuse of antibacterial agents, Mod. Vet. Pract. **56:**383, 1975.
2. Berman, D. T.: Some basic aspects of the immune response, J. Am. Vet. Med. Assoc. **155:**250, 1969.
3. Bree, M. M., Park, J. W., Beck, C. C., and Moser, J. H.: Effects of chloramphenicol on tilazol (C1-744) anesthesia in dogs, Vet. Med. Small Anim. Clin. **71:**1243, 1976.
4. Carlson, A., Rupe, B. D., Buss, D., Homman, C., and Leaton, J.: Evaluation of a new prolonged-release sulfamethazine bolus for use in cattle, Vet. Med. Small Anim. Clin. **71:**693, 1976.
5. Clark, C. H.: Penicillins in veterinary practice, Mod. Vet. Pract. **57:**1019, 1976.
6. Craig, G. R., and White, G.: Studies in dogs and cats dosed with trimethoprim and sulphadiazine, Vet. Rec. **98:**82, 1976.
7. Davis, L. E., Baggot, J. D., and Powers, T. E.: Pharmacokinetics of chloramphenicol in domesticated animals, Am. J. Vet. Res. **33:**2259, 1972.
8. Enos, L. R.: Unpublished data, 1975.
9. Pearson, R. E.: Drug evaluation data, amoxicillin, Drug Intell. Clin. Pharm. **8:**542, 1974.
10. Pierpaoli, P. G., Coarse, J. R., and Tilton, R. C.: Antibiotic use control, Drug Intell. Clin. Pharm. **10:**258, 1976.
11. Roitt, I.: Essential immunology, ed. 2, Oxford, 1974, Blackwell Scientific Publications.
12. Rossoff, I. S.: Handbook of veterinary drugs, New York, 1974, Springer Publishing Co.
13. Scott, A. J., Nicholson, G. I., and Kerr, A. R.: Lincomycin as a cause of pseudomembranous colitis, Lancet, **2:**1232, 1973.
14. Tarnawski, A., and Batko, B.: Antibiotics and immune processes, J. Am. Vet. Med. Assoc. **162:**963, 1973.
15. Thrall, M. A., Rich, L. J., and Freemyer, F. G.: Feline cryptococcosis treatment with amphotericin B, Feline Pract. **6:**15, May 1976.
16. Thornton, G. W.: Antimicrobial therapy in the dog and cat, Vet. Clin. North Am. **5:**133, 1975.

Additional readings

Abinanti, F. R.: Comments on future status of immunization procedures, J. Am. Vet. Med. Assoc. **152:**917, 1968.

Adams, H. R.: Acute adverse effects of antibiotics, J. Am. Vet. Med. Assoc. **166:**983, 1975.

Baker, L. R.: Comments on license requirements and veterinary biologicals, J. Am. Vet. Med. Assoc. **160:** 509, 1972.

Cabasso, V. J.: Comments on potency evaluation of bovine respiratory disease vaccines, J. Am. Vet. Med. Assoc. **152:**845, 1968.

Cabasso, V. J.: Comments on future status of immunization procedures, J. Am. Vet. Med. Assoc. **152:** 916, 1968.

DeGeeter, M. J., and Stahl, G. L.: Sensitivity of *Escherichia coli* after exposure to lincomycin in vitro and in vivo, Am. J. Vet. Res. **37:**531, 1976.

DeGeeter, M. J., Stahl, G. L., and Geng, S.: Effect of lincomycin on prevalence, duration, and quantity of *Salmonella typhimurium* excreted by swine, Am. J. Vet. Res. **37:**525, 1976.

Gillespie, J. H.: Comments on test requirements for bovine respiratory disease biologics, J. Am. Vet. Med. Assoc. **152:**836, 1968.

Gorham, J. R., Henson, J. B., and Dodgen, C. J.: Basic principles of immunity in cats, J. Am. Vet. Med. Assoc. **158:**846, 1971.

Gray, J. E., Purmalis, A., and Feenstra, E. S.: Animal toxicity studies of a new antibiotic, lincomycin, Toxicol. Appl. Pharmacol. **6:**476, 1964.

Kaeberle, M. L.: Do mixed bacterins and autogenous bacterins have merit? J. Am. Vet. Med. Assoc. **160:** 609, 1972.

Kaeberle, M. L.: Immune response to antigens of inactivated microbial agents, J. Am. Vet. Med. Assoc. **163:**810, 1973.

LaSalle, B.: License requirements for vaccines for bovine respiratory diseases, J. Am. Vet. Med. Assoc. **163:**845, 1973.

Myers, W. L.: Comments on the role of antibody in the "immune response," Equine disease supplement, part 2, J. Am. Vet. Med. Assoc. **155:**255, 1969.

Phillips, C. E.: Potency evaluation of vaccines used against bovine respiratory diseases, J. Am. Vet. Med. Assoc. **152:**842, 1968.

Phillips, C. E.: Progress toward improved modified live-virus vaccines, J. Am. Vet. Med. Assoc. **157:** 1864, 1970.

Quin, A. H.: Anaphylaxis a treacherous hazard, Vet. Med. **58:**164, 1963.

Todd, J. D.: Immune response to parenteral and intranasal vaccinations, J. Am. Vet. Med. Assoc. **163:** 807, 1973.

York, C. J.: Comments on license requirements for vaccines for bovine respiratory diseases, J. Am. Vet. Med. Assoc. **152:**840, 1968.

4

Infectious diseases of dogs and cats

Viral diseases
  Canine distemper
  Canine infectious hepatitis
  Canine infectious tracheobronchitis
  Feline panleukopenia
  Feline respiratory infections
  Rabies
Bacterial diseases
  Leptospirosis
  Bacterial cystitis

VIRAL DISEASES
Canine distemper

Signs. Canine distemper is caused by a virus. Frequently, the disease is complicated by secondary bacterial infection, particularly in the respiratory tract. Animals with distemper may present with signs varying in type and severity. They may have a mild skin rash or manifest severe systemic infection involving the respiratory tract, digestive system, and nervous system. Typically the animal with distemper has an upper respiratory infection. There is usually a nasal and ocular discharge. In other cases the animal may be vomiting and have diarrhea, signs primarily referable to the digestive system. Some animals manifest signs that indicate involvement of both the respiratory and digestive systems. Usually the animals have a high fever.

Frequently, animals appear to recover from the initial infection and at a later date develop signs of nervous system disease. This often occurs 3 to 4 weeks after the initial signs. Neurological signs range from mild tremors to convulsions. The neurological damage is irreversible; even if the animal recovers, signs relating to nervous system damage will remain throughout the animal's life.

Canine distemper is a highly contagious disease, spreading from one animal to another, usually through aerosols produced when animals cough or sneeze. Animals often succumb during the primary phase of the disease or from the later neurological involvement.

Prevention
Passive immunity. Puppies from immune bitches receive passive antibodies against canine distemper in the colostrum. Two products are available to artificially convey passive immunity to dogs against canine distemper: gamma globulin and anti–canine distemper serum. Generally, these products also contain antibodies to protect against other diseases such as canine infectious hepatitis and leptospirosis. In the past it was recommended that passive antibodies be administered when puppies were young to protect them until the time they had lost maternal antibodies; this procedure is no longer recommended. Both the gamma globulin

55

and anti–canine distemper serum are contraindicated in any distemper immunizing regimen.[5] The antibodies they contain interfere with the animal's ability to produce active immunity, and the protection they afford is questionable. They are mentioned here primarily for their historical significance and because they are still available on the market.

Active immunity

Distemper vaccines. Various products are available that stimulate active immunity against canine distemper in dogs. Both killed and modified live virus vaccines have been used. The modified live virus may be produced in an abnormal environment such as in ferrets, eggs, or tissue culture. The vaccine may be administered as a monovalent product, protecting only against distemper, or it may be combined with products that result in active immunity against other diseases. Commonly canine distemper vaccine is mixed with hepatitis and/or leptospirosis vaccines. One manufacturer produces a mixed vaccine that contains antigens to protect dogs against canine parainfluenza, distemper, and hepatitis. In addition, because it protects dogs against canine distemper, human measles vaccine is sometimes used to protect puppies from distemper.

To maximize the active production of antibodies in animals, animals should be healthy, free from parasites, and receiving a balanced diet. Because the effect of modified live virus vaccines on the fetus is not known, pregnant bitches should not be immunized.

When maternal antibodies are not present, modified live virus distemper vaccines are highly effective in producing immunity to distemper. However, animals with circulating maternal antibodies do not respond to canine distemper vaccine. A survey that measured the presence of maternal antibodies from 125 bitches in Great Britain revealed that the chances of puppies developing antibodies against distemper at various ages are as follows[10]:

9 weeks of age	65%
11 weeks of age	78%
12 weeks of age	87%

The American Veterinary Medical Association recommends use of modified live virus vaccine of chick embryo or tissue (cell) culture origin to immunize against canine distemper. A panel of the Association recommended the following regimen for immunizing dogs[5]:

1. If it is known that the animal did not receive maternal antibodies, it can be immunized when only 2 weeks old.

2. An animal of unknown immune status, if under 3 months of age, should be given two doses of the vaccine. One dose should be given as soon after weaning as possible and the second when the pup is between 12 and 16 weeks of age but no sooner than 2 weeks after the first dose. An alternative method, which provides maximal protection, is to give the vaccine every 2 weeks until the puppy is 16 weeks old.

3. If the puppy is more than 3 months old and of unknown immune status, only one dose of the vaccine is needed for adequate protection.

4. An alternative method is to use a nomograph. Nomographs can be used to predict the age at which puppies should be immunized. Before parturition the antibody level of the bitch is determined. This titer, or level of antibodies in the serum, is plotted on a nomograph, which indicates the time in weeks when the puppies will lose their passive antibodies and be competent to develop an active immunity. Positive assurance of immunity can be determined by testing the serum of 2 puppies from a litter 30 days after immunization. The problem with the nomograph method is that it requires a sophisticated laboratory to run the antibody determination test on the bitch. The test is not readily available to most veterinarians and is rarely used in clinical practice.

5. A dog should not be admitted to an area where it might become exposed to canine distemper virus without first being given a dose of vaccine, unless it was given modified live-virus vaccine within the previous 12 months.

Annual revaccination of dogs is recommended. The antibody level in dogs immunized against distemper decreases in time and the animal becomes susceptible unless it is either reimmunized or exposed to natural infection. Because the incidence of distemper has declined, the chance of a vaccinated dog encountering natural infection, which could restimulate antibody production, is decreased. Most vaccination breaks occur during two periods. One is 4 to 8 weeks after initial immunization, and the other is after the second year of life. The first break probably is a result of animals contracting the infection shortly before or after the initial vaccination; the second is probably a result of the natural drop in antibody level in animals that are not reexposed to the virus. A second dose of vaccine 12 months after the first is therefore indicated.[1,15]

Generally, distemper vaccine is packaged in single dose vials. The entire vial is administered to the animal regardless of body weight and should be administered according to the directions of the manufacturer. Distemper vaccine is usually administerd by the subcutaneous route.

Measles vaccine. Measles vaccine is a modified live virus vaccine prepared from human measles virus grown in canine tissue culture. The formulation is specific for use in canines.

Human measles virus and distemper virus have some similarities, just as there are similarities between features of the clinical illness and the pathologic changes produced by each virus in its natural host. The two viruses share an antigenic component.

The protection against canine distemper produced by measles vaccine is due to something other than humoral antibodies (that is, antibodies in the serum). Three modes of action have been theorized: the production of cellular antibodies, the interference phenomenon (which in theory prevents cellular infection by more than one virus at a time), or the accelerated production of canine distemper antibodies when an animal is exposed to canine distemper virus.

The efficacy of measles vaccine in protecting dogs against canine distemper can be greater than 90%.[3] However, measles vaccine is not as effective as modified live virus

canine distemper vaccine in animals from 5 to 12 weeks of age.[11,25]

Although maternal antibodies to distemper do not affect the ability of measles vaccine to produce immunity, dogs must be at least 3 weeks and preferably 4 weeks of age to respond favorably to the vaccine.[13] It has not yet been determined whether measles virus antibodies that are transmitted from bitches to offspring interfere with subsequent measles virus vaccination of the offspring.

Measles vaccine can be helpful in situations in which young puppies have enough maternal canine distemper antibody to interfere with the effectiveness of canine distemper vaccine but not enough to protect them from infection. The vaccine should be given when the puppies are 3 to 6 weeks of age. When they are 14 to 16 weeks of age, modified live-virus canine-distemper vaccine should be administered to dogs receiving measles vaccine.

Combined modified live-virus measles–distemper vaccine is available. The manufacturer states that the advantage of the product is that the measles virus will protect animals not immunologically capable of producing antibodies against distemper. However, for those animals who are ready to produce distemper antibodies, the inclusion of the modified distemper virus in the product will allow them to do so.

Treatment. Drugs are not available that kill the distemper virus. Therefore treatment of the disease is aimed at maintaining the animal in as normal a physiological state as possible to allow its own defenses to combat the virus. The administration of fluids and electrolytes is important in this regard. In addition, appropriate antibiotics are indicated to treat secondary bacterial infections. Anticholinergic drugs are often used to control diarrhea. Intestinal protectants and adsorbants such as kaopectate may be administered (Chapter 19).

Canine infectious hepatitis

Canine infectious hepatitis is caused by a specific virus that is not related to the virus causing hepatitis in humans. In dogs the virus may be relatively avirulent, resulting in subclinical infections. However, when infected by a virulent virus strain, dogs may develop severe clinical signs and even die. In severe infections the signs are typical of those associated with liver damage. In addition, the virus may cause edema of the cornea of the eye, which gives the eye an opaque bluish color.

The wild virus as well as the attenuated virus administered in the vaccine is spread from one dog to another in the urine.

Prevention

Passive immunity. Antisera, which are available for short-term protection before active immunization, may interfere with subsequent active immunization. Therefore they should not be used.

Active immunity. As with canine distemper, maternal antibodies in puppies potentially interfere with the active production of antibodies against canine hepatitis.

Two types of hepatitis vaccines are available: the modified live virus and inactivated virus vaccines. Either of these is acceptable as an immunizing agent against canine infectious hepatitis and may be combined with distemper and/or leptospirosis vaccines. Commercial combinations of canine hepatitis and canine distemper vaccines are acceptable.[5] Rarely transient opacity of the cornea may result 10 days to 3 weeks after immunization with infectious canine hepatitis modified live virus vaccines. Vaccination against canine hepatitis is recommended at the same time that dogs are vaccinated against canine distemper.

An inactivated canine infectious hepatitis vaccine has been shown to stimulate production in young puppies of active humoral immunity, regardless of the presence of maternal antibodies.[2]

Canine infectious tracheobronchitis

Canine infectious tracheobronchitis is caused by numerous viruses. The following have been implicated: canine parainfluenza virus, canine adenovirus type 2, reoviruses, and canine herpesvirus. Canine parainfluenza virus and canine adenovirus type 2 are the most frequently isolated.[9]

A vaccine containing parainfluenza virus is commercially available for dogs. Further evaluation must be made to determine the efficacy and liabilities of the vaccine.

Feline panleukopenia

Feline panleukopenia, also known as "cat distemper" or "feline enteritis," is caused by a specific virus. The disease, causing a severe enteritis and a decrease in all types of circulating white blood cells, is highly contagious and causes high mortality in the susceptible cat population. In addition to the domestic house cat, it affects other members of the feline family.

Prevention

Passive immunity. Two types of products are available for conferring passive immunity against feline panleukopenia. One is anti–feline distemper serum, which is derived from adult cats given repeated injections of feline panleukopenia virus. The other is normal serum of feline origin, which is derived from cats of undetermined immune status. Because both maternally derived antibodies and administered passive antibodies interfere with feline panleukopenia vaccines, the use of anti–feline distemper serum, normal serum, or both is not recommended in normal vaccination routines. Administration of panleukopenia vaccine to kittens at frequent intervals is a more suitable alternative.

There are only two specific indications for the use of antiserum or normal serum. Susceptible cats exposed to feline panleukopenia should be given antiserum immediately at the rate of 2.2 ml/kg of body weight. In addition, colostrum-deprived kittens should be given antiserum as soon after birth as possible. In both instances, vaccines should be given later at appropriate intervals, as defined on p. 59.[14] The merits of using antiserum in the treatment of canine feline panleukopenia have not been clearly defined.

Active immunity. The following products are available to produce active immunity against feline panleukopenia:

1. *Inactivated virus vaccine, tissue origin.* This vaccine is prepared from tissues either of cats infected with panleukopenia virus or of minks infected with mink enteritis virus. There is an antigenic relationship between the viruses of mink enteritis and feline panleukopenia. Clinically the two diseases are similar. Some of the products contain adjuvants.

2. *Inactivated virus vaccine, feline tissue culture origin.* As the name implies, the vaccine is produced from tissue cultures of feline origin infected with feline panleukopenia virus. The virus is then inactivated with formalin.

3. *Feline distemper vaccine, modified live virus, tissue culture origin.* This vaccine is produced from feline origin tissue cultures infected with modified feline panleukopenia virus.

4. *Mink enteritis vaccine, modified live virus, tissue culture origin (for use in cats).* This vaccine is developed by serial passage in feline kidney tissue culture cells until the virus is avirulent for both mink and cats. However, it retains its immunological properties.

The inactivated tissue culture vaccine for feline panleukopenia is effective in protecting cats against the disease.[4] One administration of the vaccine in cats 3 to 6 months of age results in good antibody titer formation. If a second inoculation is administered, the titer will go even higher. The immunity produced by the inactivated vaccine will last for at least a year.

Some data indicate that modified live virus panleukopenia vaccines are more effective than the inactivated vaccines. In a trial comparing the two products, the modified live virus vaccine was more effective than the inactivated vaccine against panleukopenia. When immunizing cats held by a humane society, 10% of kittens developed panleukopenia after the inactivated vaccine was administered, whereas only 1% developed panleukopenia after receiving the modified live virus.[26]

The modified live virus, tissue culture

Table 4-1. Summary of schedule for immunizing cats against feline panleukopenia[*]

	Inactivated virus (age of cat)	Modified live virus (age of cat)
First dose	9-10 weeks	9-10 weeks
Second dose	11-12 weeks	14-16 weeks
Third dose	16 weeks	Not necessary
Booster dose	Revaccinate annually	Revaccinate annually

[*]Based on data from Gillespie, J. H., and others: Report on the panel of the colloquium on selected feline infectious diseases, J. Am. Vet. Med. Assoc. **157**:2043, 1970.

origin, mink enteritis vaccine has also been shown to be highly effective in preventing feline panleukopenia.[20]

Because the feline panleukopenia virus has an affinity for cells that are dividing, the live virus vaccine should not be used in pregnant queens or in kittens less than 4 weeks of age. With these exceptions, both the inactivated and live virus feline panleukopenia vaccines are safe to use in cats.

A panel of the Colloquium on Selected Feline Infectious Diseases made the following recommendation for immunizing cats against panleukopenia (Table 4-1)[14]:

1. Use tissue culture origin inactivated or modified live virus vaccines.

2. Administer two doses of the vaccines starting at 9 to 10 weeks of age. With inactivated vaccine, give the second dose 2 weeks later. To provide maximum protection, administer a third dose of inactivated vaccine when the cat is 16 weeks old. With modified live vaccine, the second vaccination should be given at 14 to 16 weeks of age. (If kittens are older than 12 weeks of age at the time of the first vaccination, a second dose of modified live virus vaccine is not necessary.)

3. For maximum protection, annual revaccination is recommended.

4. Before introducing unvaccinated kittens into an area of possible exposure, immediate vaccination or administration of antiserum is recommended.

Feline respiratory infections

Numerous infectious organisms, most of them viral, cause respiratory disease in cats. The signs produced in these animals are similar even though the viruses responsible for the syndrome are not related.

Infected cats readily transmit respiratory diseases to other cats. Even cats showing no clinical signs but carrying the infection in their respiratory passages can transmit the disease. When cats from different households or areas are brought together in one room, such as in veterinary hospitals, pounds, or research facilities, outbreaks of respiratory infections often result. These outbreaks occur even if none of the cats showed signs of disease at the time they were brought together.

Etiology. Among the viruses that cause respiratory disease in cats are the feline pneumonitis virus, the feline caliciviruses, and a herpesvirus, which may be responsible for approximately half the clinical cases of feline respiratory infections. The syndrome caused by the herpesvirus is called "feline rhinotracheitis."

In addition to viruses, *Mycoplasma* organisms have been associated with respiratory disease in the domestic cat.

Signs. Signs of feline respiratory disease include loss of appetite, inflammation of the nasal passages (rhinitis) with possible nasal discharge, incrustations around the nose, difficult breathing, pneumonia, fever, and ulcers of the oral cavity.

Feline viral rhinotracheitis involves significant mortality, especially in young kittens. Abortion or generalized infection of newborn kittens may occur following infection with the virus of pregnant queens. The primary viral diseases can be complicated by secondary bacterial infection. In uncomplicated cases the signs usually subside within 10 days.

Prevention. Vaccines to protect cats against three viral respiratory infections are available: feline pneumonitis vaccine, feline rhinotracheitis vaccine, and calicivirus vaccine.

Feline pneumonitis vaccine. Feline pneumonitis vaccine is composed of modified live virus from chick embryos. Because cats suffer from such a wide variety of upper respiratory diseases, the efficacy of the vaccine has been difficult to determine. The use of the vaccine in pregnant animals is not recommended. Ocular contamination must be avoided because the vaccine will produce local inflammation of the eyes. When it is used, the vaccine is usually given at weaning time and repeated annually.

Feline rhinotracheitis vaccine. Feline rhinotracheitis vaccine was developed to produce immunity to the herpesvirus responsible for upper respiratory disease in cats. The vaccine is a modified live virus type. Administration results in a high production of antibodies. Challenge tests demonstrate that the vaccine has moderate efficacy in protecting cats against feline viral rhinotracheitis. Although limited studies indicate it does not cause abortion or malformed fetuses, this vaccine is not recommended for use in pregnant animals. Antibody titers are higher if a second dose is given 3 to 4 weeks after the initial dose of the vaccine. The intramuscular route results in higher antibody titers and is preferred. Generally, cats are reimmunized against the herpesvirus annually.

Feline calicivirus vaccine. It was thought at first that the large number of strains of caliciviruses would make the development of a vaccine against these organisms difficult. However, certain calicivirus strains show a high degree of antigenic relationship to others. The F-9 strain is used in a calicivirus vaccine because the manufacturer claims that according to studies, it is one of the more broadly antigenic calicivirus strains. By adapting the virus to grow at low temperatures in a tissue culture system, its virulence has been decreased. However, its antigenicity is retained. The commercial vaccine has been combined with the feline viral rhinotracheitis vaccine (FVR-C). It is moderately effective in protecting against respiratory diseases caused by caliciviruses. The manufacturer claims that it can be administered with feline panleukopenia vaccine and that immunity to all three viruses results when the combination is administered.[6] To make this vaccine, specially prepared inactivated feline panleukopenia vaccine is used as the diluent for the modified live virus bivalent respiratory vaccine (FVR-C-P).[22] The antibody titer will persist for at least 10 to 12 months.

Rabies

Rabies is the most feared disease transmitted from animals to humans. All mammals are capable of contracting the disease and transmitting it to others, although actual transmission has primarily been from carnivores, dogs, cats, skunks, raccoons, foxes, and bats. Rabies is caused by a virus with an affinity for nervous system tissue. The

normal means of infection is by way of a bite. The virus migrates along nerve trunks to the spinal cord and from there eventually to the brain. As the virus approaches the head and neck area, the salivary glands become infected, and the virus is shed in saliva. In humans, once the signs of the disease are manifested, rabies is almost always fatal.

Control of rabies. Control programs are aimed at four types of hosts: domestic pets, wild animals, domestic livestock, and humans. Table 4-2 shows the incidence of rabies in various species in the United States from 1953 to 1975. To control rabies in dogs and cats, a program of vaccination and removal of stray or unwanted animals is effective. The incidence of rabies in dogs was

Table 4-2. Incidence of rabies in United States* by type of animal, 1953-1975†

Year	Dogs	Cats	Farm animals	Foxes	Skunks	Bats	Other animals	Man	Total
1953	5688	538	1118	1033	319	8	119	14	8837
1954	4083	462	1032	1028	547	4	118	8	7282
1955	2657	343	924	1223	580	14	98	5	5844
1956	2592	371	794	1281	631	41	126	10	5846
1957	1758	382	714	1021	775	31	115	6	4802
1958	1643	353	737	845	1005	68	157	6	4814
1959	1119	292	751	920	789	80	126	6	4083
1960	697	277	645	915	725	88	108	2	3457
1961	594	217	482	614	1254	186	120	3	3470
1962	565	232	614	594	1449	1157	114	2	3727
1963	573	217	531	622	1462	303	224	1	3933
1964	409	220	594	1061	1909	352	238	1	4784
1965	412	289	625	1038	1582	484	153	1	4584
1966	412	252	587	864	1522	377	183	1	4198
1967	412	293	691	979	1568	414	250	2	4609
1968	296	157	457	801	1400	291	210	1	3613
1969	256	165	428	888	1156	321	307	1	3522
1970	185	135	399	771	1235	296	252	3‡	3276
1971	235	222	484	677	2018	465	289	2	4392
1972	232	184	547	645	2095	504	218	2	4427
1973	180	139	448	477	1851	432	170	1	3698
1974	232	121	303	302	1421	537	239	0	3155
1975	129	104	200	278	1226	514	223	3	2677

*Includes Guam, Puerto Rico, and Virgin Islands.
†From Center for Disease Control: Rabies surveillance, annual summary 1975, United States Department of Health, Education, and Welfare, Public Health Service, Aug. 1976.
‡One patient recovered.

reduced by such means in the United States from over 8000 laboratory-confirmed cases in 1946 to only 129 in 1975.

It is more difficult to control rabies in wildlife. However, since the disease is usually transmitted to humans by contact with domestic animals, controlling the disease in dogs and cats goes a long way toward protecting the human population.

In humans the disease can be prevented by minimizing exposure to rabid animals and by preexposure or postexposure immunization. Persons in high-risk groups such as veterinarians and animal health technicians should receive preexposure immunization.

A dog or cat bitten by a known rabid animal should be destroyed immediately. If the owner is unwilling, the exposed unvaccinated animal should be placed in strict isolation for at least 6 months. The animal should be immunized against rabies 1 month before being released. If a dog that has been immunized within three years with a United States–licensed, modified live virus–type vaccine or within one year with any other vaccine is subsequently exposed, it should be reimmunized immediately and restrained for at least 60 days but preferably for 90 days.

Livestock known to have been bitten by rabid animals should be slaughtered immediately. If the owner is unwilling, the animal should be immunized and placed in strict confinement for at least 6 months.

A dog or cat that bites someone should be held for rabies observation. Fortunately, dogs and cats shed the virus only a few days before the onset of signs of the disease. It is recommended that the biting animal be kept under observation 10 days after inflicting the bite. If the animal develops signs of rabies during the observation period, it should be immediately killed and the body submitted to an appropriate laboratory for rabies examination. When a wild animal bites a human, the animal should be killed immediately in such a way that the head is not damaged, and the whole body should be submitted to a laboratory for diagnosis.

To improve on control programs for rabies, a subcommittee on rabies of the National Academy of Sciences recommends the following points[17]:

1. Require the licensing of all dogs 4 months of age and older
2. Require rabies vaccination for all dogs 4 months of age or older
3. Hold rabies vaccination as a requisite to licensing
4. Require that all dogs under 4 months of age be confined to the premises of the owner or kept under physical restraint by the owner, keeper, or harborer
5. Require that local governing bodies (cities and counties) maintain or provide for maintenance of a pound system and rabies control
6. Place responsibility for holding low-cost public rabies vaccination clinics on cities and counties
7. Require that low cost public rabies vaccination fees be set by regulation adopted by the state agency responsible for administration of the law after consultation with the state veterinary medical association to ensure that uniform public clinic fees are maintained under the program
8. Require that rabies vaccination be performed only by a licensed veterinarian using only rabies vaccine approved and prescribed by the state agency responsible for administering the law
9. Restrict sale of animal rabies vaccines to licensed veterinarians, veterinary biological supply firms, or public agencies
10. Provide authority for adoption of regulations for implementation and administration of the law
11. Provide authority to local enforcement officials for the issuance of citations for violations of the law
12. Provide authority for local enforcement officials to enter upon private property for purposes of enforcement of the rabies control law

Table 4-3. Compendium of animal rabies vaccines* in United States, 1977†

Vaccine: generic name	Marketed by (product name)	For use in	Dosage (ml)	Animal's age	Revaccination recommended
Modified live virus (MLV)					
Chicken embryo origin, low egg passage, Flury strain	Schering (Rabies Vaccine)	Dogs	2	3 months and 1 year	3 years
	Fromm (Raboid)	Dogs	1	3 months and 1 year	3 years
	Haver-Lockhart (Rabies Vaccine)	Dogs	1	3 months and 1 year	3 years
Canine cell line origin, high egg passage, Flury strain	Nordan (Endurall-R)	Dogs	1	3 months and 1 year	3 years
		Cats	1	3 months	1 year
Porcine tissue culture origin, high cell passage, SAD strain	Jensen-Salsbery (ERA Strain Rabies Vaccine)	Dogs	1	3 months and 1 year	3 years
		Cats	1	3 months	1 year
		Cattle	1	4 months	1 year
		Horses	1	4 months	1 year
		Sheep	1	4 months	1 year
		Goats	1	4 months	1 year
Canine tissue culture origin, high cell passage, SAD strain	Bio-Ceutic (Neutrogen-T-C)	Dogs	1	3 months	1 year
		Cats	1	3 months	1 year
Bovine kidney tissue culture origin, high cell passage, SAD strain	Pitman-Moore (Rabies Vaccine)	Dogs	1	3 months	1 year
Hamster cell line origin, high cell passage, Kissling strain	Affiliated (Rabtect)	Dogs	1	3 months	1 year
Inactivated vaccines					
Caprine origin	Bandy (Rabies Vaccine)	Dogs	2	3 months	1 year
		Cats	2	3 months	1 year
Murine origin	Ft. Dodge (Trimune)	Dogs	1	3 months and 1 year	3 years
		Cats	1	3 months	1 year

*All vaccines should be administered intramuscularly at one site in the thigh.
†From Crawford, K. L., and others: Compendium of animal rabies vaccines, 1977, Vet. Public Health Notes, Feb. 1977.

13. Provide authority for the establishment of area quarantines in emergency situations
14. Provide a penalty clause making violations of the law a misdemeanor
15. Place responsibility for administration and enforcement of the law at the state level in an interested and concerned state agency, preferably public health or agriculture
16. Include a clause to the effect that nothing in the state law is intended to or shall be construed to limit the power of the city or county to exercise its police powers to enact more stringent requirements to regulate and control dogs within its jurisdiction

Veterinary rabies vaccines. The various rabies vaccines that were available for veterinary use in the United States in 1977 are shown in Table 4-3. Both modified live virus and inactivated vaccines are available.

The chick embryo origin Flury strain rabies vaccine, a modified live virus, was initially isolated from a human and serially passed intracerebrally in day-old chicken brains. It was then passed in chick embryos to the point at which it was lethal only when inoculated intracerebrally. This was designated "low egg passage." Later, further passages were made in chick embryos until the virus was lethal only to suckling mice inoculated intracerebrally. This level of passage was designated "high egg passage."

Generally, the modified live virus vaccines have produced adequate immunity and are safe when used in the species for which they are licensed. For example, when modified live virus rabies vaccine produced from Flury high egg passage virus grown on an established canine kidney cell is administered intramuscularly in dogs, it can produce an immunity that can last three years.[7]

Chick embryo origin modified live virus rabies vaccine has the following advantages over older products:

• Reduction of nervous tissue in the vaccine
• Elimination of chemical preservatives
• Longer duration of immunity
• Reduction in bulk
• Comparative safety and ease of manufacturing
• High effectiveness

However, chick embryo origin rabies vaccine has several disadvantages too. The vaccine contains relatively large amounts of egg protein capable of producing allergic reactions. The presence of such proteins may also interfere with the immune response. The chick embryo origin vaccine is also difficult to reconstitute with water. When low egg passage chick embryo origin vaccine is used in species other than dogs (especially cats, cattle, or wildlife), it may produce clinical rabies.

Reports vary regarding the effectiveness of killed rabies vaccines. For example, one study indicates that an inactivated hamster tissue culture vaccine provided only 70% of dogs with protection from virulent virus challenge one year after vaccination.[25] On the other hand, another study shows that killed suckling mouse brain rabies vaccine (murine origin) was 100% effective in protecting dogs three years after a single dose was given.[12]

A disadvantage of killed vaccines is that current regulations require that they be given annually to dogs, whereas modified live virus vaccines may be given every two years to dogs.

We suggest that dogs and cats should be immunized with an appropriate modified live virus vaccine. However, further research may show the suckling mouse brain rabies vaccine to be as good as or better than the modified live virus vaccine.

Simultaneous administration of rabies and other vaccines needs elucidation. One vaccine may interfere with the other. Until it is proved that antibodies against rabies will form when the vaccine is given concurrently with other vaccines, rabies vaccine should be given alone.

Accidental inoculation or other exposure may occur to individuals during the administration of animal rabies vaccines. Such exposures to inactivated vaccines constitute no known rabies hazard. The Flury low egg passage and high egg passage strains and the SAD strain vaccines (Table 4-3) appear to involve no hazard, although this is based more on empirical observation than on specific studies. However, available data on human exposure to other modified live virus rabies vaccines are inadequate. In the event of exposure to other modified live virus vaccines, public health officials should be contacted for specific recommendations.[8]

Prevention in dogs. A subcommittee on rabies of the National Academy of Sciences recommended the following immunization programs for dogs[17]:

1. All dogs between 3 and 4 months of age should be vaccinated with a vaccine licensed by the U.S. Department of Agriculture. They should be reimmunized at one year of age.

2. Adult animals immunized with modified

live virus vaccines of either chick embryo or tissue culture origin are normally protected against rabies for three years.

3. Inactivated licensed vaccines are considered safe. Nervous tissue origin inactivated rabies vaccine provides one year of immunity after a single injection. If inactivated tissue culture origin vaccines are used, two doses given 3 to 4 weeks apart are recommended for the primary immunization; annual boosters are required to maintain immunity.

4. The recommended route of administration of rabies vaccine, live or inactivated, is intramuscular.

5. Rabies vaccine should be administered to dogs under the supervision of a licensed veterinarian. (In many states this is mandatory if the animal is to be licensed.)

6. Peak rabies antibody titers are reached within 1 month after the initial vaccination. Animals should therefore be maintained on leash or confined for a month after vaccination.

Prevention in cats. For cats the following procedures should be followed:

1. All cats should be immunized annually with a rabies vaccine licensed for use in cats.

2. They should be immunized initially when they are between 3 and 4 months of age.

3. Any vaccine other than those containing the low egg passage Flury strain of virus may be used.

4. If inactivated vaccines are used, the recommendations made for dogs apply.

Prevention in wildlife. Currently no vaccine is licensed in the United States for the immunization of wildlife (nondomestic animals kept as pets) against rabies. Data on the efficacy and duration of immunity are generally lacking. If it is necessary to immunize wildlife against rabies, only inactivated vaccines should be used, since some modified live virus vaccines may produce rabies in such animals. In the absence of specific data, the dose should be based on the recommendations for immunization of dogs. Revaccination should be performed annually.[8]

Prevention in humans. Preexposure immunization of humans against rabies is recommended for personnel in high-risk occupations, such as veterinarians, animal handlers, and certain laboratory workers.

In the United States duck embryo killed virus rabies vaccine is used for rabies prophylaxis in humans. Two regimens of preexposure prophylaxis are currently recommended:

1. When rapid immunization is not important, two 1 ml doses of duck embryo vaccine are injected subcutaneously a month apart. A third dose is given 6 to 7 months after the second. Within 1 month, neutralizing antibodies will develop in 80% to 90% of those immunized.

2. When more rapid immunity is desired, three 1 ml doses of duck embryo vaccine are injected at weekly intervals. A fourth is given 3 months later. About 80% of those vaccinated by this method develop an antibody response.

The level of serum antibodies produced should be confirmed by a laboratory examination 3 to 4 weeks after the last injection.

When an immunized person who has demonstrated rabies antibody titer has a nonbite exposure to rabies, one dose of vaccine should be given. When an immunized individual with previously demonstrated rabies antibodies is bitten by a rabid animal, five daily doses of vaccine and one booster dose 20 days after the fifth dose should be administered. In an unimmunized person or a person whose immune status is unknown, antirabies serum is given to produce immediate protection while an active immunity is developing in response to the vaccine. Active immunity usually takes 2 weeks to be produced; in severe exposures the disease could develop in that time. Because it could interfere with the development of active immunity, only one dose of passive antibody should be administered.

Two products are available: antirabies serum of equine origin and antirabies serum of human origin. In 1969 approximately 8000 people in the United States received the equine serum.[24] The product provided rabies antibodies immediately as well as apparent protection from infection from 12 to 14 days. However, approximately 16% of persons who received this preparation developed an allergic response to the equine serum. For persons over 15 years of age the incidence rose to 46%. The allergic response to equine serum can be avoided by administering rabies immune globulin derived from human serum.

For postexposure treatment, human rabies immune globulin is used in conjunction with duck embryo origin rabies vaccine. The immune globulin is administered only once to a patient with the first dose of the vaccine. For postexposure immunization in nonimmune persons or persons whose immunity is unknown, twenty-one 1 ml doses of the duck embryo vaccine are given subcutaneously daily. These are followed by two booster doses, the first 10 days after the twenty-first dose and the second 10 days later.

BACTERIAL DISEASES

Dogs and cats are afflicted with many conditions caused by bacteria. Only two bacterial conditions are discussed here: leptospirosis, because a bacterin is available for its prevention, and bacterial cystitis, because there are unique factors that affect its therapy. For a discussion of anti-infective drugs used to treat other bacterial diseases, see Chapter 3.

Leptospirosis

In dogs, leptospirosis is usually caused by one of two strains of *Leptospira*: *L. canicola* and *L. icterohaemorrhagiae*. In rural areas where there is contact with wildlife reservoirs, dogs may be infected with other serotypes such as *L. pomona*. In most cases the infection causes minimal signs or is subclinical. Animals that develop a serious case of leptospirosis show signs indicating damage to various organs, especially the liver and kidney.

The disease is commonly spread through the urine. In addition to dogs, the infection can be spread to humans. However, cats are highly resistant to both natural and experimental infections caused by *Leptospira* species.[16]

Most infected dogs become renal carriers and shed *Leptospira* organisms in their urine. This contamination of urine can occur for up to a year after infection. While the leptospira are fragile and disappear rapidly from the urine if dried, frozen, or exposed to common disinfectants, they may survive for long periods if the urine falls into water or moist soil with a neutral pH. The source of most dog leptospirosis is the chronically infected renal carrier. The disease is transmitted because of the dog's habit of smelling urine for identification, which can result in an efficient intranasal inoculation of fresh *Leptospira* organisms.

Prevention. *Leptospira* bacterin is available to prevent leptospirosis in dogs. This vaccine should contain both *L. canicola* and *L. icterohaemorrhagiae* to provide maximum protection. It is sometimes combined with distemper and hepatitis vaccine.

The protection granted by the vaccine is short-lived, sometimes only 6 months. From a public health and epidemiological standpoint it is important that the vaccine not only protect against development of the clinical disease but also prevent the renal carrier state. Some research indicates that the bacterin provides excellent protection against this state. However, other investigation indicates that the bacterin does not prevent it. This issue needs clarification.[18,19]

Generally, the administration of leptospira bacterin is recommended. Because of the short duration of the immunity, in the face of an outbreak, animals should be reimmunized.

Anaphylactoid reactions can occur after administration of the bacterin.

The first dose of *Leptospira* bacterin should be administered when the puppy is 9 weeks old. By that time most dogs will have lost their passive immunity. The second dose should be given 3 weeks later or when the final dose of canine distemper–infectious hepatitis vaccine is administered. Animals should be revaccinated annually.[5]

Treatment. Penicillin administered parenterally is usually effective in treating clinical cases of leptospirosis, provided that the advanced stages of the disease have not caused irreversible organ damage. Because many clinicians believe that combinations of penicillin and streptomycin are more effective than penicillin alone in preventing the renal carrier state, that combination of antibiotics generally is administered to treat clinical cases.

Bacterial cystitis

Treatment. Bacterial cystitis is a bacterial infection of the urinary bladder. Because many antimicrobial drugs are excreted in the urine, it is easy to obtain relatively high concentrations of anti-infective drugs in the urinary bladder.

By culturing the urine, the veterinarian can determine the most ideal anti-infective drug to use. However, in addition to noting the type of infection present, the veterinarian should also monitor the pH of the urine.

Bacterial cystitis is most often accompanied by alkaline urine rather than the acidic urine normally present in dogs and cats. The pH of the urine will influence to some degree the activity of an anti-infective drug, since some are more effective in acidic urine and others are more affective in alkaline urine. For example, streptomycin, kanamycin, gentamicin, and erythromycin have increased antibacterial activity in an alkaline pH. Tetracyclines and novobiocin are more active in an acid pH. Methenamine is effective only in an acid pH. The activity of sulfonamides and chloramphenicol is greater against some organisms in an alkaline pH and greater against others in an acid pH. The activity of nitrofurantoin is unaffected by the pH of the urine.

The urinary pH may be changed to create an environment hostile to the infecting organism. However, in the absence of anti-infective therapy, merely changing the urinary pH will probably not be effective in the treatment of bacterial cystitis.

Urinary acidifiers. Because bacterial infections generally result in alkaline urine in dogs and cats, if a decision is made to change the pH, it is usually to acidify the urine. The following substances are used to acidify the urine of dogs and cats: ammonium chloride, ascorbic acid, methionine, and sodium phosphate monobasic.

Ammonium chloride, in addition to acidifying urine, acts as a diuretic. However, its effectiveness is limited to 5 to 6 days. In dogs, ammonium chloride at a dose of 200 mg/kg/24 hr given in three divided doses has been found adequate to reduce urine pH in experimental trials from a level of 6.6 to an average value of about 5.5. In dogs with acute bacterial cystitis, the same dose was effective in lowering the pH from the alkaline to acid range. At this dose, systemic acidosis was mild.[23] Generally, lower doses of 25 mg/kg have been recommended for dogs and cats.[21] The lower dose should be used first. If the urine is not adequately acidified, then a higher dose can be used in dogs.

Ascorbic acid can be administered in large doses to acidify urine without causing systemic acidosis.

Methionine, an aminio acid, is used in dogs and cats as a urinary acidifier. It is given to dogs at a dose of 25 mg/kg one to three times a day. For cats it is administered at the rate of 25 to 50 mg/kg one to three times a day.

As a 1% solution, sodium phosphate monobasic has a pH of 4.6. Its concurrent use with methenamine (Chapter 3) is not recommended because this causes methenamine to release formaldehyde in the intestinal tract rather than in the urinary bladder. However, oral doses of sodium phosphate monobasic may be followed in an hour by methenamine to achieve the desired urinary effect. In dogs and cats, sodium phosphate monobasic is given at the rate of 30 mg/kg two to three times a day to acidify the urine.[21]

In the presence of kidney or liver failure, urine acidifiers should not be used. In hepatic failure, use of urinary acidifiers may induce coma. Other potential contraindications include diabetes mellitus, prolonged diarrhea, vomiting large quantities of intestinal juices, and starvation.

References

1. Ablett, R. E., and Baker, L. A.: Periodic distemper revaccination advisable, J. Am. Vet. Med. Assoc. **145:**156, 1964.
2. Ackermann, O.: Early immunization against canine distemper and hepatitis, using combined vaccines, J. Am. Vet. Med. Assoc. **156:**1755, 1970.
3. Baker, J. A.: Measles vaccine for protection of dogs against canine distemper, J. Am. Vet. Med. Assoc. **156:**1743, 1970.
4. Bittle, J. L., Emrich, S. A., and Gauker, F. B.: Safety and efficacy of an inactivated tissue culture vaccine for feline panleukopenia, J. Am. Vet. Med. Assoc. **157:**2052, 1970.
5. Bittle, J. L., Freeman, A., Gillespie, J. H., Strating, A., Ott, R. L., Scott, F. W., Sikes, R. K., and Thornton, G. W.: Synopsis of vaccination procedures for dogs, J. Am. Vet. Med. Assoc. **162:** 228, 1973.
6. Bittle, J. L., and Rubic, W. J.: A feline calicivirus vaccine combined with feline viral rhinotracheitis and feline panleukopenia vaccine, Feline Pract. **5:**13, Nov.-Dec. 1975.
7. Brown, A. L., Merry, D. L., and Beckenhauer, W. H.: Modified live-virus rabies vaccine produced from Flury high egg-passage virus grown on an established canine-kidney cell line: three-year duration-of-immunity study in dogs, Am. J. Vet. Res. **31:**1427, 1973.
8. Crawford, K. L., and others: Compendium of animal rabies vaccines, 1977, Vet. Public Health Notes, Feb. 1977.
9. Emery, J. B., and Sweeny, W. T.: A canine parainfluenza virus vaccine, Canine Pract. **2:**26, March-April 1975.
10. Evans, J. M.: Optimal ages for canine distemper vaccination, J. Am. Vet. Med. Assoc. **151:**1455, 1967.
11. Evans, J. M., and Forrest, D. T.: Prevention of canine distemper on infected premises, J. Am. Vet. Med. Assoc. **156:**1758, 1970.
12. Fields, M., Ament, R. D., Lamb, D., and Blades, J.: Suckling-mouse-brain rabies vaccine (SMBV): duration of immunity in dogs, Vet. Med. Small Anim. Clin. **71:**37, 1976.
13. Gale, C.: Measles virus for distemper prophylaxis, J. Am. Vet. Med. Assoc. **156:**1971, 1970.
14. Gillespie, J. H., and others: Report of the panel of the colloquium on selected feline infectious diseases, J. Am. Vet. Med. Assoc. **157:**2043, 1970.
15. Howell, D. G., Floeck, A. K., and Holbrook, G.: Effect of revaccination on distemper antibody levels, Mod. Vet. Pract. **45:**81, June 1964.
16. Jones, C. K.: Cats resistant to leptospirosis, J. Am. Vet. Med. Assoc. **145:**6, Sept. 1964.
17. Kennedy, P. C., Cabasso, V. J., Davis, D. E., Sikes, R. K., and York, C. J.: Control of rabies, Washington, D.C., 1973, National Academy of Sciences.
18. Kerr, D. D.: Protection against the renal carrier state by a canine leptospirosis vaccine, Vet. Med. Small Anim. Clin. **69:**1157, 1974.
19. Kerr, D. D., and Marshall, V.: Early protection of dogs by a leptospira bacterin, Mod. Vet. Pract. **55:**430, 1974.
20. King, D. A., and Gutekunst, D. E.: A new mink enteritis vaccine for immunization against feline panleukopenia, Vet. Med. Small Anim. Clin. **65:** 377, 1970.
21. Rossoff, I. S.: Handbook of veterinary drugs, New York, 1974, Springer Publishing Co.
22. Scott, F. W.: Vaccination program, Feline Pract. **7:**34, March 1977.
23. Short, E. C., and Hammond, P. B.: Ammonium chloride as a urinary acidifier in the dog, J. Am. Vet. Med. Assoc. **144:**864, 1964.
24. Sikes, R. K.: Human-origin rabies immune globulin, J. Am. Vet. Med. Assoc. **155:**1506, 1969.
25. Strating, A., Bunn, T. O., Goff, M. T., and Phillips, C. E.: Efficacy of inactivated tissue culture rabies vaccine in dogs, J. Am. Vet. Med. Assoc. **167:**809, 1975.
26. Whitney, W. H.: Aspects of feline panleukopenia control in a human society, Vet. Med. Small Anim. Clin. **63:**1297, 1973.

Additional readings

Abelseth, M. D.: Rabies vaccination of cats, J. Am. Vet. Med. Assoc. **158:**1003, 1971.

Ablett, R. E.: Prophylaxis and clinical evaluation concerning measles virus for distemper immunization, J. Am. Vet. Med. Assoc. **156:**1766, 1970.

Anonymous: Rabies incubation time, Vet. Med. Small Anim. Clin. **65:**850, 1970.

Baer, G. M., Goodrich, W. O., Dean, D. J.: Death from anaphylactic shock in a dog vaccinated with antirabies vaccine of chicken embryo origin, J. Am. Vet. Med. Assoc. **141:**1048, 1962.

Bittle, J. L.: Feline viral rhinotracheitis (FVR) vaccine development (part I), Pract. Vet. **46:**14, July-Aug. 1974.

Bittle, J. L.: Feline viral rhinotracheitis (FVR) vaccine development (part II), Pract. Vet. **46:**9, Sept.-Oct. 1974.

Brown, A. L.: Canine distemper-measles vaccination: studies on three practical aspects, Canine Pract. **2:** 47, May-June 1975.

Brown, A. L., Vitamvas, J. A., Merry, D. L., Jr., and Beckenhauer, W. H.: Immune response of pups to modified live-virus canine distemper–measles vaccine, Am. J. Vet. Res. **33:**1447, 1972.

Croghan, D. L.: Rabies vaccines for veterinary use, J. Am. Vet. Med. Assoc. **156:**1798, 1970.

Emery, J. B., Elliot, A. Y., Bordt, D. E., Burch, G. R., and Kugel, E. E.: A tissue-culture, modified live-virus rabies vaccine for dogs: report on development and clinical trial, J. Am. Vet. Med. Assoc. **152:** 476, 1968.

Gourlay, J. A.: Comments on the use of measles virus

for distemper prophylaxis, J. Am. Vet. Med. Assoc. **156:**1769, 1970.

Hattwick, M., and Sikes, R. K.: Pre-exposure rabies prophylaxis, J. Am. Vet. Md. Assoc. **160:**136, 1972.

Hogle, R. M.: Antibacterial-agent sensitivity of bacteria isolated from dogs and cats, J. Am. Vet. Med. Assoc. **156:**761, 1970.

Humphreys, G. L.: Comments on use of rabies vaccines, J. Am. Vet. Med. Assoc. **156:**1801, 1970.

Kirk, R. W.: A decade of progress in kennel management, Mod. Vet. Pract. **42:**40, July 1961.

Lawson, K. F., and Crawley, J. F.: ERA strain rabies vaccine, intracerebral passage in dogs, Can. Vet. J. **14:**125, June 1973.

Miller, L. N.: Anaphylactic shock and allergic reaction following rabies vaccination, Vet. Med. **57:**514, 1962.

Ott, R. L.: Distemper immunization with measles vaccine, J. Am. Vet. Med. Assoc. **157:**2064, 1970.

Prydie, J., Batty, I., and Walker, P. D.: Noninterference of distemper and hepatitis viruses, Mod. Vet. Pract. **48:**68, Jan. 1967.

Scott, F. W.: Evaluation of a feline viral rhinotracheitis vaccine, Feline Pract. **5:**17, Jan.-Feb. 1975.

Scott, F. W., and Glaubert, A. F.: Aerosol vaccination against feline panleukopenia, J. Am. Vet. Med. Assoc. **166:**147, 1975.

Sikes, R. K.: Need for developing uniform rabies control practices in the United States, J. Am. Vet. Med. Assoc. **153:**1793, 1968.

Sikes. R. K.: Comments on rabies immunization for cats, J. Am. Vet. Med. Assoc. **158:**1006, 1971.

Sikes, R. K., Peacock, G. V., Acha, P., Arko, R. J., and Dierks, R.: Rabies vaccines: duration-of-immunity study in dogs, J. Am. Vet. Med. Assoc. **159:**1491, 1971.

5

Infectious diseases of cattle and sheep

Diseases of the digestive tract
  Calf scours (calf diarrhea)
  Bovine viral diarrhea
Diseases of the respiratory tract
Uterine infections
Infectious keratoconjunctivitis (pinkeye)
Mastitis
  California Mastitis Test
Diseases caused by viruses
  Blue tongue
  Ovine ecthyma (sore mouth, orf)
Diseases caused by bacteria
  Anthrax
  Clostridial diseases
    Blackleg
    Malignant edema (gas gangrene)
    Infectious necrotic hepatitis (black
      disease)
    Bacillary hemoglobinuria (red water)
    Enterotoxemia
    Tetanus
  Leptospirosis
  Brucellosis
Diseases caused by protozoa
  Anaplasmosis

Historically, some of the greatest accomplishments of the veterinary profession in the United States have been development of measures to control infectious diseases in livestock. These diseases constitute a major problem, adversely affecting the ability of cattle and sheep raisers to produce quality meat and milk at a reasonable cost.

One or more of the following processes may be used to control infectious diseases in cattle and sheep.

1. *Disease eradication programs.* Infectious livestock diseases that do not have reservoirs in the natural animal population of an area can be eradicated. For example, foot and mouth disease has been eradicated in the United States by a program of identifying animals with the virus, slaughtering them, reimbursing ranchers for their losses, and disinfecting the premises before allowing new livestock to be introduced to the ranch. Tuberculosis has been virtually eliminated from cattle in the United States through programs of tuberculin skin testing and slaughter of animals that react. Even diseases such as brucellosis with a reservoir in the natural wild animal population have been substantially reduced through programs of testing and vaccination.

2. *Evaluation of management techniques.* Examining management practices offers a good opportunity for controlling infectious diseases. The role of management is dramatically demonstrated by the different types of diseases encountered in cattle on a dairy farm as opposed to those in a beef herd. For example, dairy cattle are raised in close confinement and are far more likely to develop calf scours than beef cattle, which are spread out over a larger land area.

3. *Immunization.* Biologicals are useful tools in the control of infectious diseases.

However, it is important for those dispensing biologicals to be aware of those that are effective, those whose effectiveness is in question, and the proper methods of administration. Cattle are probably vaccinated against more diseases than any other animal species. [9] Among these are vaccines to provide protection against the following organisms:

Clostridium chauvoei	*Staphylococcus* species
Clostridium septicum	*Streptococcus* species
Clostridium novyi	*Vibrio fetus*
Clostridium haemolyti-	*Salmonella enteritidis*
cum	Infectious bovine rhino-
Bacillus anthracis	tracheitis virus
Leptospira pomona	Bovine viral diarrhea-
Leptospira canicola	mucosal disease virus
Leptospira icterohae-	Parainfluenza type 3
morrhagiae	virus
Pasteurella multocida	Rabies virus
Pasteurella haemolytica	Wart virus
Brucella abortus	*Anaplasma marginale*
Corynebacterium	*Escherichia coli*
species	*Enterobacter aerogenes*

4. *Therapy.* A wide variety of pharmaceuticals can be used in managing infectious diseases in livestock. Some are used for prevention, but most are used for therapy. Ideally, pharmaceuticals should be used only as a last resort when eradication programs, management practices, and the use of biologicals have failed to prevent the disease.

The classification of infectious diseases of cattle and sheep is difficult. Many syndromes such as scours are caused by a wide variety of organisms. However, numerous diseases of cattle and sheep are caused by specific organisms, and the management of such diseases involves specific preventive and therapeutic measures. Therefore in this chapter we will discuss conditions either as syndromes or as caused by a specific etiological agent.

DISEASES OF THE DIGESTIVE TRACT
Calf scours (calf diarrhea)

Signs. Calf scours is primarily a disease of dairy calves. The syndrome may vary from a mild diarrhea (from which the calf recovers spontaneously) to a profuse watery or blood-tinged diarrhea that can kill the infected animal. To understand the therapy of calf scours, one must understand water and electrolyte balance.

In severe cases of calf scours, extreme dehydration and a shift in the electrolyte balance result. These changes are primarily responsible for death in severe cases. [51] In addition to becoming dehydrated, calves become acidotic. The acidosis probably results from intestinal bicarbonate ion loss, increased organic acid production, and decreased hydrogen ion excretion by the kidneys. The dehydration results in a significant renal insufficiency and raised levels of blood urea nitrogen and serum inorganic phosphorus, which cause cellular malfunction and can lead to death.

Etiology. Calf diarrhea is generally caused by one or more infectious organisms. The following viruses have been implicated: a reo-like virus, a coronavirus, the virus of bovine viral diarrhea (BVD), and possibly the virus of infectious bovine rhinotracheitis (IBR). Primarily *Escherichia coli* is the bacteria associated with the syndrome. However, *Salmonella* species may also be involved. Protozoan parasites, such as coccidia, or in older calves, the nematodes, may also cause diarrhea.

Prevention
Management. When one considers the etiology of calf diarrhea, it is not surprising that dairy calves are the animals primarily affected by the disease. Dairy calves are raised in close confinement. Frequently, they are born in common maternity pens and raised in close proximity to each other. This high density of animals in a relatively confined area results in a buildup of excrement and easy contact transmission of infectious diseases (Fig. 5-1, *A*).

Calves are often administered milk replacer diets. These may be of poor quality, not providing adequate nutrition to the animals. In addition, even if whole milk is fed, calves are frequently underfed or overfed. Too much or too little of either the replacer or whole milk will predispose the calf to di-

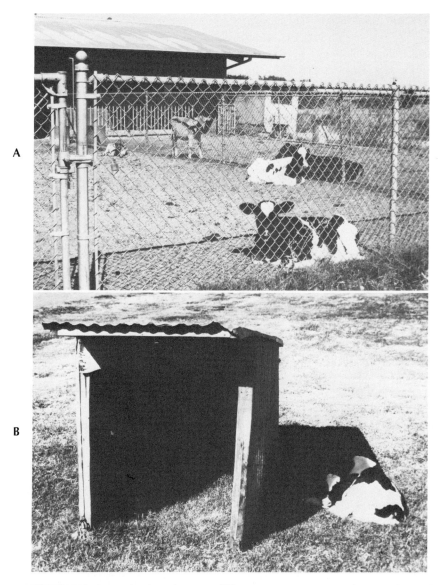

Fig. 5-1. Calves being raised under two different management schemes that will substantially affect level of pathogenic microorganisms to which animals are exposed. **A,** Many calves are penned in same area, resulting in substantial cross-contamination of microorganisms. **B,** Calf is leashed to a small shelter that is located on clean ground. Calf is not able to mix with other animals. When this calf is removed from shed, the shed will be moved to another clean area prior to housing another animal. (Courtesy Dr. Bradford P. Smith, School of Veterinary Medicine, University of California, Davis.)

arrhea. Contamination of the milk is also a common means by which calves become infected with the microorganisms responsible for calf scours.

Calves denied adequate high-quality colos-trum during the first few hours of life are far more susceptible to calf scours than those receiving antibodies by this natural route. During its first few hours of life the calf should receive 2 kg of colostrum. It is important that the manager observe the calf sucking its dam vigorously during the first 8 hours of life to be sure that the animal has received colostrum. If for one reason or another this is not possible, the calf must either be hand-fed fresh colostrum or fed colostrum from the freezer.

Vollmar[53] recommends the following management scheme to control calf scours:

1. Vigorous routine sanitary procedures should be carried out in the calf barn and maternity pens. The interior should be cleaned, disinfected, and repainted every 6 months. After each calving, maternity pens should be cleaned and disinfected.

2. Because the nutrition of the pregnant cow contributes to the health and size of the calf, particular attention should be paid to the nutritional needs of pregnant animals. They should be supplied with rations that meet their caloric and nutrient needs. (The ideal ration to supply cows with their nutrient needs will vary, depending on the feedstuffs available at the most economical price in a given community. Such information can be obtained from a standard book on animal husbandry or animal nutrition or from local farm advisors.)

3. Prior to calving, the cow's udder should be cleansed. Generally, the calf should receive colostrum within 15 to 30 minutes after birth.

4. The calf's navel should be disinfected with iodine to prevent bacteria from infecting the animal by way of the umbilical artery.

5. After the cow is returned to the milking herd (24 to 72 hours after parturition), the calf should be given reconstituted high-quality milk replacer or whole milk fed twice a day at 8% of body weight daily.

6. The calf should be administered a starter ration, a dry feed from 3 days to 3 weeks of age, and free-choice alfalfa hay after 6 weeks of age.

7. Newborn calves should be placed in individual controlled access pens to prevent contamination by and contact transmission from other calves.

8. If facilities are enclosed, a ventilation system with humidity controls should circulate air and minimize buildup of airborne pathogens. In warmer climates the calf pens may be placed outdoors in a sloping area and moved uphill each time a new calf is placed in the pen. Such a procedure assures that a calf starts out in a clean area (Fig. 5-1, *B*).*

Although these procedures seem to involve much time and effort, shortcuts only facilitate infection of calves. Unless time is taken to provide adequate facilities and husbandry practices, a successful dairy calf operation is impossible.

Use of biologicals. For vaccination to be of any value in preventing calf scours, the organism responsible for the syndrome on a particular ranch must be known. Various products have been tried for vaccination.

Currently a reolike virus vaccine is available commercially. In herds in which a reolike virus had been found in previous years, a significant decrease in rate of infection (morbidity) and death rate (mortality) resulted when an oral, modified live virus, reolike virus vaccine was used.[32]

Calves can be protected from diarrhea caused by certain *Escherichia coli* by immunizing pregnant cows.[35] The vaccine can be prepared either from a concentrated crude toxin, formalin-killed whole cells, or live nonattenuated bacteria. Cows can be immunized by either the subcutaneous or the intramammary route. There is no advantage in giving the live vaccine as compared with the killed preparation; both apparently give good protection. The live, nonattenuated organism, when given by the subcutaneous or intramammary route, does not cause any serious adverse response in the cows. It appears that the immunity resulting from the administration of the live and killed vaccines is of greater duration than the immunity brought about by the administration of the toxin vaccine. Further work will be necessary to evaluate the practical use of vaccines prepared from *E. coli.*

---

*Modified from Vollmar, R. E.: Calf diarrhea control in a dairy operation, Mod. Vet. Pract. **55:**509, 1974.

Various bovine antiserum products are commercially available. Their effectiveness in preventing calf diarrhea is unclear.

Treatment. A wide variety of preparations containing one to many active ingredients is available commercially for the treatment of calf scours. Commonly the preparations contain antibiotics, sulfas, anticholinergics that slow down gut activity, and adsorbents such as kaolin and pectin. The use of anticholinergics is discussed further in Chapter 19. There is no evidence that the anticholinergics or pectin is effective in curing the disease. As supportive measures, vitamins A, D, and B complex are often administered. Antibacterials may be beneficial; however, it is always possible that they will upset the balance of the gastrointestinal flora and further complicate the condition.

In conjunction with therapy the amount of milk or milk replacer fed to the calf is frequently reduced or eliminated. If there is severe dehydration and electrolyte imbalance, adequate fluid and electrolyte restoration is necessary if the animals are to be returned to good health. Tennant and others[51] recommend the following course of fluid and electrolyte therapy:

1. To rehydrate calves, an initial intravenous infusion of lactated Ringer's solution at the rate of 30 to 40 ml/kg of body weight should be given rapidly during the first hour of treatment.

2. Replacement of remaining fluid and electrolyte deficiencies may be accomplished slowly over a period of 24 to 36 hours. The solution administered to the animal should be isotonic (Chapter 17). Severely dehydrated calves during the first 24 hours of treatment (including the initial intravenous therapy) should receive 100 to 120 ml/kg. Of the total dose, 75% should be given as a balanced electrolyte solution, such as Ringer's solution, and the remaining 25% as 5% dextrose.

Once peripheral circulation is established, the regulation of the fluid and electrolytes will be carried on by the kidneys, lungs, and other regulatory mechanisms in the body.

The primary disadvantage of administering fluids intravenously or by other parenteral routes is that such administration takes time and skill. The oral route is more practical. The success of oral administration of fluids and electrolytes to humans suffering from severe dehydration as a result of the diarrhea of cholera led to investigation of the possible use of oral electrolyte solutions in calves.[7,18] In humans it was demonstrated that water and sodium absorption from the intestines was markedly enhanced in patients with severe diarrhea by the active transport mechanisms of glucose from the lumen of the intestine into the circulatory system. The osmotic pressure of the oral solution and the glucose concentration were critical to the efficient uptake of water and sodium by the small intestine. Later it was found that net fluid absorption was improved and the duration and volume of diarrhea decreased when a solution contained both dextrose and glycine.

The formula for calves by percentage of the powder used in trials follows[18]:

Sodium chloride	11.64
Calcium gluconate	2.20
Magnesium sulfate	0.61
Monopotassium phosphate	8.68
Glycine	21.20
Dextrose	55.67

This formula is available commercially (Ion-Aid). Each packet of the powder is mixed with 2 quarts of clean water. Two quarts of the solution are given to calves twice a day, replacing the milk replacer diet. For both mild and severe cases of diarrhea there is a significant difference in the rate of recovery and survival between groups of animals receiving the electrolyte solution and animals not so treated. The most striking effect is a lower mortality in those animals receiving the electrolyte solution.[18]

Bovine viral diarrhea

Bovine viral diarrhea (BVD) usually occurs in cattle over 10 months of age.

Prevention. Two attenuated strains of

vaccine are available for immunization against BVD: the NADL attenuated strain and the C34 V attenuated strain. These products are of similar and acceptable safety.[6] The vaccine is sometimes combined with *Leptospira* bacterin. Both fractions are compatible and produce a response equivalent to that produced by each antigen alone. The vaccine is also combined with infectious bovine rhinotracheitis (IBR) vaccine.

Effectiveness. Vaccination for BVD is highly effective.[2,16,25] A significant level of antibodies, which should confer protection against further exposures, is produced 10 to 14 days after vaccination.[16]

Safety. Despite early reports to the contrary, the vaccine has proved to be highly safe. In a survey of complications following administration of the BVD and IBR vaccine, an extremely low complication rate was observed. The maximum rate was 1 per 700 animals immunized.[42] The vaccine does not produce disease in healthy cattle, nor does disease pass from vaccinated cattle to unvaccinated animals. Because the vaccine may produce abortion, it should not be administered to pregnant animals. The vaccine should not be used as treatment for BVD.

Administration. Maternal antibodies interfere with an animal's ability to produce active antibodies against BVD. In a few animals these maternal antibodies can persist until 8 months of age. However, colostrum-deprived calves can develop immunity against BVD as early as 3 weeks of age.

To maximize protection, early immunization, with repeat immunization 6 months later, is indicated. The second immunization protects those animals that had interfering maternal antibodies when first given the vaccine. Early vaccination should not coincide with weaning but should precede weaning by several weeks. To avoid immunizing animals when they are stressed, one should not administer the vaccine when animals are shipped from the ranch to the feedlot. Open calves or heifers should be immunized at least 30 days before breeding or rebreeding. Bulls should not be immunized, since there

is evidence that attenuated virus vaccines may locate in the reproductive tracts. Because some cattle return to a serologically negative status 12 to 18 months after vaccination, annual revaccination is generally recommended.[25]

DISEASES OF THE RESPIRATORY TRACT

Etiology. Bovine respiratory diseases are caused by a number of microorganisms. Viruses causing respiratory infection in cattle include the virus of IBR, the virus of malignant catarrhal fever (MCF), infections associated with myxoviruses (parainfluenza type 3 [PI-3]), reoviruses, rhinoviruses, adenoiviruses, and psittacosis lymphogranuloma-venereum (PLV) organisms that cause pneumonias.

Respiratory diseases of bacterial origin in cattle are necrotic laryngitis, associated with *Fusobacterium necrophorum*, and pneumonia caused by *Corynebacterium pyogenes* and *Pasteurella, Haemophilus, Streptococcus, Staphylococcus,* and *Mycoplasma* species.

Both dairy and beef cattle develop respiratory infections. Dairy cattle frequently acquire respiratory disease when they are calves, frequently as a result of overcrowding in generally poor management schemes. In addition, dairy cows when confronted with the stresses of lactation in extreme climatic conditions may contract respiratory diseases.

Beef cattle are likely to develop respiratory disease when they have been stressed by shipment. Pneumonia of cattle, believed to be of viral and bacterial origin potentiated by stress, is commonly known as the "shipping fever complex" (SFC). The feedlot provides a great hazard to beef cattle. They are usually trucked to the feedlot and therefore stressed. At the feedlot, because of the crowded conditions to which the animals are subjected, they may be exposed to a wide variety of infectious organisms capable of causing respiratory disease.

Prevention

Management. In 1968 in the report of the panel for the Symposium on Immunity to the Bovine Respiratory Complex,[15] suggestions were made with regard to preventing disease in cattle. Preconditioning programs were recommended to reduce the effect of stress resulting from trucking animals from the range to the feeder. Such a preconditioning program includes the following measures:

1. Castrating, dehorning, and administering blackleg and malignant edema bacterin should occur at approximately 2 months of age. At that time, animals should be identified and records started.

2. At approximately 4 months of age, IBR and PI-3 vaccines and *Pasteurella* bacterins should be administered to all calves.[10] *Brucella* vaccine should be administered to heifer calves only.

3. At approximately 5 months of age, all animals should receive BVD and PI-3 vaccines and *Leptospira*, *Pasteurella*, blackleg, and malignant edema bacterins. They also should be treated for external and internal parasites as indicated.

4. When animals are sold at approximately 6 months of age, their records should accompany them.*

The panel recommended the following postarrival program for cattle that had no preconditioning:

1. Animals should be rested 24 to 48 hours after arrival. Nutritious, easily digested feed, adequate bedding, and clean fresh water should be provided as well as windbreaks to protect from inclement weather.

2. Close confinement in a poorly ventilated structure should be avoided. Adequate space should be provided for freedom of movement.

3. Animals should be confined so that they can be closely observed for the first 30 days.

4. Vaccines should be administered after 48 hours if cattle appear to have recovered from the stress of shipment.

5. BVD vaccine should be used at this time only if the feedlot has had previous

problems with the disease. IBR and PI-3 vaccines should be administered. These can be supplemented with inactivated *Leptospira* and blackleg bacterins plus other bacterins containing *Clostridium* species.

6. Homologous groups of cattle should be isolated for not less than 14 days.

7. Animals should be treated for internal and external parasites. However, 14 days should lapse after their arrival at the feedlot before initiation of the treatment.

8. Cattle visibly ill should be isolated and treated. Examinations should employ clinical observation, microbiological isolation, clinical pathological procedures, and necropsy, if disease conditions surpass normal expectations.*

For preconditioned animals, the panel recommended the following postarrival procedures:

1. Provide the conditions recommended in the first four points for animals that had no preconditioning.

2. Reimmunize with IBR vaccine if desirable.

3. Keep records on vaccination and illness.*

On beef-breeding ranches, replacement heifers can be handled in the same manner as preconditioned animals. They should be reimmunized against leptospirosis and *Pasteurella* species and given PI-3 vaccine before breeding.

Various management practices exist for the raising of dairy cattle. In general, these can be broken down into those involving self-contained or closed herds, in which replacements are born and raised on the premises, and those for the open herd, for which most replacements are purchased.

For self-contained herds, most deaths and illnesses occur in calves 3 to 4 months old. To provide protection against respiratory infections, colostrum should be fed within 15

---

*Modified from Gillespie, J. H., Jensen, R., McKercher, D., and Peacock, G.: Report of the panel for the Symposium on Immunity to the Bovine Respiratory Disease Complex, J. Am. Vet. Med. Assoc. **152:**713, 1968.

*Modified from Gillespie, J. H., Jensen, R., McKercher, D., and Peacock, G.: Report of the panel for the Symposium on Immunity to the Bovine Respiratory Disease Complex, J. Am. Vet. Med. Assoc. **152:**713, 1968.

minutes after birth. Animals should be immunized when 6 to 8 months of age with biologics containing immunizing agents against diseases present in the area, such as IBR, PI-3, and BVD. When indicated, IBR may be given at an earlier age. For open herds, additions should be purchased only from known healthy herds and held in isolation for a period of 30 days. They should then be immunized against the pathogens enzootic in the herd.

Use of biologicals. Biologicals can be used when the etiological agents that are likely to cause respiratory diseases in specific herds are known. The pluses and minuses of specific vaccines are discussed here.

IBR vaccines. IBR vaccine, modified live virus tissue culture origin, is highly effective in preventing IBR.[11,31,43,52] In addition to causing respiratory disease, the IBR virus can cause abortion in nonimmune cows or heifers. When nonpregnant cows are immunized with IBR vaccine, they receive a high degree of protection against abortion from the IBR virus.[43] IBR modified live virus vaccine may be administered by the intramuscular route. When it is thus administered, it must be injected intramuscularly and not subcutaneously, or the vaccine may not be effective. In addition to the intramuscular route, the intranasal route of administration has been found effective.[31,52] Not only does it provide good protection, but the intra-nasal route has the added advantage of not causing abortion when administered to pregnant cows.

Using the Cooper Isolate of IBR tissue culture origin fifth passage vaccine both intramuscularly and intratracheally, Chow[11] demonstrated that immunity can last up to 5.5 years.

Studies indicate that live attenuated IBR and BVD viruses combined in a vaccine are compatible.[3] Antibodies develop in a high percentage of animals immunized with this combination. Animals immune to one component of the product will respond to the second component.

IBR vaccine is also combined with *Leptospira* bacterin and modified live virus PI-3

vaccines. It is compatible with both of these preparations.

An inactivated IBR vaccine has been developed that is safe to administer to pregnant cows and is effective in preventing IBR.[23,29] Experimentally a combination of IBR and PI-3 modified live viruses administered intranasally has been shown to be safe to administer to pregnant cattle.[21]

The most serious side effect of immunization with IBR vaccine has been that the modified live virus, when given by the intramuscular route, may cause abortion in pregnant cattle.

PI-3 vaccines. Both killed and attenuated live virus vaccines containing the PI-3 virus have been found effective in experimental and field trials.[14]

Inactivated vaccines. Bacterins are sometimes given to prevent respiratory disease in cattle. Because the immunity they confer has a shorter duration than that of the modified live virus vaccines, at least two doses separated by a suitable interval should be given.

The antigenic type of *Pasteurella multocida* and *P. hemolytica* involved in infections of the bovine shipping fever complex is poorly understood. *Pasteurella* species play an important part in the shipping fever complex. There is some evidence that *Pasteurella* species are synergistic with PI-3 virus. The efficacy of *Pasteurella* bacterins is considered questionable.[13] This may be due to the failure to include the important antigenic type in the bacterin rather than a failure to induce an effective response.

If *Pasteurella* bacterin is used, it should be administered well in advance of shipping. At least two doses should be given, with the second dose at least 2 weeks before possible exposure to disease and conditions of stress.

If *Pasteurella* antiserum is used, it should be administered at the earliest opportunity, well before shipment as opposed to during shipment or at the time of arrival at the final destination. The disadvantages of the use of antiserum are its questionable effectiveness, the short duration of protection, and expense.

Bacterins and antisera against *Corynebacterium* species are available to prevent respiratory disease in cattle. The effectiveness of the products is questionable. In fact, whether *Corynebacterium* species are a significant cause of respiratory disease in cattle is questionable.

Treatment. Infections of the respiratory tract of cattle are generally treated either with antibiotics or sulfonamides. A common error in the administration of these drugs to large species like cattle is giving an inadequate dose for a short duration (Chapter 3). Although antibacterial drugs are not effective in treating respiratory infection caused by viruses, appropriate antibacterial drugs will be beneficial in the treatment of bacterial infections of the respiratory tract. The clinical management of the disease should be coordinated by a veterinarian.

UTERINE INFECTIONS

Signs. The primary sign of uterine infection is sterility. On beef ranches, to obtain uniform offspring to sell for meat, the bull is exposed to cows for only short periods of the year. If a cow does not conceive during the time she is running with the bull, she will be barren for the entire year. This causes economic hardship on the rancher. If large numbers of the herd do not conceive, the rancher may be driven from business.

Ewes and beef cows are exposed to the male. However, dairy cattle are artificially inseminated. Dairy cattle have more sterility problems than beef cattle. In dairy herds, cows are bred throughout the year. Ranchers aim for an average of one calf every 12 months from the dairy cow. Since gestation is 9 months in cattle, cows must conceive again within 3 months after giving birth. They lactate for approximately 9 months and then are allowed to go dry 3 months before giving birth again. Seventy-two hours after giving birth, the cows are placed on the milking string.

Not all cases of sterility result from infection. Other factors such as hormonal difficulties or poor insemination techniques can be responsible. In fact, hormonal imbalances often set up the conditions in the uterus for bacterial infection. The management of breeding failures requires the knowledge of an experienced clinician. Unfortunately many "do-it-yourself" methods have been introduced to treat breeding problems, especially in dairy cattle. Perhaps more harm than good results from these home treatments. The use of reproductive hormones for treating sterility is discussed in Chapter 16.

Etiology. Numerous types of bacteria are involved in uterine infection of dairy cattle, including *Streptococcus* species, *Corynebacterium* species, *Bacillus anthracis*, *Staphylococcus* species, *Escherichia coli*, *Proteus* species, and *Pseudomonas* species.[45]

After giving birth, cattle frequently retain the placenta. When it is retained for 24 hours or longer, conditions may be established that facilitate the establishment of bacterial infection in the uterus. More serious than the retained placenta, however, is the attempt by a lay attendant to remove it forcibly. Such an attempt can result in the introduction of numerous bacteria, particularly those contained in feces, into the vagina and uterus. Forcible removal of the placenta also often damages the internal structure of the uterus.

Treatment. Uterine infections in cattle are generally treated locally. Either a solution containing antibacterial drugs or a compressed bolus is placed in the uterus. If the drugs are to be effective, they must be delivered to the uterus by a relatively aseptic technique. This aseptic technique involves carefully washing the external genitals, the use of either sterile equipment to deliver liquids to the uterus, or the wearing of a sterile glove to place the boluses in the uterus manually.

Home treatments often fail. Frequently, ranchers unfamiliar with anatomy place the medications in the vagina where they are ineffective (Fig. 5-2). Also many ranchers unfamiliar with aseptic techniques may introduce bacteria into the uterus when they attempt to treat uterine problems.

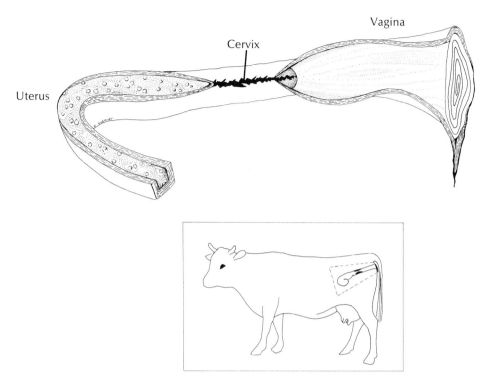

Fig. 5-2. Cow's reproductive tract. Vagina is separated from uterus by cervix. Constricted space in cervix makes it difficult to place anti-infective drugs into uterus.

In addition to antibacterials, other components are often included in medication for treating uterine infections. One of the more common preparations is the sulfa-urea bolus, which contains one or more of the sulfonamides and urea. The urea is placed in the preparation to dissolve dead tissue and/or exudates such as pus contained in the uterine cavity.

The therapeutic approach to uterine infections needs reexamination. Tightly pressed, hard uterine boluses may dissolve slowly over a period of days or even weeks and act as foreign bodies in the uterus, which delays the return of the uterus to its normal nonpregnant condition.[39] As an alternative, antibiotics can be placed into the uterus by loosely filling No. 10 gelatin capsules with 2 to 4 gm of a soluble, broad-spectrum antibiotic or by intrauterine infusion.

However, infusion of antibacterials into the uterus may damage the delicate endo-metrial lining (the surface tissue within the uterus). Seguin and others[44] found that installation of 400 ml of a 50 mg/ml solution of oxytetracycline caused superficial endometrial necrosis. It could not be determined in the study whether the endometrial changes resulted from the oxytetracycline or from other chemicals contained in the commercial product. However, the effect could be significant by adding substantially to the pathology involved in the repeat breeder syndrome. In addition to causing changes in the uterus, the oxytetracycline when administered early in estrus (on the fourth day) caused a significant shortening of the length of the estrus cycle. When administered late in estrus (on the fifteenth day), the cycle was significantly lengthened. This effect was shown to be correlated with the pathological changes caused by the drug, since when physiological saline was administered, no pathology resulted in the uterus and the length of the estrus cycle was unchanged. Compounds that appear not to cause endometriosis are 2 million units of procaine penicillin in aqueous suspension added to 0.85% saline solution and nitrofurathiazide (1 mg/ml) plus estradiol (0.1 mg/ml) in sterile peanut oil (Utonex).[37]

The uterus has great ability to clear infection. This primarily occurs in the midstage of the estrus cycle or the time when the cow is receptive to the male.

When treating uterine infections, it appears that the best results are obtained when cows are treated with an infusion of antibiotics near the time of estrus. Treating cows with antibiotics 24 hours after breeding has also produced good results.[37]

Sulfonamides, nitrofurazone, and oxytetracycline have been shown to pass from the uterus into the blood.[44] It is possible therefore to contaminate either the milk or the meat of the animal when administering intrauterine antibacterials.

INFECTIOUS KERATOCONJUNCTIVITIS (PINKEYE)

Pinkeye can involve both the cornea and conjunctiva. (See Fig. 15-1.) It is primarily a disease of white-faced beef cattle. The signs may be relatively mild, consisting of tearing and a slight inflammation of the conjunctiva. The eyes will be "bloodshot." In more severe cases, the cornea may swell, making it opaque and giving it a ground-glass appearance. Corneal ulceration may eventually occur.

The identity of the microorganisms responsible for pinkeye is not totally certain. Viruses may be involved. The bacterium *Moraxella bovis* has also been implicated. Predisposing factors include bright sunlight, dust, and the presence of flies. White-faced cattle are most susceptible because the sunlight reflects from the white fur into the eye, whereas the sun's rays are absorbed in cattle with dark faces. Flies possibly transmit the infecting organism from one animal to another.

Treatment. Many OTC preparations are available for treating pinkeye in cattle. They come in various forms, such as liquids that are squeezed from plastic bottles, powders, and sprays in aerosol cans. Generally, they contain an antibacterial and a dye to color the fur surrounding the eye. The antibacterial may be a nitrofuran, sulfonamide, antibiotic, or an antiseptic, such as methylene blue. Probably some benefit is obtained from using a medication that dyes the fur. Dying the fur reduces the glare of the sun in the animal's eyes and therefore reduces the irritation. The effectiveness of an antibacterial in spray form is questionable because of the short time it remains in the eye. Powders may further irritate an already irritated eye. Clinically, animals with mild cases often recover spontaneously. However, those with ulceration should be treated by a veterinarian. Frequently, the veterinarian will inject subconjunctivally a combination of antibiotics and corticosteroids. (See Fig. 15-4.) Although in many species, especially man, the use of corticosteroids is contraindicated in treating severe corneal ulceration, in cattle with corneal ulcers, combined use of antibiotics and corticosteroids injected subconjunctivally has proved to be effective therapy.

MASTITIS

The dairy cow, bred to produce large volumes of milk, is especially subject to injury and infection of the mammary gland. Mastitis, or inflammation of the mammary gland, is a common problem in dairy herds. Mastitis results in decreased milk production and in increased labor, drug, and veterinary costs. The yearly monetary losses to the dairy industry average approximately $100 per cow.[36]

Because each of the four quarters of the bovine mammary gland is a distinct structure separate from the other quarters, mastitis can occur in one or more of the quarters. The severity of mastitis varies widely. In subclinical infections, there is a slight decrease in milk production, and the number of cells in the milk, primarily white blood cells, increases slightly. In moderate clinical infections, the udder feels warm. It is edematous, giving it a hard feeling. A more significant drop in milk production is noted, and a higher cellular count in the milk is observed. In severe cases, the udder is extremely tender and hard. Milk production virtually stops, and in many cases only serum is expelled from the involved quarter when milked. In extremely severe cases the udder may become gangrenous, a state referred to as "blue bag." It is estimated that in most herds there are 15 to 40 cases of subclinical mastitis for every known case of clinical mastitis.[36]

Etiology. A variety of organisms have been associated with bovine mastitis. Streptococcal species are most commonly responsible, followed by staphylococcal species, and somewhat less commonly, coliform bacteria. Species of *Pseudomonas, Mycoplasma, Corynebacterium, Nocardia, Actinomycetes,* yeasts, molds, and various other organisms have also been isolated from infected glands.

Nearly all the pathogenic organisms responsible for mastitis enter the gland through the teat orifice and streak canal (Fig. 5-3). The condition and health of these structures play a major role in determining the individual cow's susceptibility to infection of the gland.

Prevention. Various management factors will influence the incidence of mastitis in a particular herd. Malfunctioning milking machines will damage and stress the teat and streak canal and encourage bacterial colonization of the udder. It is therefore essential that milking machines be properly maintained, adjusted, and handled to minimize trauma to the teat and udder.

Sanitation programs have been effective in reducing the incidence of mastitis within a herd.[40] Dips should be used to disinfect the teats after milking; many chemicals have been tried and used for this purpose. Probably the best disinfectant is either a 4% to 5% sodium hypochlorite solution or 0.5% to 1% iodophor. These preparations are effective and do not cause undue irritation to teats or udders.

Prevention is the key to minimizing mastitis in dairy herds. Each dairy operation

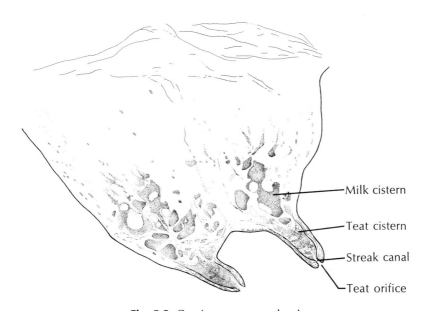

Milk cistern

Teat cistern

Streak canal

Teat orifice

Fig. 5-3. Cow's mammary gland.

should have a specifically designed program to control the incidence of mastitis. Such programs should include the following:

1. The physical plant (barns, stalls) should be designed and maintained to minimize stress to the animal and trauma and contamination of teats and udders of both adult cows and calves.

2. Animal areas should be kept dry, clean, and well bedded.

3. Milking sanitation programs, including cleaning and drying of udders and teat-dipping, should be strictly adhered to.

4. Milking machinery should be properly cleaned and maintained.

5. Adequate screening and record keeping is essential so that the extent and type of mastitis in the herd can be readily assessed.

Treatment. In an attempt to reduce the incidence of mastitis in newly freshened cows, antibiotics often are administered by the intramammary route to cows during the dry period. Dry-cow formulations may contain one of several antibiotics in a nonirritating vehicle. Frequently, procaine penicillin G and benzathine cloxacillin are used. Procaine and benzathine salts are used because they slowly dissolve and therefore remain in the gland for extended periods. The half-lives of various antibiotics in the dry udder are as follows[12]:

Benzathine cloxacillin	8.07 days
Neomycin	7.36 days
Dihydrostreptomycin	5.68 days
Spiramycin	4.27 days
Penicillin G	1.47 days
Erythromycin	Less than 1 day

The choice of an antibiotic depends on the organism involved. Penicillin G is certainly the drug of choice for use in streptococcal mastitis. Staphylococcal mastitis may sometimes be caused by penicillinase-producing strains. In these cases, cloxacillin-containing preparations are indicated.

Dry-cow treatment has been shown to be highly effective in reducing the incidence of mastitis in dairy cows.[55] This method is ex-

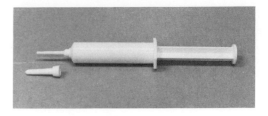

Fig. 5-4. Tube of mastitis ointment containing antibiotics used for treatment of bovine mastitis.

tremely effective against streptococcal mastitis but much less effective against staphylococcal mastitis.

In a review of the general literature, Christie and co-workers[12] concluded the following:

1. It is more effective to treat dry cows than lactating cows to eliminate udder infections.

2. Most new infections develop during the first 3 weeks of the dry period.

3. The most practical and economical means of controlling chronic mastitis is intramammary infusion of an effective antibiotic in dry cows.

4. The chance of new infections will be greatly reduced the longer the antibiotic persists in the udder at therapeutic levels.*

For clinical mastitis during the milking period, that is, in wet-cow treatment, intramammary antibiotics are used. If the animal has a fever, systemic broad-spectrum antibiotics are also administered.

The wet-cow intramammary mastitis preparations are also applied directly into the mammary gland through the streak canal (Figs. 5-4 and 5-5). The base in which the drug is contained is important. A more even distribution of antibiotics throughout the infused quarter results when water-soluble vehicles are used. Non–water-soluble ointment vehicles often adhere to the teat wall

---

*Modified from Christie, G. J., Keefe, T. J., and Strom, P. W.: Cloxacillin and the dry cow, Vet. Med. Small Anim. Clin. **69:**1403, 1974.

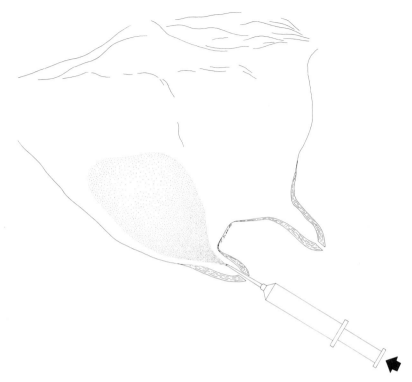

Fig. 5-5. Administration of mastitis ointment. After cleansing teat orifice with alcohol, blunt tip of container is placed through teat orifice and streak canal and placed into teat cistern. When plunger is pressed, mastitis ointment spreads through teat cistern and milk cistern and throughout quarter.

after administration. Water-soluble vehicles cover a much greater area of mammary tissue than insoluble ointments.[20]

A wide variety of antibiotics can be found in commercially available wet-cow mastitis preparations. The most common are penicillin G, sodium cephapirin, neomycin, dihydrostreptomycin, oxytetracycline, and novobiocin. In our opinion, penicillin G is the best choice in streptococcal mastitis.

In addition to antibacterials, corticosteroids are often contained in intramammary preparations for the treatment of clinical mastitis. However, corticosteroids are not routinely administered during the dry period. The rationale for using corticosteroids in acute mastitis is that they reduce the amount of scarring in the udder. It is hypothesized that the udder will then return to

near normal levels of production when the infection is cleared up. (If massive areas of scar tissue develop after the infection is cleared, the amount of milk produced by the quarter will be reduced.) Antibiotics should be given for at least 24 hours after the last corticosteroid administration.

Hydrocortisone is the corticosteroid most often employed in these preparations. One synthetic corticosteroid, dexamethasone, administered to cattle during the last trimester of pregnancy can cause abortion. The FDA requires a warning on the label of all oral and parenteral corticosteroids that abortion may occur. Since many dairy cows are pregnant when treated with hydrocortisone-containing mastitis preparations, there has been some concern about the risks of inducing abortion in these animals. Work done by

Hagg and Schlitz,[17] however, indicates that corticosteroids normally found in intramammary preparations do not pose an abortion threat to cattle.

In acute mastitis most mastitis preparations are applied at least twice daily after milking. They are usually administered for at least 24 hours after the cow has apparently recovered.

Milk taken from the cow must be withheld from human consumption for some time after the last administration of the mastitis ointment. One should always check the label of the preparation to be sure of the exact time requirement for the particular product. The cow will continue to be milked twice a day, but the milk must be discarded.

Even after milk is withheld for the proper time, residues are possible. For example, an evaluation of twenty-one commercially available intramammary infusion products used in the treatment of mastitis in lactating cows was made to determine the antibiotic milk-out rates.[34] Sixteen of the twenty-one products produced residues in milk after the prescribed withdrawal time. A correlation was found between the delay in the antibiotic excretion and low milk production, especially by cows producing less than 9 kg of milk daily. There was also a correlation between high cellular concentrations and prolonged antibiotic milk-out time. This indicated that there was prolonged antibiotic milk-out time associated with inflamed udders. Those products containing 3% aluminum monostearate in the vehicle were consistently involved with prolonged excretion of antibiotic in the milk.

In addition to contamination of milk by the excretion of intramammary-infused antibiotics, antibiotics administered orally or parenterally can result in milk residues. Several studies have detailed milk-out rates for antibiotics administered by the parenteral or intramammary routes.* There has been some concern about whether antibiotics infused into an inflamed quarter could transfer

to milk in noninflamed and therefore non-treated quarters. No direct transfer can occur because the quarters are partitioned. However, indirect transfer through the bloodstream can occur. The transfer of penicillin, streptomycin, and neomycin does occur from treated to untreated quarters. However, studies show that these drugs do not persist in the untreated quarters beyond 72 hours when normal doses are administered.[46]

The literature reports wide variation in the transfer of antibacterial drugs from infected to noninfected quarters. This variation may be attributed to many factors such as the physical form of the drug tested, the dose administered, the amount of inflammation in the mammary gland (the greater the inflammation the more likely the transfer), individual physiological differences between test subjects, the sensitivity of the test assay, and whether the test was run on the first milk obtained or a bucket sample.

California Mastitis Test

The California Mastitis Test was developed to determine the presence of subclinical cases of mastitis in a milking herd. It involves a plastic paddle containing four circular dish-like structures; into each, milk from one quarter is squirted (Fig. 5-6). A detergent solution containing an indicator is then added

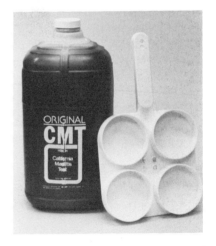

Fig. 5-6. Reagent and paddle used in California Mastitis Test.

---

*See references 4, 34, 46, 47, 56.

to the milk samples, and the entire paddle is swirled to mix the milk and test solution. When the mammary gland is free of inflammation and the milk is therefore free of cells, the combined milk and detergent remain fluid. However, when cells are present in the milk, the mixture becomes more viscous. The higher the cell count the more viscous the mixture. Estimation of the degree of inflammation can be made by the viscosity of the mixture. In addition, the indicator in the test fluid shows when milk is more acidic than normal, acidity also being an indication of mammary inflammation. Based on results of the California Mastitis Test, dairy ranchers can evaluate the level of subclinical mastitis in a herd, decide when to treat cows even before they develop clinical mastitis, and decide which cows should be exposed to dry-cow therapy.

DISEASES CAUSED BY VIRUSES
Blue tongue

Blue tongue is primarily a disease of sheep. Sheep about 1 year of age are the most susceptible. It causes inflammation in the mouth, nose, and intestinal tract and can involve the sensitive structures in the hooves. The virus is transmitted by insects.

Various strains of blue tongue virus cause the disease in sheep. At least fifteen immunological types are found throughout the world.[28]

Prevention. The only management procedure that can be employed to control the disease is protecting the animals from night-flying insects. Although the use of external parasiticide sprays may be of benefit in this regard, other measures such as housing animals indoors will usually not be practical.

A modified live virus vaccine produced in chick embryos is available to immunize animals against the disease. This is the most practical means of control. The vaccine is administered to sheep in late spring or early summer. Immunity takes approximately 10 days to develop.

A mild strain was used to manufacture the commercially available egg–modified live virus vaccine. The commercially available vaccine is effective in protecting animals challenged with the common American virus. However, it may not protect 50% to 100% of animals from the other viral strains.

Immunization of ewes is not performed during the first 60 days of gestation because deformity of the fetus can result. (The total gestation of sheep is approximately 150 days.)

Ovine ecthyma (sore mouth, orf)

Sore mouth is a highly contagious disease of sheep that results in pustules and scabs around the muzzle and lips.

Prevention. In flocks in which the disease is likely to occur, all lambs should be immunized at 6 to 8 weeks of age. The vaccine consists of a live nonattenuated virus that is scratched into an unwooled area on the inner aspect of the thigh. One week after vaccination the lambs must be checked to be sure that a lesion in the vaccination site has developed. If it has not, the animal should be revaccinated. Immunity takes approximately 3 weeks to develop and lasts for about two years.

Because ovine ecthyma vaccine consists of a live virus that can cause lesions on human skin, persons handling the product must be careful not to contaminate themselves with the product.

DISEASES CAUSED BY BACTERIA
Anthrax

Sheep and cattle may die from anthrax without showing any previous signs of disease. The carcass is often found with blood coming from the various body orifices. Because the blood contains a large population of the infective agent, autopsies should be performed on such carcasses only at the discretion of a veterinarian. It is possible to infect the premises severely by performing autopsies on animals that have died from anthrax. Because of the possibility of the infected carcass seeding the premises with the infective organism, it is important that bodies of animals suspected of having died from anthrax be incinerated.

The disease is caused by *Bacillus anthracis*. This bacteria has the ability to form spores when exposed to the atmosphere. The spores protect the bacteria against the external environment and can live in soil for many years. Any warm-blooded animals may contract the disease.

In humans it can cause a fatal pneumonia.

In cattle and sheep the disease is seen mainly in the summer·and fall months.

Prevention. In enzootic areas immunization should be performed annually. Various types of vaccines are available.

The spore vaccines consist of four separate types of varying virulence. The types are numbered 1 to 4 with 1 being the least virulent and 4 the most virulent. Spore vaccines are administered intradermally. One disadvantage of these vaccines is that intradermal injections are difficult for lay persons to administer. Because of the difficulty of administering the vaccines intradermally and because of the fear that the more virulent types of vaccines could cause the disease in animals that had not been naturally exposed, the spore vaccines have generally been replaced by other types of anthrax vaccines. However, there is no universal agreement that the spore vaccine should be discontinued. A practicing veterinarian reported that in immunizing more than 34,000 animals with live spore vaccine No. 4, only 3 animals developed minor reactions.[26]

The Sterne's South African strain vaccine is an avirulent spore vaccine. The Sterne's strain vaccine was reported successful in halting an outbreak of anthrax in Louisiana. This success supports claims of its efficacy.[22]

The Carbozo vaccine contains virulent spores adsorbed on saponin or saturated sodium chloride. Because the adsorption of the spores on an adjuvant reduces the number of virulent organisms to which the animal is exposed after vaccination, it is safe to use in susceptible cattle.

A cell-free filtrate of a culture of a nonencapsulated, spore-forming strain of *Bacillus anthracis* has been developed. It can be injected as an aqueous solution intradermally.

When absorbed onto aluminium hydroxide and injected subcutaneously, the vaccine will not cause anthrax. However, it gives a relatively short duration of immunity and therefore is not as practical as those vaccines previously listed.

Antibiotics should never be given simultaneously to animals receiving anthrax vaccine, since the antibiotics will interfere with the development of the immunity.

Clostridial diseases

The clostridial diseases are caused by a group of bacteria that are members of the genus *Clostridium*. Although each disease will be discussed separately, one should bear in mind that products to immunize against the clostridial diseases often contain bacterins to protect animals against more than one of the diseases. These diseases include the following:

1. Blackleg—*Clostridium chauvoei*
2. Malignant edema—*C. septicum, C. chauvoei, C. perfringens, C. sordellii, C. novyi*
3. Infectious necrotic hepatitis—*C. novyi*
4. Bacillary hemoglobinuria—*C. haemolyticum*

In addition, we will discuss enterotoxemia (*C. perfringens*) and tetanus (*C. tetani*) for which antitoxins and toxoids are used in biological prophylaxis.

Blackleg

Blackleg is a disease of cattle in which muscles in the leg become severely inflamed. The infection is systemic, probably resulting from ingestion of the disease-causing organism, *C. chauvoei*. Generally, the disease occurs during the months when animals are on pasture.

Infective carcasses should be destroyed by burning.

In enzootic areas, annual immunization of cattle just before the danger period is recommended. All animals 6 months to 2 years of age should be immunized. Generally, cattle over 2 years of age do not develop the disease. The bacterin consists of killed *C.*

chauvoei and frequently other clostridial organisms to protect against a wide variety of clostridial infections. Immunity does not develop until 14 days after administration of the vaccine.

Malignant edema (gas gangrene)

Malignant edema can be caused by several species of bacteria of the clostridial group. The symptoms are similar to blackleg. However, blackleg results from systemic infection, and malignant edema is always caused by the local introduction of bacteria into a wound. Although *C. septicum* and *C. chauvoei* are the most common causes of malignant edema, it can also be caused by *C. perfringens*, *C. sordellii*, and *C. novyi*. The disease is controlled by immunizing animals with malignant edema vaccine, which at a minimum should contain *C. septicum* and *C. chauvoei*. Such a bacterin would also protect against blackleg. Unlike blackleg, malignant edema may infect cattle of any age. Only individual sporadic cases are likely to be seen, since local introduction of the organism into a wound is necessary to produce the disease.

Infectious necrotic hepatitis (black disease)

Black disease is an acute toxemia (toxins in the blood) of sheep caused by *C. novyi*. These organisms reside in necrotic areas of the liver. They produce toxins that are picked up in the general circulation and kill the animal. The disease is usually associated with liver fluke infestation, which provides the necessary necrotic area in the liver for *C. novyi* to establish residence. Without areas of necrosis, the bacteria cannot produce the disease.

To control the disease in sheep the liver fluke should be eliminated. If that is not practical, animals should be immunized with a bacterin containing *C. novyi*.

Bacillary hemoglobinuria (red water)

Bacillary hemoglobinuria is caused by *C. haemolyticum*. The bacterium produces a hemolysin that ruptures red blood cells. The condition is called "red water" because the animal's urine turns red or dark brown as a result of the free hemoglobin that passes from the serum into the urine.

The disease is best prevented by annual administration of a bacterin containing *C. haemolyticum*. It is administered 4 to 6 weeks before the time that the outbreak of the disease is normally expected. It should be administered to all animals over 6 months of age in enzootic areas.

Enterotoxemia

Enterotoxemia generally occurs in very young calves or lambs. Usually the animals appear to be healthy and in fine flesh. Frequently, the only sign is sudden death. Older cattle, particularly those recently placed in feedlots, may also be affected with the condition.

The disease is caused by *C. perfringens*. Serotype C commonly causes the condition in cattle, whereas serotype D is usually responsible for the condition in sheep. However, it is possible for either serotype to be involved in these species. The bacteria reside in the gastrointestinal tract of the animals and, when conditions are right, proliferate and produce a toxin that is absorbed systemically. It is the toxin that ultimately kills the animals.

Prevention. Biological prophylaxis involves the administration of either a bacterin, a toxoid, or an antitoxin.

Cows can be vaccinated 2 to 4 months before calving with *C. perfringens*–type C bacterins or toxoids. This vaccination results in antibody and/or antitoxin development. These are passed to calves in the colostrum. A short-term passive immunity for calves is then provided during the first few critical weeks of life. To continue active immunity in cows a single annual booster dose may be given 2 to 4 months before each calving.

In feedlot cattle, *C. perfringens*–type C bacterin or toxoid should be administered at least 10 days before the animals are on full feed. During the time that animals are on full feed, they are most susceptible to the condition.

C. perfringens–types C and D antitoxin is used only during the outbreak of a disease in an unprotected herd. It is administered for rapid short-term protection, since the duration of the immunity is approximately 2 weeks.

In sheep the condition is likely to occur in suckling lambs. Immunity can be provided by immunizing the ewe at the time of breeding. The vaccination of ewes should be repeated 2 to 4 weeks before lambing. Passive immunity is then provided to the newborn lamb. Lambs should not be actively immunized until they are at least 2 months of age. Either a bacterin or toxoid is used for this purpose. If lambs are to be fed in the feedlot, they should be immunized 10 days to 2 weeks before they are started on concentrated feeds.

In trials at two feedlots using commercial *C. perfringens*–types C and D toxoid and *C. perfringens*–types C and D bacterins, no significant difference was found in the abilities of the bacterin and toxoid to protect the lambs from enterotoxemia.[38]

During outbreaks of the disease in unprotected flocks, antitoxin should be administered.

Tetanus

Tetanus is caused by *C. tetani.* Although the condition most commonly occurs in horses, it is also relatively common in sheep. The disease will be discussed in greater detail in Chapter 7. The organism establishes itself in wounds. As with other clostridial diseases, a toxin produced by the bacteria is responsible for the clinical signs, which include tetanic spasms that eventually prevent the animal from breathing.

Because tetanus is likely to follow wounds, pet sheep and sheep used in 4-H projects should be given tetanus antitoxin concurrent with any surgical procedures. Valuable sheep should be actively immunized with tetanus toxoid.

Leptospirosis

Cattle are frequently afflicted with leptospirosis. Signs of infection include sudden fever and depression, a reduction of milk flow, development of a pale yellowish color in the membranes of the eyes and mouth (icterus), elevated temperature that is persistent throughout the illness, thick blood-tinged milk, bright red or dark brown urine, and abortion in pregnant animals. In some subclinical cases the only manifestation of bovine leptospirosis is abortion. Controlling the disease through immunization can increase the conception rate in infected herds.

Commonly the disease in cattle is caused by three serotypes: *Leptospira pomona, L. grippotyphosa,* and *L. hardjo.* The organism is spread in the urine.

Prevention. Immunization with bacterins is recommended to prevent the disease in cattle. Vaccination is indicated in infected herds and in areas where leptospirosis is enzootic. Immunity is developed in a relatively large portion of vaccinated animals. In adults and calves vaccinated at the age of at least 6 to 8 months, duration of immunity is approximately 12 months. Duration is much shorter in younger animals; those less than 3 months old do not respond to the vaccine. Commercially available bacterins containing the specific strains *L. grippotyphosa, L. hardjo,* and *L. pomona* are available. To obtain the best results from the bacterin the following measures are recommended[19,57]:

1. Determine the strain causing the disease in a particular area and select the proper bacterin to protect against that strain (a bacterin containing one strain will not protect against another).

2. Do not vaccinate animals less than 6 months of age.

3. Calves and mature heifers may be immunized at any stage of reproduction.

4. In enzootic areas, repeat vaccination twice a year.

The bacterins are effective in causing an immunity that can prevent losses from death, abortion, weak offspring, and reduced milk production. Reportedly they do not cause any problems even with repeated administration.[19]

Some authorities have expressed concern about the effectiveness of the bacterins used in immunizing cattle against leptospirosis.[49] Their concern is that the bacterins are not effective in eliminating the renal carrier state. In addition, there is concern that the primary immunization with the bacterins sets up conditions that can result in anaphylaxis on a subsequent immunization.

An experimental vaccine consisting of viable cultures of avirulent *L. pomona* has been evaluated for safety, duration of immunity, and protection against both the clinical forms of leptospirosis and the development of renal leptospirosis.[48,49] The experimental vaccine induced the development of seroagglutinins and protected animals that were given a normally infecting dose of the bacteria without causing fever, leptospiremia, leptospiruria, or interruption of pregnancy.

Treatment. Leptospirosis is best treated with an effective antibiotic. Penicillin G given in appropriate dosage is normally satisfactory in eliminating the clinical signs. However, the renal carrier state should also be eliminated. There is some evidence that one dose of dihydrostreptomycin, 25 mg/kg of body weight, is effective in eliminating the renal carrier state.[50]

Brucellosis

Brucellosis in cattle is caused by *Brucella abortus*, which produces abortion in cattle. In a severe epizootic, a large number of animals can be involved, and this can raise economic havoc with ranchers. The organism is shed in the milk and with the aborted fetus and fetal membranes and readily infects humans, who may contract the disease by drinking raw milk or by handling the fetal membranes of infected cows.

In the United States the only vaccine authorized for immunizing cattle against brucellosis is the strain 19 *Brucella abortus*

vaccine. This is a relatively avirulent strain in cattle. However, the strain is virulent in humans. Accidental inoculation into an individual or the spilling of reconstituted vaccine into a person's eye are likely modes of infection. Such accidental inoculations should be immediately treated by a physician.

There has been an eradication program aimed at eliminating brucellosis from cattle in the United States. The decision whether to immunize animals against brucellosis is currently left to the owner. The attending veterinarian frequently aids in the decision by providing information on the advantages and disadvantages of a vaccination program. Only 70% of all vaccinated cattle develop immunity. The duration of immunity is six to seven years. The problem with immunizing animals is that the vaccine produces residual titers, even in animals vaccinated as early as 3 months of age. Those titers can interfere with the eradication measures, since it is impossible to differentiate titers of immunized animals from those that are infected with virulent organisms. Calves to be vaccinated should be 3 to 6 months of age.[57]

DISEASES CAUSED BY PROTOZOA
Anaplasmosis

Anaplasmosis is primarily a disease of cattle, usually affecting cattle over 2 years of age. Severe anemia is the primary clinical feature of anaplasmosis. Animals may breathe rapidly, have yellow mucous membranes, and exhibit eccentric and even aggressive behavior resulting from the decrease of oxygen delivered to their brain by the few remaining red blood cells. In enzootic areas many animals may be infected carriers, showing no clinical signs of the disease.

Anaplasmosis is caused by *Anaplasma marginale*, a protozoan parasite that infects red blood cells and results in their destruction (Fig. 5-7). The parasite is transmitted by biting insects and the use of unsterile surgical instruments or hypodermic syringes and needles. In severe infections, death may

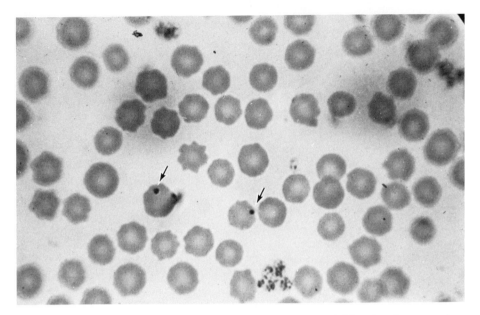

Fig. 5-7. Photomicrograph of blood smear in which two red blood cells *(arrows)* are infected with *Anaplasma marginale*. (Courtesy Dr. Bradford P. Smith, School of Veterinary Medicine, University of California, Davis.)

result. Adult animals originating in *Anaplasma*-free areas are particularly susceptible to the disease when moved to enzootic areas.

Prevention

Management. It is impossible to eliminate the insect vectors of the organism in enzootic areas. The only practical management control is to be sure that surgical procedures and injections are performed in an aseptic manner, minimizing the spread of the disease from one animal to another.

Use of biologicals. Theoretically various immunizing procedures against anaplasmosis exist. One is administration of fully virulent organisms concurrently with chemotherapeutic drugs or at an age when the animals are not normally susceptible to the disease. Another is administration of an attenuated strain of *A. marginale*. A third alternative is administration of killed organisms.

The use of a vaccine containing killed organisms in an adjuvant has been reported.[8] Although the response to the initial administration of the vaccine was small and of short duration, a second administration 6 weeks after the first resulted in an anamnestic reaction which provided an immunity that prevented serious clinical disease. Although the vaccine prevents serious clinical disease, it will not prevent the animal from becoming a carrier. It may also be incapable of preventing infections by highly virulent strains.[27]

An attenuated *A. marginale* vaccine that was developed by the serial passage of organisms in abnormal hosts is reported to be safe and effective.[27,54]

Treatment. Tetracycline, 6.6 to 11 mg/kg of body weight administered either as a single injection or as three injections daily, has been recommended for the treatment of anaplasmosis.[5]

The veterinarian must use some discretion in treating serious acute cases of anaplasmosis. If an animal has a severe anemia, the stress of restraint required to administer any medication may kill it.

Administered at the rate of 2 to 2.5 mg/kg of body weight, imidocarb dihydrochloride is highly effective in preventing clinical infections of *A. marginale* and other protozoan parasites.[1,30] Although imidocarb is effective in relieving animals of clinical signs, it cannot be relied on to free the animals of infection totally. Recovered animals may continue to be carriers of the parasite. Simultaneous administration of oxytetracycline and dithiosemicarbasone has been reported to eliminate the parasite from the animal, thereby eliminating the carrier state.[24]

There is good evidence that when latent infections result after administration of chemotherapy the animals retain immunity against further infection and the development of clinical signs.[41]

References

1. Adams, L. G., and Todrovic, R. A.: Chemotherapeutic efficacy of imidocarb dihydrochloride on concurrent bovine anaplasmosis and babesiosis, Trop. Anim. Health Prod. 6:71, 1974.
2. Bittle, J. L.: Vaccination for bovine viral diarrhea mucosal disease, J. Am. Vet. Med. Assoc. 152:861, 1968.
3. Bittle, J. L., and York, C. J.: Combination vaccines for control of bovine respiratory diseases, J. Am. Vet. Med. Assoc. 152:889, 1968.
4. Blobel, H., and Burch, C. W.: Blood serums and milk secretions, J. Am. Vet. Med. Assoc. 137:701, 1969.
5. Blood, D. C., and Henderson, J. A.: Veterinary medicine, ed. 4, Baltimore, 1974, The Williams & Wilkins Co.
6. Bordt, D. E., Thomas, P. C., and Marshall, R. F.: Bovine virus diarrhea vaccines: a comparison of two virus strains, Vet. Med. Small Anim. Clin. 70:441, 1975.
7. Braun, R. K.: Peroral use of a special dietary food as a source of electrolytes in diarrheic calves, Vet. Med. Small Anim. Clin. 70:601, 1975.
8. Brock, W. E.: Anaplasmosis vaccines and their relation to anaplasmosis control, J. Am. Vet. Med. Assoc. 147:1563, 1965.
9. Brown, A. L.: Comments on infectious bovine rhinotracheitis immunization, J. Am. Vet. Med. Assoc. 152:856, 1968.
10. Casselberry, N. H.: Present status of immunization procedures for infectious bovine rhinotracheitis, J. Am. Vet. Med. Assoc. 152:853, 1968.
11. Chow, T. L.: Duration of immunity in heifers inoculated with infectious bovine rhinotracheitis virus, J. Am. Vet. Med. Assoc. 160:51, 1972.
12. Christie, G. J., Keefe, T. J., and Strom, P. W.: Cloxacillin and the dry cow, Vet. Med. Small Anim. Clin. 69:1403, 1974.
13. Engelbrecht, J.: Present status of immunization procedures for pasteurellosis, J. Am. Vet. Med. Assoc. 152:881, 1968.
14. Gale, C.: Bovine parainfluenza-3 immunization procedures, J. Am. Vet. Med. Assoc. 152:871, 1968.
15. Gillespie, J. H., Jensen, R., McKercher, D., and Peacock, G.: Report of the panel for the Symposium on Immunity to the Bovine Respiratory Disease Complex, J. Am. Vet. Med. Assoc. 152:713, 1968.
16. Gutekunst, D. E.: Comments on vaccination for bovine viral diarrhea-mucosal disease, J. Am. Vet. Med. Assoc. 152:865, 1968.
17. Hagg, D. D., and Schlitz, R. A.: Effect of intramammary corticosteroid administration during late gestation in cattle, Mod. Vet. Pract. 54:29, May 1973.
18. Hamm, D., and Hicks, W. J.: A new oral electrolyte in calf scours therapy, Vet. Med. Small Anim. Clin. 70:279, 1975.
19. Hanson, L. E., Tripathy, V. B., and Killinger, A. H.: Current status of leptospirosis immunization in swine and cattle, J. Am. Vet. Med. Assoc. 161:1235, 1972.
20. Hueber, G., Lofgrin, C. E., Renolds, W., and Luther, G.: Vehicles for intramammary mastitis preparations, Vet. Med. 55:35, Feb. 1960.
21. Kahrs, R. F., Hillman, R. B., and Todd, J. D.: Observations on the intranasal vaccination of pregnant cattle against infectious bovine rhinotracheitis and parainfluenza-3 virus infection, J. Am. Vet. Med. Assoc. 163:437, 1973.
22. Kaufmann, A. F., Fox, M. D., and Kolb, R. C.: Anthrax in Louisiana, 1971: an evaluation of the Sterne strain anthrax vaccine, J. Am. Vet. Med. Assoc. 163:442, 1973.
23. Kolar, J. R., Shechmeister, I. L., and Strack, L. E.: Field experiments with formalin-killed–virus vaccine against infectious bovine rhinotracheitis, bovine viral diarrhea, and parainfluenza-3, Am. J. Vet. Res. 34:1469, 1973.
24. Kuttler, K. L.: Efficacy of oxytetracycline and a dithiosemicarbazone in the treatment of bovine anaplasmosis, Am. J. Vet. Res. 32:1349, 1971.
25. Lambert, G.: Bovine viral diarrhea: prophylaxis and postvaccinal reactions, J. Am. Vet. Med. Assoc. 163:874, 1973.
26. Lindley, W. H.: Anthrax vaccination, J. Am. Vet. Med. Assoc. 142:621, 1963.
27. Lora, C. A., and Koechlin, A.: An attenuated *Anaplasma marginale* vaccine in Peru, Am. J. Vet. Res. 30:1993, 1969.
28. Luedke, A. J., and Jochim, M. M.: Clinical and serologic responses in vaccinated sheep given challenge innoculation with isolates of blue tongue virus, Am. J. Vet. Res. 29:841, 1968.
29. Matsuoka, R., Folkerts, T. M., and Gale, C.: Evaluation in calves of an inactivated bovine rhinotracheitis and parainfluenza-3 vaccine combined with *Pasteurella* bacterin, J. Am. Vet. Med. Assoc. 160:333, 1972.

30. McHardy, N., and Simpson, R. M.: Imidocarb dipropionate therapy in Kenyan anaplasmosis and babesiosis, Trop. Anim. Health Prod. **6**:63, May 1974.
31. McKercher, D. G., and Crenshaw, G. L.: Comparative efficacy of intranasally and parenterally administered infectious bovine rhinotracheitis vaccines, J. Am. Vet. Med. Assoc. **159**:1362, 1971.
32. Mebus, C. A., White, R. G., Stair, E. L., Rhodes, M. B., and Twiehaus, M. J.: Neonatal calf diarrhea: results of a field trial using a reo-like virus vaccine, Vet. Med. Small Anim. Clin. **67**:173, 1972.
33. Mercer, H. D., Geleta, J. N., Schultz, E. J., and Wright, W. W.: Milk-out rates for antibiotics in intramammary infusion products used in the treatment of bovine mastitis: relationship of somatic cell counts, milk production level, and drug vehicle, Am. J. Vet. Res. **31**:1549, 1970.
34. Mercer, H. D., Geleta, J. N., and Carter, G. G.: Absorption and excretion of penicillin G from the mastitic bovine udder, J. Am. Vet. Med. Assoc. **164**:613, 1974.
35. Meyers, L. L., Newman, F. S., Wilson, R. A., and Catlin, J. E.: Passive immunization of calves against experimentally induced enteric colibacillosis by vaccination of dams, Am. J. Vet. Res. **34**:29, 1973.
36. Nicolai, J. H., Jr., Jasper, D. E., Philpot, W. N., and Schultz, L. H.: Money returns from an effective mastitis control program, Washington, D.C., 1974, National Mastitis Council, Inc.
37. Oxender, W. D., and Seguin, B. E.: Bovine intrauterine therapy, J. Am. Vet. Med. Assoc. **168**:217, 1976.
38. Pierson, R. E.: Immunization of feedlot lambs with enterotoxemia toxoid and bacterin, J. Am. Vet. Med. Assoc. **152**:380, 1968.
39. Roberts, S. J.: Postpartum antibiotic intrauterine therapy in the dairy cow, Mod. Vet. Pract. **55**:465, 1974.
40. Roberts, S. J., Meek, A. M., Natzke, R. P., Guthrie, R. S., Field, L. E., Merrill, W. G., Schmidt, G. H., and Everett, R. W.: Concepts and recent developments in mastitis control, J. Am. Vet. Med. Assoc. **155**:157, 1969.
41. Roby, T. O., Amerault, T. E., Mazzola, V., Rose, J. E., and Ilemobade, A.: Immunity in bovine anaplasmosis after elimination of *Anaplasma marginale* infections with imidocarb, Am. J. Vet. Res. **35**:993, 1974.
42. Rosner, S. F.: Complications following vaccination of cattle against infectious bovine rhinotracheitis, bovine viral diarrhea-mucosal disease, and parainfluenza type 3, J. Am. Vet. Med. Assoc. **152**:898, 1968.
43. Saunders, J. R., Olson, S. M., and Radostits, O. M.: Efficacy of an intramuscular infectious bovine rhinotracheitis vaccine against abortion due to the virus, Can. Vet. J. **13**:273, 1972.
44. Seguin, B. E., Morrow, D. A., and Oxender, W.

D.: Intrauterine therapy in the cow, J. Am. Vet. Med. Assoc. **164**:609, 1974.
45. Siddique, I. H., Grant, G. H., Blackwell, J. G., and McKenzie, B. E.: Organisms associated with abortion and reproductive problems in cattle, Mod. Vet. Pract. **57**:809, 1976.
46. Siddique, I. H., Loken, K. I., and Hoyt, H. H.: Antibiotic residues in milk transferred from treated to untreated quarters in dairy cattle, J. Am. Vet. Med. Assoc. **146**:589, 1965.
47. Siddique, I. H., Loken, K. I., and Hoyt, H. H.: Concentrations of neomycin, dihydrostreptomycin, and polymyxin in milk after intramuscular or intramammary administration, J. Am. Vet. Med. Assoc. **146**:594, 1965.
48. Stalheim, O. H.: Vaccination against leptospirosis: immunogenicity of viable avirulent *Leptospira pomona* in hamsters, swine, and cattle, Am. J. Vet. Res. **29**:473, 1968.
49. Stalheim, O. H.: Vaccination of hamsters, swine and cattle with viable avirulent *Leptospira pomona*, Am. J. Vet. Res. **29**:1463, 1968.
50. Stalheim, O. H.: Chemotherapy of renal leptospirosis in cattle, Am. J. Vet. Res. **30**:1317, 1969.
51. Tennant, B., Harrold, D., and Reina-Guerra, B. S.: Physiologic and metabolic factors in the pathogenesis of neonatal enteric infections in calves, J. Am. Vet. Med. Assoc. **161**:993, 1972.
52. Todd, J. D., Bolenec, F. J., and Paton, I. M.: Intranasal vaccination against infectious bovine rhinotracheitis: studies on early onset of protection and use of the vaccine in pregnant cows, J. Am. Vet. Med. Assoc. **159**:1370, 1971.
53. Vollmar, R. E.: Calf diarrhea control in a dairy operation, Mod. Vet. Pract. **55**:509, 1974.
54. Welter, D. J., and Woods, R. D.: Preliminary evaluation of an attenuated *Anaplasma marginale* vaccine in cattle, Vet. Med. Small Anim. Clin. **63**:798, 1968.
55. Wilson, C.: Mastitis control in Great Britain, Vet. Sci. **12**:99, 1975.
56. Wright, W. W., and Harold, L. C.: Antibiotic residues in milk after parenteral and oral administration in cows, J. Am. Vet. Med. Assoc. **137**:525, 1960.
57. Zemjanis, R.: Vaccination for reproductive efficiency in cattle, J. Am. Vet. Med. Assoc. **165**:689, 1974.

Additional readings

Abinanti, F. R.: Future requirements for prevention and control of bovine respiratory diseases in the United States, J. Am. Vet. Med. Assoc. **152**:934, 1968.
Alexander, D. C., Garcia, M. M., and McKay, K. A.: Assessment of various adjuvants in *Sphaerophorus necrophorus* toxoids, Can. Vet. J. **14**:247, 1973.
Bedford, P. G. C.: Infectious bovine keratoconjunctivitis, Vet. Rec. **98**:134, 1976.
Bordt, D. E., Thomas, P. C., and Marshall, R. F.: Bovine virus diarrhea vaccines—a comparison of two

virus strains, Vet. Med. Small Anim. Clin. **70:**441, 1975.

Brookbanks, E. O.: Dry cow mastitis therapy, N. Z. Vet. J. **16:**83, 1968.

Brown, A. L.: Comments on infectious bovine rhinotracheitis immunization, J. Am. Vet. Med. Assoc. **152:**856, 1968.

Brown, L. N., and Ramsey, F. K.: Comments on complications following vaccination of cattle against bovine respiratory diseases, J. Am. Vet. Med. Assoc. **152:**903, 1968.

Cantor, A., and Palochak, M.: The in vitro sensitivity of antibiotic resistant bacteria to intramammary antibiotic preparations, Vet. Med. Small Anim. Clin. **70:** 800, 1975.

Casselberry, N. H.: Present status of immunization procedures for infectious bovine rhinotracheitis, J. Am. Vet. Med. Assoc. **152:**853, 1968.

Christie, G. J., and Strom, P. W.: Sodium cephapirin—a new treatment for mastitis, Vet. Med. Small Anim. Clin. **71:**429, 1976.

Crenshaw, G. L.: Comments on control and management of respiratory diseases in beef cattle, J. Am. Vet. Med. Assoc. **152:**923, 1968.

Davis, W. T., Maplesden, D. C., Natzke, R. P., and Philpot, W. N.: Sodium cloxacillin for treatment of mastitis in lactating cows, J. Dairy Sci. **58:**1822, 1975.

Davis, W. T., Maplesden, D. C., Natzke, R. P., Philpot, W. N., Garrett, P., and Card, C. S.: Benzathine cloxacillin intramammary infusion for treatment of mastitis in dry cows, Vet. Med. Small Anim. Clin. **70:**287, 1975.

Dodds, J. S., Nelson, F. C., Meads, E. B., and Hebert, C.: Cloxacillin mastitis ointment in the treatment of bovine mastitis, Can. Vet. J. **10:**188, 1969.

Eberhart, R. J., Watrous, G. H., Hokanson, J. F., and Burch, G. E.: Persistence of antibacterial agents in milk after intramammary treatment of clinical mastitis, J. Am. Vet. Med. Assoc. **143:**390, 1963.

Fernelius, A. L., Classick, L. G., and Smith, R. L.: Evaluation of β-propiolactone–inactivated- and chloroform-treated virus vaccines against bovine viral diarrhea–mucosal disease, Am. J. Vet. Res. **33:**1421, July 1972.

Flack, D. E.: Comments on control and management of respiratory disease in beef cattle, J. Am. Vet. Med. Assoc. **152:**925, 1968.

Fox, F. H.: Comments on management of respiratory diseases of dairy cattle, J. Am. Vet. Med. Assoc. **152:** 932, 1968.

Fuller, D. A.: Comments on complications following vaccination against bovine respiratory diseases, J. Am. Vet. Med. Assoc. **152:**904, 1968.

Gale, C.: Rationale for application of multiple-component vaccines, J. Am. Vet. Med. Assoc. **163:**836, 1973.

Gibbons, W. J.: Management of respiratory diseases in dairy cattle, J. Am. Vet. Med. Assoc. **152:**929, 1968.

Gillespie, J. H.: Comments on bovine viral diarrhea-mucosal disease, J. Am. Vet. Med. Assoc. **152:**768, 1968.

Granston, A. E., and Welter, C. J.: A trivalent bovine vaccine, Vet. Med. Small Anim. Clin. **63:**58, 1968.

Gray, D. M., and Schalm, O. W.: Interpretation of the California mastitis test results on milk from individual mammary quarters, bucket milk, and bulk herd milk, J. Am. Vet. Med. Assoc. **136:**195, 1960.

Haigh, A. J. B., and Hagan, D. H.: Evaluation of imidocarb dihydrochloride against redwater disease in cattle in Eire, Vet. Rec. **94:**56, 1974.

Hamdy, A. H., Olds, N. L., and Roberts, B. J.: Activity of penicillin and tovobiocin against bovine mastitis pathogens, Am. J. Vet. Res. **36:**259, 1975.

Hashemi-Fesharki, R.: Studies on imidocarb dihydrochloride in experimental *Babesia bigemina* infection in calves, Br. Vet. J. **131:**666, 1975.

Hill, G. N., and Keefe, T. J.: Clinical efficacy of benzathine cloxacillin in dry-cow mastitis treatment, Mod. Vet. Pract. **55:**843, 1974.

Hiramune, T., Murase, N., Yanagawa, R.: Efficacy of antibiotic treatment in cows affected with cystitis and those affected with pyelonephritis due to *Corynebacterium renale*, J. Vet. Sci. **37:**273, Oct. 1975.

Hjerpe, C. A.: An evaluation of uterine infusion as a treatment for repeat breeding in dairy cattle, J. Am. Vet. Med. Assoc. **138:**590, 1961.

Hokanson, J. F., Watrous, G. H., Jr., Burch, G., and Eberhart, R. J.: Persistence of antibacterial agents in milk after intravenous treatment of acute bovine mastitis, J. Am. Vet. Med. Assoc. **143:**395, 1963.

Hollister, C. J.: Comments on management of respiratory diseases in dairy cattle, J. Am. Vet. Med. Assoc. **152:**931, 1968.

Holper, J. C.: Comments on bovine viral diarrhea-mucosal disease, J. Am. Vet. Med. Assoc. **152:**868, 1968.

House, J. A., and Baker, J. A.: Comments on combination vaccines for bovine respiratory diseases, J. Am. Vet. Med. Assoc. **152:**893, 1968.

Jackson, R. A.: A dry cow mastitis treatment procedure, Vet. Med. **58:**139, 1963.

Jensen, R.: Scope of the problem of bovine respiratory disease in beef cattle, J. Am. Vet. Med. Assoc. **152:** 720, 1968.

Kirkbride, C. A., and Erhart, A. B.: The effect of milking machine function on udder health, J. Am. Vet. Med. Assoc. **155:**1499, 1969.

Kirkpatrick, R. J.: Comments on combination vaccines for bovine respiratory diseases, J. Am. Vet. Med. Assoc. **152:**896, 1968.

Knight, A. P., Pierson, R. E., Hoerlein, A. B., Collier, J. H., Horton, D. P., and Pruett, J. B.: Effect of vaccination time on morbidity, mortality, and weight gains of feeder calves, J. Am. Vet. Med. Assoc. **161:** 45, 1972.

Kolar, J. R., Shechmeister, I. L., and Kammlade, W. G., Jr.: Use in cattle of formalin-killed polyvalent vaccine with adjuvant against infectious bovine rhinotracheitis, bovine viral diarrhea, and parainfluenza-3 viruses, Am. J. Vet. Res. **33:**1415, 1972.

Lambert, G., and Fuller, D. A.: Postvaccinal problems in cattle, Mod. Vet. Pract. **51**:34, April 1970.

Lambert, G., Moeller, D. J., and Welter, C. J.: Field evaluation of antiserum for prevention of the neonatal calf pneumonia-enteritis complex, Vet. Med. Small Anim. Clin. **65**:975, 1970.

Larson, K. A., and Schell, K. R.: Toxicity and antigenicity of shipping fever vaccines in calves, J. Am. Vet. Med. Assoc. **155**:49, 1969.

McCarthy, B.: Dry cow therapy as a component of mastitis control, Proc. U.S. Anim. Health Assoc. **77**:121, Oct. 1973.

McDonald, J. S.: Relationship of hygiene, milking machine function, and intramammary therapy to udder disease, J. Am. Vet. Med. Assoc. **155**:903, 1969.

McHardy, N.: Elimination of *Eperythrozoon* spp. from mixed infections with babesia and anaplasma, Int. J. Parasit. **4**:107, 1974.

McKercher, D. G., Saito, J. K., Drenshaw, G. L., and Bushnell, R. B.: Complications in cattle following vaccination with a combined bovine viral diarrhea–infectious bovine rhinotracheitis vaccine, J. Am. Vet. Med. Assoc. **152**:1621, 1968.

Morse, G. E.: Efficacy trials of two corticosteroids in the intramammary treatment of bovine mastitis, Vet. Sci. **12**:114, 1975.

Natzke, R. P., Everett, R. W., and Bray, D. R.: Effect of drying off practices on mastitis infection, J. Dairy Sci. **58**:1828, 1975.

Newbould, F. H. S.: Antibiotic treatment of experimental *Staphylococcus aureus* infections of the bovine mammary gland, Cancer J. Comp. Med. **38**:411, 1974.

Peacock, G. V.: Comments on complications that arise after vaccination against bovine respiratory diseases, J. Am. Vet. Med. Assoc. **152**:905, 1968.

Pearce, H. G., and Smith, C.: Swine dysentery, N.Z. Vet. J. **23**:183, Aug. 1975.

Peter, C. P., Tyler, D. E., and Ramsey, F. K.: Characteristics of a condition following vaccination with bovine virus diarrhea vaccine, J. Am. Vet. Med. Assoc. **150**:46, 1967.

Phillips, C. E.: Comments on combination vaccines for bovine respiratory diseases, J. Am. Vet. Med. Assoc. **152**:895, 1968.

Pierson, R. E.: Control and management of respiratory diseases in beef cattle, J. Am. Vet. Med. Assoc. **152**:920, 1968.

Postle, D. S., Dahl, J. C., Jarrett, J. A., Jr., Jasper, D. E., and Warsinske, H. E.: Recommended minimal standards of performance for practicing veterinarians who offer mastitis control programs, J. Am. Vet. Med. Assoc. **163**:375, 1973.

Postle, D. S., and Linquist, W. E.: Efficacy of an antibiotic treatment in the nonlactating udder (a field study), Vet. Med. Small Anim. Clin. **68**:1241, 1973.

Postle, D. S., and Natzke, R. P.: Efficacy of antibiotic treatment in the bovine udder as determined from field studies, Vet. Med. Small Anim. Clin. **69**:1535, 1971.

Powell, H. S., and Taul, L. K.: *Streptococcus agalactiae:* a frequent cause of high bacteria count in milk, Vet. Med. Small Anim. Clin. **62**:689, 1967.

Pugh, G. W., and Hughes, D. E.: Infectious bovine keratoconjunctivitis: experimental induction of infection in calves with mycoplasmas and *Moraxella bovis*, Am. J. Vet. Res. **37**:493, 1976.

Radostits, O. M., Rhodes, C. S., Mitchell, M. E., Spotswood, T. O., and Wenkoff, M. S.: A clinical evaluation of antimicrobial agents and temporary starvation in the treatment of acute undifferentiated diarrhea in newborn calves, Can. Vet. J. **16**:219, 1975.

Sampson, G. R., Gale, C., Elliston, N. G., Grueter, H. P., McAskill, J. W., and Tonkinson, L. V.: Clinical studies of a modified live virus bovine rhinotracheitis/parainfluenza-3 vaccine with *Pasteurella* bacterin as the diluent, Vet. Med. Small Anim. Clin. **67**:899, 1972.

Sampson, G. R., Matsuoka, T., Olson, R. D., Miyat, J. A., and Tonkinson, L. V.: Clinical appraisal of an inactivated bovine rhinotracheitis/parainfluenza-3 vaccine with *Pasteurella* bacterin, Vet. Med. Small Anim. Clin. **67**:1354, 1972.

Schipper, I. A., and Kelling, C. L.: Shipping fever prophylaxis: comparison of vaccine and antibiotics administered following weaning, Can. Vet. J. **12**:172, 1971.

Schneider, R., and Jasper, D. E.: Standardization of the California Mastitis Test, Am. J. Vet. Res. **25**:635, 1964.

Shahidi, S. A., and Marshall, R. T.: Bactericidal efficiency of penicillin G in normal and mastitic milk: tube dilution assays, Am. J. Vet. Res. **29**:1391, 1968.

Smith, P. E., and Mitchell, F. E.: Bovine virus diarrhea vaccination of young calves nursing immune dams, Vet. Med. Small Anim. Clin. **63**:457, 1968.

Steves, F. E., and Baker, J. D.: Intranasal inoculation of feedlot calves with TELC strain parainfluenza-3 virus, Vet. Med. Small Anim. Clin. **65**:333, 1970.

Studer, E.: Disease control in dairy cattle, J. Am. Vet. Med. Assoc. **163**:832, 1973.

Sweat, R. L.: Comments on bovine viral diarrhea–mucosal disease, J. Am. Vet. Med. Assoc. **152**:867, 1968.

Thomas, S. H.: Treatment of clinical mastitis, Vet. Rec. **97**:78, 1975.

Todorovic, R. A., Gonzalez, E. F., and Adams, L. G.: *Babesia bigemina, Babesia argentina,* and *Anaplasma marginale:* coinfectious immunity in bovines, Exp. Parasitol. **37**:179, 1975.

Van Os, J. L.: Treatment of clinical mastitis, Vet. Rec. **97**:40, 1975.

Watkins, J. H.: Treatment of clinical mastitis, Vet. Rec. **97**:155, 1975.

Watkins, J. H., Buswell, J. F., and Hutchinson, I.: The treatment of clinical mastitis with a combination of ampicillin and cloxacillin, Vet. Rec. **96**:289, 1975.

Wilson, A. J., Paris, J., Luckins, A. G., Dar, F. K., and Gray, A. R.: Observations on a herd of beef cattle maintained in a tsetse area, Trop. Anim. Health Prod. **8:**1, Feb. 1976.

Wilson, C.: Mastitis control in Great Britain, Vet. Sci. **12:**99, 1975.

Woods, G. T., Mansfield, M. E., Omarik, G., and Krone, J.: Effects of bovine viral diarrhea and parainfluenza-3 virus vaccines on development of respiratory tract disease in calves, J. Am. Vet. Med. Assoc. **163:** 742, 1973.

Ziv, G., Bogin, E., and Sulman, F. G.: Blood and milk levels of chloramphenicol in normal and mastitic cows and ewes after intramuscular administration of chloramphenicol and chloramphenicol sodium succinate, Zentralbl. Veterinaermed. (A), **20:**801, 1973.

Ziv, G., Shani, J., and Sulman, F. G.: Pharmacokinetic evaluation of penicillin and cephalosporin derivatives in serum and milk of lactating cows and ewes, Am. J. Vet. Res. **34:**1561, 1973.

Ziv, G., and Sulman, F. G.: Serum and milk concentrations of spectinomycin and tylosin in cows and ewes, Am. J. Vet. Res. **34:**329, 1973.

6

DRUGS FOR PREVENTION AND TREATMENT OF
Infectious diseases of swine

Swine diarrhea
Hog cholera
Erysipelas

Swine are afflicted with numerous infectious diseases. As with other species discussed in this text, the following discussion is limited to those diseases that can be prevented with an appropriate biological unique to swine or those diseases for which special chemotherapeutic drugs are available.

SWINE DIARRHEA

Diarrhea in swine can be caused by a combination of management problems and infective agents. Depending on the cause, the syndrome may be referred to as "scours," "swine dysentery," "swine colibacillosis," or "transmissible gasteroenteritis (TGE)."

Swine diarrhea is likely to be a problem during the following three periods when environmental stresses lower the animal's resistance[7]:

- The first week after farrowing when the major causes are navel contamination, dampness, and chilling
- After weaning, when the change in diet, coexisting stress, and exposure to other litters of pigs are primary causes
- In pigs ranging from 23 to 70 kg, diarrhea is associated with improper sanitary practices

Among the microorganisms responsible for diarrhea in swine are *Erysipelothrix rhusiopathiae*, *Escherichia coli*, *Streptococcus* species, *Staphylococcus* species, *Pseudomonas* species, *Clostridium perfringens* type C, *Salmonella* species, *Vibrio* species, *Treponema hyodysenteriae*, and a coronavirus responsible for TGE.

Prevention

Management. Diarrhea in the newborn can be prevented by means of management techniques that include thoroughly disinfecting the farrowing pens prior to introducing new sows to the area, thoroughly washing sows prior to placing them in the farrowing pens, cutting and disinfecting the navel shortly after birth, maintaining a warm dry environment for piglets, and assuring that each piglet receives adequate sources of iron (Chapter 17). In older animals, maintaining a sanitary environment is a key to preventing diarrhea.

Use of biologicals. In addition to management, biologicals can be used to help in the prevention of some forms of swine diarrhea.

Transmissible gastroenteritis (TGE). Because pigs are susceptible to TGE from the first day of life, immunity should be provided immediately after birth. To be effective, antibodies against TGE must be in the lumen of the gut to neutralize the virus before it penetrates the epithelial cells of the small intestine. The only practical way of delivering antibodies to the gut of piglets is to immunize sows so that appropriate antibodies will be delivered through the colostrum and milk. Even though the antibodies in the milk are not absorbed by the suckling pig, they provide protection in the gut.

It has been shown experimentally that sows can be immunized by the oral route, the natural route of infection, with virulent TGE virus or parenterally by injecting inactivated, attenuated, or virulent TGE virus. The oral route is preferred.

The results of oral inoculation and parenteral inoculation differ in the following ways. Oral inoculation results in moderate to high levels of antibody in the serum of the sow and moderate to high levels of antibody in the colostrum. Antibodies continue in the milk throughout lactation. In addition, the sow remains immune to subsequent natural infection. Parenteral inoculations result in high titers of antibody in the serum of the sow, high titers of antibody in the colostrum, and low milk antibody levels. In addition, the sow remains susceptible to natural infection with TGE virus.[11]

A vaccine is commercially available to prevent infection with the virus responsible for TGE. This modified live virus vaccine from porcine tissue culture is administered to sows intramuscularly approximately 6 weeks and then again 2 weeks before parturition. This provides passive immunity to suckling pigs. One experimental trial showed that the vaccine had only limited effectiveness, which may be related to the route by which the vaccine was given to the sows—intramuscularly rather than orally.[3]

Colibacillosis. It appears that suckling swine can be protected against *Escherichia coli* infection by immunizing sows with a live formalin-treated vaccine.[21] Sows are vaccinated three times in the periods of 24 to 31 days, 10 to 17 days, and 3 to 10 days before farrowing. In an experimental procedure, sows were immunized by both the intramammary and intramuscular routes. Both routes were highly effective in reducing the incidence of *E. coli* diarrhea in their offspring.

Piglets appear to be better protected by ingesting antibodies against *E. coli* than by having such antibodies present in their circulatory system. Generally, colostrum is the main source of antibodies for piglets. In addition, piglets continue to receive antibodies from sow's milk even after 2 days of age when they can no longer absorb the antibodies into the systemic circulation from the gut. Such antibodies remain in the intestine until they are either digested or eliminated. While in the intestine, they apparently can provide protection against *E. coli* infection.

Treatment. Many preparations are available for treating diarrhea in swine. Most of these are similar to products available for treatment of diarrhea in calves as discussed in Chapter 5. Various types of antibacterials, including antibiotics, sulfas, and nitrofurans, are popular. Among the antibacterials frequently used to treat diarrhea in swine are the following.[12]

Spectinomycin is primarily effective against gram-negative bacteria. In the United States it is only approved for treating piglets less than 4 weeks old and weighing less than 7 kg. Although it can be highly effective against *E. coli,* resistance to the antibiotic may develop rapidly. It is given orally twice a day at the rate of 110 mg/kg.[18]

Ampicillin is often used when the infection is resistant to other antibiotics. Although the manufacturer recommends an oral dose of 11 mg/kg twice a day, this dose given three or four times a day may be more effective.

Because *neomycin* has been a popular antibiotic for the treatment of colibacillosis for many years, a high percentage of *E. coli* have become resistant to the drug. In commercial preparations, neomycin is often mixed with other anti-infective medications. When given orally, neomycin is not absorbed to any significant degree from the digestive tract. Generally, when neomycin is used to treat diarrhea in newborn pigs, it is given orally at the rate of 50 mg/24 hr.[18]

In Chapter 3 the advantages and disadvantages of *lincomycin* were discussed.

When used for the treatment of diarrhea in swine, it is mixed in the feed at the rate of 100 gm/ton (110 mg/kg).[5,12]

Carbadox, a chemical antibacterial compound administered in the feed to increase weight gains and improve feed efficiency, has been shown to be effective in preventing and treating some forms of swine diarrhea.[15-17] It is mixed in the feed at the rate of 50 gm/ton (55 mg/kg). Carbadox should not be fed to swine weighing more than 35 kg or within 10 weeks of slaughter. In addition, it should not be used in feeds containing less than 15% crude protein or those containing bentonite.[18]

Among the *nitromidazole compounds* that have been tested for the treatment of swine diarrhea are dimetridazole, ipronidazole, and ronidazole. These drugs have not yet been approved by the FDA for use in food-producing animals in the United States.

Experimentally the nitromidazole compounds appear particularly effective when used to prevent and treat diarrhea caused by the spirochete bacteria, *Treponema hyodysenteriae*. For prevention of diarrhea, dimetridazole has been administered in the feed at the rate of 0.005% to 0.02% and in the drinking water at the rate of 0.003% to 0.75%.[1,4,14]

It has been shown experimentally that by the continuous feeding of 0.011% of ipronidazole in the feed (100 gm/ton), swine dysentery caused by *T. hyodysenteriae* can be prevented. In addition, animals with active infection treated with ipronidazole at the rate of from 0.005 to 0.022% in the drinking water (50 to 220 mg/liter) for 7 days can be cured of the disease.[13]

Ronidazole has been used experimentally in swine infected with *T. hyodysenteriae*. After the development of diarrhea, swine were treated with ronidazole in the drinking water for 5 days at the rates of 15, 30, and 60 mg/liter. At these rates, ronidazole was highly effective in curing dysentery.[20]

Many bacteria that cause diarrhea in swine have become resistant to antibiotics. *Sulfonamides* therefore offer an alternative, although bacteria can develop resistance to sulfonamides as well. Doses for sulfonamide drugs were given shown in Table 3-1.

In addition to anti-infectives, medications to soothe the inflamed intestine, such as Kaopectate, and anticholinergics to slow down the gut activity are often used in the treatment of diarrhea in swine (Chapter 19).

Diarrhea in swine can cause severe fluid loss and electrolyte imbalance. When it is practical, fluid therapy as discussed in Chapter 17 may be lifesaving.

HOG CHOLERA

Hog cholera is a catastrophic disease of swine that strikes large numbers of animals during an outbreak. It causes a high rate of mortality. Animals may die without showing any clinical signs or may develop signs such as high fever, vomiting, diarrhea, convulsions, and death. Stillborn deformed fetuses can result when swine are infected within the uterus.

Hog cholera is caused by a virus. There are probably various strains of the virus that result in different signs of the disease during an outbreak.

Prevention. Through a program of slaughtering infected animals, hog cholera has been eliminated from the United States. However, because the virus could be shipped in inadvertently from other countries, veterinarians must be able to recognize the disease so that they can report any suspected cases to appropriate officials. Because hog cholera vaccines are not allowed in the United States, the swine population is highly susceptible to the virus. The vaccines have been banned for the following reasons:

1. Under certain conditions the modified live virus vaccine passes through the placental barrier and may serve as a focus of new infection in a litter of pigs.

2. The modified live virus could revert to a virulent strain.

3. Immunized animals, when exposed to the field virus, may carry the virus even though they do not show clinical illness, thereby becoming reservoirs for infecting

other animals. The vaccine could therefore mask outbreaks of hog cholera. To maintain an area free of hog cholera, one must know when the virus has been introduced so that steps may be taken immediately to eradicate all infected animals.

In other countries in which hog cholera still occurs, vaccines can be effective in preventing the disease. Three general types of vaccines are used: virulent virus, attenuated virus, and inactivated or killed virus. Many vaccines used to prevent hog cholera are administered in conjunction with hog cholera antiserum.

Virulent virus vaccines. One method of preventing the disease is by the administration of virulent live virus concurrently with hog cholera antiserum. Vaccination is performed at any time after 4 weeks of age. The use of the antiserum prevents development of the disease in the animal, while the administration of the live virus allows the animal to develop an active immunity against hog cholera.

Attenuated vaccines. There are three types of attenuated vaccines:

1. *Tissue vaccine* is prepared by the treatment of infectious tissue with eucalyptol. It is slow in producing immunity, and the immunity is of short duration.

2. *Tissue culture vaccines* must be administered simultaneously with antiserum. They produce a good immunity.

3. *Lapinized vaccines* are produced by attenuating the virus through rabbit passage. Some of these vaccines must be given with antiserum, whereas others can be administered alone. They produce immunity within a few days. Some types have produced solid immunity for two years or more.

Antiserum must be used with many attenuated products because these products have not totally lost their virulence. When attenuated vaccines are administered simultaneously with appropriate doses of antiserum, active antibodies will be produced. However, if the antiserum is given in larger doses than recommended either concurrently or before the administration of the attenuated vaccine, the development of active antibodies will be blocked.[10]

Just as the virulent virus can cause death in embryos and newborn pigs by passing the placental barrier in swine, so can the virus in attenuated live virus hog cholera vaccines.[6,19]

Inactivated vaccine. Crystal violet vaccine is an inactivated (killed) product. Immunity lasts for about 12 months but does not develop until about 12 days after administration. Administration of antiserum around the time of administering the vaccine can prevent the development of active immunity.[2]

ERYSIPELAS

Swine of all ages are susceptible to infection with the bacteria *Erysipelothrix rhusiopathiae*. Adults, rather than young animals, are most likely to be affected if the strain is of relatively low virulence. Sows that have recently farrowed are particularly susceptible. With highly virulent strains, however, pigs of all ages develop the disease.

Signs. There are three forms of the disease. The acute septicemic form resembles hog cholera in that the animals have a high fever, sleepy attitude, poor appetite, and swelling of the ears, legs, and tissues around the eyes. In the subacute form, rectangular reddish patches are seen along the back of the animal. In the chronic form, arthritis may develop. Endocarditis may also occur in the chronic form. Clinically a wide variation in the virulence of the organisms is seen. This variation in virulence has been utilized in the production of living avirulent vaccines.

Prevention. Various methods of active immunization are practiced. A living organism of lower virulence than the field strain can be administered simultaneously with antiserum. Immunity lasts about 6 months. Although very young pigs are incapable of developing an immunity in response to this vaccine, animals vaccinated at 2 months of age usually develop an immunity that lasts for 3 to 5 months.

Avirulent living vaccines do not require the simultaneous administration of antiserum. Animals can be immunized at 8 to 12 weeks of age, and an effective immunity is reported to last for about 6 months.

Bacterins adsorbed onto aluminum hydroxide generally result in immunity lasting approximately 12 weeks. Booster injections are commonly given 3 to 6 weeks after the first injection. The bacterins have been shown to be effective both clinically and experimentally, although they may increase the prevalence of arthritis in swine exposed to the causative organism. Results of experiments indicate that both bacterins and attenuated vaccines increase the severity of chronic arthritis if pigs become subsequently infected.[8,9]

To prevent erysipelas, sows should be actively immunized 4 to 6 weeks before farrowing, and newborn pigs should be given antiserum monthly until they are immunized at about 12 weeks of age. However, erysipelas antiserum must be used with caution because it is usually of equine origin and may cause hypersensitivity reactions in swine. Piglets from sows that have not been vaccinated can be actively immunized at 5 to 8 weeks of age. Breeding stock should be vaccinated every 6 months.

During an outbreak all pigs on the affected premises should be given antiserum. Depending on the age of the animal, 5 to 20 ml of antiserum will provide 1 to 2 weeks of protection to animals that have been exposed to the disease during an outbreak.

Treatment. Penicillin G is the standard treatment for erysipelas. In severe cases it is administered with erysipelas antiserum.

References

1. Anderson, M. D.: Prevention and treatment of swine dysentery with dimetridazole, Am. J. Vet. Res. 34:1175, 1973.
2. Blood, D. C., and Henderson, J. A.: Veterinary medicine, ed. 4, Baltimore, 1974, The Williams & Wilkins Co.
3. Bohl, E. H., and others: Passive immunity in transmissible gastroenteritis of pigs after intramuscular injection of pregnant sows with a modified live-virus vaccine, Am. J. Vet. Res. 36:690, 1975.
4. Davis, J. W., Libke, K. G., and Osborne, J. C.: Dimetridazole for treatment and prevention of swine dysentery, Mod. Vet. Pract. 54:25, April 1973.
5. DeGeeter, M. J., Davis, L. W., and Geng, S.: Effect of lincomycin on swine dysentery, J. Anim. Sci. 42:1381, 1976.
6. Dunne, H. W., and Clark, C. D.: Embryonic death, fetal mummification, stillbirth, and neonatal death in pigs of gilts vaccinated with attenuated live-virus hog cholera vaccine, Am. J. Vet. Res. 29:787, 1968.
7. Fahrni, L. R.: Poor management the primary cause, panel report, Mod. Vet. Pract. 51:60, Nov. 1970.
8. Freeman, J. M.: Effects of vaccination on the development of arthritis in swine with erysipelas: clinical, hematologic, and gross pathologic observations, Am. J. Vet. Res. 25:589, 1964.
9. Freemen, J. M.: Effects of vaccination on the development of arthritis in swine with erysipelas: bacteriologic, immunologic, serum protein, and histopathologic observations, Am. J. Vet. Res. 25:599, 1964.
10. Gibbons, W. J.: Hog cholera antibody block, Mod. Vet. Pract. 49:54, 1968.
11. Haelterman, E. O.: Immunity to transmissible gasteroenteritis, Vet. Med. Small Anim. Clin. 70:715, 1975.
12. Kunesh, J. P.: Evaluation of drugs used in treating enteric diseases of swine, Vet. Med. Small Anim. Clin. 72:371, 1977.
13. Messersmith, R. E., Oetjen, K. B., Hussey, F. J., and Kanning, H. H.: Effect of ipronidazole on swine dysentery, Vet. Med. Small Anim. Clin. 68:1021, 1973.
14. Miller, R. L., and Fox, J. E.: Dimetridazole therapy for swine dysentery, Mod. Vet. Pract. 54:19, June 1973.
15. Rainier, R. H., Chalquest, R. R., Babcock, W. E., and Thrasher, G. W.: Efficacy of carbadox in prevention of field outbreaks of swine dysentery, Vet. Med. Small Anim. Clin. 68:171, 1973.
16. Rainier, R. H., Chalquest, R. R., Babcock, W. E., and Thrasher, G. W.: Therapeutic efficacy of carbadox in field outbreaks of swine dysentery, Vet. Med. Small Anim. Clin. 68:272, 1973.
17. Rainier, R. H., Chalquest, R. R., Babcock, W. E., and Thrasher, G. W.: Evaluation of carbadox for prophylaxis and treatment of induced swine dysentery, J. Am. Vet. Med. Assoc. 163:457, 1973.
18. Rossoff, I. S.: Handbook of veterinary drugs, New York, 1974, Springer Publishing Co.
19. Stewart, S. W., Carbrey, E. A., and Kresse, J. I.: Transplacental hog cholera infection in immune sows, Am. J. Vet. Res. 33:791, 1972.
20. Taylor, D. J.: Ronidazole in the treatment of experimental swine dysentery, Vet. Rec. 95:215, 1974.
21. Wilson, M. R.: Role of immunity in the control of neonatal colibacillosis in pigs, J. Am. Vet. Med. Assoc. 160:585, 1972.

Additional readings

Azechi, H., Terakado, N., and Ninomiya, K.: Penicillin treatment and antibody response of pigs experimentally infected with *Erysipelothrix insidiosa*, Am. J. Vet. Res. **33:**1963, 1972.

Boehm, P. N.: Antimicrobial therapy in swine, Vet. Clin. North Am. **5:**117, 1975.

Crawford, J. G., Dayhuff, T. R., and White, E. A.: Hog cholera: safety and protection studies with photodynamically inactivated hog cholera virus, Am. J. Vet. Res. **29:**1749, 1968.

Crawford, J. G., White, E. A., and Dayhuff, T. R.: Hog cholera: response of pigs vaccinated under field conditions with photodynamically inactivated hog cholera vaccine of tissue culture origin, Am. J. Vet. Res. **29:** 1761, 1968.

Culbreth, W., Simkins, K. L., Gale, G. O., Messersmith, R. E., and Alford, B. T.: Effects of chlortetracycline-sulfamethazine water medication against experimentally induced swine salmonellosis, J. Am. Vet. Med. Assoc. **160:**436, 1972.

Davis, W. T., Reynolds, W. A., and Maplesden, D. C.: Comparison of ampicillin and sulfachlorpyridazine in treatment of colibacillosis in swine, Vet. Med. Small Anim. Clin. **68:**847, 1973.

Dobson, K. J.: Letters to the editor: eradication of leptospirosis in commercial pig herds, Aust. Vet. J. **50:** 471, 1974.

Freeman, A.: All 50 states hog cholera free, J. Am. Vet. Med. Assoc. **165:**158, 1974.

Gustafson, D. P., and others: Report of the panel of the colloquium on selected infectious diseases of swine, J. Am. Vet. Med. Assoc. **160:**493, 1972.

Hamdy, A. H.: Therapeutic effect of lincomycin and spectinomycin water medication on swine dysentery, Can. J. Comp. Med. **38:**1, 1974.

Hansell, W. H.: Comments on mixed bacterins and autogenous bacterins, J. Am. Vet. Med. Assoc. **160:** 612, 1972.

Harris, D. L., Glock, R. D., Dale, S. E., and Ross, R. F.: Efficacy of gentamicin sulfate for the treatment of swine dysentery, J. Am. Vet. Med. Assoc. **161:** 1317, 1972.

July, J. W.: Influence of management and sales on disease dissemination and the need for immunizing agents, J. Am. Vet. Med. Assoc. **160:**502, 1972.

Jungk, N. K., Towey, J. P., Swangard, W. M., and Boylan, C. G.: The use of tricalcium phosphate for the adsorption and concentration of erysipelas bacterin, Am. J. Vet. Res. **21:**902, 1960.

Lee, C. H., Olson, L. D., and Rodabaugh, D. E.: Influence of medication on development of serum antibody to swine dysentery as detected with indirect fluorescent antibody method, Am. J. Vet. Res. **37:** 1159, 1976.

Messersmith, R. E., Hussey, F. J., Kanning, H. H., and Kinyon, J. M.: Further studies on the effect of ipronidazole on swine dysentery, Vet. Med. Small Anim. Clin. **71:**343, 1976.

Moscari, E., and others: Intranasal TGE vaccination of swine, Mod. Vet. Pract. **57:**464, 1976.

Moeller, D. J., and Pulliam, J. D.: Clinical field evaluation of ronidazole for the treatment of swine dysentery, Vet. Med. Small Anim. Clin. **72:**365, 1977.

Olson, L. D., and Rodabaugh, D. E.: Ronidazole in high concentrations in drinking water for treatment and prevention of diarrhea in swine dysentery, Am. J. Vet. Res. **37:**757, 1976.

Olson, L. D., and Rodabaugh, D. E.: Ronidazole in low concentrations in drinking water for treatment and development of immunity to swine dysentery, Am. J. Vet. Res. **37:**763, 1976.

Rutter, J. M., and Beer, R. J.: Synergism between *Trichuris suis* and the microbial flora of the large intestine causing dysentery in pigs, Infect. Immun. **11:** 395, 1975.

Taylor, D. J.: Ronidazole in the treatment and prophylaxis of experimental swine dysentery, Vet. Rec. **99:** 453, 1976.

Thompson, V. U.: Mixture of drugs give best results, panel report, Mod. Vet. Pract. **51:**58, 1970.

Troutt, H. F., Hooper, B. E., and Harrington, R.: Effect of carbadox in experimentally induced salmonellosis of swine, J. Am. Vet. Med. Assoc. **164:**402, 1974.

7

DRUGS FOR PREVENTION AND TREATMENT OF
Infectious diseases of horses

Viral diseases
  Equine influenza
  Equine rhinopneumonitis (equine herpes-
    virus type 1 infection)
  Equine viral arteritis
  Other equine upper respiratory diseases
  Western and eastern equine encephalo-
    myelitis
  Venezuelan equine encephalomyelitis
  Rabies
Bacterial diseases
  Strangles
  Tetanus
  Special conditions
    Equine genital infections
    Equine intestinal infections
    Miscellaneous bacterial infections

The following discussion will be limited to the infectious diseases of horses for which there are commercially available biologics or that are treated in a unique manner with anti-infective drugs.

VIRAL DISEASES
Equine influenza

In horses, influenza is manifested by a fever and a cough. It is caused by two viruses: myxoviruses IA/E1 and IA/E2. Even though these viruses are related antigenically, immunity against one will not protect against infection by the other.

Prevention. Apparently killed virus vac-

cines prepared with the two viruses produce an immunity against both viruses. When an adjuvant is added to the vaccines, a greater serum antibody titer against the equine viruses is produced than when vaccines of equal antigenic mass without adjuvant are used.[4]

Commercially available vaccines contain both viruses and an adjuvant. The vaccine is a killed virus of chick embryo origin. Initially two 1 ml doses are administered 6 to 8 weeks apart. Booster shots are given annually or during epizootics.[8] Suckling foals may be immunized.

Equine rhinopneumonitis (equine herpesvirus type 1 infection)

Signs. Primary infection by equine rhinopneumonitis generally occurs in young horses. It is manifested by the following signs: nasal discharge, fever, a decrease in the circulating white blood cells (neutropenia), mild depression, and cough.

Although subsequent infections can occur, they usually are subclinical. In pregnant mares the condition may result in an abortion in 90% of cases if the infection occurs during the last 8 months of pregnancy (The gestation period in horses is approximately 11 months.)

Prevention. The disease may be controlled by a strictly administered program of planned infections with a moderately virulent vaccine of hamster tissue origin.

The vaccine may produce disease in young foals and cause abortion in pregnant mares. Therefore its use is recommended only on breeding farms where fetal rhinopneumonitis has occurred the previous foaling period or on farms in enzootic areas. Generally, horses are bred in late winter or spring. On breeding farms the first dose of equine rhinopneumonitis should be administered in July to all horses on the premises regardless of age or sex, with the exception of mares more than 3 months pregnant. Because vaccination of mares more than 3 months pregnant may cause abortion, they should not be vaccinated but removed to isolated premises to avoid exposure to the virus vaccine. The next dose should be given in October, again removing all mares 3 months or more pregnant. After vaccination all horses should be quarantined for 3 weeks.

For horses in training the vaccine should be administered in December, January, or February. Newly vaccinated horses should not be scheduled for competition for at least 3 weeks after vaccination. In addition, because the virus vaccine can spread from one animal to another, immunized animals must not come in contact with pregnant mares for at least 3 weeks after vaccination.[4,20]

Equine viral arteritis

Equine viral arteritis is an acute viral infection of horses.

Signs. Equine viral arteritis is characterized clinically by depression, fever, decrease in white blood cell count, edema of the legs, ventral edema, lacrimation, conjunctivitis, photophobia, and nasal discharge. Infected animals may die. No specific therapy is available. Of pregnant mares, 50% to 80% will abort when infected.

Prevention. A modified live virus vaccine against equine viral arteritis has been developed and tested experimentally. It has been shown that pregnant mares can be immunized without detriment to the fetus. However, immunity is not passed to newborn foals in the colostrum.[13]

The vaccine produces a solid immunity of long duration. Unfortunately it is not yet commercially available in the United States.

Other equine upper respiratory diseases

In addition to those viruses previously listed, numerous other viruses are responsible for upper respiratory infections in horses. As in humans these infections are often referred to as "colds." Typically animals have a fever, nasal discharge, and cough. Subsequent to viral infection, bacteria can infect the sinuses or lungs.

Treatment. The animal should not be exercised during the acute phase of the disease and should have warm clean quarters available to it. Feed and clean water should be available to the animal.

When there is secondary bacterial infection, use of appropriate anti-infective drugs is indicated.

No specific medication exists to combat these viruses. However, even when pure viral upper respiratory infections exist in horses, anti-infective drugs, primarily antibiotics, are frequently administered. This practice is highly questionable, since antibiotics are not effective against these viruses.

Antibiotics and corticosteroids frequently are administered simultaneously to horses with viral upper respiratory disease. Clinical improvement after such administration is usually noted. Animals generally return to eating and cough less frequently. This results from the corticosteroids, which decrease inflammation in the respiratory tract (thereby decreasing the coughing) and give the animal a sense of well-being, with a resulting increase in appetite. Despite clinical improvements, the practice of using corticosteroids to treat horses with upper respiratory viral infection is questionable. Although they reduce inflammation, corticosteroids also reduce the animal's defense mechanisms to combat the virus. They may also predispose the animal to bacterial infections. The long-term damage that could occur from the administration of corticosteroids is not outweighed by the short-term advantage of improvement in clinical signs.

Animal species have always had to deal with upper respiratory viruses. Various evolutionary mechanisms have been developed to deal with those viruses. Corticosteroids interfere with these mechanisms. It is not wise therapeutics to employ such a drug in an attempt to improve on nature's slower process of dealing effectively with upper respiratory viruses.

Some medications, however, can be used to assist nature and to make the horse more comfortable. Expectorants can be administered to the horse to stimulate the production of mucus in the respiratory tract. This protects and reduces acute inflammatory conditions in the respiratory tract. The cough becomes more productive.

Various expectorants are used in the horse. One is etherated guaiacol, which can be administered by intramuscular injection to an adult horse at the rate of 1.5 gm.[22] Guaiacol is a constituent of creosote. When injected intramuscularly, it is absorbed and eliminated partially in respiratory secretions. Guaiacol is slightly irritating and increases the amount of respiratory secretions.

Glyceryl guaiacolate is popular in oral equine cough remedies as an expectorant and, in our opinion, is the expectorant of choice for use in horses.

Ammonium chloride given orally at the rate of 3 to 15 gm one to three times a day can be used as an expectorant in horses. Ethylenediamine dihydrochloride, an organic iodide preparation, is also administered orally to horses as an expectorant at the rate of 0.7 to 1.3 gm one to three times a day. Therapy with organic iodide should be discontinued at the end of one week.[22] Various compounds are available that contain derivatives of creosote and that are administered orally to horses as an expectorant. They should be given according to the manufacturer's instructions.

Western and eastern equine encephalomyelitis

Although eastern and western equine encephalomyelitis (EEE and WEE) are caused by two distinct viruses, they are discussed together because vaccines containing both viruses (bivalent vaccines) are available to protect animals against both diseases simultaneously.

Signs. The severity of these conditions varies, depending on the strain of virus and resistance of the infected animal. Clinical manifestations include fever and signs associated with central nervous system malfunction. Early in the course of the disease the horse may be hyperactive. Later the horse may become extremely depressed, which may progress to partial paralysis, complete paralysis, and death. Recovered horses frequently have residual nervous system damage.[2]

Etiology. The viruses of both EEE and WEE are transferred from birds (the reservoir) by mosquito vectors to mammalian species, primarily the horse. Humans can be infected with the virus; however, transmission does not occur between horses or from horses to humans. Therefore horses do not constitute a public health hazard in relation to this disease.

Prevention. Because of the serious nature of the disease and because treatment cannot be relied on to benefit an affected animal, prophylactic measures are essential for preventing the disease. The biologics available to prevent equine encephalomyelitis are monovalent (containing only one type of virus) or bivalent EEE/WEE vaccine. These are usually either chick embryo origin killed vaccine or tissue origin killed vaccine. Two doses should be administered on an annual basis. Until recently these vaccines were given only by intradermal injection. Several products are currently available, however, that can be given intramuscularly. The vaccines are inactivated with formalin. When used as directed, both the chick embryo origin and tissue culture origin inactivated vaccines are highly effective.[9]

Among unanswered questions regarding the use of the inactivated forms of WEE and EEE are the age at which foals should be immunized and whether two doses of vaccine are necessary for boosters annually or if one is sufficient. Until these questions are answered, all horses should be immunized with two doses annually, at least 15 days before the start of the insect season.

Interest in the development of attenuated vaccines against WEE and EEE has been growing. The goal has been to develop an attenuated vaccine that will produce an immunity without causing damage to the animal's central nervous system. To date apparently safe and effective attenuated products for WEE have been reported but none for EEE.[1,10] Unfortunately the attenuated WEE vaccine is not available commercially.

A disadvantage with the chick embryo origin encephalomyelitis vaccine is that it contains substantial foreign protein in addition to the inactivated virus. This foreign protein often causes noticeable local swelling after administration and may even cause fever in horses for a few days after administration. The cell culture products contain less foreign protein and therefore usually do not result in either local or systemic reaction after administration.

Lay persons should be discouraged from administering the intradermal encephalitis vaccines unless they are familiar with giving intradermal inoculations. Veterinarians and animal health technicians administering these products must be sure that they are given intradermally. For both inactivated forms, two doses are given annually at intervals recommended by the manufacturer.

Venezuelan equine encephalomyelitis

The virus of Venezuelan equine encephalomyelitis (VEE) is related to the viruses of WEE and EEE. Unlike both WEE and EEE, the Venezuelan virus can be spread from one horse to another by direct contact. In addition to direct transmission of VEE, arthropods, primarily mosquitoes, also transmit the disease.

Signs. Signs of VEE are similar to those described for WEE and EEE. VEE outbreaks occurred in the United States for the first time in July 1971. More than 1500 horses died in Texas.

Prevention. The attenuated live virus TC-83 Venezuelan equine encephalomyelitis vaccine has been well tested and shown to protect horses from the disease.[11,24] Colts that have reached 6 months of age should be free of maternal antibodies and can be immunized against VEE.[25]

Questions have been raised regarding the safety of VEE vaccine. In one experiment, animals were examined between 5 and 49 days after administration of VEE vaccine. There was no evidence of permanent gross or microscopic damage to either the brain or spinal cord.[14] In field trials, when animals are immunized with VEE vaccine, they show only slight clinical signs of disease, which probably cannot be detected by the casual observer. These signs include slight depression, decreased resistance to other diseases, and a decrease of up to 25% in circulating white blood cells. In addition, a moderate increase in body temperature can result. The animals should return to normal within 14 days after administration of the vaccine.[3,14]

Questions have been raised as to whether VEE vaccine can be administered simultaneously with WEE and EEE vaccine. Experiments tend to indicate that adequate antibodies against VEE will be formed when administered simultaneously with the first dose of bivalent WEE and EEE vaccine. However, when given to animals already containing antibodies against WEE, EEE, or both, active antibodies against VEE may not form.[12] This question is not resolved at the present time. Until it is, it is advisable to administer VEE vaccine before or simultaneous with the first dose of WEE and/or EEE vaccine. A trivalent vaccine containing WEE, EEE, and VEE is now available.

Rabies

Like other warm-blooded animals horses are susceptible to rabies. Because horses are primarily kept as pets, they can expose a large number of humans to the disease if they become infected. Although immunization of horses against rabies is not widely practiced, many newer vaccines can be used. The tissue culture vaccines are particularly appropriate. Table 4-3 shows the type of vaccines that can be used to prevent rabies in horses.

BACTERIAL DISEASES
Strangles

Strangles is caused by *Streptococcus equi.* Young animals are particularly severely affected. Any or all horses exposed may contract the disease.

Signs. Signs of the disease include severe pharyngitis accompanied by swelling and abscessation of the lymph nodes draining the head and throat. Abscesses may also occur in other parts of the body. Recovered horses are usually immune for several years. However, nonimmune stock brought onto premises infected with the organism generally will develop the disease. When one horse is infected, it is wise to take control measures to prevent the spread of the disease.

Prevention

Prophylactic antibiotics. In the face of an outbreak, animals may be prophylactically treated with penicillin G for 3 to 4 days and at the same time be immunized with a bacterin. This is in fact one of the few instances when the use of antibacterials prophylactically is of real benefit.

Immunization. Bacterins prepared from inactivated virulent encapsulated organisms are effective in preventing strangles.[6] These bacterins are effective against *S. equi,* but other streptococcal bacterins have not proved to be as effective.[7] For strangles bacterin to be safe and effective it must be administered properly. Improper administration can result in hypersensitivity allergic reactions, with varying signs from inappetence to joint inflammation or anaphylaxis. In addition, improper administration of strangles bacterin can result in a condition called "purpura hemorrhagica," which is thought to be an allergic condition that destroys the integrity of the capillary bed,

allowing serum and blood to escape into the tissues. The condition is often fatal in horses.

If proper vaccination techniques are used, the incidence of severe undesired effects need not be over 5%. However, an estimated 75% of animals immunized will develop transient stiffness and slight swelling at the site of injection.[18] There is no cross protection to strangles when horses are immunized with streptococci other than *S. equi.*

Administration. Because the incidence of strangles in foals under 3 months of age is rare, the bacterin is usually not administered to foals until they are 12 weeks old. Three milliliters can be administered aseptically into each buttock in foals. A second and third dose is then administered at 7-day intervals.

In weanlings and older horses that have neither been previously immunized nor previously had the disease, three 10 ml doses are administered 7 days apart. By dividing the dose and administering 5 ml in each site, local swelling from the injection can be reduced. Single booster immunizations of 10 ml are administered annually at least 12 months after the previous immunization period. When a horse has been given the initial series of immunizations or has been previously infected with the disease, only one 10 ml dose of the bacterin is administered annually. Two or three doses may cause allergic problems as previously noted.

Frequently, owners of a horse know nothing about the disease status or immunization history of the animal prior to the time they acquired ownership. It then becomes difficult to know whether to give the full course of strangles immunization or only to administer a booster shot. A decision can sometimes be made by a veterinarian on the basis of the reaction that occurs after an initial administration of bacterin. If the local and general effects of the first injection are comparable to those usually found in healthy young animals, the second and finally a third dose can be administered. However, if the first injection causes a general reaction or a well-defined painful swelling, it is probably advisable to discontinue the immunization and not administer a second dose. A second dose should definitely not be administered if the swelling at the injection site develops a concentric disc that is initially warm, then turns cold, becomes devoid of hair, weeps, and eventually sloughs.

Caution must be used when deciding whether to use the bacterin in animals exposed to strangles. Animals incubating the disease must not be immunized, since severe allergic reactions can result. In an outbreak, those animals appearing healthy should be separated from those with the clinical signs of the disease. Temperatures on all apparently healthy animals should be taken twice a day. If temperatures remain normal for 3 days, vaccination can be initiated. In animals exhibiting a fever, temperatures should be taken twice daily for a longer period of time. In animals that remain free of clinical signs of the disease and whose temperatures return to normal and remain normal for 3 days, vaccination can then be started.[18]

Treatment. Strangles must be vigorously treated as soon as signs are first noticed. Animals should be isolated to prevent the spread of the disease. Appropriate anti-infective drugs should be administered under the direction of a veterinarian. Penicillin G is the drug of choice in treating streptococcal infections. For a discussion on the use of penicillin G in horses, see Chapter 3.

Tetanus

Tetanus is caused by *Clostridium tetani.* The signs of the disease are caused by tetanus toxin, which is produced by *C. tetani.* Horses with tetanus develop severe muscular spasms, referred to as "tetany." Tetany results from the toxin causing "short circuiting" in the spinal cord. Stimuli such as light or noise cause severe episodes of muscular spasms. Death, which occurs in a high percentage of affected animals, is due to paralysis of the muscles of respiration.

Prevention

Passive immunization. In the past the primary mode of protecting animals against tetanus was by means of passive immunization.

Tetanus antitoxin is given shortly after an injury. Tetanus antitoxin is obtained from horses that have been immunized with tetanus toxoid. The antitoxin is periodically collected from the blood of actively immunized horses, processed, and distributed in vials containing a specified number of international units. Most commonly 1500 to 3000 IU are given subcutaneously to horses.

Effectiveness. The effectiveness of tetanus antitoxin administered in this way is questionable. Most equine practitioners do not believe that 3000 IU of tetanus antitoxin will adequately protect horses. As an alternative, active immunization of horses against tetanus should be practiced.

Toxicity. Tetanus antitoxin may produce liver damage in horses to which it is administered. Occasionally they develop severe icteris (jaundice), 27 to 160 days after administration of biologics of equine origin, indicating liver damage. Animals show neurological signs such as restlessness, excitement, aimless walking, or pressing their head or thorax against fixed objects. They may have visual impairment, tremors, and an unsteady gait. These signs are due to toxic products that build up in the blood as a result of inadequate liver function. If the disease does prove fatal, animals usually die between 12 and 48 hours after signs are first noted. The mortality has been reported to vary between 53% and 89%. Those animals that recover are generally markedly improved on the fourth or fifth day and are nearly normal after a week. Pathological studies have indicated severe liver damage.[19] Although the liver disease has not been proved to be directly related to a virus or antigen contained in biologics of equine origin, clinical evidence strongly suggests such a relationship. It is therefore highly advisable to avoid the necessity for using tetanus antitoxin by actively immunizing horses with tetanus toxoid.

Active immunization. Actively immunizing horses against tetanus is an effective means of preventing the disease.

There are some indications that in mares

immunized with tetanus toxoid, after five years the level of antibodies may drop below that which would provide protection. However, when they are reinoculated, the recall of antibodies is excellent. Higher levels of antibodies may be reached after reinoculation than the animals originally possessed with their initial inoculation.[23]

High levels of circulating antitoxins are developed in foals when they receive colostrum from toxoid immunized mares that received booster injections 2½ months before foaling.[8]

Tetanus toxoid specifically prepared for use in horses is administered intramuscularly at the rate of 1 or 2 ml, depending on the brand that is used. The first year two injections a month apart are given. Single annual booster injections should be administered after initial vaccination.

Foals can be immunized against tetanus with tetanus toxoid after they are 3 months of age. The same dose is given to foals and adult horses.

Treatment. The treatment of tetanus is most difficult, requiring skill, patience, and hard work on the part of the attending veterinarian, owners, and attendants to the animal. Generally, animals must be kept in a dark, quiet area to prevent induction of tetany by external stimuli. Depressant drugs like the phenothiazine tranquilizers are used to keep the animal quiet and to lessen excitability. In addition, antibiotics are often administered parenterally to combat organisms at the site of the wound where the *C. tetani* have set up residence.

Traditionally tetanus antitoxin has been administered to horses afflicted with tetanus. The therapeutic effectiveness of tetanus antitoxin has been questioned. However, a new method of administering antitoxin may hold out greater hope for its effectiveness. In one report, investigators believed that they increased the recovery rate from tetanus 50% to 77.5% by administering 30,000 IU of tetanus antitoxin to foals and 50,000 IU to adults in the subarachnoid space of the central nervous system after withdrawing an equal volume of cerebral spinal fluid.[17]

Special conditions
Equine genital infections

Although cases of infertility in horses resulting from infection of the genital tract by bacteria do occur, the mere presence of bacteria in the vagina, cervix, or uterus is no proof that they are causing disease.

In a recent article reviewing the use of anti-infective drugs in the uterus of mares, Davis and Abbitt[5] made the following points:

1. Frequently, mares and stallions have genital tract infections, but they remain fertile and show no evidence of disease.

2. Sometimes genital bacterial infections may be associated with lower conception rates.

3. Among the organisms commonly cultured from the genital tracts of mares are *Streptococcus* species, 50%; *Escherichia coli*, 17%; *Klebsiella pneumoniae*, 8%; *Staphylococcus* species, 8%; and *Corynebacterium* species, 3%.

4. Pathogenic fungi also cause genital infections in mares.

5. Many studies show no difference in conception rates between groups of mares treated with intrauterine anti-infective drugs and nontreated mares.

6. In Great Britain there is no significant difference between the ratios of infertile to fertile mares before and since the advent of anti-infective drugs.

7. Some anti-infective drugs cause damage to the lining of the uterus.

8. The indiscriminate use of anti-infectives in the genital tract may result in changes of the normal flora with a shift to more pathogenic bacteria, the establishment of pathogenic fungi, and/or the development of resistant strains of bacteria.

9. The best defense against most genital infections is the defense system of the animal. During estrus, mares have a high ability to clear the uterus of infection.

10. To clear infections, estrus can be induced by the uterine infusion of 500 ml sterile saline solution or by the administration of prostaglandins (Chapter 16).

11. Anti-infectives should only be used in the genital tract of mares when there are a

positive culture, clinical signs, and a history of infertility. The choice of the anti-infective should be made on the basis of clinical signs, culture, and sensitivity.*

The abuse of anti-infective agents continues in mares, and the incidence of pathogenic fungi appears on the increase. *Candida* species have been frequently encountered. Many cases of *Candida* infection are associated with infertility. For this condition the intrauterine application of nystatin, an antifungal antibiotic, has been recommended.[26]

Equine intestinal infections

Like other species, horses of any age can develop inflammation of the intestinal tract in response to infection with pathogenic bacteria. Frequently, pathogenic bacteria are present in the intestine without causing disease. When disease results, signs such as diarrhea, fever, and dehydration may occur. Severe infections can result in shock and death.

A knowledgeable skilled clinician is required to design an effective course of therapy. Although in properly selected cases the use of anti-infective therapy may be beneficial, in other cases anti-infectives will have no effect or may even do harm. Anti-infective drugs are harmful in the treatment of intestinal infections when they do not affect the pathogen but kill off normal intestinal bacteria, thereby allowing the pathogens to proliferate. In addition, it has been shown that in many infections of horses by *Salmonella* species, antibiotics that were effective against the pathogens when tested in culture had little if any effect on the outcome of the clinical infection.[15,16]

In severe infections, supportive therapy is much more important than the use of anti-infectives. In treating intestinal infections of horses the primary focus should be to prevent dehydration by means of intensive water and electrolyte therapy, as discussed in Chapter 17. Secondary anti-infectives may

be used when the experience of the clinician or results of a culture examination indicate that they might be effective. The selection, dose, and route of administration of the appropriate anti-infective depends on the nature of the infection. Drugs such as intestinal protectants and antispasmodics (Chapter 19) may also be used.

Miscellaneous bacterial infections

Horses suffer from many bacterial infections in addition to those discussed previously. Mixed bacterins containing numerous species of bacteria are commercially available to protect horses from a variety of bacterial diseases. In our opinion, mixed bacterins are of no value in protecting horses from most bacterial diseases.

Mixed equine bacterin formula No. 1. Mixed equine bacterin formula No. 1 contains *Streptococcus* (pyogenic) (30%), *Pasteurella multocida* (30%), *Staphylococcus aureus* (10%), and *Escherichia coli* (20%).

In some commercial preparations the bacteria that cause strangles, *Streptococcus equi*, may be the pyogenic streptococcus used in the bacterin. Such preparations should be avoided because allergic reactions can result if *S. equi*–containing bacterins are improperly administered. It is also better to use specific strangles bacterin rather than a mixed equine bacteria to immunize against strangles.

Effectiveness. The wisdom of including *Pasteurella multocida* in the mixed equine formula No. 1 bacterin is questionable. It has not been demonstrated that this bacteria produces clinical disease in horses. In addition, neither *Staphylococcus aureus* nor *Staphylococcus albus* are important pathogens of the horse. It is also doubtful that *E. coli* in the mixed equine bacterin offers much protection. There are various strains of *E. coli* that do not share common antigens. Selecting the appropriate serotype to protect against a natural encounter is unlikely.[21]

Mixed equine bacterin formula No. 2. The mixed equine bacterin formula No. 2 has not been produced commercially in recent years in the United States. In this formula,

---

*Modified from Davis, L. E., and Abbitt, B.: Clinical pharmacology of antibacterial drugs in the uterus of the mare, J. Am. Vet. Med. Assoc. **170:**204, 1977.

Pasteurella multocida (30%) is replaced by *Salmonella abortivioquina* (30%).

References

1. Binn, L. N., Sponseller, M. L., Wooding, W. L., McConnell, I. J., Spertzel, R. O., and Yager, R. H.: Efficacy of the attenuated westernal encephalitis vaccine in equine animals, Am. J. Vet. Res. **27**:1599, 1966.
2. Blood, D. C., and Henderson, J. A.: Veterinary medicine, ed. 4, Baltimore, 1974, The Williams & Wilkins Co.
3. Brown, D. G.: Clinical changes in burros and Shetland ponies after vaccination with Venezuelan equine encephalomyelitis vaccine, TC-83, Vet. Med. Small Anim. Clin. **67**:505, 1972.
4. Bryans, J. T., and others: Report of the panel for the Symposium on Immunity to Selected Equine Infectious Diseases, J. Am. Vet. Med. Assoc. **155**:235, 1969.
5. Davis, L. E., and Abbitt, B.: Clinical pharmacology of antibacterial drugs in the uterus of the mare, J. Am. Vet. Med. Assoc. **170**:204, 1977.
6. Engelbrecht, H.: Vaccination against strangles, J. Am. Vet. Med. Assoc. **155**:425, 1969.
7. Fallon, E. H.: The clinical aspects of streptococcic infections of horses, J. Am. Vet. Med. Assoc. **155**:413, 15.
8. Fessler, J. F.: A practical program for equine immunization, Mod. Vet. Pract. **46**:39, July 1965.
9. Hays, M. B.: Definitive efficacy and safety testing for equine encephalitis vaccine, J. Am. Vet. Med. Assoc. **150**:167, 1967.
10. Hughes, J. P.: A field trial of a live-virus western encephalitis vaccine, J. Am. Vet. Med. Assoc. **150**:167, 1967.
11. Jochim, M. M., Barber, T. L., and Luedke, A. J.: Venezuelan equine encephalomyelitis: antibody response in vaccinated horses and resistance to infection with virulent virus, J. Am. Vet. Med. Assoc. **162**:280, 1973.
12. Jochim, M. M., Barber, T. L., and Luedke, A. J.: Venezuelan equine encephalomyelitis: antibody response against eastern, western, and Venezuelan equine encephalomyelitis, J. Am. Vet. Med. Assoc. **165**:621, 1974.
13. McCollum, W. H.: Development of a modified virus strain and vaccine for equine viral arteritis, J. Am. Vet. Med. Assoc. **155**:318, 1969.
14. Monlux, W. S., Luedke, A. J., and Bowne, J.: Central nervous system response of horses to Venezuelan equine encephalomyelitis vaccine (TC-83), J. Am. Vet. Med. Assoc. **161**:265, 1962.
15. Morse, E. V., Duncan, M. A., Page, E. A., and Fessler, J. F.: Salmonellosis in Equidae: a study of 23 cases, Cornell Vet. **66**:198, April 1976.
16. Morse, E. V., Fessler, J. F.: The treatment of salmonellosis in Equidae, Mod. Vet. Pract. **57**:47, Jan. 1976.
17. Muylle, E. W., Oyaert, W., Ooma, L., and Decraemere, H.: Treatment of tetanus in the horse by injections of tetanus antitoxin into the subarachnoid space, J. Am. Vet. Med. Assoc. **167**:47, 1975.
18. O'Dea, J. C.: Comments on vaccination against strangles, J. Am. Vet. Med. Assoc. **155**:427, 1969.
19. Panciera, R. J.: Serum hepatitis in the horse, J. Am. Vet. Med. Assoc. **155**:408, 1969.
20. Peacock, G. V.: Biological requirements and control of equine rhinopneumonitis vaccine (live virus), J. Am. Vet. Med. Assoc. **155**:310, 1969.
21. Phillips, C. E.: Mixed equine bacterins, J. Am. Vet. Med. Assoc. **155**:432, 1969.
22. Rossoff, I. W.: Handbook of veterinary drugs, New York, 1974, Springer Publishing Co.
23. Scarnell, J.: Duration of protection provided by tetanus toxoid, Vet. Rec. **95**:62, 1974.
24. Spertzel, R. O., and Kahn, D. E.: Safety and efficacy of an attenuated Venezuelan equine encephalomyelitis vaccine for use in Equidae, J. Am. Vet. Med. Assoc. **159**:731, 1971.
25. Walton, T. E., and Johnson, K. M.: Persistence of neutralizing antibody in Equidae vaccinated with Venezuelan equine encephalomyelitis vaccine strain TC-83, J. Am. Vet. Med. Assoc. **161**:916, 1972.
26. Zafracas, A. M.: *Candida* infection of the genital tract in thoroughbred mares, J. Reprod. Fertil. **23**:349, 1975.

Additional readings

Byrne, R. J.: Immunity against eastern and western equine encephalomyelitis viruses, J. Am. Vet. Med. Assoc. **155**:365, 1969.
Knight, H. D.: Corynebacterial infections in the horse: problems of prevention, J. Am. Vet. Med. Assoc. **155**:446, 1969.
Knight, H. D.: Tetanus immunity in foals, Mod. Vet. Pract. **54**:21, Sept. 1973.
Morter, R. L., Williams, R. D., Bolte, H., and Freeman, M. J.: Equine leptospirosis, J. Am. Vet. Med. Assoc. **155**:436, 1969.
Roberts, S. J.: Comments on equine leptospirosis, J. Am. Vet. Med. Assoc. **155**:442, 1969.
Schroeder, W. G.: Suggestions for handling horses exposed to rabies, J. Am. Vet. Med. Assoc. **155**:1842, 1969.

8

INTRODUCTION TO DRUGS USED IN
Veterinary dermatology

There are many causes of skin disease in animals. Thus a large number of animal health products relate to diseases of the skin. Obviously before treatment is initiated, it is important for veterinarians to make the proper diagnosis and prescribe proper treatment. For example, in the treatment of flea allergy dermatitis, treatment is aimed at freeing the animal from flea infestation; in addition, some form of therapy is used to treat the lesions already present in the animal.

A primary precaution in the treatment of skin conditions is to avoid overtreatment.

DOSAGE FORMS OF TOPICAL DRUGS

In the treatment of skin conditions, a wide variety of topical preparations may be used. Some products are irritating, further inflaming already diseased skin. If fistulous tracts or denuded areas are present on the skin, some topical medications act as foreign bodies and delay healing of the lesions.

When the veterinarian decides to use topical therapy, he usually clips the hair from and cleans the affected area prior to applying medication. (An exception is in the use of external pesticides.)

Most preparations applied topically to the skin will fall into one of the following categories.

Aqueous solutions

Aqueous (water) solutions are applied to the skin in various ways. They may be simply sponged or poured onto affected areas or applied on wetted gauze sponges and left in contact with the lesion as a wet dressing for 15 minutes once or twice a day. Frequently, affected areas—particularly the feet—are soaked in containers of the solution. Solutions are usually applied for at least 15 minutes two to four times a day.

Various types of drugs are applied as solutions. The most common drugs applied in solution are astringents, antiseptics, and some antibiotics. Astringent solutions precipitate proteins on surface cells. The astringent does not kill surface cells but does reduce their permeability. This reduction of permeability of the skin restricts the passage of water to upper layers of the skin and has a drying effect on the outer layer of the skin. Thus astringent solutions reduce weeping of skin lesions. Anti-infective solutions are used topically in aqueous solutions when the clinician wishes to avoid vehicles that are oily or viscous.

Medications in solution are poorly absorbed through intact skin, and penetration into the deeper layers of skin is limited. Ideally, solutions should be sterile, particularly when applied to large lesions in which the continuity of the skin is broken by cuts, burns, or abrasions.

Topical aqueous solutions include the following.

Burow's solution (USP). Burow's solution is usually used at a concentration of 1:40 in cold water three times a day for 30 minutes. It is an astringent and somewhat antiseptic. The active ingredient is aluminum acetate.

Epsom salt (magnesium sulfate). A 1:65 solution can be made by adding a tablespoon of magnesium sulfate to each quart of warm water. The resulting solution is hypertonic, thus increasing the permeability of the skin. Frequently, hypertonic solutions of magnesium sulfate are used for their osmotic effect to draw out serum and cellular debris (exudates) in puncture wounds and superficial skin lesions.

Isotonic saline solution. An approximate isotonic saline solution can be made by adding 1 teaspoon of table salt to 1 pint of water. Because isotonic saline has the same osmotic pressure as serum and intercellular tissue fluid, it neither increases nor decreases the permeability of skin. It is an excellent solution for soothing or cleaning skin lesions. Sometimes drugs are added to isotonic saline to be used as wet dressings. For example, neomycin sulfate, 0.5% solution in normal saline, is an approximate isotonic solution used as an antibacterial soak for infections by organisms sensitive to neomycin.

Alcoholic solutions (tinctures)

Tinctures are solutions of medicinal agents, most commonly antiseptics, which usually contain 30% to 70% alcohol. Follow-ing are the most commonly used tinctures in veterinary medicine.

Iodine tincture (USP). This is a solution of 2% free iodine with 2.4% sodium iodide (NaI) in 47% ethyl alcohol. It is commonly used for superficial cuts and scratches. It is also used to disinfect the navel of newborn foals and calves.

Gentian violet (crystal violet) tincture, 3% to 5%. This tincture is used on superficial skin lesions. In addition, because of the staining properties of gentian violet, it is also used in the treatment of bovine pinkeye (Chapter 5).

Strong iodine tincture (NF). Strong iodine tincture contains 7 gm of iodine and 5 gm of potassium iodide (KI) per 100 ml of 85% ethyl alcohol. Because it is a strong irritant, it should not be used in open wounds. This tincture is used as a counterirritant in lameness (Chapter 20).

Lotions

Lotions are liquid or semiliquid, are used locally on the skin, and usually have as their base water, alcohol, glycerin, and/or propylene glycol. They contain active ingredients in solution or suspension that, after the lotion dries, are left as a powderlike deposit on the skin. Like powders, they tend not to penetrate the skin.

Lotions used in veterinary medicine include the following.

White lotion. White lotion is prepared as follows: zinc sulfate, 4.5 gm, plus lead acetate, 6 gm, plus distilled water to make 100 ml. The two chemicals react to form soluble zinc acetate and insoluble lead sulfate. The resulting suspension is commonly used as an astringent for treating minor open wounds. It is applied to the wound directly and may be covered with a bandage.

Calamine lotion. This suspension of zinc oxide and polyethylene glycol in water is used topically as a weak astringent and protective agent.

Liniments

Liniments have a water or alcoholic base in which an oily or fatty substance is emulsified and suspended. Liniments usually penetrate the skin better than lotions and are designed to be rubbed or massaged into the affected area. See Chapter 20 for a further discussion of liniments.

Soaps and detergents

Soaps and detergents are used for cleansing the coat and skin. Because many commercially available soaps and detergents that are used for laundry and dishwashing are severely irritating to the skin, they should not be used to wash animals. Only products specifically formulated for animal shampoos should be used. Generally, a shampoo is used only when the skin is intact, since shampoos are irritating to large ulcerated areas.

Sometimes medication is added to the shampoos. For example, pesticides for the treatment of flea or tick infestation and iodine preparations for the treatment of skin bacterial or fungal infections are frequently added to animal shampoos. These medicated shampoos usually are left in contact with the skin for a period of time before rinsing. All shampoos, medicated or not, should always be thoroughly rinsed from the skin.

Powders

Powder is used as a vehicle for various drugs, such as antibiotics, pesticides, and antiseptics. Insoluble powders are commonly formulated with talc, starches, or chalk. Powders have a drying effect, since they adsorb water and oils from the skin surface. They also reduce skin friction. Powders should not be used on open sores because they can be irritating and may encrust and prevent proper drainage of exudates. Some antibacterial powders are available in water-soluble bases. These can be applied to ulcerated lesions.

Ointments and creams

Classically, ointments were semisolid preparations made up in a base of fats and oils to be applied externally. Currently the term "ointment" includes a broad range of semisolid dose forms designed to be applied externally by inunction (rubbing in). Creams, semisolid preparations usually made by emulsification of both aqueous and nonaqueous substances, fall under the general category of ointments but are usually more cosmetically pleasing and often water washable.

Ointments and creams frequently are employed as vehicles in which drugs are suspended or dissolved. Anti-infective drugs, corticosteroids, and keratolytic drugs are often applied in ointment form. Ointments and creams are also used for their effects as sunscreens, protectants, or emollients.

Ointments may disrupt the horny or outer layer of the epidermis, which improves the chance of drugs being absorbed. The amount of drug absorbed increases the longer an ointment is rubbed in and the greater the pressure used. The addition of salicylic acid to an ointment increases permeability. Ointments may interfere with water loss from the epidermis, which may result in retention of water in the skin. This makes the skin softer. Because they can plug the skin's oil glands (sebaceous glands), ointments can cause inflammation of the hair follicles. Ointments should only be placed on skin after the hair has been clipped and cleaned.

Ointments are classified as follows.

Hydrophobic ointments. Hydrophobic ointments consist of oils that do not mix with water. Examples of hydrophobic oils are castor oil, white petrolatum (USP), and lard (USP), through whose oily film water will not pass. Generally, a hydrophobic ointment should not be placed over a lesion that is discharging an exudate because the ointment either will be lifted off by the exudate and thus be ineffective or it will tend to seal the lesion and prevent necessary drainage of the exudate.

Hydrophilic ointments. Hydrophilic ointments are manufactured from hydrophilic oils, which mix with water. They tend to let water pass through the film of ointment and will mix with an exudate. Examples of hydrophilic oils are hydrophilic petrolatum (USP), carbowax, and polysorbate 80 (USP).

THERAPEUTIC CLASSES OF DRUGS USED TO TREAT SKIN DISEASES
Topical anesthetics

When applied to intact skin, some topical anesthetics are absorbed. They block the conduction of nerve impulses from the region to which they are applied, thereby reducing pain or itching. Generally, they are applied in a cream or ointment base but are not used frequently because their action tends to be relatively short. The most commonly used topical anesthetics in veterinary medicine are lidocaine, tetracaine, and butacaine.

Antipruritics

Antipruritics are drugs that reduce or prevent itching. Antipruritics are important because when animals itch, they scratch or bite at their skin, which continues irritation and prevents the lesions from healing. In actual practice, corticosteroids and tranquilizers are both used more frequently than antipruritics to prevent animals from scratching and biting at skin lesions.

Trimeprazine is sometimes given parenterally or orally to dogs and cats because it is believed to be antipruritic. In dogs it is given at the rate of 2.2 mg/kg by subcutaneous or intramuscular injection followed by 1.1 to 2.2 mg/kg one to three times a day. By the third day the dose should be reduced by half.[7] It is given at the reduced rate until therapy is no longer required.

Tranquilizers

Tranquilizers are used in skin diseases to sedate the animal and to help prevent self-mutilation. Generally, they are dispensed for oral administration for small animals and for injection or oral administration for large animals. For a discussion of individual tranquilizers see Chapter 14.

Corticosteroids

The corticosteroids are a drug group with action similar to hydrocortisone, a natural hormone produced by the adrenal gland. For a discussion of corticosteroids see Chapter 16.

When used to treat skin diseases, corticosteroids reduce inflammation, decrease capillary permeability, and reduce pain and itching. Therefore their use tends to reduce self-mutilation on the part of the animal. One disadvantage of the corticosteroids is that they increase the chance of infection by reducing the body's defenses to infection. They also retard healing and may cause sodium retention.

Systemic corticosteroids should be given only under close veterinary supervision. The dose, which will vary according to the type of corticosteroid used and the condition being treated, must be carefully regulated.

To minimize their toxic effects, when corticosteroids are used to treat skin diseases, they are often applied topically. Even when the skin is abraded, the amount of corticosteroid absorbed is generally not sufficient to warrant concern.

Antibacterials

Included in the classification of antibacterials are antibiotics, sulfa drugs, and nitrofurans. (See Chapter 3 for a more detailed discussion of antibacterial drugs.) Antibacterials can be administered topically or systemically. When they are applied topically, they are usually applied in either liquid, ointment, or soluble powder formulations.

Antibiotics commonly used topically include bacitracin, gramicidin, neomycin, polymyxin B, and cuprimyxin. Nitrofurans are also commonly used topically.

In severe bacterial infections of the skin, antibiotics should be administered systemically. Common antibiotics for this purpose are the penicillins, tetracyclines, and chloramphenicol. Other antibiotics are used when culture and sensitivity tests so indicate.

Fungicides

To treat fungous infections of the skin effectively, systemic and/or topical fungicides are used.

Griseofulvin. One systemic fungicide used in veterinary medicine is the antibiotic griseofulvin (Fulvicin). After oral administration, griseofulvin is partially absorbed from the gut and is metabolized by the liver. The dose that allows effective concentrations of the drug in the skin depends on the amount absorbed from the gut and the rate of metabolism of the drug in the species to which it is administered.[3] If the particle size of the drug is decreased, absorption from the gut is increased and the dose can be decreased. For this reason, griseofulvin is available as tablets made with ultrafine or microcrystalline griseofulvin (Fulvicin UF).

Griseofulvin has an affinity for the skin. In humans it reaches its maximum concentrations in the skin after about 5 days of administration. One could therefore expect to see some improvement of the skin condition in a week. The skin acts as a reservoir for the drug. As with other reservoir systems, when the drug is discontinued, there is a shift of the drug from the skin to the plasma. When the drug is discontinued in an individual, skin levels drop to unmeasurable amounts in 2 or 3 days. If griseofulvin is administered along with topical medication, the chances of successful treatment are increased. Concurrent administration of phenobarbital may lower blood levels of griseofulvin.[1] Other potential problems caused by the drug include the following[7]: (1) it causes digestive disturbances, pruritus, and malaise in cats; (2) it may be metabolized more rapidly when given with phenylbutazone; and (3) it may produce fetal abnormalities when given to pregnant cats.

The use of griseofulvin in dogs is discussed in Chapter 9, and its use in horses is discussed in Chapter 10.

Tolnaftate. Tolnaftate (USP) is used topically, especially in small animals, for the treatment of fungal skin infections. It is a synthetic product with fungicidal activity. Tolnaftate is effective in humans against a wide variety of dermatomycotic infections, but its effectiveness against common dermatomycoses of animals is questionable (Chapter 9).

Captan. Captan is a fungicide used in shampoos or as a suspension applied to the skin. In addition to treating the animal with captan, the premises and such equipment as brushes, currycombs, and harnesses can be treated with captan to prevent the fungus from reinfecting the animal.

Miscellaneous fungicides. For topical therapy, three fatty acids—undecylenic, ca-

prylic, and propionic—have been used topically as fungistatic agents. Thiabendazole, miconazole, and organic and inorganic iodine preparations are also used topically in the treatment of fungous infections.

Emollients

Emollients are generally ointments or creams that are used to soften the skin.

Keratolytics

Keratolytics are drugs that help to soften excessive keratinized tissue so that it can be mechanically removed. Salicylic acid is an example of a keratolytic drug.

External pesticides

A wide variety of chemicals are used to treat parasitic infestations of the skin. The ideal external pesticide should be toxic to the parasite (efficacy) and nontoxic to the host (safety). In practice, none of those available meet these ideal criteria. Toxicity to both host and parasite is widely variable, and the practitioner strives to select the best possible compromise between safety and efficacy for each patient.

How toxic the preparation is to the parasite is determined by the following factors:

1. The pesticide used in the formulation.
2. The concentration of the active ingredient in the formulation.
3. The nature of the formulation (for example, powder as opposed to an oil solution or emulsion).
4. The location of the parasite. For example, a demodectic mange mite lives in the hair follicle. A normally effective compound in a suitable concentration in a powder base will not be effective against demodectic mange because the compound does not come in contact with the parasite. However, if that same product is in an oil base, its absorption into the skin will be increased, thereby increasing its effectiveness in the treatment of mange.

How toxic the preparation is to the host will be determined by the following factors:

1. The type of pesticide used in the formulation.

2. The concentration of the pesticide in the formulation.

3. The nature of the formulation, that is, whether it is in a liquid or powder form. Generally, to reduce toxicity, the drugs are developed in such a way that they are not readily absorbed from the skin.

4. The genetic and physiological state of the animal. Certain species are more likely to suffer the toxic effects of pesticides than others. For example, because cattle have lower cholinesterase levels, they are more susceptible to organophosphate toxicity than horses. Even within a species, individuals may have increased chances of developing toxic reactions. For example, Brahma cattle are so susceptible to organophosphates that they are not used in that breed. In addition, animals that are emaciated are more susceptible to the effects of parasiticides.

5. The integrity of the skin. Antiparasitic agents are more readily absorbed into the system from abraded skin.

6. Previous exposure to pesticides.

The use of external pesticides must be undertaken with concern for the possible consequences. Care must be taken to avoid toxic reactions in man and animals. Environmental consequences must be considered, and the food and water of farm animals must be kept free of pesticides so that residues in meat and dairy products do not result. This problem is discussed in greater detail in Chapter 10.

Many restrictions and regulations govern the use of pesticides. These regulations change rapidly, and the seller and user of pesticides must keep informed of these changes. Agencies involved in the control of pesticides include the Environmental Protection Agency, U.S. Department of Agriculture, FDA, and various similar agencies of state governments. Generally, university veterinary and agriculture extension departments provide up-to-date information about pesticide regulations and recommendations.

All external pesticides used in veterinary medicine fall into one of the following groups: chlorinated hydrocarbons, organophosphates, carbamates, and miscellaneous substances.

Chlorinated hydrocarbons. This group of pesticides began with DDT. (In the United States DDT is no longer used as a veterinary pesticide.) These are stable compounds that tend to persist in the environment. Chlorinated hydrocarbon compounds are fat soluble and therefore partition into body fat. For this reason they are more toxic in thin or debilitated animals with reduced amounts of body fat. The inability of these animals to store normal amounts of chlorinated hydrocarbons in fat results in higher blood concentrations of the agent. The storage of chlorinated hydrocarbons in fat and their long biologic half-lives should be kept in mind, since these characteristics permit accumulation of these compounds with repeated low level exposure. Chlorinated hydrocarbon pesticides are readily excreted in the milk.

Signs of chlorinated hydrocarbon poisoning in animals include disturbances in equilibrium, irritability, tremors, convulsions, coma, and death. Any animal suffering from chlorinated hydrocarbon toxicity should be treated by a veterinarian immediately.

Chlorinated hydrocarbons include DDT, DDD, methoxychlor, lindane, chlordane, and toxaphene. For the most part, they are not used on cats. Cats are most susceptible to the toxic effects of chlorinated hydrocarbons, a susceptibility probably resulting from their licking habits and the resultant ingestion of chemicals. In addition, cats tend to be thinner than dogs and therefore do not have the fat to pull the chemicals out of the bloodstream.

Methoxychlor. Methoxychlor is frequently used as an external pesticide. Its toxicity to mammals is about $1/25$ that of DDT. Because of this, it is often included in preparations for cats. Apparently methoxychlor is destroyed in the body before it can be deposited in any significant amounts in fatty tissue. Link[4] cites a study in which cattle were sprayed with solutions containing either 0.5% DDT or 0.5% methoxychlor. Two weeks after treatment the fat contained 11 parts per million (ppm) of DDT compared to 2.8 ppm of methoxychlor. Ten weeks later no methoxychlor was detected in the fat, whereas 5.3 ppm of DDT remained. DDT was still present in the fat at significant levels (1.7 ppm) 27 weeks after the one-time treatment.

Because it is not readily stored in the fat, methoxychlor also appears in lower concentrations in milk samples than other chlorinated hydrocarbon pesticides. However, these lower concentrations are still significant, and they prohibit the use of methoxychlor on lactating dairy cows.

Lindane (gamma isomer of benzene hexachloride). Technical benzene hexachloride contains many isomers. One is lindane, the isomer with the highest activity against external parasites. Lindane is less toxic than technical benzene hexachloride, which is as toxic to mammals as DDT. Lindane is only one-fourth as toxic to mammals as DDT.

Chlordane. Chlordane is highly residual in the environment. For this reason, its use has been discouraged. It is available as a wettable powder, a dust, an oil solution, and a concentrated solution for use as an emulsion in water. Chlordane is approximately five times more toxic to humans than DDT.

Toxaphene. Toxaphene, like most chlorinated hydrocarbon pesticides, is sold as a dust, a wettable powder, in solutions, and as an emulsifiable concentrate. It is readily stored in the fat of animals but is less likely to be excreted in the milk than DDT. Toxaphene is four times more toxic to mammals than DDT. This prohibits its use in dogs and cats. However, it has been used in beef cattle, sheep, goats, horses, and hogs.

Organophosphate pesticides. Organophosphates, far more toxic than chlorinated hydrocarbon pesticides, were originally developed as war gases. In domestic animals, organophosphate pesticides are used in the following ways:

- Topically as a dust, spray, dip, or vapor for local effect
- Systemically applied to the skin in a vehicle that is readily absorbed
- In the surroundings to reduce the number of external parasites in the environment and thus the direct damage caused by parasites or their effect as disease transmitters.
- Orally for effect against parasites em-

bedded within the skin or to treat infections of internal parasites (Chapters 11 to 13).

Some understanding of the physiology of the nervous system is necessary to understand the action of the organophosphate pesticides. The following points are important to this understanding.

The major subdivisions of the nervous system are the *central nervous system*, consisting of the brain and spinal cord, and the *peripheral nervous system*, which consists of nerves and various connections (synapses) between the central nervous system and the location where the nerve effects its action or receives information. Peripheral nerves, which send electrical impulses from the organs to the central nervous system, are *afferent nerves*. Nerves that carry impulses from the central nervous system to nervous system connections or to organs are *efferent nerves*.

Efferent nerves are classified in two major categories. Those which control voluntary movement are the *somatic efferent nerves*, and those which control the muscles and glands over which an animal has no voluntary control are the *involuntary*, or *autonomic*, *nerves* (Fig. 8-1).

Glands and muscles innervated by the autonomic nervous system are controlled by two separate divisions of the autonomic system, which have opposite effects on the target organ. One division, which in its extreme is characterized by the "fight or flight" syndrome, contains the *sympathetic nerves*. The other, which is characteristic of an animal at rest, contains the *parasympathetic nerves*. Stimulation of the sympathetic nerves tends to cause the eyes to dilate and the heart to beat faster. Stimulation of the parasympathetic nerves tends to bring about constriction of the pupil, slowing of the heart rate, increase in salivation, and movement of the intestinal tract.

Where the efferent nerves end (the neuromuscular junction), their electrical impulse causes a chemical to be released which acts on the target organ and causes a reaction. Sympathetic nerves induce their effects on target organs by causing norepinephrine to be secreted. Somatic nerves and parasym-

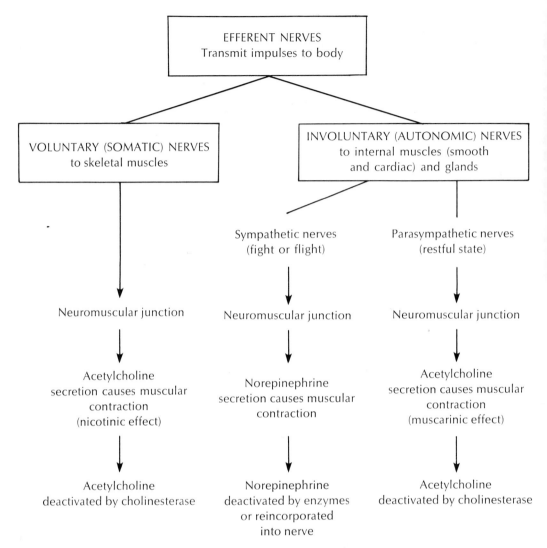

Fig. 8-1. Efferent nerve stimulation of muscular activity.

pathetic nerves bring about their effect on the target organ by causing acetylcholine to be secreted.

The effect of acetylcholine on skeletal muscles is referred to as the "nicotinic effect." Its effect on those organs innervated by parasympathetic nerves is called the "muscarinic effect." The effects of acetylcholine are then reversed by an enzyme, cholinesterase, which breaks down acetylcholine into inactive components. Muscles innervated by somatic or parasympathetic nerves can relax only if cholinesterase breaks down acetylcholine.

Organophosphate pesticides form nonfunctional complexes with cholinesterase, preventing the deactivation of acetylcholine. They thus accentuate the nicotinic and muscarinic effects of acetylcholine. These complexes are irreversible. Without therapeutic intervention the complexes are excreted from the body intact and new molecules of cholinesterase must be produced to return the animal to normal.

Toxic effects of organophosphate poisons are primarily noted by signs relating to the muscarinic effect of acetylcholine. Signs such as hyperactivity of the intestinal tract, diarrhea, increased salivation, increased tearing, constriction of the pupil, decreased heart rate, and drop in blood pressure are typical. In addition, in severe cases of organophosphate poisoning, the nicotinic effects of acetylcholine will be noted; voluntary muscles at first twitch and then become paralyzed. The causes of death from organophosphate poisoning include constriction of the bronchi, decrease in blood pressure, and paralysis of the voluntary muscles of respiration.

The poisoning of humans or animals by organophosphate preparations must be treated as an emergency by highly skilled medical personnel. In severe cases artificial respiration is necessary. Medical treatment consists of administering atropine and pralidoxime chloride. Atropine blocks the muscarinic effect of acetylcholine. It does not block the nicotinic effect such as paralysis of the respiratory muscles. Administration of pralidoxime chloride reverses the binding of the complex of organophosphate and cholinesterase and helps restore functioning of the somatic muscles (nicotinic effect).

In considering therapy for organophosphate poisoning, the following should be remembered. First, acetylcholine stimulates a response (contraction of a muscle or secretion of a gland) at the nerve endings of both somatic efferent nerves and parasympathetic nerves. That response is normally reversed by the enzyme cholinesterase.

Second, the muscarinic effect of acetylcholine can be artificially blocked by atropine. However, atropine does not block the nicotinic effect.

Third, organophosphates form a complex with cholinesterase that prevents its deactivation of acetylcholine. The muscarinic and nicotinic actions of acetylcholine are therefore exaggerated.

Finally, pralidoxime frees cholinesterase from the organophosphate-cholinesterase complex, thereby restoring its ability to deactivate acetylcholine.

When treating organophosphate poisoning, atropine sulfate should be given intravenously until signs such as decreased salivation, dilation of pupils, and increased heart beat are noted. Initial doses are as follows[2]:

Dog and cat	0.1 to 0.2 mg/kg
Cattle	0.5 to 01.0 mg/kg
Horses	0.1 to 0.2 mg/kg

If necessary, additional doses may be given as often as every 10 minutes to animals, except cattle, in which the effects of the initial dose will generally last for 1 to 2 hours.

Pralidoxime chloride is administered intravenously at the following rates[2]:

Dog and cat	20 mg/kg
Cattle	20 mg/kg
Horses	4 mg/kg

If signs persist, treatment may be repeated in 1 hour.

If the organophosphate was ingested, either an emetic or gastric lavage should be administered. If the organophosphate is absorbed from the skin, wash the skin with soap and water. In organophosphate poisoning, morphine and aminophylline are contraindicated. A brief description of some organophosphate pesticides follows.

Ciodrin. Ciodrin is used on dairy and beef cattle, sheep, goats, and hogs to control stable flies, horn flies, lice, and ticks. In cattle it is also used to control mange mites and winter ticks.

Coumaphos. Coumaphos is primarily used in beef cattle to control cattle grubs (*Hypoderma bovis*), which are the larvae of flies. During their life cycle, these insects penetrate the skin near the heel area and travel subcutaneously to the back where they mature and penetrate the skin of the back, causing damage to the hide (Chapter 10). Coumaphos is applied as a liquid to the back and is absorbed systemically, killing the migrating larva. Coumaphos is not used in milking dairy cows because it causes residues in the milk.

Dichlorvos. Dichlorvos has less toxicity than many of the organophosphates and is commonly used topically in a wide variety of animals. Dichlorvos is used in more forms and for the treatment of more conditions than any other organophosphate. It is used as a topical pesticide in flea collars (Chapter 9) and as an antihelmintic (Chapters 11 and 13).

Diazinon. Diazinon is used to control mange, lice, and ticks on cattle, dogs, and sheep. There is little absorption and good residual action on the skin. It can be used in the treatment of cattle with sarcoptic mange by pouring a 0.02% emulsion on the back at 1-month intervals or by spraying cattle with a 0.05% emulsion. Cattle and sheep with psoroptic mange can be dipped in a 0.06% Diazinon emulsion.

Malathion. Malathion is extremely toxic to insects but relatively low in toxicity to mammals. It is available as a dust, wettable powder, emulsifiable liquid, and aerosol. It is commonly contained in cat flea sprays.

Ronnel. Like coumaphos, ronnel acts systemically when applied to the skin. It is used in beef cattle to control grubs and for control of mites and ticks on dogs. It has been given orally to dogs to control fleas and mites.

Ruelene. Ruelene, like coumaphos and ronnel, can be applied to the skin to control cattle grubs.

Carbamates. Carbamates are esters of carbamic acid. They also block the action of cholinesterase. Carbamates used as pesticides are analogs of eserine or physostigmine. (Another analog of eserine is neostigmine, which is used in veterinary medicine to potentiate the effects of acetylcholine on the parasympathetic nervous system [Chapter 19].)

Like organophosphates the carbamates form nonfunctional complexes with cholinesterase. These complexes, however, are reversible, and if given enough time, the complexed molecules of cholinesterase are restored to the functional state. Pralidoxime is of no value in treatment of carbamate poisoning. Atropine is used as the antidote.

The carbamates are not broad-spectrum pesticides, and many of them are extremely toxic to mammals. The most commonly used carbamate in veterinary medicine is carbaryl (Sevin).

Naturally occurring pesticides

Pyrethrins. For mammals the least toxic pesticides are the pyrethrins, which are derived from various species of plants of the genus *Chrysanthemum.* Pyrethrins have excellent "knockdown" power for flies but have virtually no residual action because they are rapidly destroyed when exposed to air and light. Generally, piperonyl butoxide, which by itself has no insecticidal properties, is included in preparations containing pyrethrins to increase their killing power. Pyrethrins and piperonyl butoxide are often used for area fly sprays. In addition, because of their relatively nontoxic properties, they are often included in flea spray preparations and antiflea shampoos.

The mechanism and the reasons for their selective insect toxicity are not totally understood. The rapid paralysis that pyrethrins cause in insects suggests that they act on the nerves or muscles.

Rotenone. Rotenone is obtained from the root of derris plants. It is only used for external parasites such as fleas, lice, and ticks. The powdered form is relatively nontoxic because the active ingredient is not absorbed. However, when rotenone is dissolved in oil, which increases absorption, the toxic potential is increased.

Miscellaneous antiparasitic drugs

Benzyl benzoate (USP). Benzyl benzoate is often used to treat mange (mite infestation) in dogs and horses. It can be toxic to the animal if used over too large a body area for prolonged periods. Signs of toxicity include vomiting, diarrhea, and depression of the cardiac and respiratory functions.

Sulfur. Lime sulfur, a complex of sulfur with calcium and oxygen, is effective in treating some external parasites. Since the discovery of newer compounds, sulfur products have often been overlooked by veterinarians as an effective treatment for external parasites.[6] A 2% lime sulfur dip is effective in treating mange in sheep, cattle, horses, swine, and dogs. Sulfur or compounds of sulfur are also used as ointments. These preparations are safe, effective, and cheap. However, their foul odor may have caused their decline in popularity.

Oils. Most external pesticides are dispensed in oil bases. In many instances the oils themselves have some antiparasitic activity.

Mineral oil. Mineral oil can be effective in killing mites in cats' ears. However, it must come in contact with the parasite. This is often difficult because the parasites may be protected from the oil by the presence of exudates and cellular debris.

Pine oil. Pine oil is a constituent of many pesticide preparations. It is an effective insect repellent.

Tars and creosote. Tars and creosote are somewhat effective as insect repellents. They may be highly irritating to skin and mucous membranes if improperly applied.

Hormones

We have already discussed the use of corticosteroids in the treatment of the skin. Their primary action is to reduce inflammation.

Skin diseases can result when the level of certain hormones in the body is lower than normal or when there is an imbalance of various related hormones, such as the sex hormones. It requires the diagnosis of a skilled practitioner to evaluate these cases and to initiate appropriate therapy. In such instances treatment will be aimed at either replacing the deficient hormone or correcting the imbalance. The thyroid hormone and sex hormones are the ones primarily involved in skin problems.

Dietary supplements

To maintain the health of the skin as well as other organs, a balanced diet is necessary. The nutritional needs of cats and dogs have been well studied and documented. Commercial feeds are available that provide dogs and cats with proper nutrients. Problems of nutrition usually occur when dogs and cats are given insufficient food or poor quality nutrients. Cats and dogs who are overindulged by their owners may also suffer from malnutrition. These animals may be obese and receive diets concocted by their owners that are too high in calories and deficient in essential nutrients.

Instead of purchasing many dietary supplements to improve the condition of pet animals' skin, owners are well advised to feed a proper amount of a high-quality commmercial pet food. In some cases, however, improvement in the appearance of the skin and reduction of itching is obtained by oral administration of preparations containing unsaturated fatty acids. Clinically, many veterinarians have observed a response to some nonspecific itching that is accompanied by dry skin when such products are administered.[5,6]

References

1. Epstein, W. L., Shah, V., and Riegelman, S.: Dermatopharmacology of griseofulvin, Cutis **15**:271, 1975.
2. Freeman, J. I.: Diagnosis and treatment of animals poisoned with organophosphate insecticides, J. Am. Vet. Med. Assoc. **163**:368, 1973.
3. Harris, P. A., and Riegelman, S.: Metabolism of griseofulvin in dogs, J. Pharm. Sci. **58**:93, 1969.
4. Link, R. P. External antiparasitic drugs. In Jones, L. M., editor: Veterinary pharmacology and therapeutics, ed. 3, Ames, Iowa, 1965, Iowa State Press.
5. Monson, W. J.: Nutritional considerations in skin and coat maintenance, Vet. Med. Small Anim. Clin. **60:** 54, 1965.
6. Muller, G. H., and Kirk, R. W.: Small animal dermatology, Philadelphia, 1969, W. B. Saunders Co.
7. Rossoff, I. S.: Handbook of veterinary drugs, New York, 1974, Springer Publishing Co.

Additional readings

Chiou, W. L., and Riegelman, S.: Disposition kinetics of griseofulvin in dogs, J. Pharm. Sci. **58**:1500, 1969.
Civen, M., and Brown, C. B.: The effect of organophosphate insecticides on adrenal corticosterone formation, Pestic. Biochem. Physiol. **4**:254, 1974.
Clark, D. E., Wright, F. C., Radeleff, R. D., Danz, J. W., and Lehmann, R. P.: Influence of coumaphos contaminants, vitamin A, and phenothiazine-lead arsenate on certain enzymes and vitamins of cattle treated with coumaphos, Am. J. Vet. Res. **28**:89, 1967.
Failing, F., Rimer, C., and Wolley, R.: Chlordane contamination of a municipal water system—Tennessee, Morbid. Mortal. Weekly Rep. **25**:117, April 1976.
Kaplan, W., and Ajello, L.: Oral treatment of spontaneous ringworm in cats with griseofulvin, J. Am. Vet. Med. Assoc. **135**:253, 1959.
Kral, F.: Compendium of veterinary dermatology, New York, 1960, Charles Pfizer & Co.
O'Brien, R. D.: Insecticides, action and metabolism, New York, 1967, Academic Press, Inc.
Thomsett, L. R., and Rofe, P. C.: The treatment of *Microsporum canis* infection in cats with fine-particle griseofulvin, Arch. Dermatol. **81**:537, 1960.

9

DRUGS FOR PREVENTION AND TREATMENT OF
Skin diseases of dogs and cats

GENERAL INFORMATION

Dogs and cats suffer from many types of skin conditions, and some of these conditions may have similar signs but entirely different causes. Therefore a proper diagnosis is necessary before a rational course of therapy can be initiated. The veterinarian obtains a history, examines the skin, and possibly performs a variety of laboratory examinations to arrive at a diagnosis.

It is not the purpose of this chapter to review the signs associated with various skin diseases or to detail the steps that must be taken to make a diagnosis. Rather, assuming that a proper diagnosis has been made, it is our intent to highlight the more common skin conditions and discuss a rational therapeutic approach to their treatment.

BACTERIAL INFECTIONS

Whether bacterial skin infections are primary or secondary may determine the therapeutic approach. Primary skin infections are those in which one species of bacteria is isolated from an otherwise healthy skin that presents a characteristic disease pattern. Secondary skin infections have an initial cause other than bacterial infection. The initial cause increases the susceptibility of the skin to infection by a wide variety of bacteria in the animal's environment. In secondary skin infections, frequently more than one species of bacteria are present in the diseased skin, and the signs are not necessarily characteristic.

For superficial skin infections, no treatment or the administration of topical antibacterial drugs may be adequate. However, infections involving large areas of skin and those that penetrate deeply into the skin generally require treatment with systemic antibacterial drugs. The principles involved in the treatment of bacterial skin infections are similar to those for the treatment of systemic bacterial infections as discussed in Chapter 3. Of primary importance is that the anti-infective used must be one to which the bacteria are sensitive. Whether applied by the topical or systemic route or both, the antibacterial drug must reach the site of infection in adequate concentration. The best means of assuring this is to administer the drug systemically.

Pyoderma

Pyoderma is a primary or secondary infection of the skin by pus-forming bacteria (pyogenic bacteria). Commonly *Staphylococcus, Streptococcus, Proteus, Pseudomonas,* coliform, and *Corynebacterium* species are the bacteria that infect skin in either primary or secondary pyodermas.

Infections may involve only the upper layers or extend to the deep layers of the skin. Pyoderma can be secondary to such primary causes as irritated skin from self-mutilation, flea allergy dermatitis, deep folds of the skin, which set up conditions for bacterial growth, or foreign bodies.

Although primary skin infections generally can be treated successfully with topical and/or systemic antibacterials, successful treatment of secondary skin infections is only brought about when the primary insult is removed. For example, it might be necessary to remove a foreign body, initiate a flea control program (pp. 129 to 131), or surgically remove folds of the skin that predispose to infection. To reduce self-mutilation, antipruritics, tranquilizers, or corticosteroids may be administered.

In both primary and secondary pyodermic infections, fur from the infected area should be clipped and shampoos or wet dressings used to remove crusts. Topical and/or systemic antibacterials should also be administered. Among the anti-infectives commonly used topically are bacitracin, gramicidin, neomycin, polymyxin B, nitrofurazone, and cuprimyxin. A wide variety of systemic antibacterial drugs can be used to treat pyodermic skin infections. They are used as recommended for other infections in Chapter 3.

All cases of pyoderma do not necessarily respond to antibacterial therapy. The prognosis for the eventual cure of such cases is guarded.

External ear infections (otitis externa)

Because dogs' external ear canals drain poorly, the external portion of the ear and the ear canal are often involved in primary bacterial or fungal infections (Fig. 9-1). The

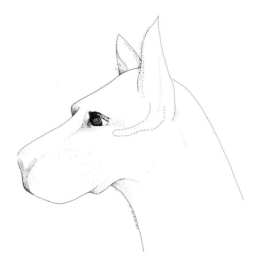

Fig. 9-1. Anatomy of dog's ear canal. Shape of dog's external ear canal does not promote drainage. Therefore ear canal is often moist and warm—a favorable environment for establishment of pathogenic bacteria.

conditions within the ear present a good environment for the growth of bacteria and fungi. Because their ears stay moist, floppy-eared breeds and water dogs are most susceptible to external ear infections.

Secondary ear infections can result when a foreign body is present in the ear. In secondary ear infections the primary cause must be removed. After removal of the initial insult, secondary ear infections are essentially treated the same as primary ear infections.

Treatment. The external ear canal should be gently and frequently cleaned to assist the body in combating external ear infections. It may be cleaned with a bland oil, mild soap, or nonirritating solution such as physiological saline. Bacterial cultures and antibiotic sensitivity tests are a useful aid in the selection of the appropriate antibacterial to treat the ear. The antibacterial may be administered topically; in a severe infection it should also be administered systemically. Frequently, corticosteroids are used along with the antibacterial medication to reduce inflammation and discomfort to the animal and prevent scratching of the ear or frequent shaking of the head. (Frequent head shaking can rupture blood vessels in the ear and cause large hematomas.) In cases that do not favorably respond to antibacterial therapy, surgery is sometimes necessary to facilitate drainage of the external ear canal. Dramatic cures often follow such surgery.

MYCOTIC DERMATOSES

Etiology. Approximately 98% of fungal skin infections in cats are caused by *Microsporum canis*. In dogs, 70% are caused by *M. canis*, approximately 20% by *M. gypseum*, and approximately 10% by *Trichophyton* species. About 1% of mycotic skin infections are caused in the dog by other species of fungi.[13] The lesions associated with dermatomycotic infections are usually small and localized. However, generalized infections can occur. Infection from *M. canis* is contagious to humans, causing the disease commonly known as "ringworm."

Treatment. Treatment of mycotic dermatosis in animals begins with clipping the hair from the infected area. This removes a substantial amount of the fungus and also allows medication applied topically to come in contact with the organisms. When treating dermatomycotic infections, it is important to clean items with which the animal comes in contact to reduce the chance of reinfection. For this purpose 0.2% to 0.25% suspensions of captan are recommended.

Shampoos with fungicides may be used on the animal daily or weekly. To gain the full effect, medicated shampoos should be left in contact with the skin prior to rinsing for a period of time specified by the manufacturer. Examples of shampoos containing fungicides are those containing organic iodines (Weladol shampoo) and those containing captan (Casteen shampoo).

Various types of topical medication can be applied to animals with mycotic dermatoses. These medications include iodine tincture (USP); 3 to 5% gentian violet tincture; ointments containing fatty acids such as undecylenic, caprylic, or propionic; thiabendazole or miconazole; and tolnaftate (USP). Although tolnaftate has been advocated

for the treatment of fungal skin infections in dogs and cats, of sixty individual *M. canis* lesions treated with tolnaftate cream daily over a period of 8 months, there was no significant decrease in the number of lesions.[2] The value of the drug in treating routine fungal skin infections in dogs and cats is therefore highly questionable.

In some cases of dermatomycotic infection, the systemic antibiotic griseofulvin is administered. Griseofulvin must be administered until the skin is free of infection. For most mycotic infections a minimum of 1 month is necessary. Frequently, several months are required for mycotic infections of the claws. Doses used in dogs and cats are currently being reevaluated. It is possible that doses recommended by the manufacturer are too low. Dogs rapidly metabolize griseofulvin in the liver. Suitable plasma concentrations and inhibiting concentrations of the antibiotic in the skin are difficult to obtain in the dog.[8] Currently it appears that the following oral doses of micronized griseofulvin are necessary[6]:

Dogs   132 mg/kg/24 hr in three or four
        doses
Cats   55 to 66 mg/kg/24 hr in three or four
        doses

Candida albicans

The fungus *Candida albicans* is a common pathogen of humans and a relatively uncommon pathogen in domestic animals. Conditions caused by *Candida albicans* are referred to as "moniliasis." In dogs *Candida albicans* can infect the oral cavity, external ear canal, nail folds, vagina, or anal mucosa.

Treatment. For these conditions, nystatin is the drug of choice. It is applied topically and in some cases is given orally. When given orally, the drug is not absorbed systemically but does reduce the number of fungi in the intestinal tract. This helps to eliminate infections in the anal mucosa and possibly in the vagina. It is administered orally to cats at the rate of 150,000 units once or twice a day and to dogs at the rate of 150,000 to 500,000 units one to three times a day.[15]

PARASITIC DERMATOSES
Mite infestation

A mite is an arachnid microscopic in size. In dogs and cats, mites affect the skin and cause a dermatitis commonly called "mange." They also attack the external ear canal. It should be noted that the term "mange" refers to a dermatitis caused by mites and is not synonomous with the term "dermatitis," even though it is often used this way by lay people.

The most common skin problems caused by mites in dogs and cats are sarcoptic mange caused by *Sarcoptes scabiei*, demodectic mange caused by *Demodex canis*, and ear mite infections caused by *Otodectes cynotis*.

Sarcoptic mange

Sarcoptic mange, which is caused by *Sarcoptes scabiei*, is primarily a disease of dogs, although rarely cats or humans can be affected. In dogs, the female mites burrow into the epidermis to lay their eggs. This burrowing, plus the depositing of fecal pellets by the mite, probably causes the severe itching that is characteristic of the disease. The skin of dogs with sarcoptic mange is so inflamed that the condition is commonly known as "red mange."

Treatment. Because the sarcoptic mange mite is located in the upper layer of the skin, treatment by applying topical pesticides or dipping the animal in solutions or emulsions of pesticides can be highly effective. Pesticides used for this purpose include 0.075% to 1% ronnel or lime sulfur suspension, supplied as a 26% calcium polysulfide (Orthorix Spray) and diluted in water at the rate of 1:20 for dogs and 1:40 for cats.

For treating sarcoptic mange there are also a variety of commercial products containing numerous pesticides. These usually include rotenone, lindane, and/or benzoyl benzoate. If necessary, saline solution or shampoos can be used to remove crusts from the skin prior to applying topical pesticides. Corticosteroids may be administered topically, systemically, or both to reduce the severe inflammation that occurs with this disease.

If sarcoptic mange results in a secondary bacterial infection of the skin, a culture and antibiotic sensitivity test should be performed and an appropriate antibacterial should be administered systemically.

Demodectic mange

Demodectic mange is caused by a cigar-shaped mite, *Demodex canis* (Fig. 9-2). This mite lives in the hair follicles and sometimes in the sebaceous glands of the skin. The mite probably is a common resident of canine skin, only infrequently causing disease. When it causes disease, the disease may occur in one of two forms, as either a local or generalized condition.

Localized demodectic mange. The local form consists of one or a few small, round, red swollen areas in which there is some hair loss. Frequently, these lesions are on the head. The veterinarian makes a diagnosis by noting the appearance of the lesion and examining a skin scraping under a microscope for the presence of demodectic mites. Generally, a skin scraping will reveal the presence of the mite.

Treatment. Approximately 90% of cases of local demodectic mange recover spontaneously.[17] However, because localized cases of demodectic mange may progress to the more generalized form, they should be treated. Treatment consists of clipping the area and applying a suitable pesticide formulation. Because the Cornell Formulation of ronnel has been highly successful in the treatment of generalized demodectic mange, it is also recommended for treating the local form. In the Cornell Formulation an 8.5% ronnel emulsion is prepared by adding 365 ml of ronnel concentrate (Ectoral Emulsifiable Concentrate) to 900 ml of propylene glycol and 150 ml of isopropyl alcohol.[16] Because ronnel can be absorbed through the skin, individuals applying the Cornell Formulation should wear rubber gloves. When applying the formulation in the region of the head, the animal's eyes should be protected with bland ophthalmic ointment.

The most common side effects of the

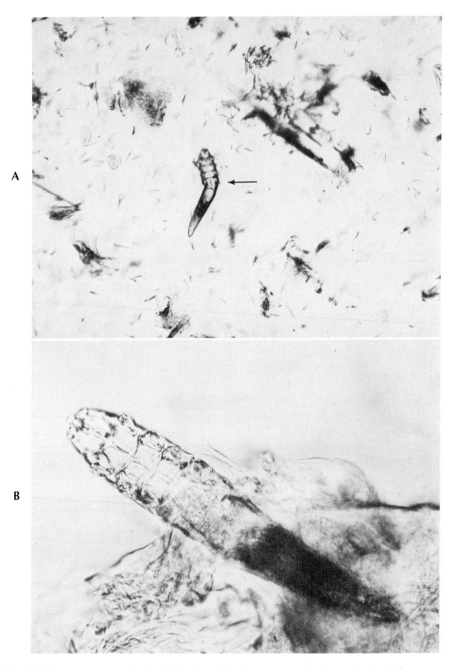

Fig. 9-2. Photomicrograph of adult demodectic mange mite *(arrow).* **A,** At low power and, **B,** at high power. (Courtesy Mr. Paul Sumner, Animal Care Facility Diagnostic Laboratory, University of California, San Francisco.)

Cornell Formulation are severe skin scaling and mild to moderate weight loss. Neither of these conditions warrant serious concern, since 4 to 6 weeks after discontinuing topical therapy animals generally return to normal. However, signs of organophosphate toxicity such as vomiting, diarrhea, and trembling are occasionally seen in young or small dogs. These signs can generally be reversed by treating one third of the body every other day rather than daily. Severe skin reactions to the Cornell Formulation, which are seen as severe redness of the skin and obvious pain and discomfort, may also be reversed by treatment every other day. Liver toxicity in animals treated with the Cornell Formulation has been reported; however, whether the liver toxicity resulted from antibiotics that were concurrently given, ronnel, propylene glycol, isopropyl alcohol, or a combination of these products is not known. If an animal stops eating or becomes depressed while on therapy, administration of the drug should be discontinued, and the veterinarian should be consulted so that he can evaluate whether there is liver damage. Animals exhibiting signs of liver damage should be removed from ronnel therapy. The Cornell Formulation should not be reapplied until the animals have completely recovered from the liver damage. Continued use of the topical medication must then be reevaluated by the veterinarian.[17]

Solutions or ointments containing rotenone or lindane have also been popular in the treatment of localized demodectic mange. The use of corticosteroids to treat localized demodectic mange is contraindicated. Corticosteroids may precipitate the conversion of the relatively mild localized form to a severe generalized infestation.[17]

Generalized demodectic mange. In the generalized form, lesions are large and may involve all areas of the body. The generalized form is far more serious than the localized form of demodectic mange. Whereas animals with the localized form appear to suffer little discomfort, the generalized form is extremely uncomfortable. Generalized demodectic mange is a serious disease requiring vigorous treatment.

It appears that animals which develop generalized demodectic mange have an immune deficiency that prevents normal resistance to the parasite.[17] Genetic predisposition may be responsible for the immune deficiency.

A major feature of generalized demodectic mange is secondary bacterial skin infection. Commonly, species of *Staphylococcus*, *Proteus*, and *Pseudomonas* are the bacteria that invade the skin.

The infections involve the deep layers of the skin. Infection by *Pseudomonas* organisms is particularly dangerous and can result in death. In addition to infecting the skin, the organisms may spread to other organs such as the liver, spleen, kidney, lung, and heart.

Treatment. In the absence of ulcerated skin surface and fistulous tracks, antibiotics can be used to treat the secondary bacterial infection concurrently with the use of pesticides directed at the demodectic mange mite. The hair should be clipped, cultures grown, and antibiotic sensitivity tests performed to select the appropriate antibiotic. The antibiotic should be administered at therapeutic levels systemically for 3 weeks.

Ulcerated skin surfaces and fistulous tracks can be caused by the secondary bacterial infection. These lesions must be healed before the application of a pesticide formulation, since they increase the absorption of the pesticide and can create a toxic condition. Animals with severe skin ulceration or deep fistulous tracks should receive whirlpool therapy until the major denuded areas are healed, which usually occurs in about 5 to 7 days. Povidone-iodine (Betadine Whirlpool Concentrate) can be added to the whirlpool solution. Once these lesions are healed, the Cornell Formulation or its variation can be applied.[17]

The Cornell Formulation should be applied to one third of the dog's body each day. One day the formulation is applied to the head, neck, shoulders, and front legs; the next day it is applied to the trunk; and the next it is applied to the hindquarters and legs. The process is repeated until treatment is discontinued.

It appears that a variation of the Cornell Formulation containing 4% ronnel (half strength) is also acceptable for the treatment of generalized demodectic mange. The half-strength Cornell Formulation is prepared by mixing 180 ml ronnel concentrate, 900 ml propylene glycol, and 150 ml isopropyl alcohol.[17]

Either the Cornell Formulation or the half-strength formulation should be used on a third of the animal's body daily for at least 3 weeks after six to ten consecutive scrapings from various parts of the body taken at the same time show no demodectic mange mites. The first negative skin scraping normally occurs 5 to 12 weeks after treatment is begun. Therefore treatment normally occurs over an 8- to 15-week period.

Over the years a wide variety of agents have been used to treat generalized demodectic mange. Among these have been oral organophosphate preparations, trypan blue, griseofulvin, and disophenol. The efficacy of these compounds is highly questionable.[13]

Corticosteroids are contraindicated in the treatment of generalized demodectic mange. They further contribute to the immune deficiency against demodectic mange mites that appears to be present in animals suffering from this disease. Corticosteroids can also increase the susceptibility of the animal to secondary bacterial infection.

Ear mites

Dogs and cats can be infected with ear mites *(Otodectes cynotis)*. These mites cause severe irritation of the external ear canal, and a collection of debris consisting of scales, crusts, and ear wax results in the canal. Frequently, a secondary bacterial infection occurs concurrent with ear mite infestation.

Treatment. Therapy aimed at treating ear mite conditions should always be directed by a veterinarian. To be effective, any drug administered into the external ear canal must come in contact with the mites. Therefore the debris in the external ear canal must be removed prior to applying the medication. This can be done by washing the ear with a mild soap or detergent solution or by using a bland oil preparation such as mineral oil.

Various pesticide preparations in an oil base are used to treat ear mite infestations. Many proprietary compounds are on the market. These may contain chlorinated hydrocarbons, organophosphates, carbaryl, or rotenone. Some preparations also contain antibiotics to treat the secondary ear infections and corticosteroids to reduce the inflammation in the ear.

A popular formula for treating ear mites involves a proprietary compound that consists of 7.5% chloroform and 0.12% rotenone (Canex). The ear mite formulation is prepared by adding one part Canex to three parts mineral oil. The solution should be shaken well prior to use. It is applied in each ear canal every 5 to 7 days.

A number of flea sprays are commonly used around the head in animals with ear mites to kill any mites that may be present in that area. Treatment should be continued for at least 2 weeks after the animals appear clinically normal.

Flea infestation

Numerous species of fleas infest dogs and cats. The most common are *Ctenocephalides canis* and *Ctenocephalides felis*. Other species of fleas that commonly infect dogs include *Pulex irritans* (the human flea) and *Echidnophaga gallinacea*.[9,10] *Pulex irritans* is capable of transmitting plague to humans.

Fleas act as an intermediate host of a small filaria worm *(Dipetalonema reconditum)*, which lives in the blood vessels of dogs. In addition, one of the major tapeworms of dogs, *Dipylidium caninum*, is transmitted by fleas (Chapter 11).

As long as no secondary complications are present, flea or tick infestation of dogs and cats is the one class of skin diseases that can be diagnosed by the animal owner and treated effectively with OTC products. Flea infestations are diagnosed by seeing the parasites on the skin. Flea excreta, which looks like dark pepper and turns red when wet, is also seen on the skin. Secondary complications to flea infestation include flea allergy dermatitis, anemia, and secondary bacterial infections. These cases should be examined and treated by a veterinarian.

Treatment

Shampoos and dips. To control fleas on pets various forms of therapy are possible. Shampoos containing pesticides are often used to treat animals with flea infestations. Such shampoos commonly contain one or more of the following ingredients: pyrethrins, piperonyl butoxide, rotenone, or lindane. Pesticide shampoos have little residual activity. Before using one of these on cats, the label should be checked to be sure that the product is safe in that species.

Dipping the animal in a water emulsion of a pesticide gives more residual action than a shampoo. Pesticide dips, generally emulsifiable concentrates, contain as their active ingredients one of the following: lindane, ronnel, pyrethrins, piperonyl butoxide, benzyl benzoate, lime sulfur, or carbaryl. It is good practice to put a bland ophthalmic ointment such as white petroleum ophthalmic ointment in the animal's eyes and cotton in the ears before dipping it in the solution. The instructions of the manufacturer should be followed.

Powders and sprays. Virtually every class of external pesticide discussed in Chapter 8 has been produced as a powder or spray for the treatment of external parasites in dogs and cats. Instructions of the manufacturer must be followed closely, especially when using a product on puppies or cats. Generally, flea powders and sprays have been the least effective means of flea control. However, a recent report indicates that newer types of flea powders may have good activity against fleas in dogs and cats. A powder containing an organophosphate (2% temephos) effectively controlled *Ctenocephalides felis* on dogs and cats for 2 weeks and partially controlled them for 3 to 4 weeks.[11] Some of the success in the use of the preparation was probably a result of the careful manner in which it was applied to the animal. Whether animal owners would apply the powder so carefully is questionable.

Flea collars. The most popular and effective way of controlling flea infestations on dogs and cats is by the use of flea collars. These collars are made of plastic impregnated with either organophosphate preparations or carbamates. Flea collars for cats generally contain lower concentrations of pesticides than those for dogs. For example, a standard dichlorvos flea collar contains about 4.5% dichlorvos for cats and 10% for dogs.

Effectiveness. Flea collars have been shown to be highly effective in controlling fleas on animals. For example, collars containing 3% dichlorvos provided at least 94% control of *Ctenocephalides felis* on cats for 14 weeks.[7]

The owners of animals sometimes report that the flea collar was ineffective. Better control often is achieved when another brand is tried. A possible explanation for this is that the second brand contains a different active ingredient to which the population of fleas are more sensitive, or if it contains the same active ingredient, that ingredient may be released more freely from the plastic impregnated collar.

Toxicity. Although flea collars are highly effective in controlling fleas, they are not without problems. The toxic effects of flea collars include signs commonly associated with organophosphate or carbamate toxicity. These include vomiting, diarrhea, and dysfunction of the skeletal muscles. In addition, flea collars can produce a mild to severe dermatitis. An animal showing any toxic signs associated with flea collar use should have their collar removed and be treated by a veterinarian. Ways of reducing the chance of flea collar toxic reactions are discussed later.

The relative incidence of toxic reactions when flea collars are properly used is low.[4] Generally, practitioners believe that the benefits derived from flea collar use far outweigh the potential toxicities.

The relative lack of toxicity of flea collars is probably a result of two factors. If either or both of these are not present, the incidence of toxicity may be dramatically increased. One built-in safety factor is the slow release of the active ingredient, although release of the active ingredient from the plastic flea collar may increase as the temperature rises. The other safety factor is the rapid destruction of the active ingredient after it is released from the collar. For example, dichlorvos is rapidly destroyed by moisture. In normal conditions of humidity, moisture in the air is responsible for breaking down most of the free dichlorvos. In addition, dichlorvos is rapidly detoxified in the liver, blood plasma, and kidneys of mammals.

Animals having impaired liver or kidney function are more likely to develop toxic reactions to flea collars.

Based on a laboratory investigation, it has been claimed that keeping cats in a hot dry environment increases the incidence of toxic reactions from flea collars.[1] However, widespread toxicity of flea collars in cats living in hot dry climates has not been reported. Further work is necessary to clarify this issue, but until further information is developed, extra careful examination of cats in hot dry climates for dichlorvos toxicity is warranted.

Some of the recommended limitations on the use of flea collars appear to have no scientific basis. For example, manufacturers of flea collars commonly recommend that they not be used in whippets, greyhounds, or Persian cats. However, there is some evidence that long-haired cats, like Persians, are less likely to suffer toxic effects than short-haired cats, which seem to be more susceptible to contact dermatitis from the flea collars.[12] Apparently this recommendation is based on economic factors rather than scientific data. Flea collars have not been extensively tested in pedigreed Persian cats because the cost of extensive testing is greater than the limited market of flea collars in such animals.[4] Companies producing flea collars overemphasize the possible danger of their use and specifically list their use for such cats as contraindicated because this is the more economical route for the companies.

Early in the use of flea collars, there was concern that using them would prolong the recovery time from barbiturate anesthesia.[18] However, it has been shown experimentally that commercially available collars with dichlorvos as the active ingredient do not affect sleeping times of dogs administered sodium pentobarbital or thiamylal anesthesia.[5,14,19] These are common intravenous barbiturate anesthetics used in veterinary practice.

Flea collar dermatitis is caused by the active ingredient in the collar.[1] Flea collar dermatitis may vary from a mild irritation to a severe dermatitis that involves secondary bacterial infection. The severity of flea collar dermatitis has been classified as follows[12]:

Grade 1: A mild irritation of the neck that clears up when the collar is removed

Grade 2: A severe irritation of the entire skin area under the flea collar; lesions heal slowly even after the collar is removed

Grade 3: A generalized involvement of the skin, especially in the head, back, tail, and sometimes the entire body that takes up to many months to heal

Grade 4: A grade 3 reaction with secondary bacterial infection

Flea collar dermatitis of grades 2, 3, and 4 must be treated by a veterinarian.

Use. To prevent direct toxic effects from flea collars and flea collar dermatitis, various preventive measures have been recommended.[3,4] Animal owners should be informed of the following when purchasing flea collars:

1. Flea collars are highly effective in the control of fleas but have certain toxic effects that should be explained. The decision whether to use a flea collar should be made by the owner of the animal.

2. The collar should be removed from the protective wrapper 24 hours (minimum) to a week before putting it on the animal.

3. Flea collars must be kept out of the reach of children.

4. Although the collar should be snug, there should be space for at least three fingers to be slipped horizontally under it.

5. Excess collar length should be cut off

and discarded after the collar is properly fitted.

6. The neck should be checked daily for signs of skin irritation, particularly during the first week of wear. Other toxic signs such as depression, loss of appetite, vomiting, diarrhea, hypersalivation, or ataxia should be watched for. If any of these occur, the collar should be removed, and, if improvement is not seen within 24 hours, a veterinarian should be called. The collar should not be reapplied for 1 week. If toxic signs recur, a flea collar should not be used on that animal.

7. The collar should be removed any time the animal is likely to get wet.

8. Organophosphates or carbamates should not be administered to the animal unless the collar has been removed for 5 days. The collar should not be put back on the animal until 5 days after administering other organophosphates or carbamate preparations to the animal.

9. Flea collars should not be used on young kittens less than 4 months of age, sick animals, or pregnant or nursing cats.

10. Cat flea collars, which generally contain ingredients that are less concentrated than those used for dogs, should be used for puppies or small dogs.

In dogs an alternative to flea collars are organophosphate flea medallions. These hang below a collar and do not come into contact with the animal's skin. Because they are relatively new, their effectiveness is still being evaluated.

Eliminating fleas. In both uncomplicated flea infestations and in those with secondary complications, the most important treatment is to eliminate fleas from the host and the environment surrounding the animal. Some pamphlets on flea control in the environment are available through agricultural extension offices and the U.S. Department of Agriculture. The government publications can be purchased in government bookstores.

If fleas are not adequately removed from the premises, reinfestation will occur. To remove fleas from the premises the following measures should be taken:

1. Vacuum all carpets and floors.

2. Wash the animal's bedding.

3. Spray the premises with one of the following: 0.5% lindane, 2% chlordane, or 0.25% dichlorvos. Because of the toxic effects of these pesticides on people, plants, and the environment, the directions of the manufacturer must be followed.

As an alternative to these measures, the services of a commercial pest control firm can be employed to rid the premises of fleas.

Secondary problems. In treating secondary problems associated with flea infestations, the removal of fleas from the animal and its environment is of primary concern. In addition, treatment must be directed at the secondary complications. For example, anemia can be so severe that blood transfusions are necessary (Chapter 18). For flea allergy dermatitis, corticosteroids are often administered systemically. Secondary pyodermic infections should be cultured, and an antibiotic sensitivity test should be performed. The infections should then be treated with appropriate systemic antibiotics.

Tick infestations

Various species of ticks affect dogs and cats. However, treatment aimed at removing one species of tick is similar to that used for any other species. Ticks cause the following problems:

1. They irritate any part of the body they bite.

2. Those that locate in animals' ears cause an inflammation of the ear canal. Secondary ear problems such as bacterial otitis or hematoma can result if the animal scratches the ears or shakes its head as a response to the tick in the ear.

3. Ticks transmit certain bacterial, rickettsial, viral, and protozoan diseases.

4. Certain species of ticks secrete a toxin that paralyzes animals. The paralysis disappears when the ticks are removed.

Treatment. In a mild infestation, ticks can be manually removed by grasping the mouth parts as near to the host's skin as possible; by applying traction the complete tick can be removed. For ear ticks, a spray with an appropriate chlorinated hydrocarbon or organophosphate is used. Most flea powders and sprays are effective in treating light infestations. However, flea collars and medallions are effective only if ticks are located near the neck. More severe infestations may require dipping dogs in emulsions of pesticides. These generally are the same types of pesticide dips described for flea control. If animals do not wander from home grounds and yet are continually being reinfected, the owner should have his premises treated. *Kerosene, gasoline, lighted matches, and cigarettes should never be used to remove ticks.* Many animals have been severely injured by these practices, and less dangerous methods are far more effective.

NONINFECTIOUS SKIN DISEASES

As described in Chapter 8, animals suffer from a wide variety of noninfectious skin diseases that are treated either with drugs specifically formulated for skin problems or that are used to treat other disease problems as well. The former are discussed in this chapter as well as Chapters 8 and 10. The others are discussed throughout the book.

References

1. Bell, T. G., Farrell, R. K., Padgett, G. A., and Leendertsen, L. W.: Ataxia, depression, and dermatitis associated with the use of dichlorvos-impregnated collars in the laboratory cat, J. Am. Vet. Med. Assoc. **167**:579, 1975.
2. Blakemore, J. C.: Dermatomycosis. In Kirk, R. W., editor: Current veterinary therapy V: small animal practice, Philadelphia, 1974, W. B. Saunders Co.
3. Doering, G. C.: Ectoparasites. In Kirk, R. W., editor: Current veterinary therapy V: small animal practice, Philadelphia, 1974, W. B. Saunders Co.
4. Editors: Flea collars: use in cats, Feline Pract. **5**:39, July-Aug. 1975.
5. Elsea, J. R., Cloyd, G. D., Gilbert, D. L., Perkinson, E., and Ward, J. W.: Barbiturate anesthesia in dogs wearing collars containing dichlorvos, J. Am. Vet. Med. Assoc. **157**:2068, 1970.
6. Enos, L. R.: Formulary, ed. 3, Davis, Calif. 1976, Veterinary Medical Teaching Hospital, University of California.
7. Fox, I., Bayona, I., and Armstrong, J.: Cat flea control through use of dichlorvos-impregnated collars, J. Am. Vet. Med. Assoc. **155**:1621, 1969.
8. Harris, P. A., and Riegelman, S.: Metabolism of griseofulvin in dogs, J. Pharm. Sci. **58**:93, 1969.
9. Kalkofen, U., and Greenberg, J.: *Echidnophaga gallinacea* infestation in dogs, J. Am. Vet. Med. Assoc. **165**:447, 1974.
10. Kalkofen, U., and Greenberg, J.: Public health implications of *Pulex irritans* infestations of dogs, J. Am. Vet. Med. Assoc. **165**:903, 1974.
11. Miller, J. E., and Baker, N. F.: Insecticidal activity of temephos against *Ctenocephalides felis* on dogs and cats, Am. J. Vet. Res. **36**:1281, 1975.
12. Muller, G. H.: Flea collar dermatitis in animals, J. Am. Vet. Med. Assoc. **157**:1616, 1970.
13. Muller, G. H., and Kirk, R. W.: Small animal dermatology, Philadelphia, 1969, W. B. Saunders Co.
14. Ritter, C., Hughes, R., Snyder, G., and Weaver, L.: Dichlorvos containing dog collars and thiamylal anesthesia, Am. J. Vet. Res. **31**:2025, 1970.
15. Rossoff, I. S.: Handbook of veterinary drugs, New York, 1974, Springer Publishing Co.
16. Scott, D. W., Farrow, B. R., and Schultz, R. D.: Studies on the therapeutic and immunologic aspects of generalized demodectic mange in the dog, J. Am. Anim. Hosp. Assoc. **10**:233, May-June 1974.
17. Scott, D. W., Schultz, R. D., and Baker, E.: Further studies on the therapeutic and immunologic aspects of generalized demodectic mange in the dog, J. Am. Anim. Hosp. Assoc. **12**:203, March 1976.
18. Small, E.: Toxicity of flea collars, Mod. Vet. Pract. **49**:20, Dec. 1968.
19. Young, R. Jr., Johnson, L. G., and Brown, L. J.: Effects of pentobarbital sodium on the sleeping time of dogs wearing placebo or dichlorvos-containing flea control collars, Vet. Med. Small Anim. Clin. **65**:609, 1970.

Additional readings

Austin, V. H.: Diagnosis and treatment of skin diseases, Friskies Res. Dig. **12**:1, Winter 1976.
Austin, V. H.: Some unusual problems involving skin of the canine ear, Mod. Vet. Pract. **57**:1008, 1976.
Blue, J. L., Wooley, R. E., and Eagon, R. G.: Treatment of experimentally induced *Pseudomonas aeruginosa* otitis externa in the dog by lavage with EDTA-tromethamine-lysozyme, Am. J. Vet. Res. **35**:1221, 1974.
Bree, M. M., Park, J. S., Moser, J. H., and Eads, F. E.: Effect of flea collars on Telazol (Cl-744) anesthesia in cats, Vet. Med. Small Anim. Clin. **72**:869, 1977.
Dawson, C. O., and Noddle, B. M.: Treatment of *Microsporum canis* ringworm in a cat colony, J. Small Anim. Pract. **9**:613, 1968.
Donovan, E. G., and Bohl, E. H.: Use of griseofulvin in the treatment of ringworm, Vet. Med. **55**:49, 1960.
Halliwell, R. E.: Pathogenesis and treatment of pruritus, J. Am. Vet. Med. Assoc. **164**:793, 1974.
Houdeshell, J. W., and Hennessey, P. W.: Gentamicin in canine otitis externa, Vet. Med. Small Anim. Clin. **67**:625, 1972.
Kaplan, W., and Ajello, L.: Therapy of spontaneous ringworm in cats with orally administered griseofulvin, Br. J. Dermatol. **76**:116, 1964.

Kissileff, A.: Relationship of dog fleas to dermatitis, Small Anim. Clin. **2**:132, March 1962.

Marshall, M. J., Harris, A. M., and Horne, J.: The bacteriological and clinical assessment of a new preparation for the treatment of otitis externa in dogs and cats, J. Small Anim. Pract. **15**:401, 1974.

Pang, W. M.: Systemic control of flea dermatitis in dogs, Vet. Med. **57**:704, 1962.

Pugh, K. E., Evans, J. M., and Hendy, P. G.: Otitis externa in the dog and cat—an evaluation of a new treatment, J. Small Anim. Pract. **15**:387, 1974.

Rose, W. R.: Otitis externa. II. Therapeutics, Vet. Med. Small Anim. Clin. **71**:755, 1976.

Saunders, E. B.: Hyposensitization for flea-bite hypersensitivity, Vet. Med. Small Anim. Clin. **72**:879, 1977.

Snyder, W. E., and Imhoff, R. K.: Cuprimyxin, a new topical antibiotic, Vet. Med. Small Anim. Clin. **70**:1421, 1975.

Snyder, W. E., and Maestrone, G.: Comparative in vitro antimicrobial activities of veterinary topical products, Vet. Med. Small Anim. Clin. **71**:585, 1976.

Thompson, W. D., and Mandy, S. H.: Benzoyl peroxide—a new topical agent for canine dermatology, Vet. Med. Small Anim. Clin. **71**:1059, 1976.

Webster, F. L., Whyard, B. H., Brandt, R. W., and Jones, W. G.: Treatment of otitis externa in the dog with gentocin otic, Can. Vet. J. **15**:176, 1974.

Youmans, B. C., and Robinson, A. K.: A successful program for treatment of demodectic mange in dogs, Small Anim. Clin. **1**:281, Sept. 1960.

10

DRUGS FOR PREVENTION AND TREATMENT OF

Skin diseases of cattle, sheep, and horses

GENERAL INFORMATION

In the course of their career, veterinarians whose specialty is large animals are likely to encounter a wide variety of skin conditions in their patients. However, a much smaller percentage of their practice is concerned with skin conditions than that of their small-animal counterparts.

BACTERIAL DERMATOSES
Bacterial skin infections

Bacterial skin infections are not as common in large animals as in small animals. How-

ever, when they do occur, they are handled in the same way as bacterial skin infections of dogs and cats. If it is a secondary skin infection, therapy is aimed at the initial condition, the one that increased the susceptibility of the skin to infection. In both primary and secondary skin infections, topical and/or systemic antibacterials are used. The choice of antibacterial drug is made on the basis of bacterial cultures and sensitivity tests or according to the clinical judgment of the veterinarian. Dosage and frequency of administration depend on the species being treated and the antibactrial drug being used. Specific recommendations are made in Chapter 3. When using systemic antibacterials in large animals such as cattle and horses, massive doses must be used to obtain concentrations in the skin that will destroy the offending bacteria, as described in Chapter 3.

Foot rot

Foot rot in cattle and sheep is an infection of the skin in the interdigital space (the space between the two claws on the feet of cattle and sheep). When animals are housed in unsanitary conditions, the interdigital space becomes easy target for bacterial infections. Commonly the disease is caused by the bacteria *Fusobacterium necrophorum.*

Treatment. Treatment consists of improving the hygienic conditions under which the animals are housed and administering sulfas

134

systemically. The following can be used:

1. *Sulfamethazine*, starting with one intravenous injection at the rate of 130 mg/kg, concurrently with the first oral administration of a prolonged-release sulfamethazine (Hava-Span) at the rate of 495 mg/kg; the prolonged-release sulfamethazine is then given every 4 days at 495 mg/kg

2. *Sulfadimethoxine*, sustained release, at the rate of 137.5 mg/kg orally every 4 days

In severe cases surgical treatment is necessary.

Thrush

In humans, thrush is an infection of the mouth caused by the fungus *Candida albicans*. In horses the term "thrush" refers to an infection of the hooves caused by a variety of bacteria, fungi, or both. The condition is analogous to foot rot in sheep and cattle, and, like foot rot, it is primarily caused by *F. necrophorum*.

Horses have only one hoof per foot. In unsanitary housing conditions, bacteria can infect the bottom of the hoof. As the infection progresses, the sensitive structures of the hoof that contain the blood vessels and nerves can become infected. When this occurs, horses become lame.

Treatment. Treatment consists of improving the hygienic conditions under which the animals live. In addition, the hoof should be cleaned out and wet dressings applied to the area. Copper naphthenate 37.5%, strong tincture of iodine, or 5% to 10% copper sulfate solutions are effective as topical therapy. An advantage of the copper naphthenate preparation is that it forms a water-resistant coating. In severe infections involving the sensitive structures of the hoof, parenteral treatment with antibacterial drugs is often necessary.

VIRAL DERMATOSES

Various viral dermatoses occur in domestic animals. Because systemic antiviral drugs are not available, the internal use of drugs to cure viral skin diseases is not possible. Antibiotics are of no value in the treatment of viral skin conditions. Various topical medications, as discussed in Chapter 8, may be used to promote healing as long as one avoids the tendency to overtreat with such drugs. Astringents such as white lotion may be applied to viral lesions to stop a continuous flow of serum from the lesion.

Corticosteroids are contraindicated in animals with viral infections because they reduce the ability of the animal to combat the offending virus.

Cattle, sheep, and horses may be infected with a wide variety of pox-causing viruses. For the most part, the spread of such diseases is prevented by the routine use of a vaccine.

Warts

Viruses specific to each species cause warts in cattle and horses. Warts usually occur on the animal's face, but in cattle they sometimes appear on the teats, which may interfere with milking. Generally, warts appear and then disappear spontaneously. Treatment therefore is usually unnecessary. When it is desirable to treat warts, commercial vaccines are commonly used.

Because separate viruses cause warts in cattle and horses, only species specific wart vaccines are used. Although some success is claimed for commercially available wart vaccines, vaccines prepared from warts of affected animals (autogenous vaccines) are preferable.

MYCOTIC DERMATOSES

Etiology. Species of *Trichophyton* are the most common fungi infecting the skin of cattle, sheep, and horses. However, infections with *Microsporum* species and others also occur. Infection commonly occurs during the winter when animals' coats are long and tend to remain damp. However, it can occur at other times of the year.

Treatment. Many animals with mycotic skin infections recover without any treatment.

During treatment, crusts from infected

areas should be removed by scraping or brushing. The scrapings and any hair that is removed should be burned. Drugs used topically should be brushed or rubbed into the area vigorously. Among those drugs used topically are iodine tincture (USP); ointments containing 10% mercury, thiabendazole, or propionic or undecylenic acids; 2% captan shampoo; and captan suspension. The captan suspension is prepared as follows: add 8 to 10 gm of captan to 4 liters of water to make up a 0.2% to 0.25% captan suspension that can be sprayed or sponged on the entire animal.

Ultrafine griseofulvin can be administered orally to adult horses at the rate of 2.5 gm/24 hr for 2 or more weeks.[13] This dose may be inadequate when the horse is heavily exercised or in hot weather. Sweating carries griseofulvin from the skin to the skin surface, thus reducing its concentration in the skin.[3]

In addition to treating the animals, it is

Table 10-1. Common North American external parasites of cattle*

Group and common names	Scientific names	Group and common names	Scientific names
Mites		*Ticks—cont'd*	
Chorioptic scab mite	*Chorioptes bovis var. bovis*	Pajaroella tick	*Ornithodoros coriaceus*
Follicle mite	*Demodex bovis*	No common name	*O. turicata*
Sarcoptic scab mite	*Sarcoptes scabiei*	Spinous ear tick	*O. (Otobius) megnini*
Ticks		Brown dog tick	*Rhipicephalus sanguineus*
Lone Star tick	*Amblyomma americanum*		
Cayenne tick	*A. cajennense*	*Lice*	
No common name	*A. imitator*	Sucking lice	
No common name	*A. inornatum*	Short-nosed cattle louse	*Haematopinus eurysternus*
Gulf Coast tick	*A. maculatum*	Cattle tail louse	*H. quadripertusus*
No common name	*A. oblongoguttatum*	Tail louse	*H. tuberculatus*
Cattle tick	*Boophilus annulatus*	Long-nosed or blue cattle louse	*Linognathus vituli*
Tropical cattle tick	*B. microplus*	Hairy cattle louse	*Solenopotes capillatus*
Moose or winter ticks	*Dermacentor albipictus, D. nigrolineatus*	Biting lice	
Tropical horse tick	*D. nitens (Anocentor nitens, Otocentor nitens)*	Common red louse	*Bovicola bovis (Damalinia bovis)*
		Flies (immature)	
Pacific Coast tick	*D. occidentalis*	Blowflies	*Chrysomya megacephala, Phormia regina*
American dog tick (wood tick)	*D. variabilis*	Screwworm	*Cochliomyia hominivorax*
Rocky Mountain wood tick	*D. venustus (D. andersoni)*	Secondary screwworm	*C. macellaria*
Bird tick	*Haemaphysalis chordeilis*	Rabbit botfly	*Cuterebra buccata*
Rabbit tick	*H. leporispalustris*	Human botfly	*Dermatobia hominis*
No common name	*Ixodes cookei*	Northern cattle grub (warble fly)	*Hypoderma bovis*
California black-legged tick	*I. pacificus*	Common cattle grub (warble fly)	*H. lineatum*
Black-legged tick (shoulder tick)	*I. scapularis*		

*Modified from Becklund, W. W.: Revised check list of internal and external parasites of domestic animals in the United States and possessions and in Canada, Am. J. Vet. Res. **25:**1380, 1964.

important to disinfect anything that comes into contact with their skin. This is especially important in horses, since transmission is possible through grooming tools, blankets, or harnesses. Tack, blankets, and other equipment should also be treated with 0.2% to 0.25% captan.

PARASITIC DERMATOSES

Most skin diseases in cattle, sheep, and horses are caused by external parasites.

These parasites are listed in Tables 10-1 to 10-3.

External parasites directly damage the skin of animals. Even when they do not cause noticeable damage, external parasites irritate the animals. Such irritation reduces the time spent by the animals eating, and therefore the amount of weight production in beef cattle and the amount of milk output by dairy cattle is reduced. External parasites also act as transmitters of other diseases.

Table 10-2. Common North American external parasites of sheep*

Group and common names	Scientific names	Group and common names	Scientific names
Mites		*Ticks—cont'd*	
Foot scab mite	*Chorioptes bovis var. ovis*	Brown dog tick	*Rhipicephalus sanguineus*
Demodectic scab mites (follicle mites)	*Demodex caprae, D. ovis*	*Lice*	
		Sucking lice	
Itch mite	*Psorergates ovis*	African blue louse	*Linognathus africanus*
Common scab mite	*Psoroptes equi var. ovis*	Sheep body louse	*L. ovillus*
		Sheep foot louse	*L. pedalis*
		Goat sucking louse	*L. stenopsis*
Sarcoptic scab mite	*Sarcoptes scabiei*	Long-nosed or blue cattle louse	*L. vituli*
Chigger	*Trombicula (Eutrombicula) alfreddugèsi*	*Biting lice*	*Bovicola caprae, B. crassipes, B. limbatus, B. ovis*
Ticks			
Lone Star tick	*Amblyomma americanum*	*Flies (immature)*	
Cayenne tick	*A. cajennense*	Cattle grub (warble fly)	*Hypoderma* species
No common name	*A. imitator*		
Gulf Coast tick	*A. maculatum*	Screwworm	*Cochliomyia hominivorax*
Tropical horse tick	*Dermacentor nitens (Anocentor nitens, Otocentor nitens)*	Secondary screwworm	*C. macellaria*
Pacific Coast tick	*D. occidentalis*	Human botfly	*Dermatobia hominis*
American dog tick (wood tick)	*D. variabilis*	Blowflies	*Chrysomyia megacephala, Phanenica sericata, Phormia regina, Protophormia terraenovae*
Rocky Mountain wood tick	*D. venustus (D. andersoni)*		
Rabbit tick	*Haemaphysalis leporispalustris*	*Louse fly*	
California black-legged tick	*Ixodes pacificus*	Sheep tick (sheep ked)	*Melophagus ovinus*
Black-legged tick (shoulder tick)	*I. scapularis*	*Flea*	
		Sticktight flea	*Echidnophaga gallinacea*
Spinous ear tick	*Ornthodoros (Otobius) megnini*		

*Modified from Becklund, W. W.: Revised check list of internal and external parasites of domestic animals in the United States and possessions and in Canada, Am. J. Vet. Res. **25**:1380, 1964.

Table 10-3. Common North American external parasites of horses*

Group and common names	Scientific names	Group and common names	Scientific names
Mites		*Ticks—cont'd*	
Chorioptic mange mite	*Chorioptes bovis* var. *equi*	Rocky Mountain wood tick	*D. venustus (D. andersoni)*
Demodectic scab mite	*Demodex equi*	No common name	*Ixodes cookei*
Psoroptic mange mite	*Psoroptes equi* var. *equi*	California black-legged tick	*I. pacificus*
Sarcoptic mange mite	*Sarcoptes scabiei*	Black-legged tick	*I. scapularis*
Chigger	*Trombicula (Eutrombicula) alfreddugesi*	Spinous ear tick	*Ornithodoros (Otobius) megnini*
		No common name	*O. turicata*
Ticks		*Lice*	
Lone Star tick	*Amblyomma americanum*	Biting louse	*Bovicola equi*
		Sucking louse	*Haematopinus asini*
Cayenne tick	*A. cajennense*	*Flies (immature)*	
No common name	*A. imitator*	Screwworm	*Cochliomyia hominivorax*
Gulf Coast tick	*A. maculatum*		
No common name	*A. oblongoguttatum*	Secondary screwworm	*C. macellaria*
Tropical cattle tick	*Boophilus microplus*	Human botfly	*Dermatobia hominis*
Moose or winter ticks	*Dermacentor albipictus, D. nigrolineatus*	Cattle grubs	*Hypoderma* species (*H. bovis, H. lineatum*
Tropical horse tick	*D. nitens (Anocentor nitens, Otocentor nitens)*	*Fleas*	
		Sticktight flea	*Echidnophaga gallinacea*
Pacific Coast tick	*D. occidentalis*		
American dog tick (wood tick)	*D. variabilis*		

*Modified from Becklund, W. W.: Revised check list of internal and external parasites of domestic animals in the United States and possessions and in Canada, Am. J. Vet. Res. **25:**1380, 1964.

Parasitic dermatoses are primarily treated with a variety of pesticidal drugs. In 1967 it was projected that livestock production would drop about 25% if pesticides were not used.[5] Because these pesticides are powerful, they are capable of producing both much good and much harm. Their proper use is determined by many factors.

The first consideration is to choose a pesticide that is effective. Second, one must consider the potential toxicity of the pesticide to the animals on which it is used and to humans. In Chapter 8 we discussed some of the properties of pesticides that influence their toxicity to man and animal.

Mange (mite infestation)

Mange in farm animals and horses is caused by a wide variety of mites. Frequently, the condition is a result of poor management. Therefore when prescribing a course of therapy, in addition to the appropriate drug regimen, the veterinarian will often recommend changes in management procedures. For example, he may encourage less crowding of the animals or improvements in the quality and quantity of the diet.

One cannot assume that a treatment which is appropriate for one species of animals will work in another. Also, drugs that are effective against one genus of mites in a given species of animals will not necessarily be effective against another genus of mites in that same species of animal. In addition, the method of applying the pesticide is as important as the kind of pesticide that is used.

Efficacious regimens of treatment are discussed for the three common types of mange in horses and other farm animals: sarcoptic, psoroptic, and chorioptic. However, the therapy recommended here may not comply with current government regulations. These regulations change so frequently that one must refer to the latest product data to be sure that the recommended pesticide and the means of applying it is cleared for the species on which it will be used.

Treatment of sarcoptic mange. All animals on the premises must be treated whether they do or do not show clinical signs. The following has been recommended for treating animals with sarcoptic mange.[2] For the treatment of sarcoptic mange in cattle, Diazinon, an organophosphate, is poured on their backs at 1-month intervals. The approximately 0.02% solution is made by adding 25 gm of Diazinon to 150 liters of water. An alternative to the recommended use of Diazinon has been suggested. A 0.05% (75 gm/150 liters) solution can be prepared and sprayed on the animals.[13]

For sheep a 0.06% (90 gm/150 liters) solution of Diazinon can be prepared. The animals are dipped in the solution.[13]

Treatment of psoroptic mange. When treating psoroptic mange, it is important to wet the animal's head thoroughly. Any of the following treatments have a high probability of success.

1. Dip the cattle or sheep in a 1.5% polysulfide suspension three times 10 days apart.[2]

2. Dip sheep in either a 0.5% toxaphene, 0.06% lindane, or 0.06% Diazinon emulsion. Dip animals for 1 minute, submerging the head two times.[7]

3. Dip cattle or sheep in a 0.1% solution of chloropyridyl-phosphorothioate (Dursban), an organophosphate.[16]

Species of psoroptic mites may infect the ears of horses. Treatment by placing 3 ml of benzyl benzoate preparation into the external ear canal every fifth day for a total of 3 treatments appears to be effective. The medication should again be applied 3 weeks after the previous treatment to kill any newly hatched mites.[8]

Treatment of chorioptic mange. Chorioptic mange is a problem primarily in cattle and horses. Ciodrin sprayed in a 0.25% concentration at a pressure of 200 to 250 psi, with the nozzle 4 to 8 inches from the hide, can be effective with one treatment. Approximately 2 liters of pesticide should be applied to each adult animal.[15] Because most other pesticides are not effective against the parasitic ova, it appears that ciodrin is the drug of choice.

Lice infestation

Animals that are infected with lice will scratch, rub, and lick their skin. This can cause damage to fleece and hide or lower the rate of weight gain or production of milk. Serious anemia as a result of heavy infestation with suckling lice may develop in cattle.

Generally, the life cycle of the louse is spent entirely on the host. However, some species of lice can survive for up to 2 weeks away from the host.

Treatment. Treatment consists of applying pesticide preparations formulated for livestock by spraying, dipping, or even dusting. Chlorinated hydrocarbons, pyrethrins, rotenone, or organophosphate preparations have been used. The recommendations of the manufacturer regarding administration of the pesticides should be followed. Complete eradication of lice in a herd can be difficult, especially since some strains of lice have developed a resistance to pesticides.

Ticks

In livestock and horses, ticks cause the following problems:

1. They are vectors and potential reservoirs of infectious disease.

2. They are active blood suckers and may cause anemia.

3. Some species cause paralysis.

4. They irritate the animals, which results in decreased rate of weight gain, feed conversion, or milk production.

A wide variety of pesticides have been used to kill ticks. These include chlorinated hydrocarbons, organophosphates, and carbamates. The recommendations of the manufacturers regarding administration of the pesticides should be followed. Many species of ticks have become resistant to various pesticide agents.

Cattle grubs (warbles)

Cattle that are infected with the larvae of flies of the *Hypoderma* species are said to have "cattle grubs," or "warbles." This parasite causes serious damage to the hides of cattle. In severe infestation, animals can be-

come systemically ill because of the large number of abscesses caused by the presence of larvae in the subcutaneous area. Attempts to remove the larvae manually sometimes result in anaphylactic reactions.

It is necessary to have some understanding of the life cycle (Fig. 10-1) of *Hypoderma* species to appreciate the methods of control and potential side reactions to chemotherapeutic regimens.

Two species of *Hypoderma* parasitize cattle, *H. bovis* and *H. lineata*. During the warmest part of summer, adult flies lay their eggs, usually on the lower portion of the legs of cattle. In about 4 days the eggs hatch, and the emerging larvae penetrate the skin. During the autumn and winter they migrate in subcutaneous tissue toward the back.

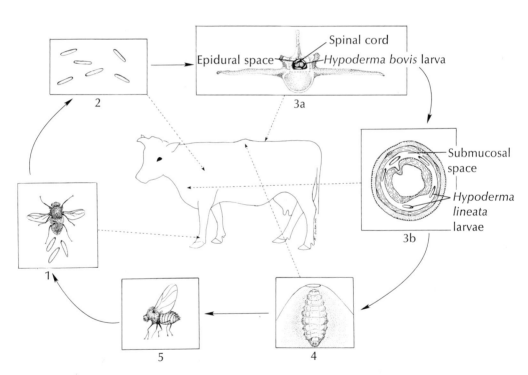

Fig. 10-1. Life cycle for cattle grubs (*Hypoderma* species). *1,* Adult fly lays eggs on fur of cattle. Larvae hatch and penetrate skin. *2,* Larvae migrate toward the back during late summer, autumn, and winter. *3,* Four months after infecting host *(3a),* *H. bovis* larvae may be located in epidural space of lumbar vertebrae and *(3b)* *H. lineata* larvae may be located in submucosa of esophagus. *4,* In spring, larvae migrate to the back and reside in abscess with breathing hole through skin. *5,* During summer, larvae emerge from abscess, fall to ground, and pupate to mature fly, completing cycle.

By early spring the larvae have reached a location on the back from which they develop a breathing pore to the exterior. There they enlarge further and in about a month perforate the skin and fall to the ground. For about 5 weeks they pupate in the ground.

One important difference between *H. bovis* and *H. lineata* is that, during the migration, *H. bovis* larvae may enter the epidural space near the spinal cord. *H. lineata* larvae commonly enter the submucosal tissue of the esophagus. They reach these sites about 4 months after the eggs have been deposited by the adult flies.

Treatment. The only practical means of killing the migrating larvae is the use of systemic organophosphate preparations once a year. These are either poured on the back or sprayed on the skin and absorbed systemically or included in the feed. For example, coumaphos is used as a 0.5% spray or as a 4% emulsifiable concentrate that is poured on the back at the rate of 15 ml/45 kg of body weight (not to exceed 120 ml per animal). Ronnel can be given as a single oral dose at the rate of 110 mg/kg.

If used at the proper time and at the proper dose, organophosphates are safe and effective for treating cattle grub infestation. However, if they are used at the wrong time, many problems can result. Timing is extremely important in treating cattle grubs. The organophosphate preparation must be administered in the autumn, after all the eggs have hatched but prior to the time that the larvae have had a chance to develop to their third stage, during which they are more resistant to the effects of the drug. At a later time, when the larvae are located in the epidural space or in the area of the esophagus, dosing can cause severe toxic reactions.

In addition to timing, it is important that the manufacturers' recommendations be followed when treating cattle grub infestation. If doses much larger than those recommended are used, toxicity can result. However, because there is a wide safety margin between the effective dose and a dose toxic to cattle, the most commonly encountered adverse effects are not due to the toxicity of the organophosphate.[9-11,14]

As previously mentioned, undesirable reactions may occur if animals are treated when the grubs are in close proximity to either the esophagus or the spinal cord. Although there is some similarity in the signs presented by animals poisoned by organophosphates and those suffering a toxic reaction from dead *Hypoderma* larvae, these can be differentiated by the veterinarian. Diarrhea and straining are usually seen in organophosphate poisoning. This sign is not seen in animals experiencing a reaction to a dead parasite. When *H. lineata* is the species causing toxic reactions because of lesions near the esophagus, the following signs will be noted: swelling of the left jugular area, gastric swelling, frothy type of salivation, and an inability to swallow in varying degrees, with animals often spitting out their partially chewed food. When the cause is *H. bovis* larvae killed in the area of the spinal cord, there will be partial to complete paralysis, particularly of the hindquarters.

It is important for the veterinarian to be able to make a differential diagnosis because, as detailed in Chapter 8, one treatment of organophosphate poisoning is atropine. This drug, however, is contraindicated when animals are undergoing a reaction to dead grubs. Atropine can further contribute to the lack of motility of the rumen and the bloat that results. When a toxic reaction to the dead grubs occurs, corticosteroids are the drug of choice. The dose depends on the specific corticosteroid that is used. Corticosteroids help to reduce the inflammatory reaction to the dead larvae.

Myiasis (fly strike)

Myiasis is the infestation of living or dead tissue of animals by larvae of certain species of flies, commonly referred to as blowflies. This infestation is usually secondary to some sort of wound.

Myiasis presents a special problem in sheep. Because the wool is thick, myiasis can be hidden and remain unnoticed in its early stages. Although myiasis does occur in horses, it is less common because horses actively keep flies away from their body.

Treatment. Treatment consists of surgically removing large portions of the area involved in the fly strike and then applying on and around the wound pesticides, such as lindane preparations or organophosphates, and fly repellents. EQ 335, developed by the U.S. Department of Agriculture, which consists of 3% lindane, a pesticide, and 35% pine oil, a repellent, has been commonly used. It is highly effective.

Before the introduction of EQ 335, preparations were used that contained one or more of the following: chloroform, oil of turpentine, bone oil, cresol, benzol, or diphenylamine. Such preparations are still commonly used in cattle and sheep; however, they should not be used in horses because they can cause severe skin irritation.

Use of pesticides on livestock

Use of the dipping vat. Cattle and sheep that are being treated for mites and lice are often put through a vat containing an appropriate concentration of a pesticide. The vat must be deep enough so that the animals can be completely submerged. Careful management of the vat is necessary so that the treatment is effective but not hazardous to the animals. The following measures have been recommended to safeguard the animals and to use the pesticides effectively[4]:

1. Before using pens or chutes, examine them for serviceability and for projecting nails, broken boards, or any object that might cause injury during treatment.

2. A gate should be near the entrance to the vat to hold animals back so that they are less likely to pile up and drown in the vat.

3. Cattle-dipping vats should be at least 33 feet long and 6 feet deep at the ⅞ full level. Vats for sheep should be at least 3½ feet deep at the ⅞ full level.

4. The capacity of each vat should be calibrated.

5. Mark the vat from its ⅞ capacity to full level in 50-gallon increments.

6. Construct the vats and draining pens so that rain and flood water will not enter.

7. Adequate help should be available to treat all livestock at a speed that is safe.

8. Lock both water inlets and outlets. They should also be leakproof.

9. Fill the vat with a known amount of water, then add the correct amount of pesticide.

10. Always mix the solution thoroughly before dipping the first animal. It is best to mix the solution with compressed air.

11. Never allow the vat to drop below the ⅞ full level.

12. Always use the correct water/pesticide ratio when replenishing the vat.

13. Remove caked mud, excessive filth, or heavy accumulations of dust from animals to increase the effectiveness of the insecticide by allowing it to reach the parasite.

14. Completely submerge the animals, including their heads.

15. When the maximum number of animals have been dipped, the maximum time has passed, or the vat becomes foul, empty and clean the vat.

16. Group animals according to size or age and dip separately.

17. Do not dip animals during rain. Wet animals will carry additional water into the vat and dilute it. After treatment, some of the dip will be washed off by the rain, and either its effectiveness will be reduced or it will concentrate on the underside of animals and perhaps cause toxic effects.

18. After dipping, keep animals in the draining pen until most of the excess pesticide has drained from them.

19. Identify each animal with a paint marker to show that it has been dipped.

20. To determine if animals are wet to the skin after dipping, examine a representative number.

21. Permit animals to dry thoroughly before allowing them to be handled or loaded for transporting.

22. Allow animals to rest and to be fed and watered after dipping. In cold weather give animals access to an open shed or windbreak. In warm weather protect them from direct

exposure to the sun. It is best to hold dipped animals overnight before they are handled.

23. Young animals should not be allowed to nurse their mothers until the dip has drained off the udder and teats.

24. Never place animals that have been recently dipped in a barn with inadequate ventilation.

25. Never allow the pesticide to contaminate feed or water.

In addition, when using pesticides in a dipping vat, be sure the formulation was manufactured for use as a *dip for livestock*. Pesticides made for plant use may not emulsify to the degree of those made for livestock. Under such conditions, large droplets of the concentrated pesticide stay in suspension and may adhere to an animal's skin. Each animal dipped could then absorb an excessive dose of pesticide, resulting in pesticide residues in meat or milk, illness, or even death.[12]

An alternative to the dipping vat is to spray pesticides on animals. Many of the precautions for using pesticides in the dipping vat also apply to pesticides that are sprayed. In addition, one should never spray animals with equipment that has been used to spray chemicals other than animal pesticides.

Pesticide residues. Improper use of pesticides can result in unacceptable residues of the pesticides in meat or agricultural products such as milk or eggs. This could cause severe economic losses because such meat, milk, or eggs will be condemned if pesticide residues exceed allowable levels. Various factors determine the level of residue in an animal. The amount of exposure is a primary contributing factor. This is influenced by the following:

- The concentration of the chemical when it is applied to the animal (the higher the concentration the greater the amount that will be absorbed)
- How the chemical is handled in the animal's body
- The chemical's persistence in the environment

Chlorinated hydrocarbons usually cause a residue problem because they are readily stored in the fat of the animal and most are not rapidly metabolized. As already mentioned in Chapter 8, methoxychlor is not as likely to cause residues as the other chlorinated hydrocarbons because it is metabolized more readily than the others.

Environmental pollution. Society has become increasingly concerned about environmental contamination by pesticides. Environmental contamination presents more consequential hazards than acute toxic reactions in animals or humans. For example, if misuse of a pesticide interrupts a food chain in a given environment, that environment can be affected for generations to come. Of total pesticides in use, about 11% are used on animals, whereas 85% are used on crops.[4] Therefore pesticides for livestock present less of a threat to the environment than those for crops. However, 11% is a substantial proportion and does present potential risk of significant environmental pollution. Users are responsible for any damage that results from misuse of pesticides, and anyone dispensing such products shares in this responsibility.

The rate at which a pesticide breaks down in the environment is a major factor in determining its potential for causing major environmental problems. That rate is usually expressed as the "half-life," or the time required for half the total amount of a pesticide to break down. For example, the half-life of DDT in soil may be as long as seventeen years, whereas other pesticides, in the presence of moisture, break down completely in 48 to 72 hours. Organophosphate preparations tend to break down readily. However, other pesticides are highly persistent, such as chlorinated hydrocarbons, DDT, aldrin, dieldrin, hepatochlor, lindane, and compounds containing arsenic, lead, or mercury. Because of their persistence in the environment, many of these chemicals have been banned from agricultural use.

Human toxicity. Human toxic reactions resulting from pesticide use in livestock result from exposure to a high concentration for short periods of time or low concentrations for long periods. There are three major routes of exposure: oral, respiratory, and dermal.[1] The chance of human toxic reaction can be greatly reduced if pesticides are purchased and used with the idea of reducing exposure.

When pesticides are being used on animals, the following measures are recommended to protect humans[4]:

1. Select the pesticide on the basis of its efficacy, safety, low probability of causing tissue residue problems, and cost.

2. Read and follow the precautions on the label.

3. When recommending or prescribing a pesticide, write down the proprietary brand name, concentration, and the amount of pesticide necessary.

4. Store pesticides only in original labeled containers in locked, ventilated, and cool facilities where children or unauthorized persons or animals cannot enter.

5. Place on the facilities appropriate warning signs indicating the type of material stored and the hazard involved.

6. Store pesticides in a manner that will prevent the contamination of food or animal feed.

7. Do not store pesticides in locations where fire hazards exist because some pesticides are flammable or explosive.

8. Do not store herbicides or defoliants in the same room with pesticides.

9. Have available the appropriate antidote as well as a supply of soap and water with which to wash. Fresh clothing should be available.

10. If symptoms of illness develop in personnel, immediately call a physician or get the individual to a hospital.

11. When handling the concentrate, wear plastic or rubber gloves and additional protective clothing.

12. Wear a respirator and goggles when spraying or dusting.

13. Avoid situations in which spray or dust will be carried by the wind.

14. Wear fresh, clean clothing every day.

15. For persons exposed to organophosphates regularly or on an intermittent basis, submit blood samples for cholinesterase determinations on a schedule recommended by a local physician or public health officer.

16. Never eat or smoke while handling pesticides or until hands and face have been washed.

17. Never use the mouth to blow out clogged lines and nozzles.

18. Empty pesticides into a sump or pit that is fenced. Identify these sites with suitable warning signs.

19. Empty containers should be considered potentially dangerous.

20. Damage empty pesticide containers so they cannot be used again and bury them at least 18 inches deep.

21. Dispose of pesticides so that they will not come in contact with animals or persons. Choose places where seepage cannot reach animal feeds, wells, or springs and where it cannot drain into ponds, streams, or underground waters.

22. Do not dispose of pesticides in sewers unless the sewer goes through a sewage treatment plant and disposal by such methods is considered safe by the manager of the sewage system.

NONINFECTIOUS DERMATOSES

Like dogs and cats, cattle, sheep, and horses are afflicted with a wide variety of noninfectious skin conditions. Because these conditions and their treatment are generally discussed in Chapter 8 and throughout the text, they will not be discussed here, except for two that have unique therapeutic needs: lower limb lacerations of horses and chemical dehorning of cattle.

Lacerations in horses

Lacerations in which there is separation of the skin surface require treatment by a veterinarian. No topical medication should be applied to lacerations, since in most instances they will be sutured by the veterinarian. The presence in lacerations of drugs, such as antibiotics in insoluble powder or ointment bases, alum, talc, or various dyes, prevents the veterinarian from suturing wounds. Healing is then unnecessarily delayed. In these cases a large amount of scar tissue may also form. Owners should be cautioned that topical therapy will do more harm than good if a laceration is going to require veterinary attention.

Minor scratches and abrasions generally do not need veterinary treatment and in fact usually do well with no treatment at all. If the owner desires to use a topical treatment, the area should be cleaned and a drying disinfectant applied. Various tinctures containing methyl violet, iodine, or acriflavine frequently are used.

In horses, lacerations below the hock (tarsus) or below the knee (carpus) require special consideration (Fig. 10-2). If such lacerations are treated improperly, the healing process continues long past the time when the skin defect is closed. A tumorlike lesion results, which is referred to as "proud flesh" by horsemen and as "exuberant granulation tissue" by veterinarians. To prevent the formation of such lesions, serious lacerations in the lower extremities should be treated immediately by a veterinarian. The area should be cleaned and shaved. The lesion may be sutured or an ointment containing antibiotics and corticosteroids and a pressure bandage may be applied. Corticosteroids retard the formation of proud flesh but permit healing of the skin, and the combination of antibiotics, corticosteroids, pressure bandage, and frequent examination by the veterinarian will permit lacerations below the knee or hock to heal properly with a minimum of scarring.

Preparations that contain astringents such as alum or copper sulfate are available for the treatment of wounds in horses. Because they are irritating and can actually stimulate the formation of proud flesh, they should not be used.

As previously mentioned, fly strike is usually not a problem in horses. However, occasionally flies will work under the pressure bandages and lay their eggs in the wound; thus it is a good idea to apply a fly repellent such as EQ 335 to the margins of the bandage. As previously noted, strong fly repellants such as preparations containing benzol, diphenylamine, and bone oil can cause skin irritation in horses. Such products should not be used on horses.

Tetanus can result from punctures or lacerations in horses. All horses should be actively immunized against tetanus (Chapter 7).

Chemical dehorning

Cattle are commonly dehorned to prevent them from injuring one another. Generally, dehorning is a surgical procedure. However, two means of chemical dehorning have been recommended. One involves the use of sodium hydroxide and calcium hydroxide; the other involves the use of calcium chloride.

Sodium hydroxide (NaOH) is a caustic material capable of burning off the horn buds on calves. A commercially available dehorning paste (Franklin Dehorning Paste) contains sodium hydroxide 44.5% and calcium hydroxide (Ca[OH]$_2$), 18.7%. To prevent skin

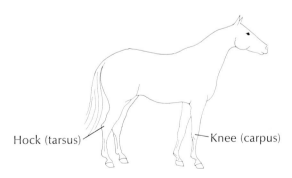

Hock (tarsus)   Knee (carpus)

Fig. 10-2. Area below carpus and tarsus. Lacerations below knee or hock in horses are more serious than lacerations in other locations.

burns, the skin around the horn buds should be protected with white petroleum jelly. Caustic dehorning paste must never be used before a rain because the paste dissolves in water and will run down the face, causing severe chemical burns.

In a continual dehorning trial involving more than 100 young calves from both dairy and beef breeds, a success rate of 70% has been achieved by injecting a solution of sterile calcium chloride ($CaCl_2$) under the horn bud. Calcium chloride kills surrounding tissue. When compared with sodium hydroxide, the calcium chloride solutions are relatively nonirritating to skin and eyes.

Hair over and around the horn buds is clipped with curved scissors. The sites are cleaned with a pledget of cotton that has been soaked in alcohol. Animals are restrained by an intramuscular injection of 10 mg of xylazine (Chapter 14). An 18-gauge 1.9 cm hypodermic needle is inserted to the hub at a site 1.9 cm dorsal and medial to the center of the horn bud so that the tip of the needle is under the center of the bud. One-half of a milliliter to 1 ml of a 50% calcium chloride solution is injected slowly under each horn, with the bevel of the needle directed toward the periosteum.

The injection results in a narrow halo of reddish swollen area around the horn bud. The area is sensitive for about 4 days. The gangrenous area separates from the surrounding normal skin along a discrete symmetrical line of necrotic tissue, and epithelization advances under the curled edges of the lesions during the next 5 weeks. Healing is complete after 6 weeks, and normal hair covers the small scar.[6]

References

1. Beat, V. B.: Human toxicosis resulting from pesticide use, J. Am. Vet. Med. Assoc. **157:**1835, 1970.
2. Blood, D. C., and Henderson, J. A.: Veterinary medicine, Baltimore, 1974, The Williams & Wilkins Co.
3. Epstein, W. L., Shah, V., and Riegelman, S.: Dermatopharmacology of griseofulvin, Cutis **15:**271, 1975.
4. Hourrigan, J. L.: Safe use of pesticides on livestock, J. Am. Vet. Med. Assoc. **157:**1818, 1970.
5. Iverson, L. G.: Pesticides, their use and misuse, J. Am. Vet. Med. Assoc. **151:**1806, 1967.
6. Koger, L. M.: Dehorning by injection of calcium chloride, Vet. Med. Small Anim. Clin. **71:**824, 1976.
7. Meleny, W. P., and Roberts, I. H.: Evaluation of acaricidal dips for control of *Psoroptes ovis* on sheep, J. Am. Vet. Med. Assoc. **151:**725, 1967.
8. Montali, R. J.: Ear mites in a horse, J. Am. Vet. Med. Assoc. **169:**630, 1976.
9. Mozier, J.: Advances in cattle ectoparasite control with a discussion of some problems related to treatment with systemic insecticides, J. Am. Vet. Med. Assoc. **154:**1206, 1969.
10. Nelson, D. L.: Toxic reactions in cattle treated with systemic organophosphate insecticides, Can. Vet. J. **11:**62, March 1970.
11. Nelson, D. L., Allen, A. D., Mozier, J., and White, R. G.: Diagnosis and treatment of adverse reactions in cattle treated for grubs with systemic insecticide, Vet. Med. Small Anim. Clin. **62:**683, 1967.
12. Ray, A. C., Norris, J. D., Jr., and Reagor, J. C.: Benzene hexachloride poisoning in cattle, J. Am. Vet. Med. Assoc. **166:**1180, 1975.
13. Rossoff, I. S.: Handbook of veterinary drugs, New York, 1974, Springer Publishing Co.
14. Scharff, D. K., Sharman, G. A., and Ludwig, P.: Illness and death in calves induced by treatments with systemic insecticides for the control of cattle grubs, J. Am. Vet. Med. Assoc. **141:**582, 1962.
15. Smith, H. J.: A preliminary trial on the efficacy of ciodrin against *Chorioptes bovis* in cattle, Can. Vet. J. **8:**88, April 1967.
16. Strickland, R. K., Gerrish, R. R., Hourrigan, J. L., and Czech, F. P.: Chloropyridyl phosphorothioate insecticide as dip and spray: efficacy against *Psoroptes ovis*, dermal toxicity for domestic animals, selective carryout, and stability in the dipping vat, Am. J. Vet. Res. **31:**2135, 1970.

Additional readings

Boyd, C. L., and Bullard, L.: Organophosphate treatment of cutaneous habronemiasis in horses, J. Am. Vet. Med. Assoc. **153:**324, 1968.
Farris, H. E., Fraunfelder, F. T., and Mason, C. T.: Cryotherapy of equine sarcoid and other lesions, Vet. Med. Small Anim. Clin. **71:**325, 1976.
Johnson, J. H.: Management of neglected lower limb wounds, Mod. Vet. Pract. **54:**47, March 1973.
Khan, M. A.: Toxicity of systemic insecticides, Vet. Rec. **92:**411, 1973.
Morris, L. S.: Effects of pesticides on embryos, Med. Trib. **10:**4, Sept. 1969.
Owen, R. R.: Use of topical enzymatic debriding agent in wounds of the equine leg, Vet. Med. Small Anim. Clin. **70:**1101, 1975.
Scharff, D. K.: Control of cattle grubs in horses, Vet. Med. Small Anim. Clin. **68:**791, 1973.
Stannard, A. A.: Some important dermatoses in the horse, Mod. Vet. Pract. **53:**31, Aug. 1972.

11

DRUGS FOR PREVENTION AND TREATMENT OF
Internal parasitic infections of dogs and cats

ANTHELMINTICS

In this chapter as well as Chapters 12 and 13 we will discuss the use of anthelmintics, which are chemotherapeutic agents that combat infestation with trematodes (flukes), cestodes (tapeworms), and nematodes (roundworms).

Characteristics of anthelmintics

Many chemicals are capable of killing parasites. Their use in clinical practice depends on certain factors, including the following:

1. *High toxicity to the parasite.* Anthelmintics should be highly toxic to the parasite. Ideally the drug should be parasiticidal, that is, it should kill the parasite.

2. *Low toxicity to the host.* The ideal anthelmintic should not injure the host in any way. Many compounds that are toxic to parasites are toxic to the host as well. A primary goal in the development of newer types of anthelmintics is to develop compounds with little or no toxicity to the host. This is especially important in livestock. When anthelmintics are used to free livestock of their parasitic burden, it is hoped that an increase in the rate of gain and feed conversion will result. However, if compounds toxic to the host are used, that desired effect will not occur. For example, if a compound is used that results in severe liver toxicity, the rate of gain and food conversion will be reduced for a long time.

3. *Consistency of effectiveness against the parasite and its toxicity to the host.* The desired effectiveness of an anthelmintic is dependent on the interrelationship among host, parasite, and drug. Generally, the greater the difference between the effective dose and the dose that is toxic to the host the greater the consistency of drug response. This consistency is important if the person administering the anthelmintic is to have any confidence regarding the expected results.

4. *Ease of administration.* The route of ad-

ministration, the volume that must be administered, and the number of times a drug must be administered determines how easy or difficult the administration of an anthelmintic is. The easier a drug is to administer the greater the chance the animal will receive it.

5. *Economics.* The more economical the anthelmintic the more likely it will be used. This is an especially important consideration in livestock because hundreds of animals may be treated at a given time. If an anthelmintic is not economical, no matter how effective, it will not be used. On the other hand, no matter how inexpensive, if the drug is ineffective, it will not be economical.

6. *Chemical stability.* The most acceptable anthelmintics are those that do not readily break down chemically and do not need special conditions of storage such as refrigeration or protection from light.

Factors that affect the efficacy of anthelmintics

It is difficult to determine which anthelmintics best fulfill the criteria of the ideal anthelmintic. Even in well-controlled studies, one investigator's data may be grossly inconsistent with another's. For example, Poole and others[31] reported that niclosamide, given at the rate of from 110 to 220 mg/kg, was 100% effective against the two common tapeworms of dogs, *Dipylidium caninum* and *Taenia pisiformis.* However, Sharp and coworkers[36] reported that in dogs, at the rate 157.1 mg/kg, niclosamide was only 18% effective against *D. caninum* and 55% effective against *T. pisiformis.* What causes such different results?

Factors that could contribute to such discrepancies include the following:

1. *Investigatory situation.* The techniques used and powers of observation of different investigating teams may vary substantially from one study to another.

2. *Interrelationship of the host, parasite, and drug.* Some factors contributing to the response of the host include the general health of the animal, its state of nutrition, its

age, its genetic resistance to a particular type of parasite, and its immune status.

3. *Resistance to the effect of the anthelmintic.* Some parasites have greater resistance to the effects of certain anthelmintics than others of the same species. In addition, during certain stages in their life cycle, parasites may not be affected by anthelmintics. For example, hookworm larvae spend a portion of their life cycle migrating through the circulatory system of the dog. When they are migrating, the larvae are not susceptible to anthelmintics that exert their effect within the gut. Therefore, even if such drugs are 100% effective in killing adults present in the intestinal tract, within a few weeks, when the migrating larvae mature and locate in the intestinal tract, the animal will be reinfected.

4. *Dose and dosage schedule used.* For example, the effectiveness of an anthelmintic may be affected by giving the entire dose all at once or by dividing it into more than one administration.

5. *Route of administration.* The maximum amount of the compound should come in direct contact with the parasite. For example, anthelmintics that are not absorbed from the gastrointestinal tract are more likely to be effective against intestinal parasites than those that are absorbed.

INTERNAL PARASITES OF DOGS AND CATS

Dogs and cats are infected with a wide variety of internal parasites. Those discussed in this text are listed in Table 11-1, but there are many other internal parasites of dogs and cats. Our discussion is limited to those which appear in the majority of clinical infections or that have public health significance.

The problems that internal parasites present to the host vary in degree. Some present relatively minor problems to the host, whereas others cause severe clinical disease and even death. For instance, the hydatid tapeworm (*Echinococcus granulosus*) presents relatively no problem to dogs, but if the eggs of the parasites are ingested by man, fatal infection may result.

Table 11-1. Selected list of internal parasites to North American dogs and cats*

Common name	Scientific name
Helminths	
Cestodes (tape-worms)	
Double-pored tapeworm	*Dipylidium caninum*
No common name	*Taenia pisiformis*
No common name	*T. taeniaeformis*
Hydatid tape-worm	*Echinococcus granulosus*
Nematodes (roundworms)	
Hookworms	*Ancylostoma braziliense*
	A. caninum
	Uncinaria stenocephala
Large round-worms (ascar-ids)	*Toxascaris leonina*
	Toxocara canis
	T. cati
Whipworm	*Trichuris vulpis*
Heartworm	*Dirofilaria immitis*
Protozoans	
Coccidia	*Eimeria caninus*
	Isospora bigemina
	I. felis
	I. rivolta

*Modified from Becklund, W. W.: Revised check list of internal and external parasites of domestic animals in the United States and possessions and in Canada, Am. J. Vet. Res. **25**1380, 1964.

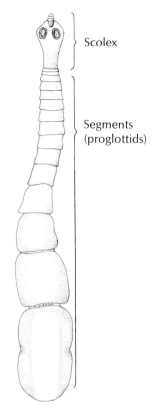

Fig. 11-1. Diagrammatic representation of a tapeworm.

We will discuss the life cycles of parasites. This is done because the life cycles influence treatment regimens.

Cestodes (tapeworms)

Tapeworms consist of a head (scolex) and numerous segments or proglottids (Fig. 11-1). The segments contain the male and female reproductive organs and ova. The posterior segments break off of many species of tapeworms and are passed from the host in the stool. Passed segments may be found around the anus of the animal and have the appearance of grains of rice.

The life cycle of all tapeworms involves an intermediate host. Direct transmission cannot occur from one host harboring the adult parasite to another host of the same species. A portion of the development of the immature tapeworm must take place in a species other than the one it infects as an adult. The species in which the immature parasite must spend part of its life prior to infecting the final host is called the "intermediate host."

Dipylidium caninum

D. caninum is the common tapeworm of the dog. It is also found in the cat and occasionally in man. In animals it is located in the small intestine. Generally, *D. caninum* infections present little problem in dogs and cats. However, in a severe infestation or in an animal of marginal health, *D. caninum* can cause abdominal distress, loss of weight, or both. Even though this parasite rarely presents

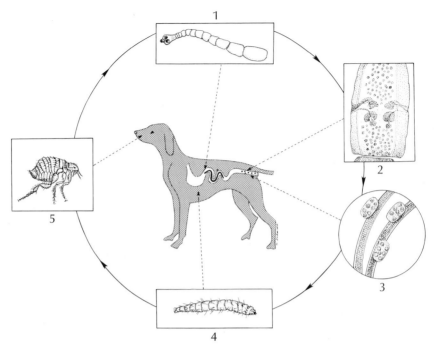

Fig. 11-2. Life cycle of *Dipylidium caninum*. *1,* Adult tapeworm lives in host's small intestine. *2,* Proglottids containing ova break off and pass out of animal through anus. *3,* Ova packets are deposited on fur and, *4,* ingested by flea larvae. *5,* Flea larvae develop to adult fleas containing immature forms of tapeworms. Infected fleas are swallowed by dog, and tapeworm matures in dog's small intestine, completing cycle.

problems to the host, most owners want their animals free of tapeworms.

The intermediate hosts of *D. caninum* are the dog flea, *Ctenocephalides canis;* the cat flea, *C. felis;* and the human flea, *Pulex irritans* (Fig. 11-2). Larvae of these fleas become infected by ingesting the tapeworm eggs. Dogs, cats, and occasionally humans acquire the parasite by swallowing infected fleas. If *D. caninum* is to be adequately controlled, the flea population of dogs and cats must also be adequately controlled (Chapter 9).

Taenia species

Like *D. caninum,* the *Taenia* tapeworms generally do not cause clinical signs in infested animals. *T. pisiformis* occurs primarily in the small intestine in dogs. The intermediate hosts are rabbits and hares, and dogs acquire the infection by eating these animals.

T. taeniaformis commonly infects cats. The parasite occurs in the small intestine. Cats acquire the infection primarily by eating rodents, the intermediate hosts. To prevent cats from acquiring the parasite, one would have to prevent them from eating wild rodents.

Treating *Dipylidium* and *Taenia* species infections. Among the drugs commercially available in the United States, the most effective for treating *Dipylidium* and *Taenia* species infestations in dogs and cats are bunamidine and niclosamide (Table 11-2).

An experimental drug, uredofos, shows high activity against both *Dipylidium* and *Taenia* species. The drug also appears to be extremely safe, safer than bunamidine, and more active against *Dipylidium* species than niclosamide. Eventually it may become the drug of choice for treating routine tapeworm infestations in dogs and cats.

Table 11-2. Effectiveness of anticestodal drugs

Drug	Dipylidium species	Taenia species	Echinococcus species
Arecoline hydrobromide	±	±	±
Arecoline-acetarsol	±	±	±
Bithional sulfoxide	?	?	+*
Bunamidine	+	+	+
Dichlorophen and toluene	±	±	?
Fospirate	?	?	+*
Mebendazole	?	?	+*
Niclosamide	±	+	−
Uredofos	+*	+*	?

Key: + = highly effective; ± = variable effectiveness; − = not effective; ? = effectiveness not clearly determined; * = further experimental trials needed before recommended for routine use.

Hydatid tapeworm (Echinococcus granulosus)

The hydatid tapeworm does not occur frequently in the United States, but when it occurs, it is of extreme public health significance. The tapeworm is found in animals of the genus *Canis*, which includes dogs. In dogs the parasite usually produces no clinical signs, although in a severe infestation, inflammation of the intestinal tract can result. The significance of the infestation in dogs is the seriousness of the infection in humans when it is acquired from dogs (Fig. 11-3).

Dogs shed eggs of the hydatid tapeworm in their feces. These eggs are ingested by the intermediate hosts, which include man and sheep. Children are readily infected from petting the animals, getting ova on their hands, and then ingesting the ova. Sheep are infected from pastures contaminated with dog feces.

Eggs of the hydatid tapeworm hatch in the intestine of the intermediate host. The embryos migrate to the circulatory system and are carried by the blood to various organs. Each embryo then has the potential for forming a large cyst (hydatid cyst), which can measure 5 to 10 cm in diameter or larger. The cysts occur in various regions of the body, including the liver, lungs, and abdominal cavity. Simply as space-occupying lesions, they may cause relatively minor clinical signs, or they may result in severe problems, such as respiratory malfunction, liver failure, and death. After about 5 or 6 months, scolices of new tapeworms can form in the lining of the cyst. These scolices may be attached to the wall of the cyst or float free. If the cysts rupture, many scolices may be expelled in the fluid and implant in other body regions, where they form new cysts. The life cycle is completed when dogs ingest viscera of animals (commonly sheep) that have hydatid cysts. The scolices mature in the dog to adult parasites, and eggs are once again shed in the feces.

Treatment. The primary control of *E. granulosus* infections is to prevent dogs from eating viscera of sheep. Once *E. granulosus* infection is diagnosed in a dog, the animal is a threat to the public health and must be either euthanized or isolated and treated until a veterinarian is sure the animal is free of infection.

Of commercially available products, only bunamidine is recommended for the treatment of *E. granulosus* infections in dogs. Experimentally the following have also been found effective: bithionol sulfoxide, fospirate, and micronized mebendazole.[12-14,35]

In humans the only treatment for the disease is to remove the cysts surgically. Care must be taken not to rupture them. Formalin is often injected into the cysts by the surgeon to kill the scolices prior to surgical removal of the cysts.

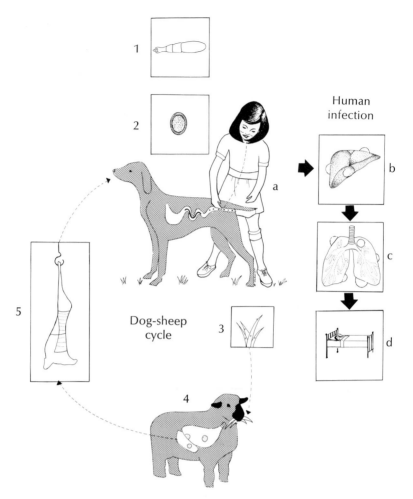

Fig. 11-3. Life cycle of *Echinococcus* species. Dog-sheep cycle: *(1)* adult tapeworm lives in dog's intestine; *(2)* it produces ova, which are passed in feces; *(3)* ova contaminate pastures; *(4)* ova are ingested by sheep and hatch to larvae, which form cysts in organs such as the lung and liver; *(5)* when viscera of infected sheep is fed to dogs, larvae mature to adult tapeworms in dog's intestine. Human infection: when humans ingest ova *(a)*, larvae hatch and form cysts in organs such as liver *(b)* or lungs *(c)*. These cysts can cause severe illness or even death *(d)*.

Cesticidal drugs

Arecoline hydrobromide. Arecoline hydrobromide stimulates the activity of the parasympathetic nervous system. As a result, it causes increased secretions in and motility of the gastrointestinal tract. Arecoline hydrobromide has been shown to exert a depressive action directly on the tapeworm. It is hypothesized that the drug acts by relaxing the muscles of the tapeworm, reducing its attachment on the intestinal mucosa; because the drug stimulates intestinal movements in the host, the detached worms are expelled. Apparently much of the anticestodal activity of the drug results from the direct action of the compound on the intestinal parasites because subcutaneous injection of arecoline hydrobromide, although causing a marked diarrhea, expels only about 0.1% of worms in the intestinal tract.[22]

Effectiveness. The effectiveness of arecoline against any species of tapeworms is highly questionable. There is no uniform agreement that the drug removes the scolices of tapeworms. The drug may give the appearance of effectiveness, since the body of the worm is passed in the feces. However, scolices that may remain in the animal grow new bodies, and the infestation continues.

Toxicity. In addition to questionable effectiveness, arecoline is more toxic than other cesticidal drugs that are at least as effective. Signs of toxicity include hypersalivation, severe intestinal cramping, vomiting, and severe diarrhea. It is especially contraindicated in small dogs or cats.

When there are severe toxic signs, the antidote for arecoline is atropine sulfate given subcutaneously at the rate of 0.04 mg/kg of body weight. This does not antagonize the action of arecoline on the tapeworms.

Dose and administration. Arecoline is dispensed as a tablet and is given orally. A dose of 0.9 mg/kg of body weight has been recommended. Studies show that this dose is nearly as effective as the more common 1.8 mg/kg dose. With the lower dose, undesirable side reactions such as discomfort, vomiting, and loss of consciousness are less likely.[22]

Dogs should be fasted approximately 12 hours before receiving arecoline. Vomiting does not reduce the effectiveness of arecoline hydrobromide as long as it occurs at least 5 minutes after dosing. After 5 minutes the drug has passed into the intestine where it is absorbed and exerts its stimulation of the parasympathetic nervous system. Diarrhea usually occurs about 15 minutes after administration of the compound and lasts for about 30 to 40 minutes. If diarrhea does not occur within 2 hours after treatment, the animal should be given a saline laxative such as epsom salt to stimulate defecation so that the paralyzed worms are removed before they recover and reattach to the intestinal mucosa.

Arecoline-acetarsol. This product is the complex of arecoline and arsenic. Adminis-

tered orally as a tablet, the drug is recommended by the manufacturer for use in dogs against *Taenia* species and *D. caninum*.

Effectiveness. It has been reported that an arecoline-acetarsol compound is 87% effective against *T. pisiformis* and 75% effective against *D. caninum* in dogs.[36]

Toxicity. The drug is contraindicated in puppies under 3 months of age and in cats. It should not be administered if there is any systemic disease. The drug may cause considerable abdominal cramping.

Dose and administration. The recommended dose of 4.4 mg/kg of body weight is high compared with that for arecoline hydrobromide. The size of the dose may be responsible for the frequent appearance of undesirable side effects. The compound is usually administered about an hour after a light meal for dogs. Ordinarily it is not necessary to give a laxative when administering the drug, but if the animal does not defecate within a couple of hours, a saline laxative (Chapter 19) or enema is indicated.

Bithional sulfoxide. Bithional sulfoxide is used primarily to treat cattle and sheep with liver fluke infestation. Its use for that purpose is discussed in Chapter 12.

The potential for using bithional sulfoxide to combat *E. granulosus* infestation in dogs has been investigated. The drug has been shown to be 100% effective when given orally in two doses 2 days apart at the rate of 50 mg/kg. Doses of over 200 mg/kg killed some dogs. When it was given twice 2 days apart at 50 mg/kg, only a small percentage of dogs showed vomiting or diarrhea.[13]

Bunamidine. Various salts of bunamidine have been used experimentally as anticestodal drugs. In the United States bunamidine hydrochloride is the salt that is marketed as a 100, 200, or 400 mg tablet.

Effectiveness. Bunamidine hydrochloride can be highly effective against *Dipylidium*, *Taenia*, and *Echinococcus* species infestations. Examples of its effectiveness are shown in Table 11-3. According to the manufacturer, a heavy mucous coat on the parasite, as may occur in an inflamed gut, can reduce the

Table 11-3. Efficacy of bunamidine hydrochloride

Method of adminis-tration and dose	D. caninum	T. pisiformis	E. granulosus	Reference
25 mg/kg	Not reported	82% of dogs completely cleared of infection	Not reported	18
Fasted 12 hours before and 3 hours after 50 mg/kg	Not reported	Not reported	85.9% of immature parasites; 100% of mature parasites	1
Overnight fast, 48-68 mg/kg	Cleared 82% of dogs of infection	Cleared 100% of dogs of infection	Not reported	32

effectiveness of the drug. Animals should be rechecked for parasites by a veterinarian and retreated if necessary.

Toxicity. Vomiting and diarrhea are commonly listed as toxic reactions to the drug. The manufacturer claims that the incidence of vomiting can be reduced by withholding feed 3 hours before administering bunamidine to animals.

In rare incidences dogs may collapse and die shortly after receiving bunamidine.[9,41] This apparently results from cardiac fibrillation (Chapter 18). Because epinephrine and related compounds appear to sensitize the heart to this effect, animals should not be allowed to exercise or become excited shortly after being given the drug.

Because liver damage may cause a high concentration of bunamidine in the blood, thus increasing the chance of toxicity, bunamidine should not be given to animals showing signs of liver pathology.

The use of bunamidine in male dogs within 1 month of breeding is contraindicated, since the drug has been shown to interfere with spermatogenesis.

Dose and administration. It is administered orally after a 3-hour fast at a rate of 25 to 50 mg/kg. Animals should be given a light meal 3 to 4 hours after receiving the drug.

Dichlorophen and toluene. A commercial product is available that contains dichlorophen and toluene. It is sold as a broad-spectrum anthelmintic that is effective against various tapeworm and roundworm species.

The product, used in dogs and cats, has limited effectiveness against *Taenia* and *Dipylidium* species. Reports in the literature cite 72% to 86% effectiveness against *Taenia* species and 52% to 85% effectiveness against *Dipylidium* species.[22,36] It is difficult to judge the actual effectiveness of the drug, however, because none of the reports states if scolices were expelled with the tapeworms.

Generally, it is administered at the rate of 264 mg toluene plus 220 mg of dichlorophen per kilogram of body weight after withholding feed and milk for 15 to 18 hours. Broth may be given during the fasting period. Animals receiving the combination should be fed 4 hours after treatment.

Fospirate. Fospirate, an organophosphate compound, may be an effective drug against *E. granulosus* infestation in dogs. In experimental trials the drug has been 100% effective in freeing dogs of *E. granulosus* infestation when given orally at the rate of 40 mg/kg in three doses 2 days apart. Doses above and below this have not been as effective.[14,35]

Toxic reactions to fospirate include vomiting and diarrhea.

Further evaluation of fospirate will be necessary before it can be recommended for the routine treatment of *E. granulosus* infestation in dogs.

Mebendazole. Mebendazole is one of a class of drugs, the benzimidazoles, primarily used against gastrointestinal nematodes in cattle, sheep, and horses. They are discussed in Chapters 12 and 13.

Table 11-4. Effectiveness of niclosamide against tapeworms

Dose	D. caninum in dogs	T. pisiformis in dogs	T. taeniaformia in cats	Reference
100-200 mg/kg	Not reported	Not reported	100%	40
110-220 mg/kg	100%	100%	Not reported	31
157 mg/kg	18%	55%	Not reported	36
154-162 mg/kg	0% of dogs totally cleared	80% of dogs totally cleared	Not reported	32

Mebendazole may be of use in dogs as a cesticidal agent for the treatment of *E. granulosus* infestation. It apparently exerts its effect on the parasite by inhibiting the rate of glucose utilization. At doses of 20 mg/kg given 2 days apart or 160 mg/kg given only once, an experimental grade of micronized mebendazole was 100% effective in freeing dogs of *E. granulosus* infestation. Single doses of 5 to 80 mg/kg were not 100% effective.[12]

The fine particle formulation was used on the theory that the increase in surface area provided by micronization increases either the dissolution rate or contact with absorptive surfaces of the parasite.

Further testing of mebendazole is necessary before it can be recommended as a routine anticestodal drug to combat *E. granulosus* infestations.

Niclosamide. Niclosamide, which is restricted by federal law to sale by or on the order of a licensed veterinarian, is dispensed in tablet form. Generally, within 6 to 48 hours after treatment, dead tapeworms are expelled. The manufacturer states that niclosamide has a disintegrating effect on tapeworms. Shortly after treatment, the discharged parasites may be intact. However, those eliminated later may be partially disintegrated. The compound kills the parasites.

Effectiveness. The effectiveness of niclosamide against various species of tapeworms in dogs and cats is shown in Table 11-4. Two reports indicate that the activity of niclosamide against *D. caninum* may be limited.[32,36]

Toxicity. At normal doses, no toxic effects from the product have been reported. The compound should not be administered to ani-

Table 11-5. Efficacy of uredofos for clearing dogs of tapeworms

Dose	D. caninum	Taenia species	Reference
25 mg/kg	73%	100%	33
50 mg/kg	100%	100%	33
50 mg/kg	100%	100%	32
100 mg/kg	100%	100%	33

mals with diarrhea, since the effect of the drug may be reduced by its rapid excretion. The product is safe to use in young puppies and kittens and in pregnant females.

Dose and administration. For dogs and cats the manufacturer recommends that niclosamide be administered at the rate of 157 mg/kg of weight. The manufacturer recommends an overnight fast prior to giving the drug.

Uredofos. An organophosphate preparation, uredofos has been tested against various intestinal parasites of dogs. In addition to activity against various nematodes (p. 168) uredofos appears to be highly effective against *D. caninum* and *Taenia* species (Table 11-5).

At doses of 25 to 100 mg/kg of body weight, uredofos appears relatively safe in dogs older than 10 weeks of age. Tests in dogs under 10 weeks of age have not yet been reported. Until proof to the contrary appears, the drug should not be used in dogs with heartworm infestation.

Nematodes (roundworms)
Hookworms

The common hookworms of dogs and cats in the United States are *Ancylostoma braziliense, A. caninum,* and *Uncinaria stenoceph-*

ala. Hookworms occur in the small intestine of the dog and cat. The species infecting dogs and cats rarely infect humans.

Hookworm ova are passed in the feces and hatch in moist environments. A infective-stage larva enters the host either through the skin or by ingestion. Larvae that enter the host through the skin reach the blood and are carried to the lungs, where the majority become trapped in capillaries. From the capillaries they move to the alveoli of the lungs and, by way of the respiratory passages, to the pharynx. They are then swallowed and pass into the small intestine where they mature. Those infective stage larvae that are not trapped in the capillaries of the lungs travel to other organs in the body, where most die. However, those that are carried to the uterus in a pregnant animal may infect the fetus. The larvae then lie dormant in the fetus until after birth when they develop into mature parasites.

When the infective-stage larva enters the host by way of the oral cavity, it commonly penetrates the wall of the intestine and migrates through the circulatory system in a manner similar to those entering through the skin.

The primary problem caused by hookworms is blood loss. In the small intestine the adult parasites attach themselves to the mucosa of the intestine and suck blood. They also inject secretions into the wound that prevent coagulation of blood. Therefore the wound continues to bleed for some time after the parasite has moved to another place. In a heavy infestation there is substantial blood loss and a resulting anemia. Infested animals often develop a severe diarrhea that is dark in color because of the blood contained in the feces. In untreated animals, death can result.

A. caninum begins to parasitize blood from the host 7 to 9 days after experimental infection. At 14 days of age, puppies that are infected in the uterus with *A. caninum* have a mixed burden of hookworms in terms of age and larval stage. At least 60% of the worms have reached the stage at which they start to draw blood. Deaths resulting from such infestations occur in 3- to 4-week-old puppies. Therefore 14 days of age appears to be the best time to treat such animals with anthelmintics.

In humans, hookworms can cause "creeping eruptions." The larvae of these nematodes enter the skin and migrate. In the skin they may cause papules, inflammation, increased thickness, and itching.

Prevention. A vaccine is available to prevent hookworm infections.

In a report on two experiments conducted in puppies that received two doses at 7 and 10 weeks of age by subcutaneous inoculation with x-irradiated *A. caninum* larvae, the number of hookworms in the gut resulting from the challenge infection were reduced by 88% to 95% in vaccinated puppies as compared with the controls.[38]

When parasites of *A. caninum* reach the intestinal tract in vaccinated animals, they do not cause significant problems. Therefore dogs benefit in two ways from vaccination: the number of worms that complete development is reduced by about 90% and the remaining 10% are apparently nonpathogenic.

Treatment. The most effective treatments for hookworm infestations in dogs and cats appear to be dichlorvos, disophenol, pyrantel pamoate, tetrachloroethylene, and uredofos. In addition, the combination of toluene and dichlorophen may be highly effective (Table 11-6). Because none of the products in use are highly effective against the larvae of the parasite, it is recommended that animals be retreated with an appropriate anthelmintic 2 weeks after the first administration.

To treat the anemia, iron-dextran (Chapter 17) can be administered at the rate of 10 to 22 mg/kg intramuscularly. If anemia is severe, blood transfusions may be necessary. If the animal is dehydrated from diarrhea, appropriate fluid therapy as discussed in Chapter 17 is indicated.

Large roundworms (ascarids)

One characteristic of ascarids is that the females produce large numbers of eggs, which are passed in the feces of the host.

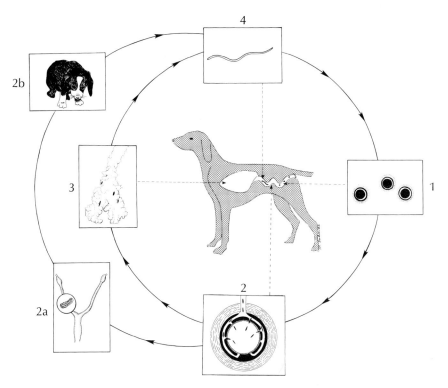

Fig. 11-4. Life cycle of *Toxocara canis*. *1,* Adult worms produce ova, which are passed in feces. Ova are ingested and hatch in intestine. *2,* In intestine, larvae migrate into blood vessels. *3,* Most larvae migrate to lungs where they are coughed up and swallowed. *4,* They then mature to adults in small intestine. Some larvae migrate to the uterus where they encapsulate *(2a).* When the bitch becomes pregnant, larvae infect pups and remain in liver until pup is born *(2b).* Larvae then migrate to lungs, are coughed up and swallowed, and mature to adults in pup's small intestine *(4).*

When the ova of *Toxocara canis* are swallowed, larvae hatch from the ova, enter the circulatory system, and penetrate the small intestine. Most migrate to the lungs and are then coughed up and swallowed (Fig. 11-4). Some larvae migrate to other organs such as the uterus. Prenatal infection of the fetus commonly occurs in the uterus. *T. canis* larvae have the ability to encapsulate themselves in the uterus of an animal that is not pregnant. When she does become pregnant, they can infect the developing fetuses.

When an animal is infected in the uterus, the larvae remain in the fetal liver until birth. When that occurs, the larvae resume migration through the lungs of the young animal. They are then coughed up, swallowed, and grow to become adults in the small intestine.

Toxascaris species occurs in the small intestine of the dog, cat, and various wild canine and feline species. When ova of *Toxascaris* species are swallowed by the dog or cat, the larvae hatches from the eggs and penetrate the mucosa of the small intestine. Usually the larvae develop in that area without migration. However, a prenatal infection of fetuses in the uterus by migrating larvae is possible.

Toxocara cati occurs in the small intestine of the cat. Generally, the larvae of this species do not migrate but rather develop in the walls of the intestine. Apparently a prenatal infection of this species does not occur.

Ascarids can cause many problems, including inflammation of the lungs, intestinal obstruction, and bile duct obstruction. Animals suffering from such parasites are often emaci-ated and may suffer from anemia. It is safe to assume that all puppies are infected with *T. canis.*

Because of the migrating habits of *Toxo-cara* larvae, many adults are immune to in-festation. However, even immune bitches can transmit the larvae prenatally to their puppies.

Visceral larva migrans is a condition in man caused by migration of the larvae of *T. canis.* This condition occurs primarily in children up to about 6 years of age. When ova are swallowed, they hatch and the larvae migrate to the liver, lungs, and sometimes other or-gans, including the brain and eye. The larvae cause inflammatory reactions in the organs. Symptoms can be serious, depending on the amount of allergic reaction in the organs.

The disease is best prevented by routinely treating puppies and kittens for ascarid in-fections. This reduces the chance that chil-dren will be contaminated with the ova of these parasites. Since the nest of a bitch with a litter of puppies is often highly contami-nated with ova of *T.* species, young children should be discouraged from playing in or visiting this area.

Treatment. The most effective drugs for the treatment of ascarid infections in dogs and cats appear to be dichlorvos, diethylcar-bamazine, dithiazanine, pyrantel pamoate, toluene, toluene and dichlorophen combina-tion, and uredofos.

Whipworms (*Trichuris vulpis*)

Members of the genus *Trichuris* are re-ferred to as whipworms because part of their body is thick and another part is narrow, giv-ing them the appearance of a whip. *T. vulpis* infests dogs. This parasite locates in the ce-cum and other parts of the dog's intestine. Animals are infected by ingestion of ova. Generally, the parasite does not cause clin-ical problems. If the cecum is inflamed, the cecum can be removed surgically. However, veterinarians usually treat whipworm infesta-tions medically.

Treatment. The most effective drugs to combat whipworms appear to be dichlorvos and phthalofyne. Mebendazole may also be highly effective in treating whipworm infec-tions.

Heartworms (*Dirofilaria immitis*)

Heartworms occur primarily in the dog. Rare cases in cats do occur.[15] The life cycle of the heartworm is shown in Fig. 11-5. The mature parasites live in the heart's right ven-tricle and the pulmonary arteries. Their pres-ence causes obstruction in small pulmonary arteries, which puts a great strain on the heart. Congestive heart failure (Chapter 18) and chronic lung disease may result. In ad-dition, secondary disease of the liver, kid-neys, and other organs is common.

A wide variety of clinical signs is seen in animals with heartworm infestation, depend-ing on the severity of the infection and the degree to which various organs are affected.

The adult parasite produces microfilariae that circulate in the bloodstream (Fig. 11-6). These microfilariae, which may circulate for as long as three years, will not mature until they have passed through an intermediate host, one of a number of mosquito species. In the mosquito the microfilariae molt. The larvae that result are inoculated into another dog when the mosquito takes a blood meal. They molt again, migrate in the dog's body, and mature in its heart. The adult parasites then produce microfilariae. The entire life cycle takes about 6 months.

Treatment. Following are the three pur-poses in using chemotherapy to combat heartworms:

• Destruction of adult heartworms
• Destruction of circulating microfilariae
• Destruction of infective larvae that have been introduced into host by mosquitos

In 1969 the *Journal of the American Vet-erinary Association* reported the recommen-dations of a panel on the treatment and pre-vention of heartworm disease in dogs.[19] The following course of therapy was recommend-ed:

1. For established infections treat with thiacetarsamide (pp. 166 and 167).

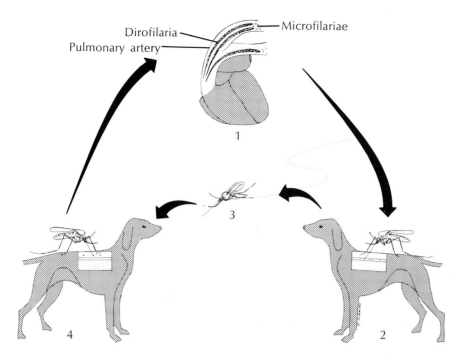

Fig. 11-5. Life cycle of canine heartworm. *1,* Adult stage *(Dirofilaria)* live in pulmonary artery and produce microfilariae, which are carried throughout circulatory system. *2,* When mosquito takes a blood meal, it withdraws some microfilariae. *3,* Microfilariae molt in the mosquito. *4,* When mosquito takes another blood meal, these microfilariae are injected under the skin, molt again, migrate into circulatory system, and travel to heart where they mature to adult stage.

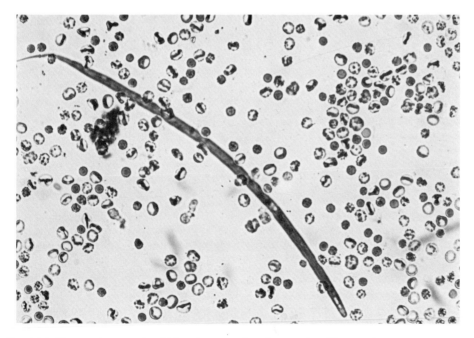

Fig. 11-6. Photomicrograph of blood smear showing a microfilaria at low power. (Courtesy Mr. Paul Sumner, Animal Care Facility Diagnostic Laboratory, University of California, San Francisco.)

Table 11-6. Relative effectiveness of antinematodal drugs*

| Drug | Hookworms | Ascarids | Whipworms | Heartworms | | |
				Circulating microfilariae	Adult	Infective larvae
Dichlorvos	+	+	+	C	C	−
Diethylcarbamazine	−	+	−	C	C	+
Disophenol	+	−	−	−	−	−
Dithiazanine	±	+	±	+	−	−
Levamisole	?	?	?	+	+ for ♂♂ − for ♀♀	−
Mebendazole	?	?	+	−	−	−
N-Butyl chloride	±	±	±	−	−	−
Phthalofyne	−	−	+	−	−	−
Piperazine	−	±	−	−	−	−
Pyrantel pamoate	+	+	−	−	−	−
Tetrachlorethylene	+	?	?	−	−	−
Thiacetarsamide	−	−	−	−	+	−
Toluene	±	+	±	−	−	−
Toluene and di-chlorophen	+	+	?	−	−	−
Uredofos	+	+	±	−	−	−

Key: + = highly effective; ± = variable effectiveness; − = not effective; C = contraindicated; ? = effectiveness not clearly determined.
*This can be used only as a guide. The susceptibility of parasites to anthelmintics varies from population to population.

2. Use dithiazanine to eliminate circulating microfilariae 6 weeks after the thiacetarsamide therapy (pp. 162 and 163).

3. To prevent heartworms either administer thiacetarsamide at therapeutic doses every 6 months starting when the dog is 1 year old or administer diethylcarbamazine in the feed starting 2 months before and continuing 2 months after the mosquito season. Diethylcarbamazine cannot be given until the animal is free of circulating microfilariae. The diethylcarbamazine prevents infective larvae from maturing to adult heartworms (p. 162).

Since 1969, other forms of heartworm therapy have evolved. Instead of dithiazanine some veterinarians prefer to use a relatively new drug, levamisole, to free the patient from microfilariae. Some practitioners and researchers also advocate administering the microfilaricide (either dithiazanine or levamisole) before using thiacetarsamide to kill the adult heartworms. It is claimed that such a schedule reduces the chances of the animal developing toxicity to the thiacetarsamide therapy.[7,10,11] In addition to freeing the patient from microfilariae, it is claimed that in low to moderate heartworm infestations the administration of levamisole will kill adult male heartworms and free the animal of the clinical signs of heartworm disease.[7,10]

Antinematodal drugs

Dichlorvos. Dichlorvos is an organophosphate preparation. Generally, it is distributed as a bead-shaped resin pellet that slowly releases the active ingredient as the pellet passes through the animal's gastrointestinal tract. Such a resin pellet is usually designed to release approximately 35% of the total active ingredient in the 24 hours it takes to pass through an animal's intestinal tract.

Dichlorvos is volatile and easily destroyed

Table 11-7. Reported effectiveness of dichlorvos

Dose	Hookworms	Ascarids	Whipworms	Reference
31.5 mg/kg	Not reported	100%	Not reported	3
35 mg/kg	100%	100%	100%	2
36 mg/kg	100%	93%	91%	36
11 mg/kg to 33- to 50-day old puppies	Not reported	87%-100%; immature parasites, 54%-100%	Not reported	16

by oxidizing agents and/or moisture. It should be stored in the refrigerator. If it becomes wet, this drug should not be used.

Effectiveness. Dichlorvos has been shown to be effective against ascarids, hookworms, and whipworms. Its effectiveness against these parasites, as reported in the literature, is shown in Table 11-7.

Generally, drug-sensitive nematodes are expelled within 3 to 12 hours after dosage. For all practical purposes, expulsion of the parasites is complete within 24 hours.

In separate studies it has been demonstrated that dichlorvos, when administered in the feed, is highly effective against all three species of hookworms. The compound was as effective when administered as a split dose of 20 mg/kg given in the evening and the following morning as it was in a single administration with the evening meal of 31.5 mg/kg. The high effectiveness of dichlorvos against ascarids has also been demonstrated.[2,3,36]

In some dogs the effectiveness of dichlorvos against whipworms may be erratic. When dichlorvos is used to combat whipworms, stool samples of all dogs should be examined 10 to 14 days after each treatment. It should be readministered to animals that show *T. vulpis* ova in their stool. These animals should have their stool rechecked in 10 to 14 days, and if whipworm ova are found, a different drug should be used (Table 11-6).

Toxicity. Generally, the reduction of cholinesterase in dogs and cats caused by dichlorvos is well tolerated. Signs of toxicity in animals resulting from dichlorvos overdosage are salivation, constriction of the pupil, retching, vomiting, and diarrhea. Toxicity can progress to such neurological disturbances as incoordination, general muscular weakness, paralysis, depressed blood pressure, and decreased respiratory rate. Toxicity to dichlorvos is treated as described in Chapter 8.

In enzootic heartworm areas, dogs over 1 year old should be examined for the presence of heartworms before the administration of dichlorvos. It should not be used in animals so infected.

Dichlorvos is not used to treat either heartworm or microfilarial infestations. When administered to dogs with heartworms, it can cause migration of heartworms into small branches of the pulmonary artery, which can compromise blood flow to the lungs. In addition, heartworms may reduce an animal's metabolic and excretory capacity for eliminating dichlorvos, which can result in blood levels high enough to cause toxicity.

Other contraindications for dichlorvos are concurrent use with other anthelmintics or muscle relaxants. It should not be administered to animals showing signs of severe constipation, mechanical blockage of the intestinal tract, impaired liver function, or circulatory failure or to animals recently exposed to or showing signs of infectious disease.

As with all cholinesterase inhibitors, it should not be used in animals simultaneously or within a few days before or after treatment with or exposure to other cholinesterase-inhibiting drugs, pesticides, or chemicals. Therefore dogs wearing flea collars should not be treated with dichlorvos until the collar has been removed for 5 days. The collar should not be put back on the animal for another 5 days after the treatment.

Dose and administration. For treatment of hookworms, large roundworms, and whipworms in adult dogs, the recommended dose is 26 to 33 mg/kg. The drug is commonly sprinkled over the animal's food. If vomiting occurs, it should *not* be assumed that the animal did not receive any dichlorvos. Instead a stool sample should be checked in 10 to 14 days, and, if necessary, the animal should be retreated at that time. One method of treatment in animals that have a tendency to vomit after receiving dichlorvos is to divide the effective dose in half and administer each half dose 8 to 24 hours apart. Efficacy of such an administration is about the same as a single administration of the total dose, and the incidence of vomiting is decreased.

For kittens and puppies 10 days to 3 months old the manufacturer recommends a dose of dichlorvos at the rate of 11 mg/kg of body weight. This dose applies only to a formulation manufactured specifically for use in kittens and puppies.

Diethylcarbamazine citrate (USP). Diethylcarbamazine citrate is a derivative of piperazine (p. 165). It is administered orally, usually as a tablet or liquid, to both dogs and cats.

Effectiveness. Diethylcarbamazine is highly effective against ascarid infestation in dogs and cats and against infective larvae of heartworms in dogs. It prevents infective heartworm larvae from becoming established.

Toxicity. Diethylcarbamazine is relatively nontoxic in dogs and cats that are free of circulating microfilariae. About the only side effect commonly noted is vomiting shortly after administration. This can be reduced by administering the drug shortly after the animal eats.

Diethylcarbamazine can cause a severe shocklike reaction in dogs with circulating microfilariae, a reaction that can be fatal. Therefore, prior to giving diethylcarbamazine to a dog with microfilariae, dithiazanine or levamisole should be administered until a blood test 2 weeks later is negative for mi-

crofilariae. Only after the patient is free from microfilariae can diethylcarbamazine be used to combat ascarid infestations or as a prophylaxis against infective heartworm larvae.

Dose and administration. For the treatment of ascarids, diethylcarbamazine is administered at the rate of 55 mg/kg of body weight for the dog and cat.[34]

For preventing infective larvae from maturing to adult heartworms, diethylcarbamazine is administered in dogs at the rate of 3.3 mg/kg/24 hr. Treatment must begin at least 2 months before and be continued for 2 months after the mosquito season. In some areas, the mosquito season is long enough to warrant year-round treatment.

Dithiazanine iodide. Dithiazanine iodide is a cyanine dye dispensed as a tablet. It is used in dogs and cats for the treatment of ascarids, hookworms, and whipworms. In addition, it is used against the microfilariae of *D. immitis.*

Effectiveness. In an experimental trial, dithiazanine was 100% effective against *T. canis* when given in the feed at the rate of 20 mg/kg of body weight daily for 7 days. At this same dose its effectiveness against hookworms and whipworms was variable.[37]

It is effective against microfilariae. However, to be sure that the blood is completely cleared, the blood should be examined 2 weeks after the last administration. If necessary, another course of dithiazanine can be given. If a blood examination indicates the presence of microfilariae 2 weeks after the second course of therapy, the use of another microfilaricide, levamisole, should be considered.

Toxicity. Vomiting and diarrhea may occasionally accompany the use of dithiazanine iodide. The owner must be warned about this, since dithiazanine will severely stain carpets and furniture. Vomiting and diarrhea can be minimized by giving the drug at or immediately after feeding. To avoid kidney toxicity, dithiazanine iodide therapy should not be continued for more than 10 days consecutively.

Dose and administration. If dithiazanine is used to treat microfilariae after a course of thiacetarsamide therapy, 6 weeks should elapse between the final treatment with thiacetarsamide and the start of dithiazanine therapy. If complications occurred during the treatment to rid the animal of the adult worms, an additional 6 weeks' rest is indicated.

Instead of giving dithiazanine *after* thiacetarsamide therapy, it can be the first drug administered in the treatment of heartworms. By eliminating the circulating microfilariae prior to initiating therapy against the adult parasites, the animal may be protected from the toxic effects of thiacetarsamide.[11]

Circulating microfilariae can be eliminated by the daily administration of dithiazanine iodide orally at the rate of 4.4 to 6.6 mg/kg for 7 days. The blood should then be checked for the presence of microfilariae 12 weeks after the last administration and the treatment repeated if necessary. For treating ascarid infestations, dithiazanine can be given orally at feeding time at the rate of 20 mg/kg for 7 days.

For hookworms and whipworms other more effective drugs are recommended.

Disophenol. Disophenol is available commercially as a 4.5% injectable solution.

Effectiveness. The drug is highly effective against all three species of hookworms.[17,22,36,42] It is used to combat mature hookworms in dogs and cats; it is not effective against immature hookworms. Its use against tapeworms and other roundworms is limited, since other drugs are preferred against these parasites.

Toxicity. Toxicity studies show that disophenol is reasonably safe at recommended doses. The formation of cataracts has been reported as a toxic effect of disophenol. However, when the recommended dosage and route of administration are used, such problems are minimal.[24]

When given in excessive dosage, disophenol can cause death. Deaths from acute disophenol toxicity have occurred with doses of 15 mg/kg subcutaneously. Doses in the range of 35 mg/kg intramuscularly commonly result in toxicosis.

Among the signs of disophenol toxicosis are panting, increased respiratory rate, higher body temperature, an increased heart rate, vomiting, and swelling of visible mucous membranes.[30] Hemoconcentration, the reduction of intravascular serum (Chapters 17 and 18), can lead to shock.

Treatments suggested for disophenol toxicosis include the following:

• Administration of parenteral fluids such as lactated ringers
• Reducing the high body temperature by using the antipyretic dipyrone

For this purpose, dipyrone can be given at the rate of 110 to 220 mg/kg of body weight intramuscularly or subcutaneously. The dosage can be repeated in 4 to 6 hours.[34] The fever can also be reduced by using alcohol rubs or ice baths.

Subcutaneous administration is recommended for disophenol. In some dogs, intramuscular administration results in signs of extreme pain. The drug has caused adverse reactions in cats. In our opinion, most of these adverse reactions result from improper dosage. The small amounts used in cats are difficult to measure accurately in syringes.

Dose and administration. The drug is administered at the rate of 10 mg/kg subcutaneously. Treatment should be repeated in 2 weeks to combat the adult hookworms that will have developed from the immature parasites, which are not affected by the drug.

Levamisole. Levamisole is a drug used to treat gastrointestinal nematode infestation in cattle, sheep, and swine.

Effectiveness. In dogs levamisole eliminates circulating microfilariae and apparently is active against adult heartworms. In separate trials, when the drug was used to kill circulating microfilariae at doses of approximately 11 mg/kg/24 hr for 10 days, 70% to 100% of dogs were cleared of microfilarial infection.[4,10,28,29]

In both clinical and experimental trials, levamisole has been given as a microfilaricide 3 to 6 weeks after animals received a full course of thiacetarsamide therapy.

There is evidence that the drug is toxic to adult heartworms.[7,10] It appears to kill male adult heartworms and to be relatively non-toxic to the females.

Toxicity. In animals free of adult heartworms or with little or moderate infestations, toxic reactions to levamisole present little problem. Such reactions normally occur after the first dose. If administration of the drug is discontinued, the animal usually recovers in 2 to 3 days. Once the animal has recovered, therapy can again be started. Toxic signs include hypersalivation, muscular tremors, vomiting, and, occasionally, incoordination. In advanced adult heartworm infestations, toxic reactions to levamisole can be severe and even result in death.

Dose and administration. Even though the drug has not yet been cleared by the FDA for use in dogs, many practitioners use levamisole in their regimen to combat heartworms. As a microfilaricide it can be given orally at the daily rate of 11 mg/kg for 10 days 6 weeks after thiacetarsamide is used to free the animal of adult parasites. As with dithiazanine it may be given to patients prior to treating them for adult heartworms. Regardless of when it is given, 2 weeks after the last administration the blood should be checked for circulating microfilariae. If these are present, the course of therapy should be repeated and the blood rechecked in 2 weeks.

If levamisole is used as a microfilaricide in animals with adult heartworms, some adult parasites will be killed. Elimination of adult heartworms that remain after the course of therapy can be elected or bypassed. If elimination is elected, thiacetarsamide should be used. If it is bypassed, the patient would be placed on diethylcarbamazine to prevent any new infection.

Mebendazole. As discussed on pp. 154 and 155, mebendazole is a potential anticestodal drug in dogs and cats. In dogs it is also apparently effective against whipworm infestations when given to each animal at the rate of 100 mg/24 hours for 3 days.[23]

N-butyl chloride. N-butyl chloride is generally administered as a soft gelatin capsule.

Effectiveness. Even though it is widely

Table 11-8. Efficacy of N-butyl chloride

Ascarids	Hook-worms	Whip-worms	Reference
100%	60%	66%	22
61%	23%	31%	36
57%	70%	19%	2

used in dogs and cats, it gives variable results as an anthelmintic (Table 11-8).

Toxicity. The drug results in relatively few toxic reactions in dogs. The most common adverse effect is vomiting. Dogs in normal health tolerate doses of N-butyl chloride up to 11 ml/kg of body weight.

Dose and administration. Following are the recommended doses of N-butyl chloride for combating hookworm and ascarid infestations:

Under 2.25 kg	1 ml
2.2 to 4.5 kg	2 ml
4.5 to 9 kg	3 ml
9 to 18 kg	4 ml
Over 18 kg	5 ml

Commonly, dogs are fasted for 12 to 18 hours before the drug is administered. For maximum effectiveness, a mild saline cathartic should be administered about 30 to 60 minutes after administration of the drug.

Phthalofyne. Phthalofyne is supplied as tablets to be given orally or as a 25% solution that is given intravenously. The intravenous solution must be kept refrigerated and is used only in dogs to treat whipworm infections.

Effectiveness. It has been reported that phthalofyne is 84% effective against whipworms when given intravenously and only 16% effective when given orally.[2]

Toxicity. In a study involving the clinical administration of phthalofyne at normal therapeutic doses to 30 dogs with whipworms, the following side effects were noted[6]:

- Vomiting in 19 dogs
- Incoordination in 1 dog after 10 minutes
- Depression in 2 dogs for a few hours
- Incoordination in 5 dogs 10 to 20 minutes after treatment followed by a period of depression that lasted 3 to 6 hours

Table 11-9. Efficacy of pyrantel pamoate against canine nematodes

Dose	Hookworms	Ascarids	Whipworms	Reference
5 mg/kg	91%-100%	100%	0.5%-1%	39
1.03 mg/kg	94%-99%	93%-96%	0%	21

Dose and administration. Phthalofyne is probably more effective when given by the intravenous route because it commonly causes vomiting and some of the oral dose is lost. When one is giving the drug orally, the animal should be fed only milk 12 hours after the last regular meal, followed 12 hours later with 200 mg/kg immediately after a small meal, with the same dose repeated 12 hours later after another light meal.

The drug is also available for intravenous administration as a 25% solution. It is administered at the rate of 250 mg/kg of body weight over a 1- or 2-minute period. Because the drug is irritating, perivascular administration, in which some of the drug is injected outside of the vein, must be avoided.

Piperazine. Piperazine is available in many forms. For example, it is available as hydrochloride, citrate, sulfate, tartrate, or adipate salts. Piperazine products are dispensed as liquids or tablets for oral administration. They are used in both dogs and cats as well as other species to treat ascarid infestations.

Effectiveness. Generally, piperazine is regarded as highly effective against ascarids. However, its effectiveness in dogs and cats has been reported to vary from 38% to 83%.

Toxicity. In ordinary use, piperazine salts are regarded as relatively nontoxic.

Dose and administration. Piperazine is usually administered at the rate of 20 to 30 mg/kg for dogs and cats.[34] A second dose should be given 2 weeks after the initial dose to kill larvae that have matured.

Pyrantel pamoate. Pyrantel pamoate is one of the tetrahydropyrimidine class of anthelmintic drugs. As a class these drugs are strong inhibitors of cholinesterase. They are used in both livestock (Chapter 12) and horses (Chapter 13). Pyrantel pamoate is also used in humans for the treatment of ascarid, hookworm, and pinworm infestation. The pamoate salt of pyrantel is the least soluble and, therefore, the least toxic.

In dogs, oral doses of 1 to 5 mg/kg of body weight of pyrantel pamoate have shown activity against hookworms and ascarids. It has little or no effectiveness against whipworms (Table 11-9). At doses of 1 to 5 mg/kg the drug does not appear to be toxic.[21,39]

Tetrachloroethylene (USP). Tetrachloroehylene is a liquid chlorinated hydrocarbon closely related to carbon tetrachloride. It largely replaced carbon tetrachloride in the 1920s as an anthelmintic because carbon tetrachloride is far more toxic than tetrachloroethylene. It has been used in dogs and cats to treat ascarid and hookworm infections but has been largely replaced by compounds that are less toxic.

Effectiveness. The effectiveness of tetrachloroethylene against various stages of *A. caninum* in young dogs has been demonstrated.[26] Uninfected puppies 8 to 10 weeks of age were inoculated with *A. caninum* larvae. A dose of 0.22 ml/kg of body weight of tetrachloroethylene was 74% effective against fourth-stage larvae, 91% effective against immature adults, and 98% effective against mature adults. In a second group of naturally infected 14-day-old puppies, a dose of 0.44 ml/kg was 39% to 64% effective against fourth-stage larvae and 94% to 96% effective against immature adult parasites. Even though the dose of 0.44 ml/kg is twice that of the recommended normal dose, no toxic effects were noted in the 14-day-old puppies; previous reports had indicated that the maximum safe dose was 0.44 ml/kg. In summary, tetrachloroethylene is highly effective against *A. caninum*. Its effectiveness against other nematodes has not been determined. Before the drug is administered to dogs and cats, they should be fasted 12 to 24 hours.

Toxicity. Tetrachloroethylene is not absorbed to any appreciable extent in the absence of fat in the intestine. However, if there is fat in the intestine, the drug will be absorbed and toxicity is likely. It is desirable to administer a saline cathartic like magnesium sulfate after the administration of the drug in small animals to remove any clumped parasites that might obstruct the bowel.

The drug should not be used if animals are suffering from any febrile disease, are extremely young or old, or are suffering from any chronic, debilitating disease such as nephritis, hepatitis, or enteritis.

Dose and administration. Tetrachloroethylene is usually dispensed in a soft gelatin capsule, to be taken orally, that often contains a cathartic (laxative). However, greater effectiveness is obtained if a saline cathartic is administered within an hour after the drug is given. The dose in dogs and cats is 0.22 ml/kg after a 12- to 24-hour fast.

Thiacetarsamide (arsinamide). Thiacetarsamide sodium is an organic arsenic compound containing about 20% arsenic. It is dispensed as a 1% solution containing 10 mg of the active compound per milliliter. The action of the drug is due primarily to its arsenic content. Generally, the concentration of arsenic in the worms is higher than in the tissues of the dog, with the exception of the dog's liver. Apparently adult worms specifically take up the arsenic when it is administered in the form of thiacetarsamide.

Thiacetarsamide is used in dogs only to combat adult heartworms. It has no effect on either the infective or circulating microfilariae.

Effectiveness. Although thiacetarsamide is effective against the adult heartworm, its effect is not immediate. Some heartworms die within a few days, but 2 to 3 weeks may be required for a complete kill.

Toxicity. Animals exhibit two general types of toxic reactions to thiacetarsamide therapy. One type of toxicity encountered is lung damage from segments of the dead worms plugging the arteries that carry blood to the lungs. The other is kidney and/or liver damage, possibly due to arsenic toxicity.

Complications resulting from plugging of vessels by dead worms are in direct proportion to the severity of the infection. When dead worms lodge in the pulmonary vessels, there is an obstruction of blood flow, an intense inflammatory reaction, and possibly an infection, all of which may interfere with pulmonary function. Coughing and fever are frequently encountered. Most veterinarians agree that appropriate supportive therapy is indicated after treatment for severe cases of heartworms to minimize such complications. Absolute rest is a necessity for at least 2 weeks after treatment, and animals should be kept in close confinement for 1 to 2 months.

Generally, during the course of therapy, animals do not show reactions to the arsenical. However, animals severely ill from the heartworm infestation may develop kidney and/or liver damage after receiving thiacetarsamide. Signs of liver or kidney damage usually show up within 8 hours of any of the four injections. These include the following:

- A depressed attitude
- Loss of appetite
- Vomiting, which occurs an hour or more after the injection
- High levels of bilirubin in the urine
- Increased bilirubin in the blood as evidenced by icterus (yellowing of mucous membranes and whites of the eyes)
- Increased blood levels of enzymes released by the damaged liver
- Increased blood urea nitrogen (BUN) levels, indicating compromised kidney function

Feeding animals 1 hour prior to treatment and careful observation for the signs just listed may minimize reactions from liver or kidney toxicity. Administration of the drug should not continue if these adverse reactions occur. Treatment may be resumed after a lapse of 6 weeks.[5,25]

It has been hypothesized that the large

number of circulating microfilariae predispose the liver to damage when thiacetarsamide is given. It has, therefore, been suggested that animals be cleared of microfilariae by the use of a microfilaricide such as dithiazanine or levamisole prior to giving thiacetarsamide. If a microfilaricide is given first, at least 3 weeks should elapse between dithiazanine and thiacetarsamide therapy. Six weeks should elapse between levamisole and thiacetarsamide therapy.

Six to 12 weeks after thiacetarsamide therapy the blood should again be checked for microfilariae and a new course of therapy with a microfilaricide given if any are present.[10,11]

Dose and administration. Because thiacetarsamide has no effect on the infective larvae, a veterinarian may decide to postpone administration of the drug until the winter when all infective larva from the previous mosquito season have matured.

In such cases a microfilaricide such as dithiazanine or levamisole is given monthly until February or March when the thiacetarsamide is given. Before the next mosquito season, the animal should once again be checked for circulating microfilariae and, if they are present, should be treated with a microfilaricide. Then the animal should be put on a prophylactic regimen of diethylcarbamazine.

The recommended dose of thiacetarsamide is 0.22 ml of a 1% solution (2.2 mg) per kilogram of body weight twice a day for 2 days. At least 6 hours should separate any two doses. The compound is administered intravenously. It is important to avoid perivascular leakage, which can result in severe inflammation of the surrounding tissues. One means of preventing such leakage is to make each of the four injections in a different site to prevent leakage of the drug through a recent venipuncture (Fig. 11-7). The injections are given into the cephalic vein, which is located on the anterior aspect of the front leg (Fig. 2-3). The first injection can be given in the lower right cephalic vein, the second in the upper right, the third in the lower left,

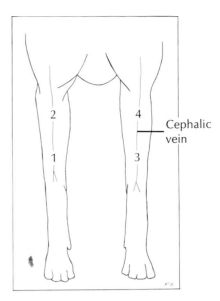

Fig. 11-7. Injection sites for thiacetarsamide. Give the four injections carefully in cephalic vein as follows: *(1)* first injection, lower right cephalic vein; *(2)* second, upper right cephalic vein; *(3)* third, lower left cephalic vein; and *(4)* fourth, upper left cephalic vein.

and the fourth in the upper left (Fig. 11-7).[8] If leakage does occur, cold compresses should be applied, and/or 1 or 2 ml of 1% procaine hydrochloride should be injected locally. The procaine injected subcutaneously reduces the pain and the resultant vasoconstriction, which reduced blood flow to the area and can result in necrosis, or death of the tissues.

Toluene. Toluene (methylbenzene) is a liquid hydrocarbon used as an anthelmintic in dogs and cats.

Effectiveness. It may be effective against ascarids. However, its effectiveness against hookworms and whipworms is variable.[20,22]

Toxicity. Toxic reactions from toluene include vomiting in about 13% of dogs treated after fasting. This occurs somewhat less frequently in cats. Shortly after dosing with the drug, temporary incoordination with muscular tremors lasting for about an hour have been observed.

168 Drugs in veterinary practice

Table 11-10. Effectiveness of toluene and dichlorophen combination

Host	Hookworms	Ascarids	Reference
Dogs	96%	93%	36
Dogs	79%	71%	2
Dogs	98%	Not re-ported	27
Cats	91%	92%	17

Table 11-11. Efficacy of uredofos against nematodes of dogs*

Dose	A. caninum	T. canis	Trichu-ris vulpis
25 mg/kg	97%	81%	30%
50 mg/kg	99%	96%	35%
100 mg/kg	100%	98%	72%
25 mg/kg two times in 24 hours	100%	Not re-ported	89%
50 mg/kg two times in 24 hours	100%	Not re-ported	99%

*Based on data from Roberson, E. L., and Ager, A. L.: Uredofos: anthelmintic activity against nematodes and cestodes in dogs with naturally occurring infections, Am. J. Vet. Res. **37**:1479, 1976.

Dose and administration. Toluene is given in a gelatin capsule. It is important to administer the capsule in such a way that it will be swallowed whole. If it breaks in the mouth, the drug will irritate the mouth and tongue. Toluene is administered orally at the rate of 0.22 ml/kg of body weight after a 12- to 18-hour fast.

Toluene and dichlorophen. This broad-spectrum combination was previously discussed in the section on anticestodal drugs. The product is dispensed in soft gelatin capsules to be administered orally to dogs and cats. It is recommended for the treatment of tapeworms, hookworms, and ascarids. Its effectiveness against hookworms and ascarids has generally been adequate (Table 11-10). For the dose and method of administration, see p. 154.

Uredofos. Uredofos, an experimental organophosphate preparation, has been tested as an anthelmintic in dogs. The effectiveness of the drug against nematodes is shown in Table 11-11. It should be noted that for uredofos to be effective against *Trichuris species*, two doses of uredofos at the rate of 50 mg/kg should be given 24 hours apart.

Protozoans
Coccidia

Coccidia are protozoa that spend some part of their life cycle in gut epithelial cells of various species of animals. The disease coccidiosis occurs more frequently in dogs than in cats. It is also seen in some farm animals (Chapter 12). Species of two genera of coccidia infect dogs and cats, *Isospora* and *Eimeria*.

The life cycle of coccidia is complicated (Fig. 11-8). For our purpose it is sufficient to know that at various stages the parasite enters the epithelial cells in the intestinal tract. Once inside the cells the parasites multiply and virtually take over the cytoplasm. Eventually they rupture the cell walls and emerge. This is an asexual stage of reproduction that may be repeated many times. Eventually the parasites form female and male cells, which unite in the lumen of the intestinal tract, forming an oocyst. The oocysts are then expelled in the feces and are capable of reinfecting the host or another animal of the same species.

In a light infection no clinical signs are seen, and an immunity to the parasites may develop. In more serious infections the intestinal tract becomes inflamed, causing diarrhea. In severe cases the feces contain a considerable amount of blood. The blood loss can be so great in young animals that anemia and death result.

Diagnosis is made on the basis of the signs that the animal presents and the presence of oocysts in the stool.

Treatment. Treatment is aimed at reducing the diarrhea, administration of fluids, and administration of appropriate chemotherapeutic drugs such as sulfonamides or nitrofurans. For example, sulfamerazine can be given orally at the rate of one dose of 130 mg/kg followed by 45 mg/kg three times a

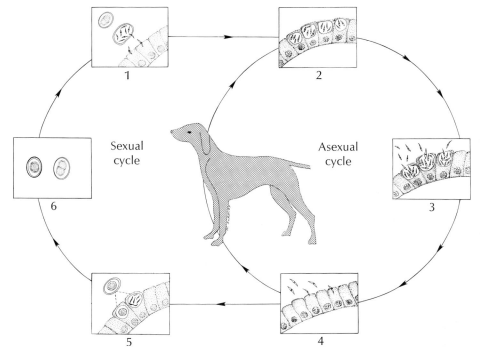

Fig. 11-8. Life cycle of coccidia. Asexual cycle: *(1)* coccidia released from an ingested oocyst invade epithelial cells of the intestine; *(2)* coccidia take over cells and multiply within them; *(3)* cells rupture releasing coccidia, which *(4)* infect other cells. This asexual cycle may be repeated many times. Sexual cycle: *(5)* eventually within the cells, male and female coccidia are produced. These unite in the intestine, forming *(6)* oocysts, which are passed in the feces.

day for 6 days. Sulfamethazine can be given at the rate of one dose of 130 mg/kg followed by 65 mg/kg twice daily for 6 days. Nitrofurazone can be given orally at the rate of 4 to 8 mg/kg three times a day for 6 days.

References

1. Anderson, F. I., Loveless, R. M., and Jensen, L. A.: Efficacy of bunamidine hydrochloride against immature and mature stages of *Echinococcus granulosus*, Am. J. Vet. Res. **36:**673, 1975.
2. Batte, E. G., and Moncol, D. J.: Evaluation of canine anthelmintics, Anim. Hosp. **3:**186, 1967.
3. Batte, E. G., Moncol, D. J., and McLamb, R. D.: Critical evaluation of an anthelmintic for dogs, Vet. Med. Small Anim. Clin. **61:**567, 1966.
4. Bradley, R. E.: Levamisole resinate as a *Dirofilaria immitis* microfilaricide in dogs, J. Am. Vet. Med. Assoc. **169:**311, 1976.
5. Carlisle, C. H., Prescott, C. W., McCosker, P. J., and Seawright, A. A.: The toxic effects of thiacetarsamide sodium in normal dogs and in dogs in-

fested with *Dirofilaria immitis*, Aust. Vet. J. **50:**204, 1974.
6. Carlos, E. R., and Directo, A. C.: Intravenous treatment of whipworm infection in dogs, J. Am. Vet. Med. Assoc. **14:**481, 1962.
7. Carr, S. H., and Bessmer, R. R.: Heartworm treatment with levamisole, Canine Pract. **2:**13, Jan. 1975.
8. Chastain, C. B.: A safe method of administering thiacetarsamide sodium for heartworm therapy, Vet. Med. Small Anim. Clin. **70:**1063, 1975.
9. Fastier, F. N.: Pharmacological aspects of bunamidine dosing of dogs, N.Z. Vet. J. **20:**148, 1972.
10. Garlick, N. L.: Canine dirofilariasis: levamisole treatment, Canine Pract. **3:**64, April 1976.
11. Garlick, N. L., Beck, A. M., and Bryan, R. K.: Canine dirofilariasis: 547 clinical cases treated first with dithiazanine iodide then with thiacetarsamide sodium, Canine Pract. **3:**44, Aug. 1976.
12. Gemmell, M. A., Johnstone, P. D., and Oudemans, G.: The effect of mebendazole on *Echinococcus granulosus* and *Taenia hydatigena* infections in dogs, Res. Vet. Sci. **19:**229, 1975.
13. Gemmell, M. A., and Oudemans, R.: The effect of bithionol sulphoxide on *Echinococcus granulosus*

and *Taenia hydatigena* infections in dogs, Res. Vet. Sci. **18**:109, 1975.

14. Gemmell, M. A., and Oudemans, G.: The effect of fospirate on *Echinococcus granulosus* and *Taenia hydatigena* infections in dogs, Res. Vet. Sci. **19**:216, 1975.

15. Harlton, B. W.: Treatment of dirofilariasis in a domestic cat (a clinical report), Vet. Med. Small Anim. Clin. **69**:1440, 1974.

16. Hass, D. K.: Critical evaluation of dichlorvos tablets in puppies, Vet. Med. Small Anim. Clin. **69**:900, 1973.

17. Hass, D. K., and Collins, J. A.: Feline anthelmintics: a comparative evaluation of six products, Vet. Med. Small Anim. Clin. **70**:423, 1975.

18. Hatton, C. J.: Teniacidal efficiency of bunamidine salts, Vet. Rec. **81**:104, 1967.

19. Jackson, R. F., Morgan, H. C., Otto, S. F., and Jackson, W. F.: Recommendations of a symposium panel: treatment and prevention of heartworm disease in dogs, J. Am. Vet. Med. Assoc. **154**:397, 1969.

20. Jordan, H. E., and Freeny, D. S.: Re-examining methylbenzene (toulene) as a treatment for *Ancylostoma caninum*, Vet. Med. Small Anim. Clin. **69**:829, 1974.

21. Lindquist, W. D.: Drug evaluation of pyrantel pamoate against *Ancylostoma, Toxocara,* and *Toxascaris* in eleven dogs, Am. J. Vet. Res. **36**:1387, 1975.

22. Link, R. P.: Internal antiparasitic drugs. In Jones, L. M., editor: Veterinary pharmacology and therapeutics, ed. 3, Ames, Iowa, 1965, Iowa State University Press.

23. Maqbool, S., Lawrence, D., and Katz, M.: Treatment of trichuriasis with a new drug, mebendazole, J. Pediatr. **86**:463, 1975.

24. Martin, C. L., Christmas, R., and Leipold, H. W.: Formation of temporary cataracts in dogs given a disophenol preparation, J. Am. Vet. Med. Assoc. **161**:294, 1972.

25. McArthy, J. J.: A practical approach to the treatment of heartworms, Vet. Med. Small Anim. Clin. **69**:1454, 1974.

26. Miller, T. A.: Anthelmintic activity of tetrachloroethylene against various stages of *Ancylostoma caninum* in young dogs, Am. J. Vet. Res. **27**:1037, 1966.

27. Miller, T. A.: Anthelmintic activity of toluene and dichlorophen against various stages of *Ancylostoma caninum* in young dogs, Am. J. Vet. Res. **27**:1755, 1966.

28. Mills, J. N., and Amis, T. C.: Levamisole as a microfilaricidal agent in the control of canine dirofilariasis, Aust. Vet. J. **51**:310, 1975.

29. Mills, J. N., and Amis, T. C.: Use of levamisole as as microfilaricide, J. Am. Vet. Med. Assoc. **167**:808, 1975.

30. Penumarthy, L., Oehme, F. W., and Menhusen, M. J.: Investigations of therapeutic measures for disophenol toxicosis in dogs, Am. J. Vet. Res. **36**:1259, 1975.

31. Poole, J. B., Dooley, K. L., and Rollins, L. D.: Efficacy of niclosamide for the removal of tapeworms (*Dipylidium caninum* and *Taenia pisiformis*) from dogs, J. Am. Vet. Med. Assoc. **159**:78, 1971.

32. Roberson, E. L.: Comparative effects of uredofos, niclosamide, and bunamidine hydrochloride against tapeworm infections in dogs, Am. J. Vet. Res. **37**:1483, 1976.

33. Roberson, E. L., and Ager, A. L.: Uredofos: anthelmintic activity against nematodes and cestodes in dogs with naturally occurring infections, Am. J. Vet. Res. **37**:1479, 1976.

34. Rossoff, I. S.: Handbook of veterinary drugs, New York, 1974, Springer Publishing Co.

35. Schantz, P. M., and Prezioso, U.: Efficacy of divided doses of fospirate against immature *Echinococcus granulosus* infections in dogs, Am. J. Vet. Res. **37**:619, 1976.

36. Sharp, M. L., Sepesi, J. P., and Collins, J. A.: A comparative critical essay on canine anthelmintics, Vet. Med. Small Anim. Clin. **68**:131, 1973.

37. Shumard, R. F., and Hendrix, J. C.: Dithiazanine iodide as an anthelmintic for dogs, Vet. Med. **57**:153, 1962.

38. Steves, F. E., Baker, J. D., Hein, V. D., and Miller, T. A.: Efficacy of a hookworm (*Ancylostoma caninum*) vaccine for dogs, J. Am. Vet. Med. Assoc. **163**:231, 1973.

39. Todd, A. C., Crowley, J., Scholl, P., and Conway, D. P.: Critical tests with pyrantel pamoate against internal parasites in dogs from Wisconsin, Vet. Med. Small Anim. Clin. **70**:936, 1975.

40. Wescott, R. B.: Efficacy of niclosamide in the treatment of *Taenia taeniaformis* infections in cats, Am. J. Vet. Res. **28**:1475, 1967.

41. Williams, J. F., and Keahey, K. K.: Sudden death associated with treatment of three dogs with bunamidine hydrochloride, J. Am. Vet. Med. Assoc. **168**:689, 1976.

42. Wood, I. B., Pankavich, W. S., Wallace, R. E., Thorson, R. E., Burkhart, R. L., and Waletzby, E.: Disophenol, an injectable anthelmintic for canine hookworm, J. Am. Vet. Med. Assoc. **139**:1101, 1961.

Additional readings

Abadie, S. H., Gonzalez, R. R., Pailet, A., and Bisso, R.: Canine heartworm infection: treatment with diethylcarbamazine, Mod. Vet. Pract. **50**:34, July 1969.

Ames, E. R.: Control of *Ancylostoma caninum* in the dog with thiabendazole, Am. J. Vet. Res. **31**:2225, 1970.

Berger, H., Burkhart, R. L., and Elliott, R. F.: Evaluation of styrylpyridinium and diethylcarbamazine as anthelmintics for dogs under field conditions, Am. J. Vet. Res. **30**:611, 1969.

Casey, H. W., Tulloch, G. S., and Anderson, R. A.: Prevention and treatment of canine hookworm disease with styrylpyridinium and diethylcarbamazine, J. Am. Vet. Med. Assoc. **159:**1003, 1971.

Congdon, L. L., and Ames, E. R.: Thiabendazole for control of *Toxocara canis* in the dog, Am. J. Vet. Res. **34:**417, 1973.

Friedheim, E. A.: Therapeutic field trial of a macro- and microfilaricidal agent in canine filariasis, Bull. W.H.O. **50:**572, 1974.

Gemmell, M. A.: Surveillance of *Echinococcus granulosus* in dogs with arecoline hydrobromide, Bull. W.H.O. **48:**649, 1973.

Gemmell, M. A., and Oudemans, G.: Treatment of *Echinococcus granulosus* and *Taenia hydatigena* in dogs with bunamidine hydroxynaphthoate in a prepared food, Res. Vet. Sci. **16:**85, 1974.

Gemmell, M. A., and Oudemans, G.: Treatment of *Taenia hydatigena* infections in dogs with bunamidine hydroxynaphthoate incorporated in food, N.Z. Vet. J. **23:**142, 1975.

Hass, D. K., and Collins, J. A.: Evolution of an anthelmintic: vincofos, Am. J. Vet. Res. **35:**103, 1974.

Henderson, J. W.: Diagnosis, treatment, and preventive therapy for heartworms, J. Am. Vet. Med. Assoc. **151:**1737, 1967.

Jackson, R. F.: Treatment of heartworm-infected dogs with chemical agents, J. Am. Vet. Med. Assoc. **154:**390, 1969.

Jackson, R. F.: Complications during and following chemotherapy of heartworm disease, Symposium on Heartworms, J. Am. Vet. Med. Assoc. **154:**393, 1969.

Jackson, R. F.: Thiacetarsamide for preventive treatment of *Dirofilaria immitis*, J. Am. Vet. Med. Assoc. **154:**395, 1969.

Jackson, W. F.: Preventative therapy with diethylcarbamazine, J. Am. Vet. Med. Assoc. **154:**396, 1969.

Otto, G. F.: Chemotherapeutic agents, J. Am. Vet. Med. Assoc. **154:**387, 1969.

Pailet, A., Abadie, S. H., Smith, M. W., and Gonzalez, R. R.: Chemotherapeutic heartworm control, Vet. Med. Small Anim. Clin. **63:**691, 1968.

Rosenberg, M. A., Wilcox, A. H., Chase, C. H., III, and Chase, C. H., Jr.: A mathematical formula as an aid in the treatment and prognosis of canine heartworm disease, Vet. Med. Small. Anim. Clin. **71:**496, 1976.

Schantz, P. M., Prezioso, U., and Marchevsky, N.: Efficacy of divided doses of GS-23654 against immature *Echinococcus granulosus* infections in dogs, Am. J. Vet. Res. **37:**621, 1976.

Schock, R. C.: Parasite control in small animals, Mod. Vet. Pract. **57:**99, Feb. 1976.

Scott, D. W.: Lungworm treatment, Feline Pract. **5:** 5, May 1975.

Simpson, C. F., Bradley, R. E., and Jackson, R. F.: Crystalloid inclusions in hepatocyte mitrochondria of dogs treated with levamisole, Vet. Pathol. **11:**129, 1974.

Trejos, A., Szyfres, B., and Marchevsky, N.: Comparative value of arecoline hydrobromide and bunamidine hydrochloride for the treatment of *Echinococcus granulosus* in dogs, Res. Vet. Sci. **19:**212, 1975.

Tulloch, G. S., Pacheco, G., Casey, H. W., Bills, W. E., Davis, I., and Anderson, R. A.: Prepatent clinical, pathologic, and serologic changes in dogs infected with *Dirofilaria immitis* and treated with diethylcarbamazine, Am. J. Vet. Res. **31:**437, 1970.

Ward, F. P., and Glicksberg, C. L.: Effects of dichlorvos on blood cholinesterase activity in dogs, J. Am. Vet. Med. Assoc. **158:**457, 1971.

Welter, C. J., and Johnson, D. R.: Effect of combined arecoline hydrobromide and N-butyl chloride complex on parasites of dogs, J. Am. Vet. Med. Assoc. **140:** 62, 1962.

Welter, C. J., and Johnson, D. R.: Anthelmintic activity of N-butyl chloride and toluene combinations in dogs and cats, Vet. Med. **58:**869, 1963.

Wilkinson, G. T.: Coccidial infection in a cat colony, Vet. Rec. **100:**156, 1977.

12

DRUGS FOR PREVENTION AND TREATMENT OF

Internal parasitic infections of cattle, sheep, and swine

RUMINANT STOMACHS

To understand the significance of intestinal parasites in sheep and cattle, one must have some knowledge of their digestive tracts. Cattle and sheep are ruminants, that is, their digestive system contains four stomachs (Fig. 12-1). The first three stomachs are actually outpocketings of the esophagus. The fourth is the true stomach and functions in a manner similar to those of simple stomach animals, as discussed in Chapter 19.

The first stomach is the rumen. It has a capacity of approximately 40 gallons in the average-size cow. It has two primary func-

tions: (1) to store large volumes of high-fiber feed and (2) to act as a "fermentation vat" in which bacteria, yeasts, and protozoa convert cellulose, sugars, and polysaccharides (fiber) to volatile fatty acids. These fatty acids can then be absorbed by the digestive tract for use as an energy source. The microorganisms present in the rumen also convert nonprotein nitrogen to free ammonia, which they use to build their own cellular protein. These microorganisms pass to the posterior part of the digestive tract where their protein is digested to amino acids. The amino acids are absorbed from the gut and used by the animal to build its proteins. The utilization of cellulose and free ammonia is not possible in animals with one stomach. Therefore ruminants make more efficient use of plant foods than do simple stomach animals.

The second stomach, the reticulum, is a pouch that lies forward of the rumen, from which it is separated by a fold rather than a valve. It is in contact with the diaphragm. When dense material is swallowed, it goes directly into the reticulum and from there into the third stomach, the omasum.

The omasum is a round structure that contains sheets of tissue that run parallel to the direction ingesta travels. It has been theorized that these sheets absorb water from the ingesta. The omasum connects the reticulum to the true stomach, the abomasum.

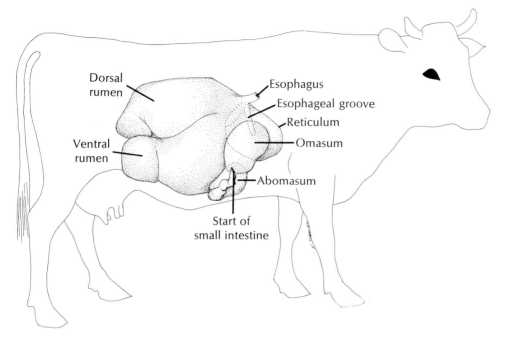

Fig. 12-1. Ruminant stomachs.

The abomasum secretes hydrochloric acid and enzymes that digest proteins. The active digestive process of the animal starts in the abomasum.

The physiology of the digestive tract of the newborn calf or lamb is essentially the same as that of an animal with one stomach. The newborn animal has not yet acquired from the environment the necessary organisms for the proper functioning of the rumen. The diet of these young animals consists almost entirely of milk, which is digested in the abomasum and intestines rather than in the rumen. To accommodate the needs of the newborn animal, suckling initiates a reflex, which forms an esophageal groove. This groove, extending from the terminal end of the esophagus to the omasum, allows ingested material to bypass the rumen and reticulum. The reflex to form the esophageal groove can also be caused by swabbing the mouth of a ruminant with a solution containing sodium or copper ions. Copper sulfate is used for sheep and sodium bicarbonate

for cattle.[63] When it is desired to deliver medication directly to the abomasum, avoiding dilution by the large volume of ingesta in the rumen, such swabbing is done. Because many parasites reside in the abomasum, it is sometimes valuable to deliver anthelmintics directly to the abomasum in this manner.

ADMINISTERING DRUGS TO FARM ANIMALS

An important factor in the selection of drugs for the treatment of internal parasites in farm animals is the method by which the drugs are administered. Animals must receive the correct dose in such a way as to ensure delivery in adequate concentration to the area in which the parasites are located. When large numbers of animals are being treated, the method of administration must be safe and efficient and require as little time as possible.

One of the most suitable methods of administration is by hypodermic injection. If injections are made properly, animals receive the dose that is correct for proper action of the drug. In addition, large numbers of animals can be treated in a relatively short period of time. Unfortunately few drugs that are effective against internal parasites can be administered by this route. Also, if the injection is performed incorrectly, severe local inflammation and/or infection can result.

The oral route is the most common route of administration for drugs effective against internal parasites of farm animals. Oral administration of a liquid is called a "drench." When oral anthelmintics are in liquid form, various methods of dosing are available. If a stomach tube is used, there is little danger of spilling any of the drug on the ground. However, there are two disadvantages to this technique. First, people untrained in the use of the stomach tube may accidentally pass the tube down the trachea and deliver the drugs to the lungs rather than the gastrointestinal tract. Such accidents are usually fatal. Second, the use of stomach tubes is very time-consuming.

In ruminants it is possible to inject drugs directly into the rumen with a large hypodermic syringe and needle. The injection can be made in the left flank area where only a thin layer of tissues separates the wall of the rumen from the skin. Because of the trauma to the animal and the probability of serious infection, this is not a common method of administering antiparasitic drugs to ruminants.

The most common method of administering liquid antiparasitic drugs by the oral route is with a dose syringe. This is a large metal syringe with a long tube that can be positioned in the rear part of the mouth (Fig. 12-2). If the drug is deposited in the correct area slowly, the animal will swallow the liquid as it is administered. When used properly, the use of the dose syringe is a highly effective technique for administering a liquid preparation orally. Problems such as the following result when attempts are made to perform the procedure too quickly:

1. If the animal's head is not properly restrained and/or if the drug is administered

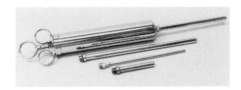

Fig. 12-2. Dose syringe. By using a dose syringe, liquid medication can be administered to cattle and sheep.

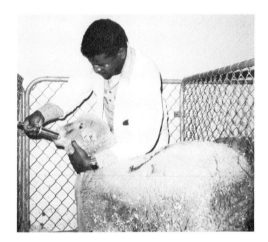

Fig. 12-3. Administering liquid medication to sheep. When sheep or cattle are given liquid medication, barrel of the dose syringe should be placed in rear of animal's mouth. Animal's head should be held high enough that medication will not fall from mouth but not so high that animal has difficulty swallowing.

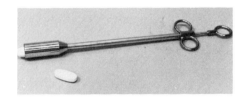

Fig. 12-4. Balling gun and bolus. Balling gun is used to administer boluses, large tabletlike dosage forms of medication, to cattle, sheep, and swine.

too quickly, a significant portion of the drug may fall from the animal's mouth. It is then impossible to know the exact dose the animal has received. Underdosing can seriously reduce the effectiveness of the drug.

2. There is the possibility that the animal will inhale the drug, resulting in a fatal pneumonia.

3. If used carelessly, the tip of the dose syringe can severely damage tissues in the mouth or pharynx.

The proper way to administer liquid medication with a dose syringe is to raise the animal's head high enough so that the medication will not fall out by gravity flow but not too high to make swallowing difficult (Fig. 12-3). The drug is then delivered slowly to the rear part of the animal's mouth. As the drug is administered, the animal should be allowed to make chewing movements and to swallow.

Probably the most common method of administering oral anthelmintic drugs to cattle, sheep, and swine is in bolus form. Boluses are large tabletlike dosage forms (Fig. 12-4). They are administered by the use of a balling gun, which has a barrel to hold the bolus and a large stem that allows positioning of the bolus in the back part of the mouth. Placement of the bolus far back in the animal's mouth ensures that the animal will swallow the bolus. If the bolus is placed too far forward in the mouth, the animal may chew and expel portions of it. When this happens, it is impossible to know exactly how much medication the animal received. For some medication such as phenothiazine, boluses may not be as effective as liquid preparations. However, there is some indication that thiabendazole is more effective as a bolus than when given as a drench.[14]

Another method of administering antiparasitic drugs orally is in paste form. A specified amount of paste is squeezed onto the roof of the mouth or gums of the animal. It adheres to the roof of the mouth or the gums, and, as animals make chewing movements, they swallow the paste. This method is safe, effective, and easy.

In addition to the methods just discussed, antiparasitic drugs can be administered in the feed. For example, powder may be mixed in with supplements such as grain, or the drug may be incorporated as a fixed percentage of pelleted feed. The primary disadvantage of this method of administration is that a sick animal sometimes will not eat its entire ration. If animals are fed as a group, some may consume a greater amount of the feed than others. If a nontoxic drug is used, those animals that received too much will not be harmed, but those that consumed less may not have received an effective dose of the antiparasitic drug.

INTERNAL PARASITES OF CATTLE, SHEEP, AND SWINE

The common, clinically significant parasites of cattle and sheep are shown in Table 12-1. Those of swine are shown in Table 12-2.

Protozoans
Coccidia

Clinically, coccidiosis is a problem in calves and lambs. It can also occur in young swine. In calves and lambs the disease is caused by various species of *Eimeria*. In swine it can be caused by various species of *Eimeria* or *Isospora suis*. The life cycle and clinical signs are similar to those described in Chapter 11 for the coccidia of the dog. It is possible for animals to harbor the parasite without showing clinical signs.

Prevention rather than treatment is the key to the control of coccidiosis in cattle and sheep. The protozoa are spread by exposure to feces containing the parasitic oocysts. Keeping dairy calves in individual pens that can be moved to clean ground before housing a new calf will effectively prevent the disease. Moving lambs and beef calves to clean pastures and housing them in uncrowded conditions will go a long way toward reducing incidence of the disease.

Drugs that prevent coccidia from multiplying (coccidiostatic drugs) are given to livestock to both prevent and treat clinical disease. Among the drugs most commonly used

Table 12-1. Internal parasites of cattle and sheep*

Group or common name	Scientific name	Infect sheep	Infect cattle	Location in host
Protozoans				
Coccidia	*Eimeria* species	X	X	Primarily small intestine
Trematodes (flukes)				
Liver flukes	*Fasciola* species	X	X	Liver Bile duct
Cestodes				
Mature common	*Moniezia* species	X	X	Small intestine
tapeworms	*Thysanosoma actinioides*	X		Small intestine, bile duct, pancreatic duct
Nematodes (round-worms)				
Stomach worms	*Haemonchus* species	X	X	Abomasum
	Ostertagia species	X	X	Abomasum
	Trichostronglyus axei	X	X	Abomasum
Intestinal worms	*Bunostomum phlebotomum*	X	X	Small intestine
	Capillaria species	X	X	Small intestine
	Cooperia species	X	X	Small intestine
	Nematodirus species	X	X	Small intestine
	Strongyloides papillosus	X	X	Small intestine
	Trichostrongylus species	X	X	Small intestine
	Oesophagostomum species	X	X	Cecum, colon
	Chaberta species	X	X	Cecum, colon
Lungworm	*Dictyocaulus* species	X	X	Bronchi
Arthropods				
Sheep botfly	*Oestrus ovis*	X		Nasal cavity and sinuses of head

*Modified from Becklund, W. W.: Revised check list of internal and external parasites of domestic animals in the United States and possessions and in Canada, Am. J. Vet. Res. **25**:1380, 1964.

Table 12-2. Internal parasites of swine*

Group or common name	Scientific name	Location in host
Protozoans		
Coccidia	*Eimeria* species *Isospora suis*	Small or large intestine
Trematodes		
Liver flukes	*Fasciola* species	Bile duct
Nematodes (roundworms)		
Large intestinal roundworms	*Ascaris lumbricoides*	Small intestine
Intestinal threadworm	*Strongyloides ransomi*	Small intestine
Nodular worms	*Oesophagostomum* species	Cecum, colon
Whipworm	*Trichuris suis*	Cecum
Lung worms	*Metastrongylus* species	Bronchi
	Hyostrongylus rubidus	Stomach

*Modified from Becklund, W. W.: Revised check list of internal and external parasites of domestic animals in the United States and possessions and in Canada, Am. J. Vet. Res. **25**:1380, 1964.

are amprolium, nitrofurazone, and sulfona-mides. Decoquinate and monensin may also be of value.

In addition to coccidiostatic drugs, other drugs are used to treat the secondary problems associated with the diarrhea caused by the coccidial infection. To reduce the diarrhea and soothe the inflamed gut, adsorbents such as kaolin and pectin may be administered orally. Drugs that block the action of acetylcholine (anticholinergic drugs) are often administered to slow down the movement of the intestine and thereby reduce the diarrhea. Specific anticholinergic drugs are discussed in Chapter 19.

Fluids and solutions of electrolytes, particularly sodium ions, can be used in severe cases of diarrhea. The use of these preparations is discussed in detail in Chapters 5 and 17.

Amprolium. Amprolium is a coccidiostatic drug used in poultry that is being tested rather extensively in lambs and calves. In cattle and sheep it appears to be effective for both prevention and treatment of infections.[11,44,69,74]

Amprolium is a thiamine antagonist. However, in cattle, toxic doses appear to be well above normal therapeutic doses.[69]

For cattle, a prophylactic dose of 5 mg/kg daily given in feed for 21 days and a therapeutic dose of 10 mg/kg daily given in the feed for 5 days have been recommended.[69] For sheep, a prophylactic dose of 50 mg/kg a day for 21 days appears effective.[11]

Decoquinate. Decoquinate is a coccidiostatic drug used in chickens. It has been tested in calves for preventing coccidiosis. At a dose of 0.5 to 0.8 mg/kg given in the feed 3 days before and 28 days after an experimental infection, it was effective in preventing oocyst discharge and bloody diarrhea. Signs of infection did not occur in animals until they were off the medication for 28 days.[68] Further clinical evaluation of decoquinate to determine its effectiveness in lambs and calves is necessary.

Monensin. Monensin is an antibiotic with coccidiostatic activity. It has been tested ex-perimentally for use in lambs and calves. When given in feed at doses of 0.36 to 1.6 mg/kg/24 hr, it has been effective in preventing coccidiosis.[21,22,39,64]

Once lambs have developed signs of coccidiosis, monensin is moderately effective in treating the disease when given at the rate of 2 mg/kg.[64]

Nitrofurazone. Nitrofurazone is used as a coccidiostat in lambs and pigs. It is given in the feed at a concentration of 0.104% or at the rate of 11 mg/kg for 7 days.[24]

Sulfonamides. Sulfonamides have been widely used in the treatment of coccidiosis. In calves, sulfamethazine, sulfamerazine, sulfaquinoxaline, and sulfaguanidine have been used. Probably the most effective compound is sulfamethazine, a coccidiostat, which is administered at a dose of 130 mg/kg of body weight orally on the first day, followed by 65 mg/kg twice a day on each of the 3 ensuing days. This regimen should be repeated on the first, third, and fifth week for adequate therapeutic effect. Sulfamethazine can also be given at the rate of 198 mg/kg for 5 days intravenously.[74]

Sulfamerazine can be administered at the rate of 130 mg/kg of body weight orally for the first day, followed by 45 mg/kg three times a day.

In sheep and swine, sulfa drugs can be administered at the same dose as in calves. Sulfaguanidine can be administered in the feed at the rate of 0.5%.

Trematodes (flukes)
Liver flukes

Liver flukes that infect cattle, sheep, and swine are members of the genus *Fasciola*. Cattle, sheep, and swine are the primary hosts, that is, they are infected by the adult fluke. Clinically the most important species are *F. hepatica* and *F. magna*. Liver fluke infestation results in the condemnation of 1 to 1.5 million bovine livers annually. This amounted to a rate of 3.73% in 1973. The prevalence of these parasites is particularly high in the western United States and Florida. For example, the percentage of bovine livers condemned in 1975 in states with serious fluke problems was as follows[41]:

California	11.8%
Florida	22.2%
Nevada	25.0%
Oregon	17.4%
Utah	17.6%

Adult flukes live and lay eggs in the bile duct. Eggs that enter the duodenum with the bile and leave the primary host in feces eventually hatch to an intermediate stage called the "miracidium." The miracidium can live free for only about 24 hours. For further development it must enter an intermediate host, numerous species of snails. After entering the snail, the miracidium forms a sporocyst. From each of these sporocysts, many more intermediate flukes are developed. These leave the snail 4½ to 7 weeks from the time of initial infection. After leaving the snail, they usually settle on plants and form cysts. At this stage they are infectious. When they are swallowed by the primary host, they escape from their cyst in the duodenum and burrow into the intestinal wall. The usual route to the liver is through the abdominal cavity. After about a week, the fluke enters the liver by penetrating through the liver capsule. It is at this stage, 1 to 5 weeks after infection, that the fluke causes most damage. For about a month or more it grows and wanders in the liver, eventually reaching the bile duct. The fluke reaches maturity in the bile duct 8 to 12 weeks after entering the primary host.

Since it is the migration of the immature parasite in the liver that causes the main damage to the primary host, killing the parasite from 1 to 5 weeks after the initial infection is essential to prevent extensive liver damage. Killing adult flukes in the bile duct is important only in that it reduces contamination of the pasture areas with fluke eggs.

Many compounds are effective against the mature stages of liver flukes but are relatively ineffective against the immature forms when administered at recommended doses. This may be caused by greater susceptibility of

Table 12-3. Efficacy of flukicide drugs

Drug	Immature flukes	Mature flukes
Bithional	+	+
Carbon tetrachloride	?	+
Clioxanide	+	+
Diamphenethide	+	+
Hexachloroethane	−	±
Mebendazole	?	+
Menichlophalan	+	+
Oxyclozanide	−	±
Rafoxanide	+	+
Sulfoxide of bithional	+	+

Key: + = effective; ± = variably effective; − = not effective; ? = effectiveness not determined.

flukes that reach the bile ducts as opposed to those in liver tissues.

Liver fluke disease can be eliminated from an area if the intermediate hosts, various snails, are eliminated or if animals are prevented from grazing on pastures in which these snails are located. The application of copper sulfate to pastures has been recommended to eliminate the snails. Although this may work, such an application can result in copper toxicity in sheep and cattle. In addition, fish in streams that drain the pasture can be severely affected by the copper sulfate. Fencing those areas of a pasture that are most likely to contain snails harboring the parasites can be an effective measure in reducing infection. For example, cattle and sheep should be fenced out of swampy areas.

For treating fluke infestations, the following drugs are apparently the most effective: bithional, clioxanide, diamphenethide, menichlophalan, rafoxanide, and sulfoxide of bithional (Table 12-3).

Drugs used to kill liver flukes

Bithional. Bithional is a phenolic compound almost completely insoluble in water. It has substantial bacteriostatic activity and is effective in killing various tapeworms of dogs, cats, sheep, and chickens. It can be used in cattle and sheep to kill liver flukes.

Effectiveness. Both bithional and sulfoxide

of bithional are used to kill liver flukes. When administered orally as a dry powder in a gelatin capsule at the rate of 220 mg/kg, bithional was 84% effective against immature and 100% effective against mature *F. hepatica* in naturally infected sheep.[85]

In a natural infection in sheep, sulfoxide of bithional was 100% effective against both immature and mature flukes when given at the rate of 200 mg/kg.[85]

Toxicity. Sheep treated with bithional and sulfoxide of bithional may develop diarrhea after treatment. When the dosage to sheep is 200 mg/kg, no other toxicity is expected. However, when sulfoxide of bithional is given at the rate of 300 mg/kg, toxic signs such as poor appetite, loss of weight, difficulty in walking, and even death may result. This rather narrow margin of safety dictates that calculation of weight and accuracy of dose be carefully performed when using this drug.

Dose and administration. To combat fluke infestation in sheep, it appears that effective doses are 220 mg/kg for bithional and 200 mg/kg for sulfoxide of bithional.

Carbon tetrachloride. Carbon tetrachloride is an organic liquid. For injection it is usually mixed with mineral or vegetable oil with or without a local anesthetic and with emulsifiers. It can also be administered orally in gelatin capsules or through a stomach tube.

Effectiveness. There is some question as to whether carbon tetrachloride is effective against immature forms of liver flukes. Therefore it has been largely replaced by safer and potentially more effective compounds.

Toxicity. Carbon tetrachloride is generally regarded as a highly toxic substance. When it is used to kill liver flukes, the type of poisoning seen usually results from the drug's toxic effect on the liver. Absorption of large amounts of carbon tetrachloride kills liver cells. If small numbers of cells die, the animal will recover and the liver will return to normal function. However, if large numbers of cells in the liver are killed, the animal will eventually die of liver failure. Cattle appear

to be more susceptible to carbon tetrachloride poisoning than sheep.

Various factors predispose the animal to poisoning from carbon tetrachloride. Large amounts of fat in the feed promote greater absorption of carbon tetrachloride and therefore increase toxicity. In a like manner, accumulation of fat in the liver leads to a greater accumulation of carbon tetrachloride there, resulting in greater damage. On the other hand, a liver with large deposits of glycogen, a stored carbohydrate, has a greater resistance to the toxic effects of carbon tetrachloride than one with no glycogen reserve. A ration high in carbohydrates and low in fats is therefore desirable before carbon tetrachloride is administered.

The toxic effects of carbon tetrachloride are variable when it is used to kill liver flukes. This variability is perhaps due to varying degrees of liver damage already present from the flukes. Those animals with large amounts of liver damage are far more susceptible to toxic effects than those with minimal liver damage.

One should keep in mind that in clinical practice the toxic effects of carbon tetrachloride will be erratic, and fatalities, even at therapeutic doses, can be expected. Therefore it is recommended that, if carbon tetrachloride is to be used, a small portion of the flock should be dosed 48 to 72 hours prior to treating the main group of animals. If toxic reactions occur in the small group, carbon tetrachloride should not be considered for use in the remainder of the animals.

Dose and administration. Because it is highly irritating when given subcutaneously, carbon tetrachloride should always be given by the intramuscular route. When given by injection, only commercial products specifically prepared for injection should be used.

In sheep 3 ml of carbon tetrachloride can be given orally in a gelatin capsule or through a stomach tube.[81] Generally, carbon tetrachloride is diluted with mineral oil for oral administration. (*Note:* Even though fats and oils increase the toxicity of carbon tetrachlo-

Table 12-4. Efficacy of clioxanide against fluke infestations

Host	Species	Dose	Route	Immature	Mature	Reference
Bovine	F. hepatica	50 mg/kg	Orally	Not reported	99.5%	76
Ovine	F. hepatica	40 mg/kg	Orally	99.5%	100%	85
Ovine	F. hepatica	40 mg/kg	Orally	85%	Not reported	28
Ovine	F. hepatica	20 mg/kg	Orally	Not reported	96%	28

ride, mineral oil does not because it is not appreciably absorbed from the gastrointestinal tract.) Four milliliters of a 50% carbon tetrachloride–50% mineral oil mixture can be given intramuscularly per lamb.[24]

Cattle can be administered pure carbon tetrachloride by intramuscular injection at the rate of 1 ml/9 kg of body weight, up to a maximum of 30 ml per animal and a maximum of 15 ml at any one injection site.[24]

A second treatment may be administered in a month to kill flukes that are not killed by the first treatment.

Clioxanide. Experimental trials indicate that clioxanide is highly effective against fluke infestations in cattle and sheep (Table 12-4).

Contrary to previous reports, it has been shown experimentally that the drug is less effective when it is delivered directly to the abomasum rather than the rumen. Although clioxanide has been shown to be highly effective against immature *F. hepatica* in sheep at the rate of 40 mg/kg given by either the oral or intraruminal route, it is not significantly effective at the same dose when placed directly in the abomasum.[28] Unfortunately when liquid is swallowed, it may be shunted to the omasum and abomasum, bypassing the rumen. When this occurs, clioxanide will be less effective against immature flukes.

The dose for sheep is 40 mg/kg orally and for cattle, 50 mg/kg orally.

Diamphenethide. Diamphenethide is effective against *F. hepatica* in cattle and sheep. In contrast to other flukicides, diamphenethide is most effective against immature flukes. Experimentally it has been shown that diamphenethide was 99% to

100% effective against 1- to 8-week-old infections and 83% to 85% effective against 9- to 11-week-old infections in sheep, when given orally at the rate of 100 mg/kg.[52,54,55] At the same dose the drug was 80% effective against a 3-week-old infection in cattle. Because flukes develop slower in cattle than in sheep, a 3-week-old infestation in cattle is essentially like a 1-week-old infestation in sheep.

At 100 mg/kg in cattle and sheep, toxicity is apparently not a problem.

Hexachloroethane. Hexachloroethane is used in treating both sheep and cattle for liver fluke infestation. It occurs as white crystals that are insoluble in water. This drug is usually dispensed as a water suspension prepared with 5% bentonite, a clay used as a suspending agent.

Hexachloroethane is absorbed in the intestinal tract, and most of the drug is removed from the blood by the liver and excreted in the bile. Some is also excreted by the kidneys. Hexachloroethane is excreted into the bile in large enough concentrations to be lethal to mature flukes in the bile ducts.

Effectiveness. Hexachloroethane has been shown to be 89% effective against mature *F. hepatica* in cattle.[41] However, it is not effective against the immature flukes in the liver. At a dose of 120 mg/kg it apparently has no effect against *F. magna*.[41]

There is some evidence that hexachloroethane is not as effective as either carbon tetrachloride or menichlophalan in treating animals with liver flukes.[62] It is not as effective as diamphenethide.

Toxicity. Apparently hexachloroethane causes some liver damage. Animals seem less susceptible to the toxic effects of hexachloroethane if they have adequate glycogen stores in the liver. It is best to try the drug on a few animals and wait a day or two to see if toxic signs develop before treating the whole herd or flock.

Dose and administration. Hexachloroethane is administered orally, usually as a drench. The following doses have been recommended[81]:

Adult cattle	60 gm
Calves	10 gm/45 kg of body weight but not to exceed 30 gm
Sheep and goats	15 to 20 gm
Large kids and lambs	7 to 10 gm
Swine	400 mg/kg

Mebendazole. Mebendazole, a benzimidazole anthelmintic, has been shown to be effective against mature *F. hepatica* in sheep when given orally at a dose of 100 mg/kg.[53]

Menichlophalan (Bayer 9015, ME 3625). Menichlophalan is supplied as a liquid solution or suspension and as granules or tablets. It is administered by injection or orally. When it is given orally, ruminants' mouths should be swabbed with a solution of sodium bicarbonate or copper sulfate to close the esophageal groove because it is necessary that the drug be delivered directly to the abomasum if the full potential of the compound is to be realized. Granules or tablets should be coated by the manufacturer so that they are insoluble until they reach the abomasum.

Effectiveness. In sheep with natural infections, menichlophalan has been shown to be relatively effective against immature forms of liver flukes and highly effective against mature forms. For example, in one study,[85] when given at 4 mg/kg subcutaneously, menichlophalan was 91% effective against immature flukes and 100% effective against mature flukes. When given orally at 6 mg/kg, it was 83% effective against immature flukes and 100% effective against mature flukes.

Toxicity. Menichlophalan apparently causes slight liver damage.[58,62] However, it probably causes less liver damage than carbon tetrachloride.

Dose and administration. Menichlophalan should be administered as follows[81]:

Cattle	3 to 6 mg/kg body weight orally
Sheep	3 to 10 mg/kg of body weight orally or 1 to 3 mg/kg subcutaneously

The higher doses should probably be used to kill the immature forms of the parasite.

Oxyclozanide. Oxyclozanide is available in many countries as a 3% suspension, but it is not available in the United States. It is given to sheep and cattle orally as a flukicide. This drug has poor activity against immature flukes and variable activity against mature flukes.[29,60] Recommended doses are 10 mg/kg for cattle and 15 mg/kg for sheep.[81]

Rafoxanide. Rafoxanide is used in many countries as a flukicide, but it is not yet available in the United States. When given orally, it appears to be highly effective against both immature and mature flukes in sheep and cattle.[28,29,52,59] Although rafoxanide generally works well, strains of flukes with apparent resistance to the drug have been reported.[87] When such strains are encountered, another flukicide should be used.

Rafoxanide is given either orally or through a stomach tube. An appropriate dose for both sheep and cattle appears to be 8 mg/kg.

Cestodes (tapeworms)

For the most part the mature tapeworms of sheep and cattle do not cause a significant clinical problem. Lambs and calves under 6 months of age are usually the only animals that show signs of infection when infected by *Moniezia expansa* and *M. benedini.* When *Moniezia* tapeworms do cause disease, the disease may be due to the tapeworms' rapid growth and prolific production of ripe segments, which compete for nutrients with the host animal. In addition, tapeworms produce a large quantity of waste products, which may be partially absorbed by the host. A diagnosis of *Moniezia* species infection is made by the presence in the feces of ripe segments, which resemble cooked grains of rice. *Moniezia* ova can be identified in these segments.

The fringed tapeworm, *Thysanosoma actinioides*, occurs in the bile ducts, pancreatic ducts, and small intestines of sheep and cattle. Generally, it does not cause a disease problem. However, it may partially obstruct the flow of bile and pancreatic juice, cause digestive disorders, and interfere with utilization of feed.

Cesticidal drugs

Benzimidazoles. The benzimidazoles are a class of drugs used in livestock and horses primarily to treat gastrointestinal nematode infestation. Some of the benzimidazoles also have cesticidal activity. The experimental drug albendazole given orally at the rate of 10 and 15 mg/kg has been 100% effective in clearing lambs of *Moniezia* species infestations.[91] In addition, cambendazole is apparently effective against cestodes (*Monieza* species) in cattle and sheep when given at the rate of 20 to 25 mg/kg.[30,47]

Bithional. Bithional, discussed as a flukicide on pp. 178 and 179, is also used to combat *T. actinioides* and *Moniezia* species in sheep. For *T. actinioides* infestations, bithional is administered at the rate of 200 mg/kg and for *Moniezia* species infestations, at the rate of 100 mg/kg.

Bunamidine. Bunamidine, a cholinesterase inhibitor, is discussed as a cesticide in Chapter 11. It is highly effective against *M. expansa* in sheep. In sheep it is given at the rate of 25 mg/kg.[81]

Dichlorophen. Dichlorophen is discussed as a cesticide in Chapter 11. Its value in combating tapeworm infections in farm animals is questionable.[65] In sheep it is given at the rate of 200 to 400 mg/kg.

Lead arsenate. Lead arsenate contains 59.7% lead and 21.6% arsenic. Generally, it is dispensed as a liquid suspension along with phenothiazine. Phenothiazine is used to treat stomach and intestinal worms of farm animals. After administration, the lead arsenate probably reacts with water in the digestive tract to release both lead and arsenic.

Effectiveness. The effectiveness of lead arsenate against tapeworms other than *Moniezia* species is questionable.[65]

Toxicity. Because of the high toxicity of both lead and arsenic, the product probably should not be administered to lambs less than 2 months of age. Although debilitated animals may be more susceptible to the effects of lead arsenate, adult sheep can tolerate significantly more than the recommended dose.

Even though toxicity from lead arsenate is cumulative, adult sheep can receive about nineteen treatments at a normal dose of 22 mg/kg before fatal levels of arsenic accumulate.[16] Even if treatment were given every 3 months, five years would be required to reach lethal levels, a longer period than a sheep's life span in a normal management routine. If given at the rate of 22 mg/kg to adult sheep on successive occasions, death will result when the total dose reaches about 417 to 475 mg/kg. Death results primarily from accumulation of arsenic. Sheep pass almost all the lead in the feces. However, a substantial amount of arsenic is retained in the liver.[16]

Dose and administration. Lead arsenate is dosed at the rate of 500 mg for lambs weighing approximately 20 kg and 1 gm for adult sheep 27 kg and over. The dosage is 500 mg to 1.5 gm for young cattle; for adult cattle no more than 2 gm should be administered.[81]

Niclosamide. Niclosamide is discussed in Chapter 11. It is highly effective against *Moniezia* species when given at the rate of 75 mg/kg. Very young lambs need 1 gm regardless of their weight. Generally, the expense of niclosamide precludes its use in farm animals.

Nematodes

Gastrointestinal nematodes of cattle and sheep

Family Trichostrongylidae. The major stomach and intestinal worms of cattle and sheep belong to the family Trichostrongylidae. Generally, the animals are infected with several of the following species.

Trichostrongylus species. Members of the genus *Trichostrongylus* may be located in either the abomasum or the small intestine. Eggs that are laid by the adult parasites are passed in the feces and contaminate pastures. After 3 to 4 days, under suitable conditions, eggs reach the infective stage. Only 3 weeks are required from infection to the development of mature parasites, which shed a new generation of ova.

The parasites penetrate and disrupt the mucosa of the abomasum and intestines. This damage can be extensive in heavy infestation. The parasites also suck blood but do not harm the hosts significantly in this way.

In a severe infection, rapid death without the development of any significant signs may result. In more chronic cases, however, animals may lose their appetite, become emaciated, and develop diarrhea. If anemia is present, it is mild.

Ostertagia species. When the infective larvae of *Ostertagia ostertagia* are ingested by the host, they penetrate the mucosa of the abomasum and cause the formation of small circular raised areas, about 1 to 2 mm in diameter. In severe cases, swelling (edema) of the mucosa of the abomasum results. Because the worms suck blood, anemia may be present in heavy infestations. Such infections result in a state of general illness, malnutrition, weakness, and death.

Cooperia species. The various *Cooperia* species penetrate into the mucosa of the small intestine and suck blood. A light infection causes no significant clinical signs. However, young cattle and sheep can become heavily parasitized on wet pastures. Such infections cause severe signs similar to infection with *Trichostrongylus* species. The anemia is more severe.

Nematodirus species. In otherwise healthy lambs, infestations of *Nematodirus* species usually can be tolerated without producing clinical signs. Infestation of sheep in poor condition or with concurrent disease or heavy infestations will produce signs similar to those of *Trichostrongylus* species infestation. Phenothiazine has little effect on *Nema-todirus* species. Therefore, when it is used for the removal of other species of stomach worms, it may remove competitors of *Nematodirus* species, which may enable the *Nematodirus* organisms to multiply and seriously affect the host by damaging the mucosa of the small intestine.

Haemonchus species. Species of the genus *Haemonchus* cause the most serious damage in the gastrointestinal tract of ruminants. Strains of the parasite have developed that are highly resistant to many anthelmintics.

In the abomasum the fourth-stage larva sucks blood and causes the formation of small blood clots on the mucosa. Adult worms live free in the abomasum. They pierce the mucosa with lancets in their mouths and suck blood. It is likely that they inject into the wound a substance to prevent clotting of the blood. This deprives the host of a larrge quantity of blood. In severe infestations the contents of the abomasum are bloody, and the abomasal mucosa becomes severely irritated. In addition, *Haemonchus* species infestation decreases the ability to digest and absorb protein, calcium, and phosphorus.

In severe cases, animals become anemic and may die rapidly without showing much in the way of signs. A classical sign of *Haemonchus* infestation is edema under the jaw (bottle jaw) and along the abdomen; this is caused by a decrease of protein in the serum.

Family Rhabditidae
Strongyloides papillosus. *Strongyloides papillosus* infects the small intestine of sheep, cattle, and other ruminants. Fully developed embryos rather than ova are passed in the feces of the host. A severe infestation in lambs results in erosion of the intestinal mucosa, watery intestinal contents, loss of appetite, loss of weight, diarrhea, and moderate anemia.

Family Ancylostomatidae (hookworms)
Bunostomum phlebotomum. *Bunostomum phlebotomum*, the hookworm of cattle and sometimes sheep, has a life cycle similar to that of the hookworms of dogs and cats. Infection of the small intestine by adult para-

sites can result in diarrhea, anemia, and weakness, especially in calves.

Family Trichinellidae

***Capillaria* species.** Parasites of the genus *Capillaria* occur in the small intestine of cattle and sheep. Although they are widely distributed, there is no evidence that *Capillaria* species produce clinical disease in the animals.

Family Trichonematidae

***Oesophagostomum* species.** *Oesophagostomum* species occur in the large intestine, where the larvae pass into the submucosa, causing localized inflammation. The inflammatory process results in the larvae becoming encased in a nodule. Thus *Oesophagostomum* is often called the "nodular worm."

When nodules occur in large numbers, they may interfere with intestinal movement (peristalsis) and the processes of digestion and absorption.

When young worms leave the nodule and return into the lumen of the intestine, they cause an intense irritation of the mucosa, resulting in diarrhea. Typically, sheep with a chronic infestation are extremely emaciated. The infestation can lead to complete prostration and death. A similar condition is caused in cattle by *Oesophagostomum radiatum.*

Family Strongylidae

Chabertia ovina. *Chabertia ovina* can occur in both sheep and cattle. It is commonly referred to as the "large-mouthed bowel worm." Animals become infested by ingesting the larvae. These attach themselves to the mucosa of the colon. The adjoining areas of the mucosa become congested and swollen. The presence of the parasites also causes small hemorrhages in the colon. In severe infestations, sheep may become anemic and die.

Treatment of cattle and sheep with gastrointestinal nematodes. Because it is common for sheep and cattle to have mixed infestation of various species of stomach and intestinal worms and because for the most part the same drugs are used to destroy the various species, we will discuss the treatment of the entire group of parasites.

Husbandry plays an important role in the control of gastrointestinal worms in sheep and cattle. To minimize and control infections the following management practices are important.

1. Throughout the year animals should be maintained on a well-balanced diet. As a result of genetic selection, which causes meat-producing animals to gain weight rapidly and milk-producing animals to produce a larger volume of milk than would normally be the case, such livestock have great nutritional demands. If these nutritional demands are not met, susceptibility to parasitic infections is increased. On many ranches, good quality pasture is available some part of the year, whereas at other times the naturally available feed is of inferior quality. When animals are not supplied from their pasture with a full range of nutrients, the feed must be supplemented.

2. Do not overstock pastures. Overstocking pastures results in gross contamination with parasitic ova. Some animals that are resistant to a clinical infection by a relatively small number of parasites may develop serious clinical disease when exposed to an overwhelming number of parasitic ova.

3. Treat animals with an appropriate anthelmintic when they show clinical signs of gastrointestinal nematode infestations. In addition, because stomach and intestinal worms are almost universally present in livestock, routine schedules for treatment should be established. These schedules will vary depending on the locale and management practices. Schedules should be established on the recommendation of local veterinarians, agricultural advisors, or both. To reduce the probability of the development of strains resistant to particular anthelmintics, it is a good practice to change frequently from one effective anthelmintic to another. Furthermore, to increase the effectiveness of anthelmintics and to reduce the possibility of the development of resistant strains, the highest recommended dose levels should be used. The only exception to this is in severely debilitated animals, in which lower doses may be indicated to reduce the possibility of toxic reaction.

4. House dairy calves separately in clean

areas. Beef calves and lambs should be housed separately from adults as soon as possible after weaning.

5. If possible, do *not* house animals on wet or moist pastures. Such pastures are ideal environments for parasitic ova and infective larvae of gastrointestinal worms.

6. Feed stabled animals from raised troughs and hayracks to prevent contamination of the feed with ova or infective larvae of gastrointestinal worms.

In our opinion, the following are the drugs of choice to treat sheep and cattle infected with stomach and intestinal parasites: the benzimidazoles, coumaphos, haloxon, levamisole, and phenothiazine.

Gastrointestinal nematodes of swine

Ascarids (large intestinal roundworms). Ascarid infection of swine can cause serious problems. The life cycle of the parasite and the course of the disease are similar to that described for the dog and cat. Unlike dogs, prenatal infection does not appear to occur in swine. Swine are infected with *Ascaris lumbricoides.* Digestive disturbances and poor growth occur in infected animals. Serious damage can also be caused by migration of the immature parasites through the liver and lungs. *A. lumbricoides* is not transmissible to humans.

When ova of parasites are ingested by hosts, they hatch quickly in the small intestine. The larvae then penetrate the intestine and are transported to the liver through the portal vein. From the liver they are transported by the circulatory system to various parts of the body, but most end up in the lung. The larvae are coughed up and swallowed. They mature in the intestine. It requires approximately 3 to 4 weeks after infection for the worms to reenter the intestine. About 8 to 9 weeks after infection, the parasites mature and begin to lay eggs. In the intestine, second-stage larvae irritate the mucosa. Mature worms compete for feed substances with the host. Large numbers of larvae migrating through the liver can cause inflammation, death of the tissue, and formation of large amounts of scar tissue. Thus

severe infection can greatly compromise liver function. Irritation of the lungs can also result from migration.

Strongyloides ransomi. *Strongyloides ransomi*, the intestinal threadworm, occurs in the small intestine of swine. In severe infections, young pigs become weak and their growth may be stunted.

Oesophagostomum species. Species of *Oesophagostomum*, the nodular worm, live in the cecum and colon of swine where they cause a condition similar to that described for *Oesophagostomum* in ruminants (p. 184).

Trichuris suis. *Trichuris suis*, the whipworm, lives in the cecum of swine. Usually it causes no clinical disease. However, in severe infections or in debilitated animals, it may result in diarrhea and loss of body condition.

Hyostrongylus rubidus. *Hyostrongylus rubidus* occurs in the stomach of swine. In the stomach the parasites burrow into the mucosa and suck blood. In healthy animals they seem to cause no problem. However, if the animal's resistance is lowered by such factors as pregnancy or lactation, marked disease can result. Such diseased animals become weak, incoordinated, thin, and have diarrhea.

Prevention and treatment of swine gastrointestinal nematodes. Many of the methods discussed for the prevention of parasites in ruminants are applicable to the prevention of parasites in swine. In addition, because baby pigs acquire ascarid infections from adults, the separation of sows into clean quarters prior to farrowing is highly desirable. If the sow is cleared of ascarid infection and washed before she gives birth and nurses her young, infection of young pigs can be prevented. Such husbandry practices also help to prevent scours caused by microorganisms in piglets (Chapter 6).

A wide variety of drugs are available for killing intestinal parasites in swine. Some of these are narrow-spectrum drugs, that is, they are effective only against one parasite, whereas others possess activity against all the common internal parasites of swine.

For treatment of ascarid infestation in

swine the following appear to be the drugs of choice: fenbendazole, parbendazole, levamisole, and pyrantel tartrate. For *Oesophagostomum* species infestations the drugs of choice are cambendazole, fenbendazole, parbendazole, levamisole, phenothiazine, and pyrantal tartrate. For *Strongyloides* species infestations, parbendazole and levamisole are the drugs of choice. Parbendazole and levamisole (when injected subcutaneously) are also preferred for *Trichuris suis* infestations. Cambendazole is the drug of choice for treatment of infestation by *Hyostrongylus rubidus*.

It appears that parbendazole and levamisole are the most versatile anthelmintics for swine.

Lungworms

Cattle and sheep are infected with *Dictyocaulus* species, and swine are infected with *Metastrongylus* species. Sheep are primarily infected with *D. filaria*. This parasite occurs in the bronchi of sheep, goats, and some wild ruminants. Animals acquire the infection by the oral route. Within 3 days, larvae penetrate the intestine and pass by way of lymph vessels to the lungs, where they lodge in the capillaries and break through to the air passages. Some larvae pass through the capillaries of the lung into the general circulation and establish prenatal infections in the fetus. In the host, the parasites develop to maturity in about 6 weeks.

The parasites produce a bronchitis by residing in the small bronchi where they suck blood and irritate the mucosa. The resulting exudate may pass into the bronchioles and alveoli, and pneumonia may then develop. As the young larvae pass through the intestine, they may irritate the mucosa and cause diarrhea.

Primarily young animals are infected. However the disease may occur at all ages and is usually chronic. Mucus drips from the nostrils, and animals may cough. However, a cough is not always present. Frequently, animals have difficulty breathing.

Cattle are primarily infected with *D. vivi-*

parus. Its life cycle is similar to that of *D. filaria*. Generally, only calves are infected. The disease produced is similar to that in sheep.

In swine, two species of lungworm occur, *M. apri* and *M. salmi*. The life cycle of *M. apri* involves an intermediate host, any of a number of species of earthworm. Pigs usually become infected by eating infected earthworms. In swine the development of lungworms is similar to that described for sheep.

The signs of lungworm infection in swine are similar to those described in sheep. However, disease caused by lungworms in swine is generally less serious than in ruminants. Primarily the worms cause a loss of body condition and retard growth. Since they carry the virus that causes swine influenza, swine lungworms can spread that disease.

Treatment. The elimination of lungworm infestations by drug therapy in cattle, sheep, and swine is more critical than it is for gastrointestinal parasites. Effective anthelmintic therapy can rid the animals of their gastrointestinal parasites, and with proper nutrition, reduction in further exposures to parasitic ova, and/or periodic treatment, the animals will gain weight and return to a normal state. However, if the lungs are severely damaged by lungworms, drug therapy, even if effective in killing the parasites, will not return the lungs to normal. It is important therefore that animals with lungworm infection be treated early.

In some areas where the disease is present (enzootic), animals can acquire a natural resistance by being exposed to an extremely low level of lungworm larvae. On the other hand, exposures to massive numbers of larvae result in fatalities. To prevent severe infestations, young susceptible animals should not be grazed on pastures that have been contaminated by older animals. In areas where cattle are pastured during the winter, older animals and especially yearlings, primary carriers of the infection, should have an appropriate anthelmintic administered before being turned out to pasture.

The drug of choice to combat lungworms

in swine appears to be levamisole. In cattle and sheep, albendazole, cambendazole, fenbendazole, and levamisole appear to be effective.

A vaccine has been developed, consisting of irradiated lungworm larva. However, it has a short shelf-life, that is, it deteriorates rapidly and loses its effectiveness. Because it is necessary to combine sophisticated management procedures and chemotherapeutic treatment when using the vaccine, it should only be used under the close supervision of a veterinarian.

ANTHELMINTICS

The benzimidazoles. The benzimidazoles are an extremely successful class of anthelmintics and enjoy wide use in livestock and horses. Certain members of the class may be used in dogs (Chapter 11) and in man. Their popularity results from their high level of effectiveness against a wide variety of internal parasites and their high degree of safety. A measure of the success of the benzimidazoles is the large number that have been developed, tested, and marketed by various drug companies.

Thiabendazole. Because it was the first benzimidazole commercially available in the United States and because it shares many of the characteristics of the other benzimidazoles, thiabendazole is discussed first.

Thiabendazole is manufactured in various forms for oral administration to sheep and cattle. It is dispensed in the following forms: a drench, granules or powder for top dressing on feed, combined in alfalfa pellets, a paste, or a bolus.

Effectiveness. Thiabendazole is used to kill stomach and intestinal parasites in cattle and sheep, in which it is highly effective in destroying most of the stomach and intestinal worms that have been discussed.[20,23,40]

However, some strains have developed varying degrees of resistance to the drug. There is some experimental evidence to indicate that resistance of a strain of parasites to thiabendazole may also result in resistance to other benzimidazole anthelmintics.[93]

Such cross-resistance is often seen when drugs have similar structures. Cross-resistance usually does not occur between drugs of dissimilar chemical structures.[49] If resistance to thiabendazole is encountered, one option is to switch therapy to a drug from a totally different class of drugs, such as levamisole, which is not a benzimidazole.

Sometimes increasing the dose in sheep from the normal 40 mg/kg to 150 mg/kg will greatly increase the effectiveness of thiabendazole against resistant strains of parasites.[93]

Generally, thiabendazole is considered to have greater effectiveness against stomach and intestinal parasites of cattle and sheep than phenothiazine.[14] The superiority of thiabendazole, however, will not always hold up. For example, the effectiveness of thiabendazole administered once a month in the feed to naturally infected lambs at the rate of 27.5 mg/kg of body weight was compared with the monthly administration of a commercial fine particle–size formulation of phenothiazine at the rate of 25 gm per animal as a drench. Although thiabendazole was more effective than phenothiazine against *T. colubriformis* and *S. papillosus*, phenothiazine had greater activity against *H. contortus*.[61]

The form in which thiabendazole is administered may influence its effectiveness. For example, in sheep there is evidence that the administration of thiabendazole boluses is more effective than the administration of the thiabendazole as a drench.[14]

Thiabendazole has been shown to be highly effective against a wide variety of gastrointestinal nematodes of cattle when administered in protein blocks at the rate of 110 mg/kg over a 3-day period.[2]

Toxicity. A primary advantage of the use of thiabendazole is its relatively low toxicity in sheep and cattle. It is much safer than levamisole or phenothiazine. The toxic dose is many times greater than the dose necessary to obtain the desired therapeutic effect. For this reason, increasing the normal dose two or three times to increase its effectiveness against resistant strains is a rational approach. This is not the case with levamisole or phenothiazine, since these drugs do not enjoy such a wide margin of safety.

The first sign of toxicity in sheep normally occurs at doses greater than 600 mg/kg and in cattle at the 1.6 gm/kg dose.[67] In a sheep receiving a fatal dose of thiabendazole (1.2 gm/kg) autopsy findings indicated that there was damage to the liver and kidneys.[14]

Dose and administration. The commercial manufacturer of thiabendazole recommends a normal oral dose of 40 mg/kg in sheep. In severe infections, doses of 60 to 150 mg/kg given orally are recommended. In cattle, oral doses of 60 to 111 mg/kg are recommended.

Albendazole. Albendazole is an experimental benzimidazole that has been tested against various internal parasitic infestations in sheep and cattle.

At doses of 2.5 to 10 mg/kg, albendazole was effective in trials against a variety of gastrointestinal nematodes in sheep.[91] In cattle at doses of 5 to 10 mg/kg given orally, albendazole was highly effective against a wide variety of larvae and adult gastrointestinal parasites.[92] At doses of 10 mg/kg it is also effective against *D. filaria* (lungworm) in cattle.

Before it is released for clinical use, albendazole needs further study regarding its safety and effectiveness.

Cambendazole

Effectiveness. Cambendazole, which is closely related to thiabendazole, has been shown to be highly effective against a wide variety of gastrointestinal nematodes of cattle.[10,18,27] Apparently the compound is also effective against a wide variety of gastrointestinal nematodes of sheep.

In swine, cambendazole is highly effective against adult *H. rubidus* and *Oesophagostomum* species infestations. Its effectiveness against larval stages of these same species is variable.[88] In addition, when given in the feed to swine at the rate of 0.03% of the diet, cambendazole may be effective in preventing infection with ascarids.

Cambendazole was shown to be 95% effective against a 22-day-old experimental infection of *D. viviparus* (lungworm) at a dose of 40 mg/kg in cattle.[10,83]

Cambendazole is approximately equally effective given as a feed premix, in feed pellets, as a suspension, or as a bolus. However, one trial showed cambendazole to be less effective against *O. ostertagi* when given in feed pellets as compared with other forms.[18]

Toxicity. At normal doses the drug appears to be nontoxic.

Dose and administration. Cambendazole should be administered to sheep at the rate of 20 mg/kg and to cattle at the rate of 20 to 40 mg/kg.[81] The higher dose in cattle is to ensure effectiveness against more resistant strains.[12]

Cambendazole can be given at the rate of 7.5 mg/kg for the treatment of *Strongyloides* species infestations in swine.[81] However, to be effective against larvae in swine, doses of approximately 40 mg/kg may be required.[88]

Fenbendazole. Fenbendazole is a relatively new benzimidazole anthelmintic.

Effectiveness. Experimentally and in field trials, it has been shown to be highly effective against gastrointestinal parasites of sheep and cattle and against ascarids and *Oesophagostomum* species in swine. Oral doses of from 5 to 10 mg/kg were used.*

In sheep, doses as low as 5 and as high as 80 mg/kg have been 100% effective against the lungworm *D. filaria.*[37] Doses up to 80 mg/kg given orally to sheep have proven effective against various species of thiabendazole-resistant gastrointestinal parasites.[46]

Toxicity. When used at therapeutic doses of 7.5 mg/kg no toxic signs were noted in debilitated sheep.[56] The drug is apparently extremely safe, with the toxic dose much higher than the therapeutic dose. For example, one dose of 5 gm/kg caused no ill effects in sheep.[5]

Mebendazole

Effectiveness. Mebendazole, at a dose of 12.5 mg/kg, has been shown to be highly

---

*See references 5, 56, 57, 80, 94.

effective against *Haemonchus, Ostertagia, Trichostrongylus, Oesophagostomum,* and *Strongyloides* species in sheep.[53]

Toxicity. The drug is low in toxicity. It has been reported that the lethal dose that will kill 50% of the animals to which it is administered (LD-50) in sheep is above 320 mg/kg.[98]

Parbendazole. Parbendazole is used to treat gastrointestinal nematode infestations of sheep, cattle, and swine.

Effectiveness. Experimentally, parbendazole has been shown to be effective against a wide variety of gastrointestinal parasites of sheep when given orally or intraruminally (injected directly into the rumen) at the rate of 12.5 to 15 mg/kg. It has been shown to be highly effective against *Haemonchus, Ostertagia, Trichostrongylus, Strongyloides, Cooperia, Bunostomum, Nematodirus, Oesophagostomum,* and *Chabertia* species. Parbendazole has had limited effectiveness against *Trichuris* species in sheep.[89]

In cattle, parbendazole is effective against a wide variety of gastrointestinal parasites at doses from 10 to 40 mg/kg.[17,25,82,89]

Trials in swine have shown parbendazole to be highly effective against ascarids, *Oesophagostomum, Trichuris,* and *Strongyloides* species when administered at the rate of 20 to 30 mg/kg.[13,31,90]

In all species, parasites resistant to other benzimidazole anthelmintics are likely to be resistant to parbendazole. However, increasing the dose from the normal of 15 mg/kg to 60 mg/kg in sheep may result in effective control of benzimidazole-resistant strains of parasites.[93] Frequently, parbendazole is effective against strains resistant to phenothiazine.[15]

Toxicity. Parbendazole, like other benzimidazoles, appears to be relatively nontoxic. For example, the drug was well tolerated in growing pigs when given at 500 mg/kg and 1000 mg/kg, which are about sixteen and thirty-three times the normal therapeutic dose.[90]

Dose and administration. Parbendazole is given orally. Recommended doses are 15 mg/kg in sheep and 30 mg/kg in swine. In cattle it is given at the rate of 30 to 40 mg/kg. To ensure effectiveness against the widest variety of parasites the 40 mg/kg dose is probably indicated in cattle.[81] In swine the drug can be given as a drench or mixed in the feed at the rate of 0.06%.

Hygromycin B. Unlike other anthelmintics, hygromycin B is an antibiotic. Used only in swine, it is not administered as a single dose but rather is included over a period of time in the feed.

Effectiveness. Hygromycin B is used for the control of ascarids. In swine it also has activity against nodular worms and whipworms. The assumption is made that swine are continuously exposed to ascarid ova, and thus hygromycin B is added to the feed to reduce infections. On infected ranches, animals receiving hygromycin B in the feed would be expected to have fewer parasites and less liver damage than untreated pigs grown under the same conditions.

Toxicity. Hygromycin B can be fed to pregnant sows; it has no effect on their reproductive ability. Because of the cost, however, it is not fed to animals over 35 to 40 kg.

Hygromycin B must be discontinued in swine 48 hours before slaughter. Because the compound has been associated with the formation of cataracts in dogs and deafness in dogs and swine, it should be kept away from dogs who might be tempted to eat the medicated feed. Humans should avoid direct contact with the product on skin or eyes. Hygromycin B has been reported to depress weight gains when continually fed to animals over 45 kg.[81]

Dose and administration. Hygromycin B is administered in the feed at the rate of 12 gm/ton of finished feed. It should be fed for at least 6 weeks, from the time piglets receive solid feed until the animals have reached 35 to 45 kg.[81]

Levamisole. Levamisole is available for sheep and cattle as a soluble powder that is added to water for drenching and as boluses and feed pellets. In addition, an 18.2% sterile solution for subcutaneous injection is available for cattle.

Effectiveness. Levamisole has been shown to be highly effective against common gastrointestinal parasites in sheep in experimental and field trials.[8,96,97] It is also highly effective in sheep against the lungworm *D. filaria.*[78,95]

In cattle, levamisole has been shown to be highly effective against gastrointestinal roundworms and the lungworm *D. vivipara.**

Results are sometimes poor against *T. axei.* When such failures occur, other effective anthelmintics such as the benzimidazoles or phenothiazine are indicated.

Levamisole has been shown to be highly effective in swine against ascarids, *Oesophagostomum* species, *Strongyloides* species, and the lungworm *Metastrongylus.*†

When injected subcutaneously at the rate of 7.5 mg/kg, levamisole is effective in treating *T. suis* infestation in swine. However, at the same dose orally its effect has been variable.[48] It is probable that strains of gastrointestinal parasites resistant to benzimidazole anthelmintics will be susceptible to levamisole.[49]

Toxicity. At normal doses the side effects of levamisole are minor. Muzzle foam may form after animals receive the drug. However, it usually disappears within a few hours.

When levamisole is injected in cattle, swelling may develop at the injection site. The swelling usually subsides in 7 to 14 days.

The drug has not been approved in the United States for use in dairy cattle of breeding age, probably to prevent contamination of milk.

It is important to calculate the dose of levamisole carefully when giving it to animals because the margin of safety that exists between the therapeutic and toxic doses is not as high for levamisole as it is for the benzimidazoles. For example, sheep receiving 40 mg/kg can be expected to demonstrate the

following signs: extension of the head, excitability, mild spastic movements when walking, continuous chewing and grinding of the teeth, and diarrhea. These signs normally pass within 1½ hours after administration of the drug. At levels of 160 mg/kg, death in lambs can be expected.[7]

Levamisole is relatively nontoxic in swine when administered at therapeutic doses. When levamisole was given to pigs at three times the recommended dose, only occasional vomiting resulted. A threefold overdose given twice within 7 days, either early or late in gestation in pregnant sows, did not cause adverse effects with regard to the size of the litter or the weight, appearance, or vigor of the baby pigs. Twenty-four hours after treatment with 8 mg/kg of body weight, fat, skeletal muscle, and blood specimens collected from swine were free of drug residues. Kidneys were clear in 48 hours and the liver in 72 hours.[51]

In swine, salivation or muzzle foam may be observed after administration. This reaction usually disappears within a short time. Coughing and vomiting after administration usually indicates that the animals were infected with mature lung worms. When the drug is injected subcutaneously in swine, swellings 1 to 15 mm in diameter may be seen at the injection site. These are expected to disappear totally within 10 days.[71]

Dose and administration. The drug can be given orally or by subcutaneous injection. When it is given in the drinking water, the suggestion has been made that water be withheld for 15 to 16 hours prior to administration. Levamisole is then dissolved in about half of the daily water ration so the animals will consume the full dose over a short period of time.

The dose for sheep, cattle, and swine is approximately 8 mg/kg. The manufacturer prints instructions for calculating this approximate dose in the labeling of the product. The instructions should also be consulted for the time that should elapse between the administration of the drug and the slaughtering of the animals.

*See references 1, 9, 26, 33, 66, 77, 79, 84.
†See references 38, 51, 70-72, 75.

Organophosphates. Various organophosphate preparations have been tested for treating gastrointestinal nematodes of sheep, cattle, and swine. Because of their high toxicity, great care must be taken to follow the directions on the label of commercial products. Because cattle have low blood cholinesterase levels, organophosphates must be used with great caution. They are not used in brahman cattle, which are the most susceptible to the toxic effects of the drug.

Coumaphos. Coumaphos can be placed in the feed of cattle to treat gastrointestinal nematode parasitism. This organophosphate is effective against the major gastrointestinal parasites when given at the rate of 2 mg/kg of body weight mixed in feed for 6 consecutive days.[32,99]

Haloxon. Haloxon has been shown experimentally to be effective against *Haemonchus, Cooperia, Ostertagia,* and *Trichostrongylus* species in sheep and cattle.[3,6,19] The drug may be given orally or by injection. For cattle and sheep the recommended dose is 50 to 60 mg/kg, and for swine, 35 to 80 mg/kg.[81]

Phenothiazine. Until the introduction of thiabendazole in the 1960s, phenothiazine was the most effective anthelmintic to combat gastrointestinal nematodes in ruminants. It is still highly effective against many strains of gastrointestinal nematodes in ruminants and nodular worms in swine.

The compound is best known in human medicine as the substance from which a whole class of tranquilizers and antihistamines is derived.

Phenothiazine is available in two states of purity and various average particle size. These factors contribute significantly to the degree of effectiveness of the drug. The two levels of purity available are phenothiazine (NF) (approximately 85% phenothiazine) and purified phenothiazine (approximately 99% phenothiazine).

As the size of the particle decreases, the effectiveness increases. Generally, the particle size is shown on the label. It is measured in microns (μ), which are each 1/1000 of a millimeter. Phenothiazine is referred to as micronized when its average particle is 10 μ or less. Those micronized forms of phenothiazine having an average particle size as small as 2 to 3 μ are obviously more effective than those of larger size. The various formulations of phenothiazine are listed in order of decreasing effectiveness as follows[65]:

1. Micronized purified phenothiazine
2. Micronized (average particle size 2.6 μ) phenothiazine (NF)
3. Purified phenothiazine (average particle size 14.4 μ)
4. Micronized (85% of the particles less than 10 μ) phenothiazine (NF)
5. Phenothiazine (NF)

It has been shown experimentally how important the particle size and purity of phenothiazine is. For example, in an experiment in which sheep were infected with a phenothiazine-resistant strain of *H. contortus,* phenothiazine (NF) was only 44.1% effective when given at a dose of 24.5 gm per animal. However, 25 gm per animal of phenothiazine having an average particle size of 2 to 3 μ was 99% to 100% effective against the same parasite.[45]

Phenothiazine is available in various dosage formulations. The powdered form, which can be suspended in water, is not recommended because some individuals develop hypersensitive skin reactions from the material. Drenches are available that usually contain about 12.5 gm/30 ml. These suspensions of phenothiazine usually also contain bentonite as a suspending agent.

Phenothiazine boluses are also available. The clinician should keep in mind two factors regarding use of the boluses: (1) the particle size of boluses is usually higher than that of the drench; and (2) many boluses do not disintegrate easily after administration to the animal.

Effectiveness. Even though phenothiazine has a wide spectrum of activity against gastrointestinal nematodes, resistant strains have developed.

Toxicity. One must be careful in using the liquid preparation of phenothiazine in light-colored horses or sheep. If any of the drug is spilled, it is oxidized to a product that dyes the hair or wool red. After oral administration, two phenothiazine derivatives, phenothiazone and thionol, are passed in the urine. Both are red and capable of staining fur or wool. When practical, such urine should be covered with straw, wood shavings, or dirt to prevent it from staining the animal. The milk of a treated animal often is discolored for a few days after treatment. The milk is nontoxic to animals but cannot be used for human consumption. The label of any phenothiazine product should be checked to determine the number of hours that milk must be withheld from human consumption after administration of the drug.

In animals there is a wide variety of susceptibility to the toxicity of phenothiazine. Generally, birds, sheep, and goats seem to be the most resistant. Cattle are more susceptible to the toxic effects than other ruminants. However, phenothiazine is a safe anthelmintic in cattle. Swine are more susceptible to toxicity than cattle, and horses are more susceptible than other farm-type animals. The product is not used in carnivores such as dogs and cats because generally it is not effective against their parasites, and it is highly toxic to carnivorous species. Phenothiazine is not used in humans. However, derivatives of phenothiazine are used as tranquilizers and antihistamines in both man and animals.

The reactions that can result from the toxicity of phenothiazine are inflammation of the cornea, destruction of red blood cells, abortion, incoordination, paralysis, and destruction of the kidneys.

In the intestinal tract, some phenothiazine is converted to phenothiazine sulfoxide. Once absorbed it is primarily metabolized by the liver. When metabolism of phenothiazine sulfoxide by the liver is not complete, some reaches systemic circulation and diffuses into the anterior chamber of the eye (aqueous humor). The phenothiazine sulfoxide causes the cornea to become inflamed and sensitive to light. This results in excessive tearing, squinting, and some cloudiness of the cornea. Animals so affected should be moved out of direct sunlight.

Phenothiazine can cause abortion if administered in late pregnancy. It may cause incoordination or paralysis in swine or young lambs. In sheep that are dehydrated or otherwise refuse water, normal doses of phenothiazine can cause destruction of the kidney cells. To prevent toxic reactions from phenothiazine, some judgment should be exercised in its application. Phenothiazine should not be administered to animals that are extremely ill, debilitated, anemic, or emaciated. The drug should not be administered to animals that are constipated because the likelihood of toxicity increases with the slowed passage of the drug through the digestive tract and the resulting increase in absorption. It should not be administered during the last month of pregnancy.

Generally, it is recommended that phenothiazine and organophosphates not be given together. Theoretically phenothiazine increases the toxicity of organophosphates. However, there is evidence that questions the theory.[86] Phenothiazine was administered as a single dose and as continuous low level doses in amounts recommended for control of internal parasites in 6- to 8-month-old calves. In addition, the calves were treated with numerous organophosphate insecticides at doses and treatment regimens recommended by the manufacturer. There did not appear to be any potentiation of toxic effects of the organophosphates by phenothiazine.[86]

Dose and administration. The following doses are recommended for phenothiazine in animals[81]:

Cattle	275 to 440 mg/kg (a maximum of 60 gm of micronized products and 80 gm for the other forms should be administered per animal)
Sheep	500 to 800 mg/kg
Swine	4 to 23 kg, 8 gm; 45 kg and over, 10 gm/45 kg of body weight, with total dose not to exceed 30 gm

The piperazines. Various salts of piperazine (Chapter 11) can be used to treat swine for infestations with ascarids or nodular worms. The effectiveness of piperazine against ascarids in swine is questionable. As the base, piperazine can be administered at 0.3% to 0.4% in feed for at least 1 day or 0.1% to 0.2% in the drinking water for 1 to 2 days.

Diethylcarbamazine. Diethylcarbamazine is used in sheep, cattle, and swine to combat lungworms. It has a narrow spectrum of activity in cattle and sheep. This drug is only effective against lungworms and not against the gastrointestinal nematodes of ruminants.

Effectiveness. How effective diethylcarbamazine is in the field is questionable. Experimentally a dose of 20 mg/kg injected intramuscularly was effective against 15-day-old experimental infections in calves. However, at 31 days there was no apparent benefit from use of the drug.[50]

Toxicity. The drug is remarkably nontoxic to calves. It requires at least 440 mg/kg of body weight to observe transient toxic signs.[73]

Dose and administration. The following doses are recommended.[81] For cattle, give 20 to 40 mg/kg intramuscularly once a day for 2 or 3 successive days. Orally give twice the intramuscular dose. For sheep, give 20 mg/kg intramuscularly once a day for 3 days. Orally, give 60 mg/kg. For swine, give 20 mg/kg intramuscularly once a day for 3 successive days or 100 mg/kg once intramuscularly.

Sodium fluoride. Sodium fluoride in its pure form is a fine white powder that unfortunately can be confused with flour or powdered sugar. To avoid the confusion, it should be colored and well labeled. It has been used at the level of 1% in feed to rid swine of ascarid infection. This is fed over a 24-hour period.

Toxicity. The product is highly toxic to all forms of life. Sodium fluoride must be administered in dry ground feed. If water is added to the feed, it will become too palatable, and animals may consume toxic amounts of the sodium fluoride. The addition of water to the ration will also increase the absorption of the sodium fluoride from the stomach.

After 24 hours, the remaining feed should be discarded. Because sodium fluoride makes the feed unpalatable, the calculated dose should be mixed with about $^1/_3$ the amount of feed consumed daily. To ensure that some animals are not overdosed and others underdosed, sodium fluoride must be thoroughly mixed throughout the feed, preferably by mechanical mixing. If it is mixed with the feed manually, the drug should be mixed with an equal volume of ground feed. After that is thoroughly mixed, it is combined with an equal volume of untreated feed and mixed. This is continued until the sodium fluoride has been mixed with all of the feed to be fed. Animals should be fasted overnight before receiving the drug. More prolonged fasting will perhaps increase the amount of food the animals eat and thereby result in toxic levels being consumed. Fresh nontreated water should be made available throughout the day to animals being treated.

Because a 4% to 5% mixture of sodium fluoride in the feed is fatal to swine, sodium fluoride has largely been replaced by the other anthelmintics discussed previously. The other disadvantage is its narrow spectrum of activity against parasites.

Dose and administration. It is safe to worm pigs shortly after weaning according to the previously given schedule. Sows should not be given the drug during the last half of pregnancy. Sodium fluoride is fed as 1% of the ration for 24 hours using the precautions just mentioned.

The tetrahydropyrimidines

Morantel tartrate. Morantel tartrate is effective against various gastrointestinal nematodes in sheep and cattle. It is a strong inhibitor of cholinesterase.

Effectiveness. When this drug was given in experiments to cattle as boluses or as top dressing on grain, morantel tartrate was highly effective against adult stages of *Haemonchus*, *Trichostrongylus*, *Cooperia*, *Oesophagostomum*, and *Ostertagia* species. In general the drug has not been effective against larval stages of gastrointestinal parasites.[34-36]

A dose of 10 mg/kg has been highly effective against *Haemonchus*, *Ostertagia*, *Trichostrongylus*, and *Nematodirus* in sheep.[43]

Toxicity. The maximum tolerated dose has been reported to be in excess of 200 mg/kg in calves.[36]

Dose and administration. Recommended doses for cattle and sheep are 10 mg/kg.

Pyrantel tartrate. Pyrantel tartrate can be used in swine to prevent the establishment of ascarid or nodular worm infections or to remove the infections once they are established. To prevent infections, 96 gm of the compound is mixed with a ton of feed (0.0106% of ration).

For treating infections, 800 gm of the compound is mixed with a ton of feed (0.0881% of ration). This is fed in measured amounts to deliver 22 mg/kg of active ingredient. Experimentally, pyrantel tartrate has been shown to be effective in the removal of ascarids and *Oesophagostomum* species when administered to swine in this manner.[4]

ARTHROPODS
Oestrus ovis (sheep botfly)

Sheep are infected with the larva of a fly (botfly) that causes problems in the nasal and sinus cavities. The flies deposit larvae around the nostrils of the host. The larvae then crawl upward, entering cavities next to the turbinate bones or frontal sinuses. As they grow, they are unable to leave these cavities because of the small openings. Therefore they die in the cavities and produce a foreign body reaction. Some larvae develop in areas where, after they mature, they are able to leave the host. After leaving the animal, they pupate on the ground for 3 to 6 weeks during the cold season before adult flies emerge. The full grown larva is about 3 cm long.

The flies annoy the animals when they attack them to deposit larvae. Animals may shake their heads or press their noses against the ground or between other sheep. When flies are plentiful, they may interfere with

animals' feeding. In addition, the larvae irritate the mucosa of the nasal and sinus surfaces. This results in the secretion of a viscid mucous exudate. Infected animals have a nasal discharge and frequently sneeze. They may quickly become emaciated. Erosion of the bones of the skull can occur. Even injury to the brain can result from infection by *O. ovis*.

Treatment. Treatment primarily consists of organophosphate preparations. It has been demonstrated that ruelene is highly effective against the various stages of *O. ovis* when administered orally to sheep at the rate of 125 to 150 mg/kg of body weight.[42]

References

1. Alicata, J. E., and Furumoto, H. H.: Efficacy and safety of l-tetramisole hydrochloride in experimental *Cooperia punctata* infection of dairy calves, Am. J. Vet. Res. **30:**139, 1969.
2. Ames, E. R., and Hutchinson, H. D.: Safety and efficacy of thiabendazole (TBZ) in protein blocks, Vet. Med. Small Anim. Clin. **68:**1376, 1973.
3. Andersen, F. L., and Christofferson, P. V.: Efficacy of haloxon and thiabendazole against gastrointestinal nematodes in sheep and goats in the Edwards Plateau area of Texas, Am. J. Vet. Res. **34:** 1395, 1973.
4. Arakawa, A., Conway, D. P., and DeGoosh, C.: Therapeutic efficacy of pyrantel tartrate against *Ascaris* and *Oesophagostomum* in swine, Vet. Med. Small Anim. Clin. **66:**108, 1971.
5. Baeder, C., Bahr, G., Christ, O., Duwel, D., et al.: Fenbendazole: a new highly effective anthelmintic, Experientia **30:**753, 1974.
6. Baker, N. F., Douglas, J. R., and Fisk, R. A.: Anthelmintic activity of haloxon in calves with parasitic gastroenteritis, Am. J. Vet. Res. **30:**2233, 1969.
7. Baker, N. F., and Fisk, R. A.: Levamisole as an anthelmintic in calves, Am. J. Vet. Res. **33:**1121, 1972.
8. Baker, N. F., Fisk, R. A., and Douglas, J. R.: Study of *dl*-tetramisole in lambs: anthelmintic efficacy and toxicity, Am. J. Vet. Res. **31:**977, 1970.
9. Baker, N. F., Fisk, R. A., and Douglas, J. R.: Administration of the anthelmintic levamisole in drinking water for cattle, Am. J. Vet. Res. **33:**1395, 1972.
10. Baker, N. F., and Walters, G. T.: Anthelmintic efficacy of cambendazole in cattle, Am. J. Vet. Res. **32:**29, 1971.
11. Baker, N. F., Walters, G. T., and Fisk, R. A.: Amprolium for control of coccidiosis in feedlot lambs, Am. J. Vet. Res. **33:**83, 1972.
12. Baker, N. F., Walters, G. T., and Hjerpe, C. A.:

Experimental therapy of *Dictyocaulus viviparis* infection in cattle with cambendazole, Am. J. Vet. Res. 33:1127, 1972.

13. Batte, E. G., and Moncol, D. J.: Evaluation of parbendazole, a new broad spectrum anthelmintic for swine and sheep, Vet. Med. Small Anim. Clin. 63:984, 1968.

14. Bell, R. R., Galvin, T. J., and Turk, R. D.: Anthelmintics for ruminants. VI. Thiabendazole, Am. J. Vet. Res. 23:195, 1962.

15. Bennett, D. G.: Comparative anthelmintic efficiencies of parbendazole, thiabendazole, and phenothiazine in lambs, Am. J. Vet. Res. 29:2325, 1968.

16. Bennett, D. G., and Schwartz, T. E.: Cumulative toxicity of lead arsenate in phenothiazine given to sheep, Am. J. Vet. Res. 32:727, 1971.

17. Benz, G. W.: Efficacy of parbendazole in the treatment of natural gastrointestinal parasitisms in cattle, J. Am. Vet. Med. Assoc. 153:1185, 1968.

18. Benz, G. W.: Anthelmintic activities of cambendazole in calves, Am. J. Vet. Res. 32:399, 1971.

19. Benz, G. W.: Anthelmintic activity of haloxon in calves, Am. J. Vet. Res. 33:1273, 1972.

20. Benz, G. W.: Evaluation of paste form of cambendazole and thiabendazole for administration to calves, Am. J. Vet. Res. 34:35, 1973.

21. Bergstrom, R. C., and Maki, L. R.: Effect of monensin in young crossbred lambs with naturally occurring coccidiosis, J. Am. Vet. Med. Assoc. 165:288, 1974.

22. Bergstrom, R. C., and Maki, L. R.: Coccidiostatic action of monensin fed to lambs: body weight gains and feed conversion efficacy, Am. J. Vet. Res. 37:79, 1976.

23. Bliss, D. H., and Todd, A. D.: Milk production by Wisconsin dairy cattle after deworming with thiabendazole, Vet. Med. Small Anim. Clin. 69:638, 1974.

24. Blood, D. C., and Henderson, J. A.: Veterinary medicine, ed. 4, Baltimore, 1974, The Williams & Wilkins Co.

25. Bradley, R. E.: Evaluation of parbendazole as an anthelmintic in cattle, Am. J. Vet. Res. 29:1979, 1968.

26. Broome, A. W. J., and Lewis, J. A.: Activity of levamisole against developmental stages of *D. viviparus* in experimentally infected calves, Vet. Rec. 94:563, 1974.

27. Cairns, G. C., Holmden, J. H., Feringa, A., and Murray, J.: The efficacy of cambendazole against gastrointestinal nematodes and lungworms in cattle, N.Z. Vet. J. 23:28, March 1975.

28. Campbell, N. J., and Brotowidjoyo, M. D.: The efficiency of clioxanide and rafoxanide against *Fasciola hepatica* in sheep by different routes of administration, Aust. Vet. J. 51:500, 1975.

29. Campbell, N. J., and Richardson, N. J.: A controlled test of oxyclozanide and rafoxanide against *Fasciola hepatica* in calves, Vet. Rec. 91:647, 1972.

30. Campbell, W. C., and Butler, R. W.: Efficacy of cambendazole against tapeworms and roundworm infections in lambs, Aust. Vet. J. 49:517, 1973.

31. Chang, J., and Wescott, R. B.: Anthelmintic activity of parbendazole in swine, Am. J. Vet. Res. 30:77, 1969.

32. Ciordia, H.: Activity of a feed premix and crumbles containing coumaphos in the control of gastrointestinal parasites of cattle, Am. J. Vet. Res. 33:623, 1972.

33. Ciordia, H., and Baird, D. M.: Efficacy of two levo-tetramisole formulations in controlling nematodes of cattle, Am. J. Vet. Res. 30:1145, 1969.

34. Ciordia, H., and McCampbell, H. C.: Anthelmintic activity of morantel tartrate in calves, Am. J. Vet. Res. 34:619, 1973.

35. Conway, D. P., DeGoosh, C., and Arakawa, A.: Anthelmintic efficacy of morantel tartrate in cattle, Am. J. Vet. Res. 34:621, 1973.

36. Cornwell, R. L., Jones, R. M., and Pott, J. M.: Controlled anthelmintic trials of morantel tartrate against experimental infections in calves, Br. Vet. J. 129:518, 1973.

37. Eslami, A. H., and Anwar, M.: Activity of fenbendazole against lung worms in naturally infected sheep, Vet. Rec. 99:129, 1976.

38. Ferguson, D. L., and White, R. G.: Anthelmintic activity of levamisole against *Ascaris*, *Trichuris*, and *Metastrongylus* infections in swine, J. Anim. Sci. 40:838, 1975.

39. Fitzgerald, P. R., and Mansfield, M. E.: Efficacy of monensin against bovine coccidiosis in young Holstein-Friesian calves, J. Protozool. 20:121, 1973.

40. Flack, D. E., Frank, B. N., Easterbrooks, H. L., and Brown, G. E.: Thiabendazole treatment: effect upon weight gains, feed efficiency and cost of gain in commercial feedlot cattle, Vet. Med. Small Anim. Clin. 62:565, 1967.

41. Foreyt, W. J., and Todd, A. C.: Liver flukes in cattle: prevalence, distribution and experimental treatment, Vet. Med. Small Anim. Clin. 71:816, 1976.

42. Galvin, T. J., Turk, R. D., and Bell, R. R.: Anthelmintics for ruminants. IV. Further studies on ruelene in sheep, Am. J. Vet. Res. 23:185, 1962.

43. Gibson, T. E., and Parfitt, J. W.: The action of morantel tartrate against nematodes in sheep, Vet. Rec. 93:423, 1973.

44. Hammond, D. M., Fayer, R., and Miner, M. L.: Amprolium for control of experimental coccidiosis in cattle, Am. J. Vet. Res. 27:199, 1966.

45. Hasche, M. R., and Todd, A. C.: Selection of nematodes resistant to anthelmintics—the effect of micronized purified phenothiazine on a resistant strain of *Haemonchus contortus*, Am. J. Vet. Res. 24:670, 1963.

46. Hogarth-Scott, R. S., Kelly, J. D., Whitlock, H. V., Thompson, H. G., James, R. E., and Mears, F. A.: The anthelmintic efficacy of fenbendazole

against thiabendazole-resistant strains of *Haemonchus contortus* and *Trichostrongylus colubriformis* in sheep, Res. Vet. Sci. **21**:232, 1976.

47. Horak, I. G., Snijders, A. J., and Pienaar, I.: The efficacy of cambendazole against cestodes and nematode infestations in sheep and cattle, J. S. Afr. Vet. Assoc. **43**:101, March 1972.

48. Jacobs, D. E., Lean, I. J., and Oakley, G. A.: Levamisole: efficacy against *Trichuris suis*, Vet. Rec. **100**:49, 1977.

49. Jambre, L. F., Southcott, W. H., and Dash, K. M.: Resistance of selected lines of *Haemonchus contortus* to thiabendazole, morantel tartrate and levamisole, Int. J. Parasitol. **6**:217, 1976.

50. Jarrett, W. F. H., McIntyre, W. I., and Sharp, N. C.: A trial of the effect of diethylcarbamazine on prepatent and patent parasitic bronchtis in calves, Am. J. Vet. Res. **23**:1183, 1962.

51. Johnson, W. P. Eggert, R. G., Poeschel, G. P., and Wang, G. T.: Levamisole as an anthelmintic for swine, J. Am. Vet. Med. Assoc. **161**:1221, 1972.

52. Kadhim, J. K.: The comparative efficacy of diamphenethide and rafoxide against *Fasciola gigantica* in sheep, Tropenmed. Parasitol. **26**:201. 1975.

53. Kelly, J. D., Chevis, R. A., and Whitlock, H. V.: The anthelmintic efficacy of mebendazole against adult *Fasciola hepatica* and a concurrent mixed nematode infection in sheep, N.Z. Vet. J. **23**:81, May 1975.

54. Kendall, S. B.: Chemotherapy of infection with *Fasciola hepatica* in cattle, Vet. Rec. **97**:9, 1975.

55. Kendall, S. B., and Parfitt, J. W.: The effect of diamphenethide on *Fasciola hepatica* at different stages of development, Res. Vet. Sci. **15**:37, 1973.

56. Kennedy, T. J., and Todd, A. C.: Efficacy of fenbendazole against gastrointestinal parasites of sheep, Am. J. Vet. Res. **36**:1465, 1975.

57. Kirsch, R., and Duwel, D.: Laboratory investigations on pigs with the new anthelmintic fenbendazole, Res. Vet. Sci. **19**:327, 1975.

58. Knapp, S. E., Nybert, P. A., Dutson, V. J., and Shaw, J. N.: Efficacy of Bayer 9015 against *Fasciola hepatica* in sheep, Am. J. Vet. Res. **26**:1071, 1965.

59. Knapp, S. E., and Presidente, P. J.: Efficacy of rafoxanide against natural *Fasciola hepatica* infections in cattle, Am. J. Vet. Res. **32**:1289, 1971.

60. Knapp, S. E., Schelegel, M. W., Presidente, J. A., and Armstrong, J. N.: Effect of oxyclozanide on feed efficiency in cattle with chronic fascioliasis, Am. J. Vet. Res. **32**:1583, 1971.

61. Knight, R. A., Morrison, E. G., and McGuire, J. A.: Anthelmintic activity of thiabendazole in feed compared with phenothiazine orally in Mississippi lambs, J. Am. Vet. Med. Assoc. **151**:1438, 1967.

62. Kuttler, K. L., Matthew, N. J., and Marble, D. W.: Comparative therapeutic efficacy of carbon tetrachloride, hexachloroethane, and ME 3625 in *Fasciola hepatica* infections of sheep, Am. J. Vet. Res. **24**:52, 1963.

63. Lapage, G.: Monnig's veterinary helminthology and entomology, ed. 5, Baltimore, 1962, The Williams & Wilkins Co.

64. Leek, R. G., Fayer, R., and McLoughlin, D. K.: Effect of monensin on experimental infections of *Eimeria ninkohlyakimovae* in lambs, Am. J. Vet. Res. **37**:339, 1976.

65. Link, R. P. In Jones, L. M., editor: Veterinary pharmacology and therapeutics, ed. 3, Ames, Iowa, 1965, Iowa State University Press.

66. Lyons, E. T., Drudge, J. H., LaBore, D. E., and Tolliver, S. C.: Controlled test of anthelmintic activity of levamisole administered to calves via drinking water, subcutaneous infection, or alfalfa pellet premix, Am. J. Vet. Res. **36**:777, 1975.

67. Michaud, L.: Thiabendazole—an anthelmintic of cattle, Can. Vet. J. **8**:85, April 1967.

68. Miner, M. L., and Jensen, J. B.: Decoquinate in the control of experimentally induced coccidiosis of calves, Am. J. Vet. Res. **37**:1043, 1976.

69. Norcross, M. A., Siegmund, O. H., and Fraser, C. M.: Amprolium for coccidiosis in cattle: a review of efficacy and safety, Vet. Med. Small Anim. Clin. **69**:459, 1974.

70. Oakley, G. A.: The anthelmintic activity of levamisole administered subcutaneously to pigs at 7.5 mg/kg, Br. Vet. J. **130**:36, 1974.

71. Oakley, G. A.: Activity of levamisole hydrochloride administered subcutaneously against *Asuum* infections in pigs, Vet. Rec. **95**:190, 1974.

72. Oakley, G. A.: Efficacy of levamisole hydrochloride administered subcutaneously against *Metastrongylus apri* infections in pigs, Vet. Rec. **97**:498, 1975.

73. Parker, W. H.: Lungworm infection in cattle-control and treatment, J. Am. Vet. Med. Assoc. **142**:743, 1963.

74. Peardon, D. L., Bilkovich, F. R., Todd, A. C., and Hoyt, H. H.: Trials of candidate bovine coccidiostats: efficacy of amprolium, lincomycin, sulfamethazine, chloroquine sulfate, and di-phenthane-70, Am. J. Vet. Res. **26**:683, 1965.

75. Poeschel, G. P., and Emro, J. E.: Evaluation of levamisole against *Metastrongylus* spp. in swine, J. Am. Vet. Med. Assoc. **160**:1637, 1972.

76. Presidente, P. J., Knapp, S. E., Schelegel, M. W. and Armstrong, J. N.: Anthelmintic efficacy of clioxanide against experimentally induced *Fasciola* hepatic infections in calves, Am. J. Vet. Res. **33**:1593, 1972.

77. Presidente, P. J., Schlegel, M. W., and Knapp, S. E.: Efficacy of levamisole in alfalfa pellets against naturally occurring gastrointestinal nematode infections in calves, Am. J. Vet. Res. **32**:1359, 1971.

78. Presidente, P. J., and Worley, D. E.: Efficacy of levo-tetramisole against experimental *Dictyocaulus filaria* infections in lambs, Am. J. Vet. Res. **30**:1625, 1969.

79. Ronald, N. C., Bell, R. R., and Craig, T. M.: Evaluation of less than recommended dosages of levam-

isole phosphate for the treatment of gastrointestinal nematodes in cattle, J. Am. Vet. Med. Assoc. **170:**317, 1977.

80. Ross, D. B.: The effect of fenbendazole on nematode parasites in experimentally infected lambs, Vet. Rec. **96:**357, 1975.

81. Rossoff, I. S.: Handbook of veterinary drugs, New York, 1974, Springer Publishing Co.

82. Rubin, R.: Efficacy of parbendazole against *Ostertagia, Trichostrongylus,* and *Cooperia* spp. in cattle, Am. J. Vet. Res. **29:**1385, 1968.

83. Rubin, R.: Efficacy of cambendazole against lungworm (*Dictyocaulus viviparus*) of cattle, Am. J. Vet. Res. **33:**425, 1972.

84. Rubin, R., and Hibler, C. P.: Effect of the levo form of tetramisole on *Ostertagia, Trichostrongylus,* and *Cooperia* in cattle, Am. J. Vet. Res. **29:**545, 1968.

85. Samson, K. S., Wilson, G. I., and Allen, R. W.: Sheep liver fluke anthelmintics: preliminary experiments with eight compounds against mature and immature *Fasciola hepatica,* Am. J. Vet. Res. **30:** 807, 1969.

86. Schlinke, J. C., and Palmer, J. S.: Combined effects of phenothiazine and organophosphate insecticides in cattle, J. Am. Vet. Med. Assoc. **163:**756, 1973.

87. Snijders, A. J., and Horak, I. G.: Trials with rafoxanide. VII. Efficacy against *Fasciola hepatica, Haemonchus placei* and *Bunostomum phlebotomum* in cattle, J. S. Afr. Vet. Assoc. **46:**265, 1975.

88. Taffs, L. F.: The effect of oral cambendazole against 10-day-old *Hyostrongylus rubidus* and *Oesophagostomum* spp. larvae in experimentally-infected pigs, Br. Vet. J. **132:**105, 1976.

89. Theodorides, V. J., Laderman, M., and Pagano, J. F.: Methyl-5(6)-butyl-2-benzimidazolecarbamate in the treatment of gastrointestinal nematodes in ruminants, Vet. Med. Small Anim. Clin. **63:**257, 1968.

90. Theodorides, V. J., Laderman, M., and Pagano, J. F.: Parbendazole in treatment of intestinal nematodes of swine, Vet. Med. Small Anim. Clin. **63:** 370, 1968.

91. Theodorides, V. J., Nawalinski, T., and Chang, J.: Efficacy of albendazole against *Haemonchus, Nematodirus, Dictyocaulus,* and *Moniezia* of sheep, Am. J. Vet. Res. **37:**1515, 1976.

92. Theodorides, V. J., Nawalinski, T., Murphy, J., and Freeman, J.: Efficacy of albendazole against gastrointestinal nematodes of cattle, Am. J. Vet. Res. **37:** 1517, 1976.

93. Theodorides, V. J., Scott, G. C., and Laderman, M.: Strains of *Haemonchus contortus* resistant against benzimidazole anthelmintics, Am. J. Vet. Res. **31:**859, 1970.

94. Todd, A. C., Bliss, D., Scholl, P., and Crowley, J. W., Jr.: Controlled evaluation of fenbendazole as a bovine anthelmintic, Am. J. Vet. Res. **37:**439, 1976.

95. Turton, J. A.: Anthelmintic efficiency of levamisole against lungworm (*Dictyocaulus filaria*) in lambs, Vet. Rec. **93:**108, 1973.

96. Turton, J. A.: Controlled trials to determine the anthelmintic efficacy of levamisole against *Ostertagia circumcincta* and *Trichostrongylus colubriformis* in lambs, Res. Vet. Sci. **16:**152, 1974.

97. Turton, J. A.: An evaluation of the anthelmintic activity of levamisole against *Chabertia ovina* in lambs using the improved controlled test, Br. Vet. J. **130:** 510, 1974.

98. Varga, I., and Janisch, M.: Anthelmintic activity of mebendazole against naturally acquired gastrointestinal nematodes in sheep, Acta Vet. Acad. Sci. Hung. **25:**105, 1975.

99. Zeakes, S. J., Mozier, J. O., White, R. G., and Hansen, M. F.: Efficacy of coumaphos crumbles and naftalofos boluses against nematodes of cattle, Am. J. Vet. Res. **37:**709, 1976.

Additional readings

Allen, R. W.: Preliminary evaluation of levamisole, parbendazole, and cambendazole as thysanosomicides in sheep, Am. J. Vet. Res. **34:**61, 1973.

Anderson, N., Morris, R. S., and McTaggart, I. K.: An economic analysis of two schemes for the anthelmintic control of helminthiasis in weaned lambs, Aust. Vet. J. **52:**174, 1976.

Arakawa, A., Kohls, R. E., and Todd, A. C.: Lincomycin therapy for experimental coccidiosis in calves, with special reference to macroscopic and microscopic observation, Am. J. Vet. Res. **29:**1195, 1967.

Baker, N. F., Tucker, E. M., Stormont, C., and Fisk, R. A.: Neurotoxicity of haloxon and its relationship to blood esterases of sheep, Am. J. Vet. Res. **31:**865, 1969.

Bennett, D. G., and Todd, A. C.: Efficiency of phenothiazine of varying purity and particle size against a phenothiazine-resistant strain of *Haemonchus contortus,* Am. J. Vet. Res. **25:**450, 1964.

Bliss, D. H., and Todd, A. C.: Milk production by Vermont dairy cattle after deworming, Vet. Med. Small Anim. Clin. **71:**1251, 1976.

Borgers, M., DeNollin, S., DeBrabander, M., and Thienpont, D.: Influence of the anthelmintic mebendazole on microtubules and intracellular organelle movement in nematode intestinal cells, Am. J. Vet. Res. **36:**1153, 1975.

Bris, E. J., Dyer, I. A., Howes, A. D., Schooley, M. A., and Todd, A. C.: Anthelmintic activity of 2,2-dichlorovinyl dimethyl phosphate in cattle, J. Am. Vet. Med. Assoc. **152:**175, 1968.

Brooker, P. J., and Goose, J.: Dermal application of levamisole to sheep and cattle, Vet. Rec. **96:**249, 1975.

Bryan, R. P.: Helminth control in Queensland beef cattle: comparison of part paddock and whole paddock treatment in the Wallum of South Eastern Queensland, Aust. Vet. J. **52:**267, 1976.

Ciordia, H., and McCampbell, H. C.: Activity of levamisole (1 form of tetramisole) in control of nematode parasites and body weight gains of feedlot cattle, Am. J. Vet. Res. **32**:545, 1971.

Connan, R. A.: The efficacy of thiabendazole against the arrested larvae of some *Trichostrongylidae* and *Chabertia ovina* in sheep, Res. Vet. Sci. **20**:13, 1976.

Cornwell, R. L., Jones, R. M., and Pott, J. M.: Anthelmintic treatment with morantel of cattle yarded for the winter, Br. Vet. J. **129**:526, 1973.

Davis, L. E., Wescott, R. B., and Musgrave, E. E.: Influence of pH on uptake of thiabendazole by the nematode *Haemonchus contortus*, Am. J. Vet. Res. **30**:1015, 1968.

Eichler, D. A.: The anthelmintic activity of thiophanate in sheep and cattle, Br. Vet. J. **129**:533, 1973.

Galvin, T. J., Bell, R. R., and Turk, E. D.: Anthelmintics for ruminants vs. the organic phosphorus compounds, Bayer L 13/59 and Bayer 22/408, Am. J. Vet. Res. **23**:191, 1961.

Galvin, T. J., Turk, R. D., and Bell, R. R.: Anthelmintics for ruminants. I. Studies on the toxicity and efficacy of Bayer 21/199 as an anthelmintic, Am. J. Vet. Res. **21**:1054, 1960.

Hascke, M. R., and Todd, A. C.: Selection of nematodes resistant to anthelmintics—the effect of micronized purified phenothiazine on a resistant strain of *Haemonchus contortus*, Am. J. Vet. Res. **24**:670, 1973.

Hass, D. K.: Anthelmintic efficacy of dichlorvos against *Hyostrongylus rubidus* and *Oesophagostomum dentatum* in swine at timed intervals after exposure to infective larvae, Vet. Med. Small Anim. Clin. **70**:187, 1975.

Hass, D. K., and Young, R., Jr.: Anthelmintic efficacy of multiple-dose dichlorvos therapy in pregnant swine, Am. J. Vet. Res. **34**:195, 1973.

Hentschi, A. F.: Experimental use of amprolium as an anticoccidial agent in feedlot cattle, Vet. Med. Small Anim. Clin. **66**:248, 1971.

Herrick, J. B.: Some points to remember regarding deworming of cattle, Vet. Med. Small Anim. Clin. **71**:950, 1976.

Horak, I. G., and Pienaar, I.: The efficacy of thiabendazole against immature and adult *Dictyocaulus filaria* in sheep, J. S. Afr. Vet. Assoc. **43**:107, 1972.

Horak, I. G., Snijders, A. J., and Louw, J. P.: Trials with rafoxanide—efficacy studies against *Fasciola hepatica*, *Fasciola gigantica*, *Paramphistomum microbothrium* and various nematodes in sheep, J. S. Afr. Vet. Assoc. **43**:397, 1972.

Kirsch, R., and Duwel, D.: Laboratory investigations in sheep with a new anthelmintic, Vet. Rec. **97**:28, 1975.

Kistner, T. P., and Lindsey, J. B.: Efficacy of cambendazole against naturally occurring *Nematodirus helvetianus* and *Cooperia oncophora* infections in calves, Am. J. Vet. Res. **35**:1405, 1974.

Knapp, F. W., and Drudge, J. H.: Efficacy of several organic phosphates against botfly of sheep, Am. J. Vet. Res. **25**:1686, 1964.

Leland, S. E.: Effect of hygromycin B on migrating and adult *Strongyloides ransomi* in weanling pigs, J. Am. Vet. Med. Assoc. **160**:58, 1972.

Leland, S. E., Caley, H. K., and Ridley, R. K.: Efficacy of levamisole (1-tetramisole) and thiabendazole in reduction of helminth egg counts in cattle, J. Am. Vet. Med. Assoc. **158**:1373, 1971.

Leland, S. E., Neal, F. C., and Plummer, C. B.: Treatment of *Strongyloides ransomi* infection of pigs with thiabendazole and dichlorvos, Am. J. Vet. Res. **29**:1235, 1968.

Lyons, E. T., Drudge, J. H., and Knapp, F. W.: Controlled test of anthelmintic activity of trichlorfon and thiabendazole in lambs, with observations on oestrus ovis, Am. J. Vet. Res. **28**:1111, 1967.

Lyons, E. T., Drudge, J. H., Labore, D. E., and Tolliver, S. C.: Field and controlled test evaluations of levamisole against natural infections of gastrointestinal nematodes and lungworms in calves, Am. J. Vet. Res. **33**:65, 1972.

Lyons, E. T., Drudge, J. H., and Tolliver, S. C.: Controlled tests of parbendazole and thiabendazole against natural infections of gastrointestinal helminths of lambs, Am. J. Vet. Res. **35**:1065, 1974.

McKenna, P. B.: The anthelmintic efficacy of thiabendazole and levamisole against inhibited *Haemonchus contortus* larvae in sheep, N.Z. Vet. J. **22**:163, Sept. 1974.

Mullee, M. T., Cox, D. D., and Allen, A. D.: Effect of naphthalophos, phenothiazine, and thiabendazole on gastrointestinal nematode egg counts in feedlot cattle, Am. J. Vet. Res. **31**:1203, 1970.

Panitz, E., and Knapp, S. E.: In vitro effects of certain anthelmintic drugs on histochemically demonstrable cholinesterases and succinate oxidase of *Fasciola hepatica*, Am. J. Vet. Res. **31**:763, 1969.

Partosoedjono, S., Drudge, J. H., Lyons, E. T., and Knapp, F. W.: Evaluation of naphthalophos against *Oestrus ovis* and a thiabendazole-tolerant strain of *Haemonchus contortus* in lambs, Am. J. Vet. Res. **30**:81, 1969.

Poeschel, G. P., and Todd, A. C.: Controlled evaluation of formulated dichlorvos for use in cattle, Am. J. Vet. Res. **33**:1071, 1972.

Reid, J. F., Duncan, J. L., and Bairden, K.: Efficacy of levamisole against inhibited larvae of *Ostertagia* spp. in sheep, Vet. Rec. **98**:426, 1976.

Roe, C. K., Stockdale, P. H., and Wilson, M. R.: The efficacy of dichlorvos against *Oesophagostomum* spp. in swine, Can. Vet. J. **11**:72, April 1970.

Ross, D. B.: Controlled trials with morantel tartrate plus diethylcarbamazine given to lambs infected experimentally with *Haemonchus contortus*, *Ostertagia circumcincta*, *Nematodirus battus*, *Trichostrongylus colubriformis* and *Dictyocaulus filaria*, Vet. Rec. **93**:359, 1973.

Schock, R. C.: Nematode parasitism in cattle, Mod. Vet. Pract. **57**:273, 1976.

Shelton, G. C.: Some critical evaluations of anthelmintics of ruminants, Am. J. Vet. Res. **23**:506, 1962.

Sinclair, K. B.: The effect of promezathine hydrochloride on the development and pathogenicity of *Fasciola hepatica* in the sheep, Br. Vet. J. **130:**577, 1974.

Sinclair, K. B., and Prichard, R. K.: The use of disophenol in studies of the pathogenicity of the arrested fourth-stage larvae of *Haemonchus contortus* in the sheep, Res. Vet. Sci. **19:**232, 1975.

Smalley, H. E., and Radeleff, R. D.: Enhancement of insecticide toxicity by the antidiuretic agent, diazoxide, Am. J. Vet. Res. **32:**345, 1971.

Smith, H. J.: Anthelmintic activity of tetramisole against lungworms, roundworms, nodular worms, threadworms and whipworms in a natural mixed infection of swine, Can. Vet. J. **13:**40, Feb. 1972.

Smith, H. J.: The effects of anthelmintic treatments on the development of gastrointestinal parasitism in calves, Can. J. Comp. Med. **38:**139, 1974.

Smith, H. J., and Archibald, R. M.: Controlled trials on the efficacy of tetramisole and thiabendazole against nematode parasites in calves, Can. Vet. J. **10:**136, May 1969.

Smith, J. P., and Bell, R. R.: Toxicity of the levo form of tetramisole in angora goats, Am. J. Vet. Res. **32:** 871, 1971.

Stewart, T. B., Ciordia, H., and Utlev, P. R.: Anthelmintic treatment of subclinical parasitism of feedlot cattle in Georgia, Am. J. Vet. Res. **36:**785, 1975.

Stewart, T. B., Hale, O. M., Marti, O. G.: Efficacy of two dichlorvos formulations against larval and adult *Hyostrongylus rubidus* in swine, Am. J. Vet. Res. **36:**771, 1975.

Todd, A. C.: Summary of swine anthelmintics, J. Am. Vet. Med. Assoc. **151:**1446, 1967.

Todd, A. C., and Thacher, J.: Suppression and control of bovine coccidiosis with Aureo-S-700 medication in the feed, Vet. Med. Small Anim. Clin. **68:**527, 1973.

Tumbleson, M. E., and Wescott, R. B.: Serum biochemic values in piglets from sows fed dichlorvos prior to farrowing, J. Comp. Lab. Med. **3:**67, 1969.

Williams, J. C., and Knox, J. W.: Effect of nematode parasite infection on the performance of stocker cattle at high stocking rates on coastal bermuda grass pastures, Am. J. Vet. Res. **37:**453, 1976.

13

Intestinal parasitic infections of horses

GASTROINTESTINAL PARASITES OF HORSES

Horses are infested by a wide variety of gastrointestinal parasites. Chemotherapy is primarily aimed against ascarids, large strongyles, small strongyles, pinworms, and larvae of botflies. The scientific names of these parasites are listed in Table 13-1.

Nematodes
Ascarids (Parascaris equorum)

The life cycle of *P. equorum* in horses is similar to the life cycle of *Toxocara canis* in

dogs, except that prenatal infection does not occur with *P. equorum* (Fig. 13-1). It takes about 3 months from the time of infection to the appearance of mature parasites in the gut.

P. equorum is primarily a problem in young horses 3 to 9 months of age. Depending on the severity of the infestation the parasites can cause serious disease, manifested by an elevated temperature, cough, loss of weight, exhaustion, and digestive disturbances. Large masses of parasites may obstruct the intestine. Severe infestations can kill the animal.

As infested animals mature, they develop a relative or complete immunity to the parasite.

Treatment. Drugs that are most effective against adult ascarids in horses are cambendazole, mebendazole, the organophosphates, the piperazines, and pyrantel tartrate.

Large strongyles

Three species of large strongyles reside in the large intestine of horses: *Strongylus equinus*, *S. edentatus*, and *S. vulgaris*. The adult large strongyles may irritate the large intestine and suck blood from the host. The larvae of *S. vulgaris* cause the most significant clinical problems. An understanding of the life cycle of this parasite is therefore important (Fig. 13-2).

After ingestion, larvae penetrate the in-

Table 13-1. Common internal parasites of horses*

Group and common names	Scientific names	Location in host
Nematodes (roundworms)		
Ascarids	*Parascaris equorum*	Small intestine
Large strongyles	*Strongylus edentatus*	Large intestine
	S. equinus	Large intestine
	S. vulgaris	Large intestine
Small strongyles	*Craterostomum* species	Large intestine
	Cyathostomum species	Large intestine
	Cylicobrachytus species	Large intestine
	Cylicocercus species	Large intestine
	Cylicocyclus species	Large intestine
	Cylicodontophorus species	Large intestine
	Cylicostephanus species	Large intestine
	Cylicotetrapedon species	Large intestine
	Gyalocephalus species	Large intestine
	Oesophagodontus species	Large intestine
	Poteriostomum species	Large intestine
	Triodontophorus species	Large intestine
Pinworms	*Oxyuris equi*	Cecum and colon
Arthropods (flies)		
Nose botfly	*Gasterophilus hemorrhoidalis*	Stomach, rectum, anus
Horse botfly	*G. intestinalis*	Stomach
Throat botfly	*G. nasalis*	Stomach, small intestine

*Modified from Becklund, W. W.: Revised check list of internal and external parasites of domestic animals in the United States and possessions and in Canada, Am. J. Vet. Res. **25**:1380, 1964.

testinal wall and then the blood vessels of the intestine. They migrate in the blood vessels toward the anterior mesenteric artery (the artery supplying the small intestine), where they are found from the fourteenth day after ingestion. In addition to the anterior mesenteric artery, larvae of S. *vulgaris* may be found in arteries from the aortic valve of the heart to the branches of the iliac arteries (which supply the hind legs). Larvae may cause a number of serious lesions in arteries. Initially they cause inflammation, which sets up a condition in the arteries leading to the formation of thrombi (blood clots). Pieces of the clots may break off and plug the blood supply to various organs, and these are called "emboli." If the blood flow is compromised in the iliac arteries, temporary or permanent lameness can result. Emboli in the mesenteric arteries (those supplying the intestine) can result in severe abdominal pain (colic).

Fatality can result if a major branch is plugged.

In addition to the formation of thrombi, a thickening of the mesenteric artery walls can occur. This progresses to a dilation of the artery due to degeneration of the elastic fibers. Ultimately a large dilated mass (aneurysm) occurs. Such an aneurysm is a weak spot in the artery, which can rupture and cause death from internal bleeding.

Colic, or the manifestation of abdominal pain, is common in horses. It has been hypothesized that a large percentage of all colics result from infection with larvae of S. *vulgaris*.[18]

Small strongyles

The term "small strongyles" refers to a large number of genera (Table 13-1). Larvae of these parasites do not cause serious illness to the horse. However, the adult stage

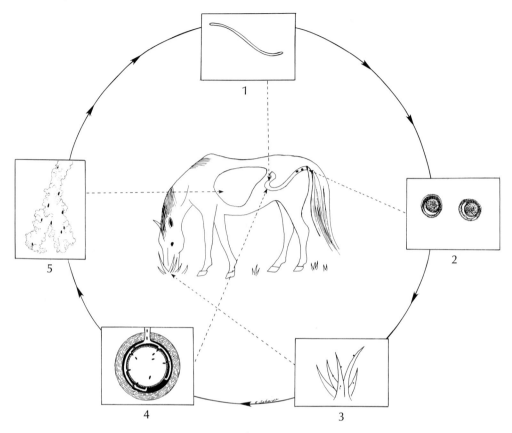

Fig. 13-1. Life cycle of *Parascaris equorum*. *1,* Adult parasites reside in small intestine, where they produce ova. *2,* Ova are shed in feces and contaminate surroundings. *3,* Horses ingest ova from contaminated feed. *4,* Ova hatch in the intestine, and larvae migrate from intestine into circulatory system and are carried to lung. *5,* In lung, larvae penetrate into alveolar spaces. They are then coughed up, swallowed, and mature to adults in small intestine.

organisms can be responsible for a variety of clinical signs. Large numbers of these parasites may be present in foals. In light infections no clinical signs may be apparent, but in heavy infections the feces may become soft and have a bad odor. Later, the animals may develop diarrhea or constipation; they become emaciated and easily exhausted, and their hair coat may become rough. Because many of the strongyle species are blood suckers, anemia may also develop.

Treatment of strongyle infestations. The drugs that are most effective against both small and large strongyle species are the benzimidazoles, pyrantel tartrate, and combinations of phenothiazine and piperazine.

To depress egg production by female strongyle parasites and suppress the development of infective larvae from eggs that are produced, low-level phenothiazine can be administered (p. 208).

Pinworms (oxyuris equi)

Pinworms, *O. equi*, inhabit the cecum and colon of horses. Mature females containing fertile ova travel to the rectum and crawl out through the anal opening. They then deposit ova in clusters on the skin. The ova drop off after about 3 days and are ingested by horses with food or water. The primary problem presented by pinworms is the extreme itching caused by the ova-depositing females, which results in horses backing up to objects and vigorously rubbing in an attempt to re-

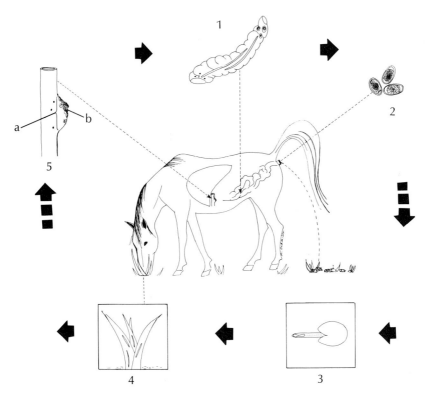

Fig. 13-2. Life cycle of *Strongylus vulgaris*. *1,* Adult parasites reside in large intestine, where they produce ova. *2,* Ova are passed with feces and contaminate surroundings. *3,* Larvae hatch from ova and contaminate feed, such as pasture grass. *4,* Larvae are ingested by horse. *5,* Larvae migrate to arteries where they can cause *(a)* aneurysms and *(b)* thrombi. Larvae migrate to large intestine where they mature to adults.

duce the itching. The activity may be so intense that a large area of hair is worn off the upper surface of the tail. In addition, many fences have been destroyed by the rear ends of pruritic, pinworm-infested horses.

Treatment. Usually effective in the control of pinworms are dichlorvos resin, trichlorfon, and the benzimidazoles.

Arthropods
Botflies (Gasterophilus species)

It is the larvae of botflies that infect horses. Adult flies are present in the summer and deposit their eggs on the hair of horses. The eggs may be seen as small, cream-colored spheres near the end of the hair. Generally, the eggs are laid either around the mouth or

on the chest and upper part of the forelegs of the horse. Those laid near the mouth hatch spontaneously. However, those on the chest and upper forelegs require licking or rubbing to hatch.

Before developing into an adult, the immature bot goes through various stages of development (instars). When the first-stage instars enter the mouth, they penetrate the tissues and gradually migrate toward the pharynx in the submucosal tissue. The first-stage instars of *G. intestinalis* and *G. haemorrhoidalis* locate in the mucosa of the tongue before migrating to the stomach.

Bots remain in the stomach of the horse for approximately 10 to 12 months. They then pass through the intestines, are expelled,

Table 13-2. Guide to efficacy of equine anthelmintics

Drug	Parasite				
	Ascarids	Large strongyles	Small strongyles	Pinworms	Bots
Benzimidazoles					
Cambendazole	+	+	+	+	−
Fenbendazole	±	+	+	+	−
Mebendazole	+	+	+	+	−
Thiabendazole	−	+	+	+	−
Carbon disulfide	±	−	−	−	+
Organophosphates					
Butonate	+	±	±	±	+
Dichlorvos resin	+	±	+	+	+
Dichlorvos gel	+	−	−	−	+
Trichlorfon	+	−	−	+	+
Phenothiazine	−	±	±	−	−
Piperazine	+	−	+	±	−
Pyrantel	+	+	+	±	−

Key: + = highly effective; ± = variably effective; − = not effective.

pupate in the ground for 3 to 5 weeks, and then emerge as flies. The cycle is complete.

Apparently, during the migration in the tissues of the mouth, no damage is done. However, when bots attach in the stomach, inflammation develops around the site of attachment. Ulcers may develop, and occasionally perforations of the stomach have occurred. Clusters of larvae around the pylorus (the area where material leaves the stomach) may interfere with the action of the pyloric sphincter and the passage of food to the intestine. Usually clinical signs that can be attributed to bots do not occur. Therefore many people believe that the parasite does not harm horses. However, their presence in no way helps and could possibly cause serious damage. It is thus advisable to use an effective drug to destroy bots when they are present either in the mouth or stomach.

Treatment. Organophosphates are highly effective against the second- and third-stage instar in the stomach and intestines. Carbon disulfide is also highly effective against the second- and third-stage instar.

Dichlorvos gel has been shown to be effective against first-stage instars of *G. nasalis* and *G. intestinalis* during their 3-week migration period in the tissues of the mouth.[9]

ANTHELMINTICS

To establish an effective equine parasite control program, one must be familiar with the properties of the various drugs used. These will be discussed next. At the end of this chapter the proper utilization of these drugs to treat internal parasitism of horses is discussed. The general effectiveness of equine anthelmintics is shown in Table 13-2.

Benzimidazoles

Generally, the benzimidazoles are highly effective against pinworms and small and large strongyles. Some are effective against ascarids at normal doses, whereas others are not. They are not effective for treating bot infestation.

As in other species the benzimidazoles tend to be free from toxic side effects at normal clinical doses.

Cambendazole. Cambendazole appears to be more effective against equine ascarids and immature pinworms than are either thiabendazole or fenbendazole. The reported effectiveness of cambendazole is shown in Table 13-3. Cambendazole may be given by stomach tube, in feed pellets, or as a paste. It is given at the rate of 20 mg/kg. Although toxic reactions are generally not observed at 20

Table 13-3. Efficacy of cambendazole

	Study	
Parasite	Bello and others[2]	Drudge and others[12]
Immature and adult ascarids	100%	100%
S. vulgaris		
Adult	100%	82%-100%
Immature	70.6%	*
Small strongyles		
Adult	99.5%	87%-99%
Immature	69.8%	*
Adult pinworms	100%	100%

*Not reported.

Table 13-4. Efficacy of mebendazole against equine parasites

Parasite	8.8-9 mg/kg by stomach tube	9 mg/kg in feed	8.8 mg/kg in paste
Ascarids	99%-100%	100%	100%
S. equinus	100%	100%	100%
S. edentatus	64%-98.6%	71-98%	99.5%
S. vulgaris	89%-100%	100%	100%
Small strongyles	81%-99.46%	73%-99.37%	98.5%
Pinworms (adult)	100%	100%	100%
Bots	0%-21.2%	0%-8.2%	0.2%-2.8%
Reference	3, 5, 11	3, 5	22

mg/kg, cambendazole is not recommended for use in pregnant mares.

Fenbendazole. When given by stomach tube at the rate of 5 mg/kg, the following efficacies have been reported for fenbendazole[13]:

S. vulgaris	100%
S. edentatus	99%
S. equinus	87%
Pinworms	
Mature	100%
Immature	50%
Ascarids	
Mature	86%
Immature	3%

In horses, toxic reactions to fenbendazole have not been reported.

Mebendazole. A summary of the effectiveness of mebendazole is shown in Table 13-4. Mebendazole is available commercially both as a paste and as a drench for use in horses and is given as one dose at the rate of 8.8 mg/kg.

Table 13-5. Efficacy of thiabendazole in horses

	Dose	
Parasite	44 mg/kg	88 mg/kg
Ascarids	10%-46%	32%-100%
S. equinus	*	100%
S. edentatus	90%-100%	89%-100%
S. vulgaris	95%-100%	100%
Small strongyles	90%-100%	*
Adult pinworms	90%-100%	100%
Reference	18, 20	20

*Not reported.

Thiabendazole. The effectiveness of thiabendazole in combating parasitic infestations in horses is shown in Table 13-5. Thiabendazole, even in very large doses, is not a consistently effective anthelmintic against ascarids. However, when given with a normal dose of piperazine, good activity against ascarids can be obtained.

The normal dose for thiabendazole in

horses is 44 mg/kg. It is administered in many forms, including as a liquid via a stomach tube, as a paste, or in the feed. As with all anthelmintics, when it is placed in the feed, a check must be made to see that the animal consumes the entire ration.

Carbon disulfide

Carbon disulfide is a highly volatile liquid with an unpleasant odor. Although it is only moderately soluble in water, it is very soluble in fat. The vapor is highly explosive.

It is dispensed either in its pure form, as a liquid complexed with piperazine, or in the form of a bolus prepared by adsorbing carbon disulfide on magnesium carbonate.

Effectiveness. Carbon disulfide is effective against only two equine parasites, bots and ascarids. It is effective only against the second- and third-stage instars of bots and is not active against the first-stage instar in the mouth. The effectiveness of carbon disulfide has been reported as 90% to 100% for bots and 50% to 100% for ascarids.[18] Carbon disulfide is often added to other anthelmintics to include bots in the product's spectrum of activity. For example, when carbon disulfide, 2.5 ml/45 kg of body weight, is combined with mebendazole given at the rate of 9 mg/kg of body weight, the following efficacy has been reported[3]:

Ascarids	100%
S. edentatus	98%
S. vulgaris	98%
Small strongyles	99%
O. equi (adults)	100%
G. intestinalis	98%
G. nasalis	98%

Dose and administration. The liquid is administered either by way of a stomach tube or in a hard gelatin capsule. Care must be taken in administering the capsule, because if it breaks in the mouth, severe irritation of the tissues in the mouth will result. If this happens, the mouth should be irrigated with mineral oil to protect the mucosa and remove as much of the carbon disulfide as possible.

Generally, carbon disulfide is not adminis-

tered to mares during the last 30 days of pregnancy. Horses are usually fasted for 18 hours before administration of the drug and for 4 hours afterward. It is administered at the rate of 2.5 ml/45 kg. Dosage should not exceed 25 ml.

Morantel tartrate

Currently morantel tartrate has not been cleared for use in horses in the United States. Reports indicate that its range of effectiveness is similar to pyrantel tartrate (p. 209).[6,7]

Organophosphates

Generally, the organophosphates have a high degree of activity against bots and ascarids. They produce variable results against the other internal parasites of horses.

Because of their potential toxicity, one must exercise caution when using organophosphates in the horse. Even though signs of toxicity do not usually occur when correct doses are given, substantial reductions in blood cholinesterase levels can be expected.[1] If other drugs are given that further reduce cholinesterase, toxicity is likely to occur. Because of the potential toxicity resulting from interaction with other drugs, the following precautions should be observed when using organophosphate parasiticides in horses:

1. Do not use in mares within 30 days of foaling.

2. Do not use in animals weighing less than 227 kg.

3. Do not retreat with organophosphates within 30 days.

4. Do not treat animals with diarrhea, constipation, respiratory distress, or infectious diseases.

5. Do not use in severely debilitated animals.

6. Provide a substantial time (at least a month) between the administration of organophosphates for internal parasites and that for external parasites. In addition, provide substantial time (at least a month) between giving organophosphates and muscle relaxants (such as succinylcholine, which is inactivated by cholinesterase), phenothia-

zine-derived tranquilizers, or depressants of the central nervous system.[17,23]

Butonate. Butonate is an organophosphate equine anthelmintic.

Effectiveness. When administered in the feed at the rate of 39 mg/kg after feed has been withheld 24 hours, the following efficacies were reported[27]:

Ascarids	92%-100%
Bots	88%-100%
Large strongyles	0%-100%
Small strongyles	0%-64%
Pinworms	0%-100%

Toxicity. Some horses may develop mild diarrhea when given therapeutic doses of butonate. However, the feces should return to normal within 24 hours. Doses of 55 to 100 mg/kg may cause toxic signs.[24]

Dose and administration. A dose of approximately 45 mg/kg of body weight is recommended by the manufacturer. It is not necessary to withhold feed or water before giving butonate.

Butonate is only given through a stomach tube. The concentrated (13%) commercial solution is mixed with water (3 ml of the concentrate per 250 ml to 2 liters of water) before administration. The solution should be prepared immediately prior to administration. Once the concentrate is mixed with water, it should not be stored in that form.

Dichlorvos. Dichlorvos is available for use in horses in two forms: a resin pellet and a gel. The form will determine the range of activity and safety of the drug.

Resin-pellet dichlorvos. The resin-pellet formulation (Equigard) is designed for oral administration, being fed to horses in their grain. The product is relatively slow in releasing its active ingredient. This property of the formulation decreases the toxicity by reducing the amount of drug absorbed and increases the antiparasitic activity by making dichlorvos available as it passes through the digestive tract. As the drug is gradually released, it is rapidly metabolized in the intestinal tract to nontoxic materials. Therefore only minimal toxic effects are observed in the host.

Effectiveness. Single doses administered in the feed at the rate of between 33 and 43 mg/kg have been reported to be 90% to 100% effective against bots (*G. intestinalis*, *G. nasalis*), ascarids, *S. vulgaris*, small strongyles, and pinworms. However, the same regimen was only 65% to 75% effective against *S. edentatus*.[8]

Toxicity. At normal doses the only toxic effect of the resin pellet is softening of the feces in some horses, a condition usually corrected without treatment. The treatment of breeding stock does not have a demonstrable effect on pregnancy or fertility.[8] The resin formulation is not recommended for use in suckling or newly weaned foals because the amount of grain consumed is so variable.

Dose and administration. The resin formulation should be administered immediately after opening the package in a limited amount of the normal grain ration. Some horses may be reluctant to eat grain containing dichlorvos. Although fasting before or after administration of the drug is neither necessary nor recommended, water should be withheld 12 hours before and 4 hours after administration. The drug should not be given by a stomach tube because the water in which it would be dissolved would inactivate the drug. The dose of dichlorvos must be given by closely determining the weight of the horse. It is given at the rate of 37 mg/kg or 16.6 gm/450 kg horse.

Dichlorvos gel. Another form of dichlorvos is a gel preparation (Equigel). Release of the drug from the gel is more rapid than from the resin. This permits effective concentrations to be achieved in the mouth and upper portions of the gastrointestinal tract.

Effectiveness. The gel is effective only against bots and ascarids.[16] Dichlorvos gel, when administered to ponies at doses of 10 or 20 mg/kg of body weight, has been shown to be effective against first instars of *G. nasalis* and *G. intestinalis* during their 3-week migration period in the tissues of the mouth.[9]

Toxicity. Because dichlorvos gel can be absorbed from the skin, it should be washed off with soap and water if it accidentally comes in contact with the skin of either humans or animals.

Dose and administration. When given to combat both bot and ascarid infestation, it is dosed at the rate of 20 mg/kg, repeated every 30 days. For control of bots only, it is given at the rate of 10 mg/kg every 30 days only during the fly season.

When treating nursing foals, fasting is neither recommended nor necessary. When treating adult animals and weaned foals, however, it is advisable to withhold feed overnight and for 4 to 6 hours after dosing.

Trichlorfon. Trichlorfon is a widely distributed equine anthelmintic that appears under a variety of brand names (Appendix I).

Effectiveness. Primarily effective against bots, ascarids, and pinworms, trichlorfon has only limited activity against either large and small strongyles.[10,14,18] When given in the grain, trichlorfon appears to be more effective against bots and potentially less toxic than when given as a liquid by stomach tube.[10]

Toxicity. At the recommended dose trichlorfon usually causes no toxic side effects.

Dose and administration. The dose in horses is 40 mg/kg, usually with a small portion of the grain ration.

Piperazines

Effectiveness. The piperazines are highly effective against ascarid parasites. Their effect against strongyles is similar to that of phenothiazine. They are effective against small strongyles but only marginally effective against large strongyles.

The following efficacy for piperazine at the rate of 88 mg/kg has been reported[18]:

Bots	0%
Ascarids	95%-100%
S. vulgaris	40%-60%
S. edentatus	0%-10%
Small strongyles	90%-100%
Mature oxyurids	40%-60%

Dose and administration. The piperazines are generally administered orally to horses at the rate of 88 mg of piperazine base per kilogram of body weight. To increase the spectrum of effectiveness, piperazine is often mixed with other anthelmintics. These combinations are discussed later in this chapter.

Phenothiazine

Phenothiazine is used in two ways to combat internal parasitic infections of horses.

Low-level method. In the low-level phenothiazine method, the drug is administered in the grain at the rate of 2 gm/24 hr per animal for the first 21 days of each month on a year-round basis. This results in depression of egg production by female strongyle parasites and suppression of the development of infective larvae from any eggs that are produced. All horses on the premises must be treated.

High-level method. In the high-level method the drug is used in therapeutic doses to kill strongyle parasites.

Effectiveness. For many years phenothiazine had been the drug of choice for strongyle control. Compared to the benzimidazoles, it is not highly effective against the large or small strongyles when administered alone. Phenothiazine is highly useful when combined with other drugs such as the piperazines or organophosphates, increasing their activity against both large and small strongyles.

The comments made in Chapter 12 about the increased effectiveness of phenothiazine when it is administered in more purified or micronized forms holds true for its use in horses. For this reason, the exact dose of phenothiazine may vary according to the purity and amount of micronization. The recommendations on the label of a particular product concerning dosage in horses should be followed.

Toxicity. Of the species of animals in which phenothiazine is used, horses are the most susceptible to its toxic effects. Phenothiazine may cause destruction of the red blood cells and thus anemia in horses in a poor state of nutrition or that have excessively high parasitic burdens.

Dose and administration. When phenothiazine is used at full therapeutic dose, it is usually administered by way of a stomach tube. When administered with either piperazines or organophosphates, the dose is 12.5 gm/450 kg horse (27.5 mg/kg). When the drug is administered alone, therapeutic doses are 25 to 30 gm per mature 450 kg horse.

Pyrantel tartrate

Pyrantel tartrate is an analog of morantel tartrate. Other salts of pyrantel seem to be equally effective. Examples are pyrantel hydrochloride and pyrantel pamoate.

For horses, pyrantel tartrate is dispensed as a powder in packets containing 1.13, 2.83, and 5.66 gm of the active ingredient. The product is designed to be mixed with the animal's grain ration for oral administration.

Effectiveness. Pyrantel tartrate has been shown to exhibit the following efficacy against equine internal parasites[19]:

S. *vulgaris*	92%-100%
S. *edentatus*	42%-100%
S. *equinus*	100%
Small strongyles	69%-99%
Pinworms	7%-100%
Ascarids	86%-100%

The drug is ineffective against bots but is compatible with carbon disulfide.

Toxicity. The manufacturer claims a good margin of safety for the drug.

Dose and administration. Pyrantel tartrate is administered to horses in feed at the rate of approximately 10 to 12.5 mg/kg. The drug should be thoroughly mixed in the grain ra-

tion. Fasting animals before or after treatment is not necessary. As with all compounds administered in the feed, each individual animal must consume the proper amount of grain, neither too much nor too little. Reports in the literature show that the drug can be given by stomach tube.[14]

Combination equine anthelmintics

No single equine anthelmintic is effective against all the common internal parasites of horses. By combining certain equine anthelmintics, the probability of reducing an animal's entire gastrointestinal parasitic load is increased.

Ideally when treating horses for internal parasites, the nature of the infection is determined and specific drugs to combat the type of parasites present are used. In certain mixed infestations, for example, large strongyles and bots, no one drug will be effective. In such a case more than one drug must be used. These might be given together or separately. If they are given together, three conditions must be met:

1. The combination should be effective against the entire parasite population.

2. The combination must be physically and chemically compatible (Chapter 2).

3. Neither drug should add to the toxicity of the other.

The safest approach when using combinations is to use commercially prepared products or those that have been well documented experimentally and in clinical practice.

The reported effectiveness of the combina-

Table 13-6. Guide to efficacy of combined equine anthelmintics

	Parasites				
Compound	Ascarids	Large strongyles	Small strongyles	Pinworms	Bots
Mebendazole-trichlorfon	+	+	+	+	+
Piperazine–carbon disulfide	+	−	+	±	+
Piperazine–carbon disulfide–phenothiazine	+	+	+	NR	+
Thiabendazole-piperazine	+	+	+	+	−
Trichlorfon-piperazine-phenothiazine	+	+*	+	+	+

Key: + = highly effective; ± = variably effective; − = not effective; NR = not reported.
*Except low activity against S. *edentatus*.

Table 13-7. Efficacy of thiabendazole (44 mg/kg) and piperazine (55 mg/kg) in horses*

Parasite	In feed	Via stomach tube
Bots	12.7%	7.9%
Pinworms	85.5%	80%
S. edentatus	100%	82.3%
S. vulgaris	100%	100%
Small strongyles	99.02%	99.8%

*Based on data from Bradley, R. E., and Radhakrishnan, C. V.: Critical trials with morantel tartrate against *Parascaris equorum*, Res. Vet. Sci. **14**:134, 1973.

Table 13-8. Effectiveness of trichlorfon-piperazine-phenothiazine in horses*

Parasite	
Bots (second and third instars)	90%-100%
Ascarids	95%-100%
S. vulgaris	95%-100%
S. edentatus	30%- 50%
Small strongyles	90%-100%
Pinworm	90%-100%

*Based on data from Drudge, J. H., and Bello, T. R. In Kester, W. O.: *Strongylus vulgaris* — the horse killer, Mod. Vet. Pract. **56**:569, 1975.

tions discussed in this section is shown in Table 13-6.

Mebendazole-trichlorfon. When mebendazole and trichlorfon are combined, the activity of mebendazole against the common equine nematodes and the effectiveness of trichlorfon against bots are maintained. This combination is given at the rate of 8.8 mg/kg mebendazole and 40 mg/kg trichlorfon as a single dose mixed in the feed or by stomach tube.[21]

Piperazine–carbon disulfide. To broaden the effectiveness of piperazine, one commercial product was developed that includes carbon disulfide complexed with piperazine (Parvex). Although it has some activity against bots (approximately 78% to 85%), this compound is not as effective against bots as carbon disulfide given alone. Its effectiveness against other parasites is essentially the same as piperazine alone. It is active against ascarids and small strongyles but has little activity against large strongyles. The product is available as a liquid to be given by a stomach tube or a bolus given orally. It is given at the rate of 88 mg/kg of the piperazine base.

Piperazine–carbon disulfide–phenothiazine. To further increase the spectrum of the piperazine–carbon disulfide complex, phenothiazine can be added at the rate of 27.5 mg/kg of body weight. The administration of the piperazine–carbon disulfide complex with phenothiazine has been reported to be 96% to 97% effective in re-

moving both large and small strongyles. One caution should be kept in mind about the combination of the three drugs. When they are administered in combination, there may be a decrease in ova production while the adult worms survive in the gastrointestinal tract. Evaluation of efficacy by fecal examination and ova count may often lead to falsely optimistic appraisals.

By combining pretreatment fasting and the supplemental administration of 600 ml of 0.5% hydrochloric acid to free the carbon disulfide, efficacy against bots is increased to 80% to 100%. Fasting and the use of hydrochloric acid do not affect the high rate of effectiveness against strongyles or ascarids. The effect of these variables on the efficacy of the mixture against pinworms is inconclusive.

Thiabendazole-piperazine. A commercial product containing thiabendazole and piperazine is intended to deliver 44 mg/kg of thiabendazole and 55 mg/kg of piperazine. It can be administered in the feed or suspended in water and administered by stomach tube. The efficacy of the compound when administered in the feed and by way of a stomach tube at the normal dose rate is shown in Table 13-7. The combination is also effective against ascarids.

Trichlorfon-piperazine-phenothiazine Trichlorfon is available commercially in combination with phenothiazine and piperazine. The combination is dispensed so that it delivers 18.2 gm of trichlorfon, 12.5 gm of micronized phenothiazine, and 40 gm of piperazine dihydrochloride per 450 kg of body weight. The dose for piperazine given with trichlorfon is the same as when given alone. The amount of phenothiazine given with trichlorfon is half that of the normal dose. Piperazine is added primarily to increase the effectiveness of the compound against species of both large and small strongyles. The reported efficacy of the combination is shown in Table 13-8.

TREATMENT OF HORSES WITH INTERNAL PARASITES

It is common for the internal parasitic burden of horses to consist of a wide variety of nematodes and one or more species of bots. Because treatment is usually aimed at the entire internal parasitic burden of a horse, we shall discuss treatment in general.

Before a rational approach to the prevention and treatment of equine internal parasites can be begun, the types of parasites infecting the population must be determined. The selection of the appropriate anthelmintic is then made.

To prevent the development of resistant strains of parasites, anthelmintics should be periodically changed. Use only those preparations that indicate on the label that they are safe to use in horses. Just because a chemical is acceptable for use in horses does not mean that all preparations containing that compound are safe.

The primary means a veterinarian has to determine the nature of gastrointestinal parasitism is to examine samples of the feces under the microscope for the presence of parasitic ova. By using quantitative techniques, the number of ova per gram of feces can be determined. Although the number of ova shed in the feces may vary in a given level of infestation, veterinarians usually interpret a drop in the number of ova in the feces to mean either that the adult population of parasites has been reduced or that the fertility of the females has decreased. By performing fecal egg counts, the veterinarian can evaluate the effectiveness of anthelmintics.

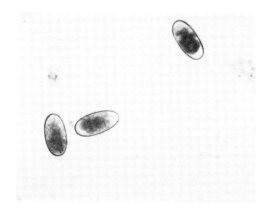

Fig. 13-3. Photomicrograph of strongyle ova. (Courtesy Mr. Paul Sumner, Animal Care Facility Diagnostic Laboratory, University of California, San Francisco.)

The large strongyles, S. *vulgaris* and S. *edentatus*, are the most pathogenic strongyle parasites and the most difficult to remove from the host. Small strongyles, which usually occur in greater number, are far easier to remove. Because the parasitic ova of the large and small strongyles appear identical (Fig. 13-3), evaluating the effectiveness of drugs against the strongyle infection can be misleading when only the fecal egg counts are considered. For example, if the egg counts are reduced by 90% but the remaining 10% of the parasites are all large strongyles, the infection remains significant.

Large strongyles cause their most serious problems during the larval stages. However, anthelmintics are effective only against the adult stages of the parasite. Because the commonly used anthelmintics are not effective against the larval stages of large strongyles, the only successful way to eliminate the damage caused by the larvae is to prevent infection. This can be accomplished by the following means:

- Maintaining a high level of sanitation
- Using drugs to minimize the adult strongyle population
- Using drugs to sterilize female strongyle worms

In any attempt to control equine gastrointestinal parasites, the program must include all horses in the group. Failure to include only one animal can result in massive seeding of the area with infective ova or larvae, destroying the benefit of the therapy. New arrivals must be isolated from the group and treated until free of infection. Because infection with internal parasites occurs by way of the feces, sanitation is an essential part of a parasite control program. For stabled horses the manure should be removed every 24 hours and either be composted or disposed of in an area where animals do not graze.

Although eliminating *S. vulgaris* from horses is difficult, it is possible by improved sanitation alone. Five days are required for strongyle eggs to develop into infective larvae. Therefore removing all fecal material from a horse's environment every 24 hours will prevent infection with *S. vulgaris*. It has been demonstrated that, if mares and foals are kept isolated from all other horses and all fecal material is removed every 24 hours, foals can be raised free of strongyles.[4]

Rotating pastures helps to reduce infection. It is best to alternate horses with cattle or sheep. Because cattle and sheep do not share common gastrointestinal parasites with horses, they will not seed the pasture with infectious ova while time helps to clean the pasture from the last equine population. In a like manner, cattle and sheep benefit from this alternating arrangement.

If pasturing cannot be rotated, the newborn foals should receive the cleanest pasture. It has been shown experimentally that pastures can be made relatively free of infective larvae of various equine nematodes by treating the population with effective anthelmintics monthly.[15]

Perhaps the least understood aspect of any control program using equine anthelmintics is frequency of treatment. The frequency for a particular population can be decided only when the nature of the parasitic infection is known. However, guidelines can be established. The goal of therapy is to free the animal of ascarids, pinworms, second- and third-stage bot instars, and strongyle larvae and adults.

For treating and preventing mixed infec-

tions the periodic administration of anthelmintics according to a rationally set schedule can be highly effective. Treatments limited to once or twice a year will have little effect.

Because foals commonly eat their mothers' feces, it is highly recommended that mares be treated for gastrointestinal parasites during the last 2 weeks of gestation and again within 24 hours after foaling. A relatively nontoxic anthelmintic such as thiabendazole and piperazine should be used. Treatments of foals for ascarids and strongyles can be started when foals are 8 weeks old and should be continued every 2 to 8 weeks. All other horses should also be treated every 2 to 8 weeks. The length of time between treatments will be determined by the rate at which ova return in the feces. When treatment is more frequent than every 4 weeks, one must remember not to use organophosphate anthelmintics more frequently than every 30 days.

Even though anthelmintics are not effective against strongyle larvae, horses can be freed of strongyles through anthelmintic administration every 2 to 8 weeks.[15,25,26] It may take from two to three years to eliminate worms by using treatment.

Horses should be treated for bots every 30 to 60 days during the fly season. Because the parasites migrate for 3 weeks before they reach the stomach, horses should be treated again 30 days after the first killing frost.

To be sure the parasite control program is effective, a veterinarian should make fecal examinations at least twice a year.

As an alternative to the frequent use of therapeutic anthelmintics, if the total population consists of adult horses and the primary concern is strongyles, low-level phenothiazine mixed in the feed the first 21 days of each month will reduce the output of strongyle ova and, over a period of time, reduce and eventually eliminate the infection (p. 208).

When giving anthelmintics, an important consideration is the method of administration. The easiest way for owners to give an

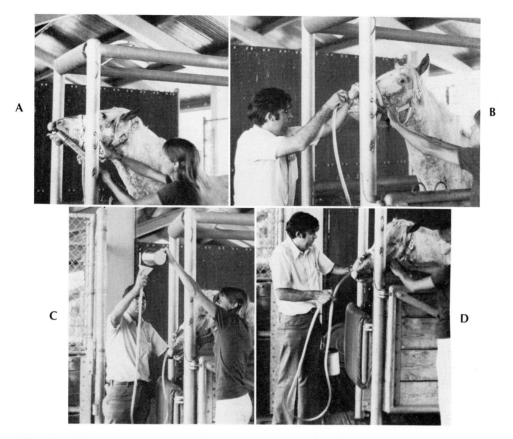

Fig. 13-4. Placing nasogastric tube in horse. Horses are commonly administered liquid medication by means of nasogastric tube that passes through nose to stomach. It is necessary for two people to perform this procedure. **A,** Horse must first be restrained. **B,** Tube is then carefully passed through nose and down esophagus. **C,** Medication is then poured through tube into stomach. **D,** Tube is then carefully withdrawn.

anthelmintic is to mix it in a portion of the animal's grain ration. This must be given individually, and the animal must consume the entire dose.

Another easily administered dose form is the paste or gel, which is squeezed into the horse's mouth. It adheres until swallowed. Boluses should be used with extreme caution because they can lodge in the upper part of the cervical esophagus. When boluses are caught in the esophagus, they can cause various degrees of inflammation or even death of surrounding tissues. One way to prevent this is to lubricate the bolus. However, the effect of lubrication on the disintegration time is unknown. In addition, the person ad-

ministering the bolus should be at the left side of the horse's head so that the passage of the bolus down the esophagus can be observed. If a bolus stops, the operator should give it a quick push to start it on its way again.

When veterinarians treat horses for internal parasites, they often administer the anthelmintic by way of a stomach tube (Fig. 13-4). Either a solution or suspension of the anthelmintic is used. An attendant holds the horse, and the veterinarian passes a tube through the horse's nose to the pharynx. As the horse swallows the tube, by reflex action, it is gently moved down the esophagus to the stomach. When the tube reaches the stomach, the anthelmintic is either pumped or allowed to flow by gravity into the stomach. The advantage of "tube worming" is that one can be sure the horse receives the entire dose. There are disadvantages too. The procedure is time-consuming. Two people, one of whom must be highly skilled in the use of a stomach tube, are required. Great caution must be used when placing the stomach tube. The tube must be lubricated and correctly placed in the nose, or damage to the turbinate bones can result; such damage is usually accompanied by severe nasal hemorrhage. If the tube is passed down the trachea rather than the esophagus and if the medication is administered, a fatal chemically induced pneumonia will probably result.

References

1. Bello, T. R., Amborski, G. F., and Torbert, B. J.: Effects of organic phosphorus anthelmintics on blood cholinesterase values in horses and ponies, Am. J. Vet. Res. 35:73, 1974.
2. Bello, T. R., Amborski, G. F., Torbert, B. J., and Greer, G. J.: Anthelmintic efficacy of cambendazole against gastrointestinal parasites of the horse, Am. J. Vet. Res. 34:771, 1973.
3. Bennett, D. G.: Efficacy of mebendazole as an anthelmintic in horses, Vet. Med. Small Anim. Clin. 68:604, 1973.
4. Bennett, D. G.: Predisposition to abdominal crisis in the horse, J. Am. Vet. Med. Assoc. 161:1189, 1972.
5. Bradley, R. E., and Radhakrishnan, C. V.: Critical test evaluation of mebendazole against gastrointestinal parasites of horses and ponies, Am. J. Vet. Res. 34:475, 1973.
6. Cornwell, R. L., Jones, R. M., and Pott, J. M.: Critical trials with morantel tartrate against *Parascaris equorum*, Res. Vet. Sci. 14:134, 1973.
7. Cornwell, R. L., Jones, R. M., and Pott, J. M.: Critical trials of morantel tartrate in equine strongylosis, Vet. Rec. 93:94, 1973.
8. Drudge, J. H., and Lyons, E. T.: Critical tests of a resin-pellet formulation of dichlorvos against internal parasites of the horse, Am. J. Vet. Res. 33:1365, 1972.
9. Drudge, J. H., Lyons, E. T., and Swerczek, T. W.: Activity of gel and paste formulations of dichlorvos against first instars of *Gasterophilus* spp., Am. J. Vet. Res. 33:2191, 1972.
10. Drudge, J. H., Lyons, E. T., and Taylor, E. L.: Critical tests and safety studies on trichlorfon as an antiparasitic agent in the horse, Am. J. Vet. Res. 37:139, 1976.
11. Drudge, J. H., Lyons, E. T., and Tolliver, S. C.: Critical and clinical test evaluations of mebendazole against internal parasites of the horse, Am. J. Vet. Res. 35:1409, 1974.
12. Drudge, J. H., Lyons, E. T., and Tolliver, S. C.: Critical tests of suspension, paste, pellet formulations of cambendazole in the horse, Am. J. Vet. Res. 36:435, 1975.
13. Drudge, J. H., Lyons, E. T., and Tolliver, S. C.: Critical tests of the benzimidazole anthelmintic, fenbendazole, in the horse, Vet. Med. Small Anim. Clin. 70:537, 1975.
14. Drudge, J. H., Lyons, E. T., and Tolliver, S. C.: Critical and controlled tests of the antiparasitic activity of liquid and paste formulations of trichlorfon in the horse, Vet. Med. Small Anim. Clin. 70:957, 1975.
15. Frerichs, W. M., Holbrook, A. A., and Allen, P. C.: Effect of antiparasitic medication in ponies on pasture, J. Am. Vet. Med. Assoc. 168:53, 1976.
16. Hass, D. K., Albert, J. R., Pillow, B. G., and Brown, L. J.: Dichlorvos gel formulation as an equine anthelmintic, Am. J. Vet. Res. 34:41, 1973.
17. Himes, J. A., Edds, G. T., Kirkham, W. W., and Neal, F. C.: Potentiation of succinylcholine by organophosphate compounds in horses, J. Am. Vet. Med. Assoc. 151:54, 1967.
18. Kester, W. O.: Strongylus vulgaris—the horse killer, Mod. Vet. Pract. 56:569, 1975.
19. Lyons, E. T., Drudge, J. H., and Tolliver, S. C.: Critical tests of three salts of pyrantel against internal parasites of the horse, Am. J. Vet. Res. 35:1515, 1974.
20. Lyons, E. T., Drudge, J. H., and Tolliver, S. C.: Critical tests of anthelmintic activity of a paste formulation of thiabendazole in horses, Am. J. Vet. Res. 37:701, 1976.
21. McCurdy, H. D., Sharp, M. L., and Kruchkenberg, S. M.: Critical and clinical trials of mebendazole and trichlorfon in the horse, Vet. Med. Small Anim. Clin. 72:245, 1977.
22. McCurdy, H. D., Sharp, M. L., and Sweeny, W. T.: Evaluation of mebendazole in paste formulation in the horse, Vet. Med. Small Anim. Clin. 71:97, 1976.
23. Nelson, D. L., White, R. G., Mozier, J. O., and Allen, A. D.: Margin of safety of succinylcholine chloride in horses treated with anticholinesterase pesticides, Vet. Med. Small Anim. Clin. 62:436, 1967.
24. Rossoff, I. S.: Handbook of veterinary drugs, New York, 1974, Springer Publishing Co.
25. Round, M. C.: Some aspects of naturally acquired helminthiasis of horses, Equine Vet. J. 3:31, 1971.
26. Smith, H. J.: Strongyle infections in ponies. I. Response to intermittent thiabendazole treatments, 40:327, 1976.
27. Voss, J. L., and Hibler, C. P.: Critical tests of an orally administered butonate as an anthelmintic in horses, Am. J. Vet. Res. 34:1209, 1973.

Additional readings

Albert, J. R., and Stearns, S. M.: Safety toxicity of a gel formulation of dichlorvos in the foal, Am. J. Vet. Res. **34:**1359, 1973.

Bello, T. R., Gaunt, S. D., and Torbert, B. J.: Critical evaluation of environmental control of bots (*Gasterophilus intestinalis*) in horses, J. Equine Med. Surg. **1:**126, 1977.

Bello, T. R., and Torbert, B. J.: Toxicity of an organic phosphate anthelmintic (Shell SD 15803) at excessive dosages in two-month-old pony foals, Am. J. Vet. Res. **33:**329, 1972.

Cook, T. F.: The anthelmintic efficiency of haloxon in horses, N.Z. Vet. J. **21:**82, May 1973.

Cook, T. F.: The efficiency of a mixture of haloxon and trichlorfon against strongyles and bots in horses, N.Z. Vet. J. **21:**157, Aug. 1973.

Drudge, J. H.: The use of anthelmintics for parasite control in the horse, Vet. Med. Small Anim. Clin. **60:**243, 1965.

Drudge, J. H., and Lyons, E. T.: Control of internal parasites of the horse, J. Am. Vet. Med. Assoc. **148:**378, 1966.

Drudge, J. H., and Lyons, E. T.: Activity of dichlorvos against horse bots, Mod. Vet. Pract. **51:**45, Dec. 1970.

Drudge, J. H., and Lyons, E. T.: Treatments for equine parasitism, J. Am. Vet. Assoc. **158:**2042, 1971.

Drudge, J. H., Lyons, E. T., and Szanto, J.: Critical tests of piperazine–carbon disulfide complex and phenothiazine mixtures against internal parasites of the horse, Am. J. Vet. Res. **30:**947, 1969.

Duncan, J. L.: The anthelmintic treatment of horses, Vet. Rec. **98:**233, 1976.

Gibbons, W. J.: Administration of boluses, Mod. Vet. Pract. **44:**78, Aug. 1963.

Gibbons, W. J.: Some problems in toxicology, Mod. Vet. Pract. **45:**74, March 1964.

Glenn, M. W., and Burr, W. M.: Toxicity of a piperazine–carbon disulfide–phenothiazine in the horse, J. Am. Vet. Med. Assoc. **160:**988, 1972.

Howell, L. M.: Verminous colic in horses, **72:**857, 1977.

Olsen, R. E., and Phillips, T. N.: Effects of phenothiazine and carbon disulfide on liver function in the horse, J. Am. Vet. Med. Assoc. **149:**400, 1966.

Schooley, M. A., Marsland, W. P., and Fogg, T. J.: Monthly distribution of *Gasterophilus* spp. in horses in the United States–implications on treatment schedules, Vet. Med. Small Anim. Clin. **66:**400, 1971.

Slocombe, J. O., and McCraw, B. M.: Suppression of the pathologic effects of *Strongylus edentatus* larvae with thiabendazole, J. Comp. Med. **39:**256, 1975.

Smith, H. J.: Strongyle infections in ponies. II. Reinfection of treated animals, Can. J. Comp. Med. **40:**335, 1976.

14

The central nervous system

ANTICONVULSANT DRUGS

Convulsions can be defined as a syndrome resulting from a central nervous system disturbance that is manifested by one or more of the following:

- Abnormal body movements
- A loss or disturbance of consciousness
- Abnormal behavior
- Involuntary urination and defecation

For the purpose of this text the term "convulsion" could be interchanged with epilepsy, seizure, or fit.

The animal may be in a continuous state of convulsions (status epilepticus) or may recover from an episode spontaneously and experience varying periods, from hours to many days, of normal activity prior to another convulsive episode. The therapy indicated in each of these two situations is different. In status epilepticus, therapy is aimed at stopping the continuous seizure activity and saving the animal's life. For intermittent seizures, therapy is aimed at preventing recurrence of seizures but leaving the animal alert to pursue its daily activities.

Animals are presented to veterinarians in convulsions resulting from a variety of causes. By taking a thorough history and performing a physical examination and clinical pathological studies, the veterinarian will arrive at a diagnosis and initiate the appropriate therapy. The drugs discussed here are used to treat convulsions produced by disorders in the central nervous system. Generally, they are used during a prolonged course of therapy.

Anticonvulsant therapy does not cure the condition that produces the seizures. The basic pathology responsible for the seizures remains. However, by using appropriate anticonvulsants, a complete or partial remission of seizures can be achieved. In fact, success of anticonvulsants is measured by the absence of seizures. Because several days are required to achieve effective tissue levels of certain anticonvulsant drugs, animals may continue to have convulsions during the initial part of the treatment. When one drug does not effectively control the seizures, another one or combinations of anticonvulsant drugs are tried.

Initially, standard dose recommendations are used, then adjustments are made to meet the specific needs of the individual animal. Once effective doses are determined, they must be maintained at suitable intervals to keep central nervous system tissue levels at an appropriate concentration for the desired effects. Reducing the dose or extending the time period between administration of the drugs can result in recurrence of the seizures. If one is taking animals off anticonvulsant drugs or reducing the dose, the dosage should be reduced gradually rather than discontinued abruptly. Rapidly decreasing the daily dose can precipitate seizures.

In veterinary medicine the most commonly used drugs for treating intermittent seizures are phenobarbital (a barbiturate closely related to sodium pentobarbital) and primidone.

In status epilepticus, drugs are administered intravenously to immediately eliminate seizure activity. Sodium pentobarbital, a general anesthetic, is often administered intravenously slowly until the seizures cease. When used to terminate the seizures of status epilepticus, sodium pentobarbital should not be given at normal anesthetic dose but just at a level to achieve the desired results.

There are problems relative to the use of sodium pentobarbital to arrest convulsions in animals in status epilepticus. The mortality for such canine patients is unknown. However, in humans, mortality has been reported to be 10% to 30%.[1] A patient in status epilepticus usually lacks adequate tissue levels of oxygen. This endangers cardiac and respiratory function. Sodium pentobarbital adds further strain to the heart and lungs. When high levels of sodium pentobarbital are used, a deep surgical anesthesia may be produced. This is undesirable because it further reduces oxygen levels, prevents neurological examination, and makes both physical examination and oral administration of other anticonvulsant drugs difficult.

Diazepam sodium has been used for several years to treat status epilepticus in humans. As discussed on p. 218, it can also be used to treat dogs in status epilecticus.

Phenothiazine tranquilizers, which will be discussed later in this chapter, are contraindicated in animals prone to seizures because these drugs lower the animals' resistance to seizures. In addition to phenothiazine tranquilizers, some antibiotics given in large doses can also precipitate seizures. Chloramphenicol and penicillin have been reported to do this.[16]

Diphenylhydantoin

Diphenylhydantoin is used much less in dogs and cats for preventing seizures than are phenobarbital and primidone. However, diphenylhydantoin is commonly used in humans. Its limited use in dogs and cats is probably due to the manner in which these species metabolize the drug. Relatively small doses of diphenylhydantoin result in high plasma concentrations and toxicity in cats. This is probably caused by the relative inability of cats to metabolize the drug. On the other hand, dogs given massive doses of diphenylhydantoin, in comparison to doses used in humans, show relatively low plasma concentrations.

To use diphenylhydantoin safely in cats it is necessary to establish a maintenance dose that would provide effective plasma concentrations without reaching toxic levels. For example, in cats, diphenylhydantoin might be given at intervals as long as 1 week. Dogs must receive multiple daily doses to obtain effective tissue concentrations of the drug. Because of this, current dosage recommendations for use of diphenylhydantoin in both dogs and cats are probably incorrect.[18,19] In both species, doses based on the human dose are totally inappropriate.

When animals are under-dosed, convulsions continue. When they are overdosed, incoordination, depression, or gastric irritation may result. Until adequate regimens for diphenylhydantoin in dogs and cats are worked out, the drug should only be used in those patients in which other anticonvulsants fail to control seizures. In addition, the drug should only be used by experienced clinicians who have been able to titrate effective and safe doses.

Diazepam

Diazepam is commonly used in humans as a tranquilizer and anticonvulsant. Only limited reports of its use in veterinary medicine exist. In clinical cases of status epilepticus in dogs, diazepam sodium has been used according to the following regimen[1]. A 5 mg dose per dog is administered slowly intravenously. If convulsions do not cease in 1 or 2 minutes, another 5 mg is given. If still no response occurs, pentobarbital is administered slowly intravenously at the rate of 16.5 mg/kg. If convulsions occur again, 2 to 4 hours after the first treatment the regimen is repeated. Once seizures stop, other oral anticonvulsants can be given to prevent a recurrence. Because diazepam can seriously aggravate digitalis-induced cardiac arrhythmias, the drug must be used with caution in animals receiving digitalis or digitalis-like drugs.[17]

Paramethadione

Paramethadione has been used experimentally in the treatment of epileptic disorders in dogs. It has not yet been cleared by the FDA for veterinary use.

Effectiveness. Early reports indicate that paramethadione is approximately 65% effective in cases that do not respond to other medication and approximately 70% effective in routine epileptic disorders.[15]

Toxicity. Liver and kidney diseases are contraindications to the use of paramethadione. Vomiting during the first week of therapy has been eliminated by providing a little food with each pill. Initial reports on the veterinary use of the drug are confined to dogs. Paramethadione should not be used in cats until it is proved that the drug is not toxic to that species.

Dose and administration. The drug is available in small capsules of 150 and 300 mg. The dose ranges used to date have been 10 to 60 mg/kg, with most dogs needing between 15 and 30 mg/kg.[15]

Phenobarbital

Phenobarbital, a barbiturate, is not used as a general anesthetic. However, of the barbiturate drugs, it is the best to treat sporadic seizures. When used at clinically effective doses, the drug may cause drowsiness. As an anticonvulsant it is generally given to cats at the rate of 3.5 to 7 mg/kg and to dogs at the rate of 7.5 to 15 mg/kg.[17]

Phenobarbital is often administered concurrently with diphenylhydantoin. However, those using such combinations should be aware that phenobarbital may increase the metabolism of diphenylhydantoin, decreasing the effectiveness of that drug. (See Table 2-2.)

Primidone

Primidone is probably the most popular anticonvulsant used in dogs. It acts on the central nervous system to raise the seizure threshold.

Toxicity. When given to dogs at normal doses, the drug is apparently well tolerated. Side effects such as staggering and drowsiness may infrequently occur. Such side effects usually disappear with downward adjustment of the dose. The dose recommended for dogs can cause neurotoxicity in cats.[17]

Dose and administration. Primidone is normally administered to dogs at the rate of 55 mg/kg orally. When convulsions occur every few days or less, the daily dose is given at one time. However, when convulsions are frequent, the daily dose must be divided and administered at 6 to 12 hour intervals.[17] Doses for cats have not yet been clearly defined.

TRANQUILIZERS

Tranquilizers are central nervous system depressant drugs. They are distinguished from the sedative-hypnotics because at clinical doses tranquilizers do not produce unconsciousness or depress cardiac or respiratory function.[3] Tranquilizers are used to reduce aggressive or defensive behavior patterns but ideally do not interfere with voluntary movement.

Phenothiazines

This group of tranquilizers are all derivatives of phenothiazine, which in veterinary medicine is used as an anthelmintic (Chapters 12 and 13). The phenothiazine tranquilizers exert their action by depressing the brain stem and its connections to the cerebral cortex. In addition to the desired tranquilizing action of these drugs, the following effects are produced:

- Potentiation of analgesics, sedatives, and general anesthetics
- Slight antihistamine activity
- Moderate to marked fall in blood pressure

Phenothiazine tranquilizers should not be used with epinephrine hydrochloride because the action of epinephrine, which normally raises the blood pressure is reversed so that a drop in blood pressure results. However, when used with the phenothiazine tranquilizers, norepinephrine does not cause a further reduction in blood pressure. Phenothiazine tranquilizers can precipitate seizures in epileptic dogs. They should therefore be used with caution in these animals.

One use of phenothiazine tranquilizers in animals has been as preanesthetics. When so used, they facilitate the administration of anesthetics and reduce the dose necessary to produce surgical anesthesia. They have also been used to reduce fear and excitability in animals, prevent motion sickness, and increase weight gain in livestock.

One phenothiazine derivative, trimeprazine, is not used so much for its tranquilizing effects but rather to reduce itching, nausea and coughing and as an antihistamine. Its use to reduce itching was discussed in Chapter 8.

Acetylpromazine. Acetylpromazine is used in dogs, cats, and horses as a tranquilizer.

Dose and administration. Acetylpromazine is available as tablets for use in small animals and as an injectable solution that can be given by either the subcutaneous, intramuscular, or intravenous routes. Some clinicians believe that the doses of acetylpromazine recommended by the manufacturer (0.55 to 2.2 mg/kg) are ten times higher than necessary, particularly when used as a preanesthetic medication. When giving the drug by the parenteral route, the following doses can be used, depending on the degree of tranquilization required: dogs, 0.55 to 1.1 mg/kg; cats, 1.1 to 2.2 mg/kg; and horses, 2 to 4 mg/45 kg. When given orally, the following doses are used: dogs, 0.55 to 2.2 mg/kg, and cats, 1.1 to 2.2 mg/kg.

Chlorpromazine. Chlorpromazine is not as popular in veterinary use as acetylpromazine or promazine. It should not be used in horses because some horses react by dropping to their hocks and then suddenly lunging forward.[2] For dogs and cats, doses should not exceed those in the following list[17]:

Cats	1 mg/kg intramuscularly
	2 mg/kg orally
Dogs	1 mg/kg intravenously
	2 mg/kg intramuscularly
	3 mg/kg orally

Perphenazine. Perphenazine is better at preventing vomiting than either chlorpromazine or promazine. It is effective in preventing motion sickness in the dog if administered orally 20 to 30 minutes before the beginning of a journey. The drug should not be used in horses because it causes excitation in that species. Generally, the tranquilizer is acceptable in the dog, cat, and swine and is particularly potent in producing tranquilizing effects in cattle. However, because they produce more predictable results, promazine and acetylpromazine are preferred by most practitioners. Subcutaneous injections of perphenazine should not be used because severe reactions can result.

Doses for cattle under 360 kg are 10 mg/45 kg intravenously or intramuscularly. For cattle weighing 360 to 700 kg, 75 to 125 mg can be given intravenously or 100 to 150 mg intramuscularly. In cats 2 mg/kg can be given orally or 1 mg/kg intravenously or intramuscularly. In dogs 1 mg/kg can be given orally or 0.5 mg/kg intravenously or intramuscularly.

Piperacetazine. Piperacetazine was recently introduced as a tranquilizer in veterinary practice. To date there appears to be no advantage to using this drug in place of more traditional veterinary tranquilizers.

Toxicity. Piperacetazine can markedly potentiate hypotension produced by central nervous system depressants, general anesthetics, and hypnotics. It should not be used with epinephrine because it can reverse the action of epinephrine and produce severe hypotension. Because this drug may potentiate their toxicity, it should not be used with various anticholinesterase drugs, procaine, or other phenothiazines.

Dose and administration. In dogs and cats, peak effects are obtained as follows[17]: oral administration, 1 to 3 hours; intravenous administration, within 15 minutes; and subcutaneous and intramuscular administration, within 45 minutes.

Doses for dogs and cats are as follows[17]:

1. For tranquilization, give 0.1 mg/kg orally two to four times a day, with the dosage reduced after 2 to 3 days; or 0.1 mg/kg subcutaneously or intramuscularly twice to three times a day.

2. For sedation, give 0.4 mg/kg subcutaneously, intramuscularly, or intravenously.

Promazine

Use. Promazine has been a popular tranquilizer in veterinary medicine. In addition to its use in dogs and cats, it is a satisfactory tranquilizer for use in horses. Promazine can be used in farm animals such as cattle as long as adequate precautions are taken with respect to residues in meat. The label should be consulted regarding mandated withdrawal times. Because milk can be contaminated with promazine, it cannot be used on lactating dairy cattle.

Toxicity. When used in horses, some animals develop an allergic response following intravenous use or some local swelling after intramuscular use. In treating such animals, epinephrine is contraindicated because it potentiates the hypotensive effect of promazine. As with other phenothiazine tranquilizers, norepinephrine should be used to treat the allergic response to promazine without creating an hypotensive episode.

Dose and administration. Doses are as follows: Cattle, horses, sheep, and swine should receive 0.4 to 1 mg/kg intramuscularly or intravenously. The oral dosage to tranquilize cattle or horses to facilitate handling or shipment is 1 to 2.5 mg/kg. Cats and dogs should be given 2.5 to 6.5 mg/kg orally, intramuscularly, or intravenously.

Propiopromazine. Propiopromazine was an extremely potent and popular tranquilizer that was generally withdrawn from the American market by the FDA in 1969. It is assumed that this drug was withdrawn from the market because it caused paralysis of the retractor peni muscle in stallions. It has been reintroduced as an approved product for oral use in dogs and cats. In dogs the drug can be administered at the rate of 1.1 to 4.4 mg/kg orally.

Xylazine

Xylazine is a relatively new (about 1970) veterinary tranquilizer. Not a phenothiazine, xylazine is a thiazine derivative. The effects of xylazine differ substantially from those of the phenothiazines. For example, it produces a sleeplike state in dogs and in cattle. The dosage and effects of this drug also differ greatly between species. Great care must be exercised in the use of this drug in species of animals in which the veterinarian has not previously used the drug. Xylazine is available in the United States for use in small animals (dogs and cats) and horses only. It is supplied as an injectable solution in both 20 and 100 mg/ml concentrations.

Toxicity. The effects of xylazine on blood pressure are variable between species. In dogs and cats, blood pressure drops to about 80% of normal for about 1½ hours. In horses there is an initial rise in blood pressure to about 125% of normal. This effect lasts about

5 minutes, then blood pressure drops to approximately 85% to 90% of normal. Xylazine also results in a slowing of the heart rate by 20% to 30%. Cardiac arrhythmias may occasionally occur in animals receiving xylazine. Administration of atropine sulfate in conjunction with xylazine will help prevent arrhythmias and slowing of the heart rate.

Xylazine is contraindicated in animals with significantly depressed respiration, heart disease, advanced liver or kidney disease, severe shock, and extreme stress conditions. The safety of the drug in pregnant animals is uncertain. It is contraindicated in cattle during the last month of pregnancy.

Use in small animals. In dogs and cats the effects of xylazine develop within 10 to 15 minutes after intramuscular or subcutaneous injection. These effects persist for 1 to 2 hours. An occasional animal may require 5 to 8 hours for recovery. Onset after intravenous administration is 3 to 5 minutes. Xylazine produces a sleeplike state in dogs and cats. Its use in dogs and cats is in our opinion not without risk. Vomiting nearly always occurs in cats, and convulsions are not uncommon in both dogs and cats. The dosages recommended in small animals are 8.4 mg/kg intramuscularly or 1 mg/kg intravenously.[17]

Use in horses. In horses, xylazine produces an awake but very relaxed and calm state. The head hangs near the ground, and in male animals the penis becomes relaxed and partially extended. There seems to be little or no loss of coordination. It is important that horses maintain adequate coordination so that falling, stumbling, thrashing, and panic are avoided. An intravenous dose of 0.5 to 1 mg/kg in the horse produces its effect in 1 to 2 minutes, and tranquilization lasts 30 to 40 minutes. An intramuscular dose of 1 to 2 mg/kg produces its effect in approximately 15 to 20 minutes, and the duration is 30 to 60 minutes. Xylazine injectable solution is irritating and should not be given subcutaneously to horses.

Use in cattle. Although not officially recommended for use in cattle and other ruminants, xylazine appears to be a valuable drug

for use in these species. In cattle, in particular, the drug produces a light sleep with excellent relaxation. Cattle generally lie down in sternal recumbancy under the effects of xylazine. Minor surgery and cesareans can be accomplished after administration of xylazine and local anesthetics. The dosage in cattle is one tenth that of the horse, 0.05 to 0.1 mg/kg intravenously or 0.1 to 0.2 mg/kg intramuscularly.

ANALGESICS AND ANTIPYRETICS

Analgesics are drugs that alleviate pain. Frequently, analgesics have antipyretic activity, that is, they reduce fever.

Analgesics are not used in veterinary medicine to the degree that they are used in human medicine. The primary reason for this is that animals are often unable to communicate pain, and it is often difficult for the owner or the veterinarian to determine when analgesics are indicated. Animals certainly experience pain. For example, a horse that limps may do so because it is reacting to painful stimuli. When external manifestations of pain are evident, the use of analgesics should be considered. Analgesics are also indicated after surgical procedures likely to result in pain.

Aspirin

Chemically, aspirin is acetylsalicylic acid. Although this is probably the most commonly used drug in humans, it has enjoyed only limited use in veterinary medicine.

Effectiveness. Aspirin is an effective analgesic and antipyretic. For example, it has been reported that arthritic cattle treated with aspirin improved a few hours after receiving the drug.[11]

Toxicity. One reason that aspirin has not been popular in veterinary medicine is that many problems have been associated with its use. The relatively minor problem of gastric irritation caused by aspirin is recognized in animal species as well as man.

Cats are particularly susceptible to aspirin toxicity. Persons working in veterinary hospitals need to be alert to the possibility that owners may administer aspirin to sick cats and produce serious aspirin toxicity. Clinical signs of aspirin intoxication include poor appetite, vomiting, weight loss, and staggering. Hypersensitivities also occur. Animals that die from aspirin intoxication show anemia, severe ulceration, and hemorrhage throughout the upper gastrointestinal tract, hepatitis, and suppression of red cell production in the bone marrow.[13,22]

To prevent aspirin toxicity, doses specific for each species must be used. Even though there are numerous reports in the literature of aspirin toxicity in cats, the drug apparently has no special toxicity for the tissues of the cat. Rather doses used in the past have been too high, producing toxicity. The toxicity is caused by high serum concentrations that result from the slow metabolism of aspirin by cats. Therefore it is necessary to give cats smaller doses of aspirin at greater intervals than those given to other species. These reduced doses maintain serum concentrations that are effective without being toxic.

In humans, serum salicylate concentrations between 10 and 30 mg/100 ml are effective and safe. It is probably correct to assume that such a range would also be effective and safe in the cat.[21] However, compared to man, a much smaller dose per kilogram must be given to cats to obtain these serum levels. Experimentally a dose of 25 mg/kg of body weight given once daily to cats maintained serum salicylate content between 10 and 25 mg/100 ml of serum. When given for 15 days, no clinical evidence of salicylate toxicity was detected.[21] Other work indicates that therapeutic concentrations of aspirin in humans are 5 to 20 mg/100 ml of serum and that the proper dose in cats to achieve this level is 10 mg/kg of body weight every 52 hours.[6]

Dose and administration. In cattle, aspirin can be given at the rate of 100 mg/kg of body weight every 12 hours to maintain concentrations greater than 30 mg/100 ml of serum.[11]

In dogs, doses of 25 mg/kg every 8 hours maintained adequate serum salicylate concentrations within the desired range of 10 to 30 mg/100 ml without producing vomiting. Twenty-five to 35 mg/kg every 8 hours appears to be the optimal dose of aspirin in the dog.[20]

Doses between 10 mg/kg every 52 hours to 25 mg/kg once daily appear to be safe in cats.

Dipyrone

Dipyrone is an analgesic and antipyretic. It has been used primarily in the treatment of hyperactivity of the equine gastrointestinal tract (spasmodic colic).

Dipyrone can be used in dogs and cats as an analgesic and antipyretic. It is supplied in 100 ml multidose vials for injection and as tablets for oral use.

Cattle and horses can be administered the drug intramuscularly, subcutaneously, or intravenously at the rate of 2.5 to 10 gm. In sheep and swine, 2.5 gm given intramuscularly or subcutaneously may be administered. Cats and dogs may be administered 110 to 220 mg/kg intramuscularly or subcutaneously. Doses may be repeated in 4 to 6 hours as necessary.[17]

Fentanyl

Fentanyl is a narcotic analgesic. Its action is similar to morphine. It is reported by the manufacturer to be over 100 times more potent on a weight basis than morphine as an analgesic. Unlike morphine, however, fentanyl does not produce vomiting when administered to dogs. This drug can be given as an analgesic to dogs at the rate of 0.02 mg/kg intravenously.

Fentanyl-droperidol

A combination of fentanyl and droperidol is supplied for use in dogs as an analgesic tranquilizer. The commercial product (Innovar-Vet) is supplied as an injectable solution containing a 0.4 mg of fentanyl and 20 mg of droperidol in each milliliter. By combining droperidol, a sedative tranquilizing agent, with fentanyl, a product is produced that provides both sedative and analgesic properties.

Effectiveness. According to the manufacturer, droperidol potentiates the analgesic effect of fentanyl.

The product has been indicated for various procedures, including the following:

- Diagnostic manipulations such as vaginal examinations and radiographic examinations
- Orthopedic procedures such as setting and casting of fractures
- Dental procedures such as the scaling of teeth
- Minor surgical procedures of relatively short duration
- Therapeutic manipulations such as the irrigation and packing of anal sacs, cleaning of ears, and treatment of eyes and ears
- Grooming
- Preoperative and postoperative medication for sedation and relief of pain
- As a preanesthetic with barbiturates or gaseous anesthetics
- For major surgery in conjunction with local anesthetics

Droperidol produces a reduced responsiveness to environmental stimuli. It tends to block the effects of adrenalin, combat nausea, and potentiate the action of pentobarbital. By itself it has little effect on respiration or cardiac output but does reduce blood pressure.

Because it sedates animals, if used in conjunction with pentobarbital, the dose of pentobarbital must be reduced.

Toxicity. A decreased heart rate may occur due to the stimulation of the vagal nerve caused by fentanyl. This can be prevented by administration of a standard dose of atropine.

The fentanyl-droperidol combination has produced undesirable central nervous system stimulation in cattle, sheep, cats, and horses.

Fentanyl, alone or in combination with droperidol, can cause severe respiratory depression. Nalorphine hydrochloride or naloxone, both antagonists of morphine, reverse the respiratory depression. For this purpose, nalorphine may be given intravenously, intramuscularly, or subcutaneously in a dose of 0.44 to 1.1 mg/kg and naloxone at a rate of 0.04 mg/kg intramuscularly, subcutaneously, or intravenously. If the combination of fentanyl and droperidol is given intravenously, the dose of nalorphine should be reduced by about one third. The use of these drugs will immediately reverse all the effects of fentanyl, including the analgesia. They do not, however, reverse the effects of droperidol.

Dose and administration. For analgesia and tranquilization of dogs the recommended intramuscular dose of the combination product is 1 ml/7 to 9 kg of body weight. Intravenously it can be administered at the rate of 1 ml/11 to 27 kg of body weight. The actual dose given is determined by the response desired. Administration of 0.04 mg/kg of atropine sulfate prevents hypersalivation and decreased heart rate induced by fentanyl.

Flunixin meglumine

Flunixin meglumine (Banamine) is being marketed as a nonnarcotic, nonsteroidal drug that has analgesic, anti-inflammatory, and antipyretic activity in the horse. The manufacturer claims that the drug inhibits the synthesis of prostaglandin and modifies its activity as a mediator of pain, fever, and inflammation. It is believed that prostaglandins either cause pain at the site of injury by direct action or sensitize pain receptors to other stimulants. It is also believed prostaglandins are involved with pain transmission in the central nervous system.

Use. Flunixin meglumine is recommended by the manufacturer for use in horses for the management of pain from musculoskeletal disorders and colic.

Toxicity. To date toxic effects at recommended doses have not been reported. Flunixin meglumine does not cause the usual corticosteroid side effects of adrenal suppression, immunosuppression, sodium retention, or electrolyte imbalance.

Dose and administration. Flunixin meglumine can be administered intravenously or intramuscularly. Onset and duration of activity appear to be uninfluenced by the route of administration.[12] When given parenterally at the rate of 1.1 mg/kg, onset of activity occurs within 2 hours, and peak response is seen 12 hours after administration. Activity can persist for 30 hours. For musculoskeletal disorders the recommended dose is 1.1 mg/kg intravenously or intramuscularly once daily. Treatment may be repeated up to 5 days. For the relief of pain associated with equine colic, 1.1 mg/kg are given intravenously. Treatment may be repeated when there is a recurrence of the signs of colic.

Meperidine

Use. Meperidine is a narcotic analgesic that is used primarily in horses, dogs, and cats as a preanesthetic agent and for relief of severe pain. Meperidine potentiates a number of phenothiazine tranquilizers. It also reduces the amount of barbiturate required to produce general anesthesia. Because cats metabolize meperidine so rapidly, its usefulness in this species is limited. Even if given at high doses that are potentially toxic, meperidine may have an extremely short plasma half-life of 42 minutes in cats.[7]

Toxicity. If meperidine contacts the oral mucosa of cats, an undesirable reflex salivation may result. Given in high doses or with barbiturate anesthetics, it can depress respiratory function. The depression caused by meperidine can be reversed with naloxone.

Dose and administration. Meperidine is administered as meperidine hydrochloride. In cats the drug is normally administered at the rate of 11 mg/kg subcutaneously or intramuscularly. It should not be administered in doses that exceed 11 mg/kg in cats. Larger doses may result in signs that vary from incoordination and mild excitement to convulsions and death. The simultaneous administration of promazine hydrochloride at the rate of 4.4 mg/kg greatly enhances the sedative and analgesic effects of meperidine.[5]

In dogs meperidine hydrochloride may be given at the rate of 10 to 15 mg/kg intramuscularly or subcutaneously.

Cattle and horses may be administered 150 to 200 mg/45 kg intramuscularly, subcutaneously, or intravenously.[17]

Morphine

Morphine is a highly addictive narcotic derivative of opium.

Use. Morphine has excellent analgesic and antispasmodic properties. Apparently the analgesic properties are by direct action of the central nervous system, whereas its antispasmodic properties are by direct action on the smooth muscle of the intestinal tract. Perhaps its greatest use in veterinary medicine is as a preanesthetic agent in dogs. Most commonly it is employed with atropine as a preanesthetic agent. Animals that have been premedicated with morphine are easier to handle and therefore easier to administer anesthetics to. Use of morphine reduces the amount of anesthetic that is used to reach a surgical plane of anesthesia.

One advantage of the use of morphine in dogs as a preanesthetic agent is that it causes dogs to defecate and vomit. Ideally animals enter major surgical procedures with empty gastrointestinal tracts. If food is present in the upper gastrointestinal tract, vomiting can occur during anesthesia, resulting in inhalation of the vomitus, which can cause a fatal inhalation pneumonia. Dogs with full lower gastrointestinal tracts commonly defecate either during the excitement stage of anesthesia or when they are under full surgical anesthesia. Normally, vomiting and defecation during surgery is prevented by withholding feed from animals before surgical procedures. However, if the surgery is an emergency and such withholding of food is not possible or if dogs accidentally receive food prior to surgery, the administration of morphine will clear the upper and lower gastrointestinal tracts. Shortly following vomiting and defecation, dogs become sedated. Morphine is also an excellent analgesic to administer to animals postsurgically after they have recovered from the general anesthesia.

Toxicity. Animals suffering from tetany due to strychnine poisoning or tetanus need to be sedated to block the spasms. Although morphine does sedate animals, it is not an appropriate drug for this purpose. Strychnine and tetanus toxins produce tetany by stimulating activity in the spinal cord. Morphine stimulates spinal cord activity as well. Therefore, if used in the treatment of tetanus or strychnine poisoning, morphine will potentiate tetanic spasms.

Even though morphine is a sedative, it can produce excitation under certain circumstances. Historically, because it produced excitation in cats, morphine was not recommended for that species. However, there is evidence that the observed excitation may be due to improper dosing in cats. Cats do not conjugate or detoxify morphine as readily as dogs and other species. Therefore clinically safe and effective doses in cats must be much smaller than those used in dogs. Evidence exists that a dose of 0.1 mg/kg of morphine sulfate in cats produces analgesia with no excitation. The analgesia produced by this dose of morphine should last in excess of 4 hours. When given at this dose, morphine may serve as an appropriate and effective preanesthetic agent in the cat.[7]

Similarly, morphine is not used in horses because it produces hyperexcitation. Whether this is due to improper dosing as in the cat, or a basic phenomenon of the drug in that species needs further study.

In overdosage, morphine can cause severe respiratory depression. When animals are exhibiting toxic reactions to morphine, the effects of the drug can be reversed with nalorphine or naloxon. Doses are given on p. 223.

Dose and administration. The dose of morphine in cats is 0.1 mg/kg intramuscularly.[17] In dogs the dose is about 0.5 to 2 mg/kg subcutaneously or intramuscularly.[10]

Phenylbutazone

Use. Phenylbutazone is used as an anti-inflammatory analgesic and antipyretic. It is commonly used to relieve pain associated with musculoskeletal disorders. These include conditions such as arthritis, bursitis, and common lamenesses. The drug produces an anti-inflammatory response in the involved tissues and at the same time apparently produces an analgesic effect by its action on the central nervous system.

Toxicity. Because phenylbutazone inter-

acts with other drugs, its use must be considered in that light (Chapter 2). It prevents the plasma binding of sulfonamides, increasing their serum levels and antibacterial effectiveness. Phenylbutazone also can increase the anticoagulant effect of coumarins. When given orally, it can cause gastric upsets and ulcers. Because the drug can accumulate in animals with severe cardiac, renal, or hepatic pathology, it should not be used in the presence of such conditions. Prolonged oral doses have caused the development of hepatic portal vein phlebitis and blood dyscrasias.

Phenylbutazone is metabolized slowly in cats. Doses of 44 mg/kg/24 hr administered to healthy cats have resulted in deaths after 13 to 20 days. Signs preceding death included progressive loss of appetite, decrease in body weight, dehydration, and severe depression.[4] In dogs, anemias have been reported following its use.

Dose and administration. Phenylbutazone is supplied as 100 mg tablets for oral administration to small animals, 1 gm and 2 gm tablets for oral administration to large animals, and a 20% solution (200 mg/ml) for parenteral administration.

Recommended doses of the drug should be carefully followed. Increasing the doses does not appear to increase the effectiveness of the drug but does greatly increase the possibility of toxic reactions.

If the drug is to be used in cats, the dose should be approximately 6 to 12 mg/kg of body weight daily. If inappetance or depression occurs or speedy clinical improvement does not result, the drug should be withdrawn.[4]

Because the dog metabolizes phenylbutazone twenty-five times faster than man, it has been suggested that oral doses in the range of 15 mg/kg four times a day are required to reach therapeutic concentrations in that species.[14] Normal recommended doses for dogs are 10 to 15 mg/kg three times a day with a maximum dose of 800 mg daily.

When given orally, doses of 2 to 4 gm/450 kg one to three times daily are recommended in horses. When given intravenously, 1 to 2 gm/450 kg are used.

Meclofenamic acid

Meclofenamic acid (Arquel) is a recently marketed anti-inflammatory, analgesic, and antipyretic drug for use in horses. The mechanism of action of meclofenamic acid, like those of other analgesic-antipyretic agents, is not known. The manufacturer recommends the use of this drug in horses suffering from a variety of inflammatory musculoskeletal conditions.

It should not be administered to horses with active gastrointestinal, hepatic, or renal diseases. This drug should be discontinued at the first signs of intolerance as demonstrated by colic, diarrhea, decrease in appetite, or change in stool consistency. When used at doses higher than recommended, blood appears in the feces and anemia results. In animals with heavy bot infestations, mild colic and change in stool consistency have been observed when the drug was used.

The drug is given orally in the grain. The manufacturer recommends a dose of 2.2 mg/kg of body weight once daily for 5 to 7 days for both acute and chronic conditions. If treatment is indicated beyond the initial 5 to 7-day period, a maintenance dosage level should be individualized for each animal and may be repeated at appropriate intervals. Ideally the lowest reasonable dosage that provides the desired effect is recommended.

Meclofenamic acid has not been available long enough to comment on its eventual place in the therapy of horses.

Naproxen

Naproxen is another new anti-inflammatory analgesic antipyretic. Like meclofenamic acid, it is intended for use in horses. The drug is available in granulated form for oral administration in feed. The dosage recommended by the manufacturer is 10 mg/kg orally twice daily. This drug is also too new at this time to comment on its eventual place in equine therapy.

Pentazocine

Pentazocine (Talwin) is a strong analgesic, effective in humans against both visceral and musculoskelatal pain. In horses it appears to be useful for alleviating abdominal pain from a variety of causes.[9] It seems to have a minimum effect on depressing either gut motility or arterial blood pressure.[8] The only toxic side effect reported in horses to date is mild transient incoordination.

For the treatment of colic in horses, a combination of the intravenous and intramuscular routes appears to be the best method of administration. The best analgesic effects are obtained after an initial intravenous dose of 0.33 to 0.44 mg/kg is given, followed 10 minutes later by a similar dose intramuscularly.[9]

References

1. Averill, D. R.: Treatment of status epilepticus in dogs with diazepam sodium, J. Am. Vet. Med. Assoc. **156:**432, 1970.
2. Booth, N. H.: Tranquilizers (ataractics). In Jones, L. M., editor: Veterinary pharmacology and therapeutics, Ames, Iowa, 1965, Iowa State University Press.
3. Bowman, B. M.: Piperacetazine: a clinical survey, Pract. Vet. **48:**30, Winter 1975.
4. Carlisle, C. H., and others: Phenylbutazone in cats, Br. Vet. J. **124:**560, 1968.
5. Clifford, D. H., and Soma, L. R.: Meperidine in cats, Fed. Proc. **28:**1482, 1969.
6. Davis, L. E.: Clinical pharmacology of salicylates, Clin. Pharmacol. Newsletter **1:**7, 1976.
7. Davis, L. E., and Donnelly, E. J.: Analgesic drugs in the cat. J. Am. Vet. Med. Assoc. **153:**1161, 1968.
8. Donawick, W. J.: Metabolic management of the horse with an acute abdominal crisis, J. Afr. Vet. Assoc. **46:**107, March, 1975.
9. Dresher, K., Kind, R. E., and Miller, R. M.: Clinical assessment of pentazocine in treatment of equine colic, Vet. Med. Small Anim. Clin. **67:**683, 1972.
10. Enos, L. R.: Formulary, Veterinary Medical Teaching Hospital, University of California, 1976.
11. Gingerich, D. A., Baggot, J. D., and Yeary, R. A.: Pharmacokinetics and dosage of aspirin in cattle, J. Am. Vet. Med. Assoc. **167:**945, 1975.
12. Houdeshell, J. W., and Hennessey, P. W.: A new nonsteroidal, anti-inflammatory analgesic for horses, J. Equine Med. Surg. **1:**57, 1977.
13. Larson, E. J.: Toxicity of low doses of aspirin in the cat, J. Am. Vet. Med. Assoc. **143:**837, 1963.
14. Nielsen, C. K., and others: Dosage of phenyl-

butazone in the dog, Dtsch. Tieraerztl. Wochenschr. **76:**378, 1969.

15. Parker, A. J.: A preliminary report on a new antiepileptic medication for dogs, J. Am. Anim. Hosp. Assoc. **11:**437, 1975.

16. Redding, R. W.: The diagnosis and therapy of seizures, Anim. Hosp. **5:**79, May 1969.

17. Rossoff, I. W.: Handbook of veterinary drugs, New York, 1974, Springer Publishing Co.

18. Roye, D. B., Serrano, E. E., Hammer, R. H., and Wilder, B. J.: Plasma kinetics of diphenylhydantoin in dogs and cats, Am. J. Vet. Res. **34:**947, 1973.

19. Tobin, T., Dirdjosudjono, S., and Baskin, S. I.: Pharmacokinetics and distribution of diphenylhydantoin in kittens, Am. J. Vet. Res. **34:**951, 1973.

20. Yeary, R. A., and Brant, R. J.: Aspirin dosages for the dog, J. Am. Vet. Med. Assoc. **167:**63, 1975.

21. Yeary, R. A., and Swanson, W.: Aspirin dosages for the cat, J. Am. Vet. Med. Assoc. **163:**1177, 1973.

22. Zontine, W. J., and Uno, T.: Acute aspirin toxicity in a cat, Vet. Med. Small Anim. Clin. **64:**680, 1969.

Additional readings

Davis, L. E., and Westfall, B. A.: Species differences in biotransformation and excretion of salicylate, Am. J. Vet. Res. **33:**1253, 1972.

Dunn, P. S.: Symposium: (1) A clinician's view on the use and misuse of phenylbutazone, Equine Vet. J. **4:**63, April 1972.

Ebert, E. F.: Clinical use of phenylbutazone in large animals, Vet. Med. **57:**33, 1962.

Finco, D. R., Duncan, J. R., Schall, W. D., and Prasse, K. W.: Acetaminophen toxicosis in the cat, J. Am. Vet. Med. Assoc. **166:**469, 1975.

Garner, H. E., Amend, J. F., and Rosborough, J. P.: Effects of BAY VA 1470 on respiratory parameters in ponies, Vet. Med. Small Anim. Clin. **66:**921, 1971.

Herrgesell, J. D.: Aspirin poisoning in the cat, J. Am. Vet. Med. Assoc. **151:**452, 1967.

Hopes, R.: Symposium: (2) Uses and misuses of anti-inflammatory drugs in racehorses—I, Equine Vet. J. **4:**66, April 1972.

Huebner, R. A., Edens, J. D., and Morton, J. D.: Promazine hydrochloride peletized in alfalfa in large animals, Vet. Med. **58:**883, 1963.

Lev, R., Siegel, H. I., and Glass, G. B.: Effects of salicylates on the canine stomach: a morphological and histochemical study, Gastroenterology **62:**970, 1972.

Moss, M. S.: Symposium: (3) Uses and misuses of anti-inflammatory drugs in racehorses—II, Equine Vet. J. **4:**69, April 1972.

Muir, W. W., III, and Hamlin, R. L.: Effects of acetylpromazine on ventilatory variables in the horse, Am. J. Vet. Res. **36:**1439, 1975.

Rowe, E. T., and Christian, C. W.: Clinical experiences with use of methocarbamol to control muscular spasms in treatment of spinal lesions in dogs, Vet. Med. Small Anim. Clin. **65:**1082, 1970.

15

DRUGS FOR TREATMENT OF
Diseases of the eye

ANATOMY

For one to understand the use of drugs in treating diseases of the eye, a basic knowledge of the physiology and anatomy of the eye is necessary. The anatomy of the eyes of domestic animals discussed in this text have many similar features. However, the management of specific disease conditions of the eye may be unique to a particular species.

Fig. 15-1 shows the basic structures of the eye. The conjunctiva is a membrane that lies over the anterior surface of the eye and the inner aspects of the upper and lower lids. The sclera encompasses the entire globe of the eye with the exception of the small area covered by the cornea. The sclera is white.

The cornea is transparent. It occupies the area over the pupil and iris. The cornea gains its transparency from cells being lined up in columnlike fashion. In corneal edema, the columnlike arrangement is disrupted, and the cornea develops a milky appearance that makes it opaque.

The iris acts as the diaphragm of the eye, regulating the amount of light that is allowed to enter the structure. It is dilated by muscles controlled by the sympathetic nervous system and constricted by muscles controlled by the parasympathetic nervous system. Behind the iris is a lens, which focuses the beam of light entering the eye onto the retina in such a way that the image is clear.

Posterior to the lens the entire globe of the eye is filled with a clear substance called the "vitreous body." This largely contributes to the shape of the eye and the pressure within the eye.

Both the iris and the lens attach directly or indirectly to a structure referred to as the "ciliary body." The ciliary body is involved in the producton of aqueous humor. Aqueous humor is contained in two chambers, which are separated by the iris. These two chambers communicate through the pupil. Aqueous functions as the system by which nutrition is provided to the lens and part of the cornea. Aqueous flow removes metabolic waste products of the structures it bathes. It is also responsible in part for the distention of the globe.

Internally the posterior aspect of the globe

228

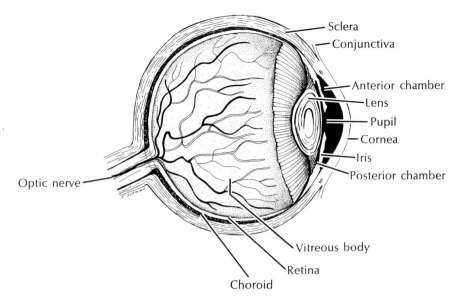

Fig. 15-1. Anatomy of eye.

is lined by the retina. The image is projected on the retina and conducted to the brain through the optic nerve. The choroid lies between the retina and the sclera. It contains the blood vessels that nourish the eye. The vessels extend from the choroid to the ciliary body and iris. These three structures make up the vascular coat, or uvea. The uvea is often described as having an anterior segment, the iris and ciliary body, and a posterior segment, the choroid.

The region in front of the lens that is bound by the lens posteriorly and the posterior surface of the iris anteriorly is referred to as the "posterior chamber." The anterior chamber has the anterior surface of the iris at its posterior boundary and the interior surface of the cornea at its anterior boundary. In the anterior chamber the junction of the cornea and iris base forms the angle through which aqueous humor is removed. This angle is referred to as the "drainage angle."

AQUEOUS HUMOR

In the posterior chamber, aqueous is produced by the ciliary body and ciliary processes. The aqueous fills the posterior chamber and then enters the anterior chamber through the pupil. At the drainage angle the aqueous humor flows into veins and back into the general circulation (Fig. 15-2).

As with the production of urine in the kidneys, the production of aqueous humor depends on both an active and a passive process. The passive process is that of osmosis. The active process is secretion. By enzymatic action, secretion is accomplished with an active transport of sodium ions from the blood to the aqueous humor. The increased osmolality, resulting from the sodium ion shift, causes water to flow in the direction of the highest sodium ion concentration, that is, to the aqueous. In addition to sodium, the active transport of other ions may influence the transport of water. Two that may be important, depending on the species, are bicarbonate ion (HCO_3^-) and chloride ion (Cl^-). Drugs referred to as "carbonic anhydrase inhibitors" are sometimes used to decrease aqueous production. These drugs probably function by decreasing the amount of bicarbonate and/or chloride ion secreted into the aqueous humor. This also decreases the amount of water that follows such ions. (The use of

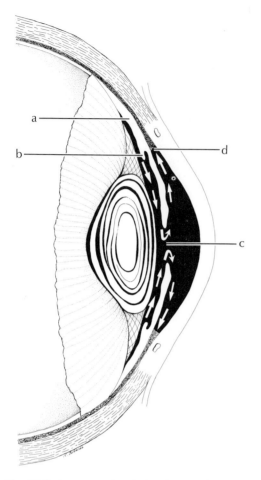

Fig. 15-2. Aqueous circulation in eye. Aqueous is produced in posterior chamber by the ciliary body *(a)* and ciliary processes *(b)*. It flows to anterior chamber through pupil *(c)* and flows into blood vascular system at drainage angle in anterior chamber *(d)*.

carbonic anhydrase inhibitors as diuretics is discussed in Chapter 18.)

Glaucoma

Normally the eye has a certain fluid pressure. When that pressure within the eye exceeds the normal range, a condition referred to as "glaucoma" exists. Glaucoma is simply a description of a sign, that of increased intraocular pressure. Various conditions can cause glaucoma.

The drugs used in glaucoma therapy fall into three categories: those which improve the outflow of aqueous (miotics), those which reduce aqueous production (carbonic anhydrase inhibitors), or those that reduce the volume of intraocular structures, primarily the vitreous body (hyperosmotic agents). Each category is discussed in this chapter.

OPHTHALMIC DRUGS
Administration of ophthalmic drugs

Ophthalmic drugs are administered by either topical instillation, by subconjunctival injection, or systemically. Other methods of administration of ophthalmic drugs, which are beyond the scope of this text, are retrobulbar injection and intraocular injection.

Topical administration. For treating disease of the eyelids, conjunctiva, and anterior segment, topical administration of ophthalmic products is the most frequently used route of administration. Diseases of the posterior segment are primarily treated by systemic administration.

When drugs are placed topically in the eye, they may exit through the nasolacrimal duct and then be either swallowed or removed through the mouth, diffuse into conjunctival blood vessels, or penetrate the cornea. Drugs more readily diffuse into conjunctival blood vessels when the conjunctiva is inflamed and the vessels are more permeable. Ophthalmic drugs are more readily absorbed through the cornea in the presence of keratitis or corneal ulceration.

Solutions, suspensions, and ointments are most frequently used for the topical administration of ophthalmic products in veterinary medicine. As topical solutions or suspensions are placed in the eye, the eye or eyelids should not be touched with droppers or dropper bottles in order to maintain sterility of the drugs. Rather a drop should be allowed to fall into the eye (Fig. 15-3).

The advantages of solutions and suspensions are (1) they are easy to administer, and (2) they produce less interference with healing of the cornea than ointments. Because solutions and suspensions have a

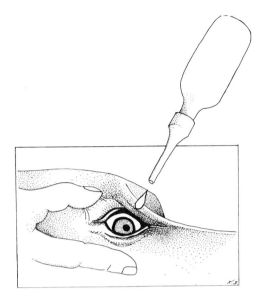

Fig. 15-3. Placing drops in eye. When placing drops in eye, hold container above eye and let drop fall into eye. Container should not contact eye.

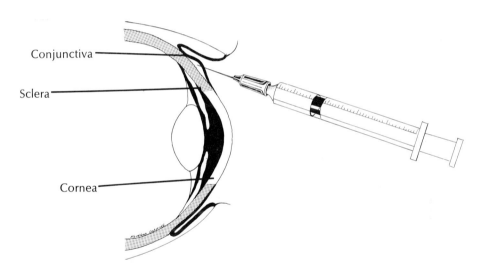

Conjunctiva

Sclera

Cornea

Fig. 15-4. Subconjunctival injection. Medication can be injected under conjunctiva to obtain higher drug levels in eye.

short corneal contact time, they require frequent instillation. This is a substantial disadvantage.

Ophthalmic ointments provide longer corneal contact time than solutions or suspensions. In addition, ointments are less likely to be lost through the nasolacrimal duct. Ointments are particularly good vehicles for antibiotics. However, they blur vision and tend to hold exudate, like pus, in the con-

junctival sac. Ointments retard healing of the cornea more than do solutions.

Subconjunctival injections. Subconjunctival injections (Fig. 15-4) are used to obtain high drug levels inside the eye. The technique is especially useful when maximum levels of a drug are needed quickly and when frequent topical applications are impractical. Subconjunctival administration of ophthalmic drugs is used in treating acute anterior uveitis, panophthalmitis, episcleritis, pannus (infiltration of the cornea with vessels), and corneal burns. Potential side effects from subconjunctival drug administration are conjunctival necrosis and/or fibrosis at the injection sites.

Systemic administration. Drugs are administered systemically to treat diseases of the eyelids, orbit, and posterior and anterior segments. Other routes of drug administration may be combined with systemic medication. Among the ophthalmic drugs given systemically are anti-infectives, corticosteroids, diuretics, hyperosmotic agents, and enzymes. Drugs enter the eye by active transport or simple diffusion through the ciliary processes. They must pass through what is known as the "blood-aqueous barrier." Generally, when there is active ocular inflammation, drug penetration through the blood-aqueous barrier is increased.

Miotics

Miotics cause the pupil to constrict. This increases the drainage angle and facilitates the removal of aqueous, which tends to cause a decrease in the intraocular pressure. There are both short-acting reversible, and long-acting irreversible miotics. They are generally applied to the external surface of the eye in ointments or as solutions.

Short-acting miotics

Pilocarpine. An example of the short activity of miotics is pilocarpine in concentrations of 1% to 4%. Pilocarpine exerts its action by direct parasympathetic action. It reduces aqueous pressure by three actions:
1. Facilitating aqueous outflow by removing the iris tissue from the drainage angle
2. Increasing the outflow of aqueous by the action of the drug on longitudinal muscles, which open the portals through which the aqueous exits from the eye
3. Inhibiting the active secretion of aqueous by the ciliary epithelium

Dose and administration. When used in acute glaucoma, 2% pilocarpine should be administered in the eye once every 5 minutes for the first half hour and then every 3 to 4 hours. Once the desired effects are obtained, a higher concentration of 4% can be administered twice daily rather than administering the 2% four times daily.[6]

Long-acting miotics. Long-acting miotics are irreversible cholinesterase inhibitors. Included in this group are echothiophate, isoflurophate, and demecarium. They reduce intraocular pressure primarily by improving outflow of aqueous. These drugs are not recommended in acute glaucoma because they may cause a severe iritis (inflammation of the iris) and increase vascular congestion. This can result in further reducing the drainage angle. Therefore these drugs are only used after control of acute glaucoma has been achieved with pilocarpine. The anticholinesterase drugs are potent and have prolonged action. These drugs are a convenience to the owner because they may only be administered once a day.

Because these drugs are extremely toxic, owners must be informed of the dangers involved if some of the animal's medication is ingested by children.

Echothiophate 0.06% is used twice daily for 3 to 4 days. Once the pressure in the eye becomes normal, animals may be maintained by decreasing the drug to once daily. If pressures do not stabilize, the concentration of the drug may be increased to 0.12%.[7]

Miotics should not be given in combination. If one drug does not control the condition, another drug should be substituted.

Mydriatics

Mydriatics are drugs that dilate the pupil. They function in one of two ways. One class, which consists of epinephrine and related sympathomimetics, directly stimulates the muscles in the eye controlled by the sympathetic nerves. These muscles dilate the pupil. The other class of drugs, parasympatholytics, blocks the action of acetylcholine on the muscles that would constrict the pupil. The pupil therefore dilates.

In the presence of anterior synechia or

narrow drainage angles, mydriatics are generally contraindicated.

Sympathomimetic mydriatics. In selective cases, sympathomimetic mydriatics such as epinephrine can reduce ocular pressure. This occurs by a reduction in the rate of aqueous production and improving the outflow of aqueous. However, the exact mechanism is unknown. These drugs can only be used in glaucoma in which the angle of drainage is not closed off by the mydriatic effect. For this effect, 1% to 2% epinephrine is administered as a topical drug two or three times daily.[6]

Chemically, phenylephrine is similar to epinephrine. At a 10% concentration, phenylephrine hydrochloride is a potent direct-acting mydriatic. Its action, unlike the parasympatholytics, can be reversed by the instillation of miotics.

In some conditions, adhesions form between the iris and lens (posterior synechia) or between the iris and the cornea (anterior synechia). To prevent these from forming, some veterinarians attempt to keep the iris in motion by alternating miotic and mydriatic drugs. Phenylephrine is an excellent mydriatic for this purpose.[4]

Phenylephrine is also used to dilate the pupil to facilitate ophthalmoscopic examination of the eye.[2]

Parasympatholytic mydriatics. The parasympatholytic mydriatics include atropine, scopolamine, and tropicamide. The drugs of this class paralyze the ciliary body and are referred to as "cycloplegic drugs." Ciliary spasm is an important source of pain in iritis, uveitis, and corneal lesions such as corneal ulceration or keratitis (inflammation of the cornea). One of the most important uses of the parasympatholytic mydriatics is to stop the ciliary spasm associated with these conditions and thereby alleviate pain. When used for this purpose, cycloplegic drugs are far more effective in alleviating pain than local anesthetics. In addition, they do not share the disadvantages of local anesthetics discussed later in this chapter.

Atropine. Atropine, which exerts a my-driatic effect by blocking acetylcholine, is one of the most popular mydriatic drugs. Atropine produces a mydriasis of long duration. After the instillation of one drop of 1% atropine sulfate, mydriasis occurs within an hour and may last up to 5 days in dogs. It is therefore used when prolonged mydriasis is desired.

Once inflammation of the iris and ciliary body occurs in horses and dogs, atropine must be applied frequently to obtain the desired effects. Atropine 1% in dogs may be administered six to eight times daily until dilation occurs. Once mydriasis occurs, the dosage frequency can be reduced. Atropine 3% is often used to treat conditions in horses.

As an alternative to keeping the iris in motion, atropine can be used to keep the iris as far away from the lens as possible to prevent posterior synechia.

A paradoxical profuse salivation may occur in small animals after the instillation of atropine into the eye. This is probably a reflex action occurring when the drug reaches the mouth by way of the nasolacrimal duct.

Tropicamide. A synthetic anticholinergic that can be used as a mydriatic is tropicamide. Tropicamide has a rapid onset of action and short duration. It is an excellent drug for dilating the pupil for examination purposes. In normal eyes, tropicamide usually produces mydriasis within 15 minutes after administration and seldom lasts for more than 8 hours.

Tropicamide does not produce salivation in dogs. In cats it will sometimes produce salivation when the 1% solution is used. However, when a 0.5% concentration is used, salivation rarely occurs.[4]

Hyperosmotic agents

Hyperosmotic agents have higher osmotic pressure than serum. Hyperosmotic agents include 20% mannitol, 30% urea, and glycerol. They are given to increase the osmotic pressure of serum to increase fluid flow from the eye, thereby reducing intraocular pressure. Hyperosmotic agents are used in acute glaucoma only on an emergency basis and are not effective in long-term control. Water must be withheld 2 to 3 hours after administration. Intraocular pressure is primarily reduced by the vitreous (the largest intraocular structure) being markedly dehydrated as a result of the increased serum osmolarity. The effect is usually noted 30 to 35 minutes after administration.

The most widely used hyperosmotic agent in veterinary medicine is glycerol. Most dogs and cats tolerate it well and can be redosed in 4 to 5 hours if necessary. Glycerol is given at the rate of 1 to 2 gm/kg orally as a 50% solution. It can cause vomiting due to gastric irritation.

Mannitol can be administered intravenously as a 20% solution at a dose of 2 gm/kg it should be warmed to body temperature before administration. Urea is administered intravenously at a dose of 1 gm/kg as a 30% solution.

Carbonic anhydrase inhibitors

Another class of drugs that can be used to reduce intraocular pressure are the carbonic anhydrase inhibitors. These include acetazolamide, dichlorphenamide, and ethoxzolamide. The reduction in intraocular pressure is brought about not by the effect of these drugs on the kidney but rather by a direct effect in the eye. In fact, other diuretics, including furosemide and the chlorothiazide diuretics, are not effective in reducing aqueous production and should not be used for glaucoma therapy.

The carbonic anhydrase inhibitors work by directly decreasing aqueous production. They probably act by decreasing the bicarbonate and/or chloride secretion in the eye, thus decreasing the production of aqueous. For a more detailed discussion of the carbonic anhydrase inhibitor diuretics see Chapter 18.

Dose and administration. To reduce intraocular pressure, acetazolamide may be administered at the rate of 7 to 11 mg/kg three times daily; dichlorphenamide may be administered at the rate of 5.5 mg/kg two to three times a day; and ethoxzolamide may

be administered at the rate of 3 to 7 mg/kg three times daily.[6]

Anti-infective drugs

Various anti-infective drugs are used to treat bacterial or fungal infections of the eye. Superficial infections of the cornea or conjunctiva are most easily treated because of their accessibility to topical anti-infective therapy. Structures deeper in the eye, however, are less accessible than other tissues in the body. Anti-infective drugs in general do not penetrate into aqueous as readily as into other body tissues. Because it is essential to get adequate levels of these drugs into the eye when infections are internal, a therapeutic regimen must be designed that will provide effective inhibitory concentrations at the site of infection. Adequate doses must be given systemically to maximize the diffusion of the anti-infective from the blood into the aqueous. If given topically, one must consider how well the drug will diffuse through the cornea. Generally, anti-infective drugs more readily penetrate an abraded or ulcerated cornea than an intact one.

In addition to the ability of a drug to penetrate either the blood aqueous barrier or the cornea, the irritation that can be produced by repeated topical administration of anti-infective drugs must be considered.

When used to treat eye infections, anti-infective drugs are administered either topically, subconjunctivally, or systemically. The ability of a particular anti-infective drug to achieve effective concentrations in the eye varies from one species to another. Unfortunately, data are lacking in veterinary ophthalmology as to which drugs penetrate best in each of the various domestic animal species. When selecting a drug, veterinarians must use their knowledge, primarily based on experience, for the selection of an appropriate anti-infective.

Several ophthalmic preparations contain anti-infectives available for the topical treatment of eye infections. Both ophthalmic drops (sterile solutions in aqueous vehicles) and ophthalmic ointments (sterile ointments usually in mineral oil bases) are available that contain anti-infective drugs. The amount of the preparation applied to the eye and the frequency at which it is applied depends primarily on the condition being treated, the specific anti-infective, and the nature of the topical formulation. Generally, drops must be applied more frequently than ointments. The manufacturer's recommendations regarding dose and frequency of administration should be consulted. The drugs most commonly employed in topical therapy of eye infections follow.

Chloramphenicol. Chloramphenicol provides a broad spectrum of antibacterial action, including many gram-positive and gram-negative bacteria and some rickettsia and viral-like agents. Chloramphenicol is supplied in drop and ointment form. It is most often used in combination with polymyxin B to include antipseudomonal activity in the preparation.

Gentamicin. Gentamicin is available in two different veterinary ophthalmic preparations for topical administration, both with and without dexamethasone, an antiinflammatory corticosteroid. Gentamicin provides a broad spectrum of activity including *Pseudomonas* organisms. Although many gram-positive cocci are sensitive to gentamicin, several stains of streptococci and staphylococci are not. Serious streptococcal infections of the eye have occurred during gentamicin therapy.

Penicillin G. It has been shown that when given intramuscularly at a dose of 20,000 units/kg of body weight, potassium penicillin G reaches low concentrations within the aqueous humor of dogs within 30 minutes. The concentrations of the antibiotic increase and last for at least 2 hours. When 5000 units of penicillin G are administered subconjunctivally, high concentrations of antibiotic are obtained in aqueous humor that last for approximately 6½ hours. When 10,000 units of penicillin G are applied topically to normal corneas, the aqueous humor concentrations reach a peak 30 minutes after in-

stillation. However, the quantity in the aqueous humor is low. When 5000 units of potassium penicillin G are instilled in an eye with abraded cornea, high concentrations result in the aqueous humor within 15 minutes and are detectable 2 hours after instillation.[3] Penicillin G ophthalmic ointment is no longer available for humans, and its availability on the veterinary market varies. It is the antibiotic of choice for streptococcal eye infections in animals.

Neomycin. Neomycin is a broad-spectrum antibiotic commonly used in ophthalmic preparations. Available in both drops and ointment preparations, neomycin is usually in combination with gramicidin or bacitracin to increase effectiveness against gram-positive cocci and polymyxin to include activity against pseudomonal species.

Tetracyclines. The tetraclines, most commonly oxytetracycline, are used topically in the eye. Their spectrum includes many gram-positive and gram-negative organisms, rickettsia, chlamydia, and some large viruses.

Polymyxin B. Effective against most strains of *Pseudomonas*, polymyxin B is often included in ointments and drops containing other antibiotics to prevent growth of *Pseudomonas* organisms in both the eye and the preparation.

Idoxuridine. Idoxuridine is an antiviral agent for topical application. Available in both ointment and drops, idoxuridine is useful in the treatment of keratitis caused by herpesviruses. To be effective the drops should be applied every hour during the day and every other hour during the night. An alternate method is to instill one drop every minute for 5 minutes, repeating this procedure every 4 hours.

For a further discussion of ocular anti-infective drugs see Wyman.[7]

Anti-inflammatory drugs

Corticosteroids are commonly used to treat various eye disorders. Corticosteroids are used in ocular disease to reduce inflammation, prevent vascularization of the cornea, and reduce scarring of the cornea. Both scarring and vascularization of the cornea can interfere with vision. As with anti-infective drugs, it may be necessary to obtain levels of corticosteroids in the aqueous if the drug is to be effective in treating conditions of the internal eye.

Topical instillation of corticosteroids only affects the superficial structures of the eye. These include the conjunctiva, sclera, and cornea. To treat the deeper structures, systemic and/or subconjunctival injection is necessary.[2] The dose and frequency of administration depend on the condition being treated and the corticosteroid being used.

Toxicity. When using corticosteroids in the eye, one must keep in mind that certain dangers are inherent in the use of corticosteroids. Corticosteroids can increase the susceptibility of the eye to viral, bacterial, and fungal infections. Use of corticosteroids in early corneal ulcers sometimes results in superinfection with destruction of the cornea and rupture of the eye. For this reason, corticosteroids should not be used in early corneal ulcers in dogs, cats, and horses. However, as discussed in Chapter 5, the general rule does not apply to cattle. Even in the presence of corneal ulcers in keratoconjunctivitis of cattle, corticosteroids are administered subconjunctivally.

As corneal ulcers heal, corticosteroids are sometimes indicated to prevent vascularization and scarring of the cornea. However, the therapeutician must keep in mind that their use increases the eyes' susceptibility to viral, fungal, or bacterial infection. Safeguards against infection must be taken. Therefore broad-spectrum antibacterials are commonly used with corticosteroids. However, antibacterials usually do not protect the eye from fungi or viruses. Some clinicians believe that the incidence of fungal infections of the eye is increasing as a direct result of indiscriminate use of ophthalmic corticosteroid preparations.

Local anesthetics

In veterinary ophthalmology only a few topical anesthetics are used. They are primarily used to facilitate the performance of minor procedures in the eye. Those most commonly used are tetracaine, proparacaine, and benoxinate. Two percent butacaine, 2% piperocaine, 1% phenocaine, and 0.1% dibucaine cause excessive irritation and toxicity and, therefore, should not be used.

The best way to obtain prolonged topical anesthesia in the conjunctiva and cornea is by repeated instillation. For example, repeated instillation of tetracaine, proparacaine, or benoxinate for 5 minutes increases the duration of anesthesia to approximately 2 hours as opposed to approximately 10 to 20 minutes from a single application.[1]

Toxicity. Because tetracaine is an ester of *p*-aminobenzoic acid, which interferes with the therapeutic action of sulfonamides, it should not be used in combination with sulfonamide therapy.

A disadvantage to the use of topical anesthetics in the eye is that they retard corneal healing. Mild irritation and damage to the normal cornea may result from the use of topical anesthetics. Prolonged application may further intensify the damage. When used over a long period of time the possibility of local hypersensitivity of the eyelids and conjunctiva to the drugs is increased. When tetracaine and benoxinate are used, transient corneal edema may occur. Topical benoxinate may produce an extensive sloughing of the corneal epithelium in dogs with glaucoma and corneal edema. Use of topical anesthetics can increase inflammation in an eye that is already inflamed.

When anesthesia of the cornea and conjunctiva is complete, there is a loss of the protective eyelid reflex, increasing the hazard of exposure keratitis. The insensitive cornea may also be accidently damaged.

Miscellaneous ophthalmic drugs

Synthetic tears. In certain conditions, animals fail to produce tears, and the conjunctiva and cornea become dry. Methylcellulose as a 0.5% to 1% solution is available for use as synthetic tears. Methylcellulose in the artificial tears increases the corneal contact time over nonmethylcellulose solutions.

Synthetic tears must be applied frequently.

When tear production decreases but the tear glands are intact, pilocarpine can be used to increase tear flow. It has been shown experimentally in both dogs and cats that at least 3.75 mg of pilocarpine orally, subcutaneously, or subconjunctivally results in increased tear flow. In dogs, doses of 2 to 4 mg orally resulted in an increase in tear flow. Signs of intoxication include salivation, vomiting, increased heart rate, and, in extreme cases, heart block and pulmonary edema.[4,5]

Fluorescein. Fluorescein is a dye that is used to delineate lesions on the cornea, primarily corneal ulcers and abrasions. Either a solution is applied to the eye or a sterile paper is impregnated with fluorescein and applied to the eyeball for a long enough period for the tears to dissolve the fluorescein. Because the papers are disposable and sterile, they are preferred over the use of a multidose solution. It is easy to contaminate the solution, which serves as a good culture media for *Pseudomonas* species. Subsequent use could produce a disastrous pseudomonal infection in the eye.

References

1. Gelatt, K. N.: Veterinary ophthalmic pharmacology and therapeutics. II. Topical anesthetics, Vet. Med. Small Anim. Clin. **63:**751, 1968.
2. Magrane, W. G.: Canine ophthalmology, Philadelphia, 1965, Lea & Febiger.
3. Rowley, R. A., and Rubin, L. R.: Penetration of penicillin into the aqueous humor of the dog, Am. J. Vet. Res. **30:**1945, 1969.
4. Rubin, L. F.: Applications of adrenergic drugs in ophthalmology, Anim. Hosp. **41:**250, 1968.
5. Rubin, L. F., and Aquirre, G.: Clinical use of pilocarpine for keratoconjunctivitis sicca in dogs and cats, J. Am. Vet. Med. Assoc. **151:**313, 1967.
6. Wyman, M.: Applied anatomy and physiology of the anterior chamber angle, Vet. Clin. North Am. **3:**439, 1973.
7. Wyman, M.: Anti-infectives in ophthalmology, Vet. Clin. North Am. **5:**71, 1975.

Additional readings

Miller, G. K.: Gentamicin for canine and feline eye infections, Vet. Med. Small Anim. Clin. **71:**1577, 1976.
Schmidt, G. M.: Problem oriented ophthalmology. II. Anterior uveitis, Mod. Vet. Pract. **57:**516, 1976.
Schmidt, G. M.: Problem oriented ophthalmology. III. Chronic superficial keratitis, Mod. Vet. Pract. **57:**812, 1976.
Schmidt, G. M.: Problem oriented ophthalmology. IV. Corneal ulceration, Mod. Vet. Pract. **58:**25, 1977.

16

Hormones

ENDOCRINE SYSTEM

The endocrine system consists of glands that secrete hormones. Hormones are chemical substances, produced in a gland, that have an effect on other organs or tissues. Hormones are carried by the blood from their site of secretion to the target organ that they affect.

An example of a hormone is follicle-stimulating hormone (FSH) produced in the pituitary gland, which is located at the base of the brain. FSH stimulates development of follicles in the ovaries of females and production of sperm in the testicles of males.

Hormones are generally administered to animals for one of two purposes. First, when an animal fails to produce sufficient quantities of hormones, therapy is directed at correcting the deficiency. Second, when no deficiency exists, hormones are used to obtain a desired effect. For example, a synthetic progesterone, used as a birth control agent, may be administered to normal bitches.

To fully appreciate the rational use of hormones in veterinary medicine, one must appreciate some basic concepts regarding the endocrine system.

Pituitary gland

The pituitary is the master gland of the endocrine system (Fig. 16-1). It is located at the base of the brain beneath the hypothalamus. The hypothalamus controls the pituitary.

The pituitary gland consists of the anterior pituitary and posterior pituitary, with each portion secreting different hormones. The hormones secreted by the pituitary may produce a direct or an indirect effect. Those with an indirect effect (tropic effect) stimulate the secretion of hormones from other glands. They are secreted by the anterior pituitary. They include thyroid-stimulating hormone (TSH), adrenocorticotropic hormone (ACTH), and the gonadotropic hormones, FSH, and luteinizing hormone (LH). In the male, LH is sometimes referred to as "interstitial cell–stimulating hormone" (ICSH).

Hormones secreted by the anterior pitu-

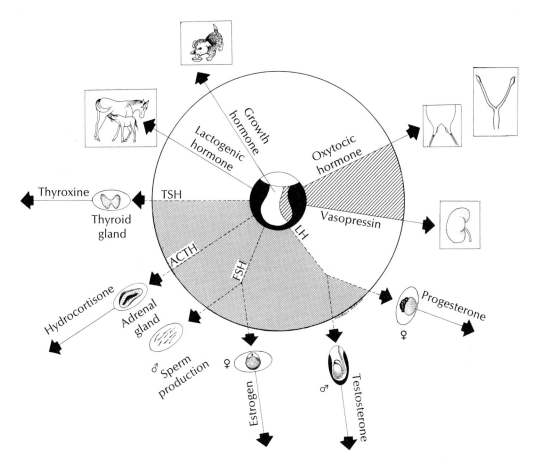

Fig. 16-1. Pituitary gland function. Anterior pituitary gland secretes growth hormone, which is necessary for normal growth; lactogenic hormone, which is necessary for milk production; thyroid-stimulating hormone (TSH), which causes thyroid gland to secrete thyroxine; adrenocorticotropic hormone (ACTH), which causes adrenals to secrete hydrocortisone; follicle-stimulating hormone (FSH), which in male causes sperm production and in female causes development of Graafian follicle and estrogen production; and luteinizing hormone (LH), which in male causes testosterone production in testicles and in female causes development of corpus luteum and production of progesterone. Posterior pituitary gland secretes oxytocic hormone, which causes milk let-down and uterine contractions, and vasopressin, which increases water resorption in kidney.

itary that have direct actions in the body are growth hormone and lactogenic hormone. The posterior pituitary secretes two direct-acting hormones. These are oxytocic hormone and vasopressin, the antidiuretic hormone.

Other endocrine glands

The *thyroid gland* is located in the neck. Under the influence of TSH, it secretes the thyroid hormone, thyroxine. Thyroxine aids in regulation of metabolism in the body. The term "metabolism" is used to refer to all the chemical and energy transformations that occur in the body. When one speaks of a specific metabolism such as carbohydrate metabolism, one is referring to all the transformations that occur in the body involving carbohydrates. Animals oxidize carbohydrates, proteins, and fats, producing principally carbon dioxide, water, and the energy necessary for life processes. In the body this occurs step by step in a process referred to as "catabolism," which liberates energy in small usable amounts. The body also stores energy in the form of proteins, fats, and complex carbohydrates synthesized from simpler molecules. As the substances are formed, they take up rather than liberate energy. This is called "anabolism."

Alongside the thyroid are the *parathyroid glands*, which secrete parathyroid hormone. Parathyroid hormone regulates calcium and phosphorous metabolism.

The *islets of Langerhans* in the pancreas secrete insulin, which controls sugar metabolism.

The *adrenal glands*, which lie near the kidneys, consist of two zones, each secreting different hormones. The center of the glands, the medulla, secretes epinephrine and norepinephrine, which stimulate activity of the sympathetic nervous system. The adrenal cortex surrounds the medulla. Under the influence of ACTH from the anterior pituitary gland, the adrenal cortex secretes hydrocortisone. In addition, ACTH stimulates production of the male sex hormones (androgens) and the female sex hormones (estrogens and progestogens) in the adrenal cortex. All three sex hormones are produced in the adrenal cortex in both sexes. The adrenal cortex also produces aldosterone, which is concerned principally with the control of water and electrolyte metabolism. It acts on the kidney to conserve sodium and excrete potassium. Rather than being influenced by ACTH, aldosterone production and secretion are influenced by the levels of serum sodium and potassium and the degree of hydration.

Although sex hormones are produced by the adrenal cortex, the glands primarily responsible for their production are the *gonads*. In the female, depending on the stage of the estrus cycle, the ovaries produce primarily estrogen or progesterone. In the male under the influence of ISCH the interstitial cells of the testes produce the androgens, primarily testosterone.

The clinical use of pituitary hormones, corticosteroids, sex hormones, and thyroid hormone is discussed in this chapter. Parathyroid hormone and insulin are discussed in Chapter 17.

CLINICAL USE OF HORMONES

When hormones are used clinically, either the natural hormone from the glands of animals or hormones manufactured synthetically are used.

Corticosteroids

Although there is some overlapping of function, corticosteroids are divided into two groups. The mineralocorticoids primarily influence how electrolytes are handled in the body. They cause retention of sodium and facilitate the excretion of potassium. Glucocorticoids make up the second group. In animals the primary glucocorticoid, hydrocortisone, is formed and secreted in response to stimulation of the adrenal cortex by ACTH. In a feedback mechanism, hydrocortisone levels affect the release of ACTH by the pituitary. ACTH secretion is inhibited or prevented when the hydrocortisone level reaches a certain critical point. This has an important therapeutic consequence. When glucocorticoids are administered therapeutically, ACTH is suppressed, and the adrenal cortex may become seriously depleted of hydrocortisone. If therapeutic steroids are suddenly withdrawn after chronic administration, the adrenals may be unable to respond when natural steroids are needed. This can place the animal in a severe crisis. To prevent this, prolonged courses of therapy are often gradually withdrawn over a 2-week period. Suppression of the adrenal glands may be reduced if corticosteroids are given only every other day. This allows therapeutic levels of the corticosteroid to drop and allows ACTH to stimulate the adrenals to produce more hydrocortisone. Another good idea is to administer corticosteroids at the time of day when natural secretion is highest. In humans this is in the morning. In animals this is assumed to be at the beginning of *their* "day."

For daytime animals like dogs and horses, it is in the morning and for nocturnal animals like cats, in the evening.

The glucocorticoids decrease inflammation. In addition, they initiate metabolic processes that break down tissue proteins, converting them to glucose (gluconeogenesis). Administration of corticosteroids results in increased blood glucose levels and increases the storage of glucose in the liver in the form of glycogen. Because of their tendency to break down proteins if high doses of glucocorticoids are administered over long periods of time, muscle mass is reduced and brittle bones result.

It has been theorized that glucocorticoids reduce inflammation by the following mechanisms[14]:

- Maintaining normal permeability of the vascular bed, thus preventing edema
- Stabilizing and maintaining the integrity of the microcirculation in the involved area
- Decreasing resistance in the vascular bed and improving venous return
- Exerting antiallergic action by modifying the effects of histamine on the cells

The commonly used glucocorticoids vary in their activity in terms of potency, relative activity, rate of absorption, and amount of ACTH suppression.

Types. Various synthetic corticosteroids have been developed by drug companies. Commercially produced corticosteroids are primarily used for their anti-inflammatory and gluconeogenic effects. Among those currently in use in veterinary medicine are the following:

Betamethasone	Methylprednisolone
Desoxycorticosterone	acetate
acetate (USP)	Prednisolone
Desoxycorticosterone	Prednisolone sodium
pivalate	succinate
Flumethasone	Prednisone
9-Fluoroprednisolone	Triamcinolone
acetate	acetonide
Hydrocortisone	

For parenteral use two types of corticosteroid preparations are available: water soluble and water insoluble. When intravenous administration is desired such as in shock, water-soluble corticosteroids are used. For nonemergency situations such as arthritis and dermatitis, sterile suspensions of water-insoluble products are used. These suspensions can be given intramuscularly, subcutaneously, or intralesionally and are generally absorbed slowly.

Use. We have already discussed a wide variety of conditions in animals for which corticosteroids are administered to combat inflammation. Corticosteroids may be used topically or systemically in various skin conditions. Their use as anti-inflammatory agents in traumatic musculoskeletal and arthritic conditions is discussed in Chapter 20. As has been noted, they are used in ophthalmology to reduce inflammation and prevent scarring of the cornea. We discussed their value in the treatment of acute mastitis in cattle to prevent scar formation in the udder.

The glucocorticoids are also used in bovine ketosis to restore normal blood glucose levels (Chapter 17) and in the treatment of shock (Chapter 18).

The dose is dependent on the steroid that is used, the condition for which it is used, and the species in which it is used. Recommendations of the manufacturer should be consulted.

Toxicity. Excessive use of corticosteroids can result in some or all of the following toxic effects:

- Sodium and water retention
- Potassium depletion
- Excessive protein breakdown
- Gastric bleeding
- Suppression of the immune system (with large doses)
- Decreased calcium absorption
- Suppression of ACTH secretion by the anterior pituitary
- Development of brittle bones that fracture easily
- Aggravation of diabetes by increasing blood sugar
- Decreased immune response, which

may increase susceptibility to infectious diseases

• Retarded bone and wound healing

Depending on the type of corticosteroid and the dose and time when it is administered to pregnant cattle, abortion or early calving can result. Steroids that have been reported to cause either abortion or early calving are dexamethasone, betamethasone, flumethasone, and 9-fluoroprednisolone acetate.[13,20] Parturition can be induced during the last 3 months of pregnancy. If delivered during the last 14 days of gestation, the calf will generally be healthy. However, inducing parturition as late as 1 month before full term can result in the delivery of a calf that is too immature to survive. The risk of uterine in-

fections and retained placenta is increased when corticosteroids are used to induce the parturition of immature calves. When induced by the use of corticosteroids, parturition generally occurs within 24 to 48 hours after the administration of the drug. Doses used to induce parturition in cattle are 15 to 20 mg of dexamethasone or the equivalent.[19]

Cushing's syndrome. Many side effects of corticosteroids occur naturally when animals overproduce the corticosteroid hormones. This is referred to as "Cushing's syndrome," which occurs in dogs as well as in humans.

Treatment. Cushing's syndrome in dogs has been treated effectively using *o,p*-DDD.[21,26] The drug is an isomer of the insecticide DDT. It has been used in humans for

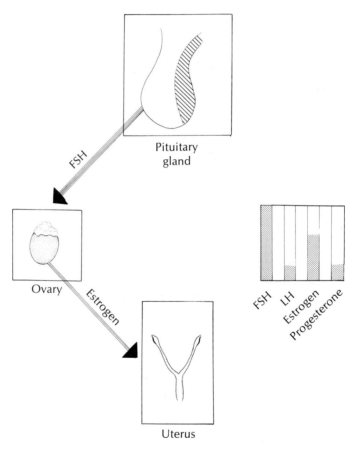

Fig. 16-2. Proestrus. Under influence of FSH, ovary develops Graafian follicle, which secretes estrogen. Estrogen causes uterus to become more vascular.

the treatment of Cushing's syndrome and for prolonging the useful life of humans with inoperable adrenocortical carcinoma.

Side effects in dogs directly related to *o,p*-DDD are depression, loss of appetite, and hyperpigmentation of the fur. When treatment is discontinued, the depression and loss of appetite should completely reverse. Because of the toxic potential,

o,p-DDD should only be used under close supervision by the attending veterinarian.

Good results have been obtained in dogs when an initial daily dose of 50 mg/kg was administered until adequate response or adverse side effects are noticed. The daily dose is given for 4 to 13 days. Following the daily dosage, 50 mg/kg are administered once a week indefinitely.[26]

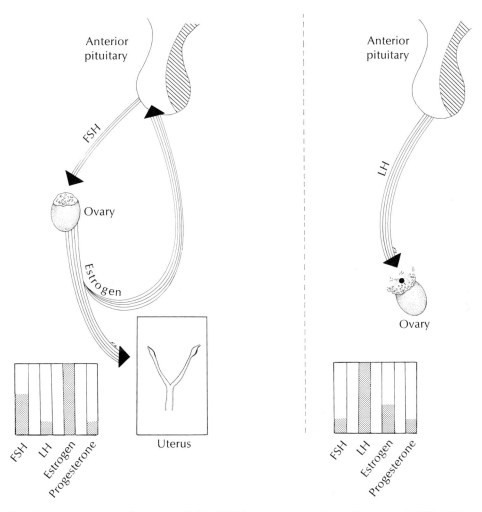

Fig. 16-3. Estrus. In early estrus *(left)*, follicle matures under influence of FSH. High levels of estrogen cause female to become receptive to breeding and cause uterine changes. Uterus becomes highly vascular, mucosa grows, and uterine and vaginal mucus increase. High blood levels of estrogen block further release of FSH. In most species during late estrus *(right)*, there is sudden surge of LH produced in pituitary, which causes ovulation.

Sex hormones

Normal estrus cycle

To understand the use of the various sex hormones in veterinary medicine, one must understand the female estrus cycle. The female sexual cycle of domesticated animals is different from that of animals in the order of primates, of which the human is a member.

The estrus cycle in all animals is regulated by hormones from the anterior pituitary gland, FSH and LH. The release of these hormones is under control of the hypothalamus, which lies above the pituitary.

FSH stimulates development of Graafian follicles in the ovary. In the Graafian follicle the ovum is developed and the hormone estrogen is secreted.

LH stimulates rupture of the Graafian follicle and release of the ovum into the reproductive tract (ovulation). It also stimulates development of the corpus luteum in the ovary. The corpus luteum secretes the hormone progesterone.

The estrus cycle of animals can be roughly divided into the following phases: proestrus, estrus, metestrus, diestrus, and anestrus.

1. *Proestrus* (Fig. 16-2). During proestrus the pituitary gland secretes high levels of FSH. This stimulates growth of the Graafian follicle in the ovary. As the Graafian follicle grows, it begins to secrete the hormone estrogen. Progesterone levels are low. The uterus during proestrus becomes more vascular.

2. *Estrus (heat)* (Fig. 16-3). In animals the period of estrus is defined as that period when the female is receptive to breeding. The behavior probably results from high levels of blood estrogen secreted by the Graafian follicle. As the level of estrogen rises, it blocks further release of FSH from the pituitary. During estrus the Graafian follicle is large and mature. It secretes estrogen. The uterus becomes highly vascular; the lining of the uterus, the mucosa, grows rapidly; and large amounts of uterine and vaginal mucus are present. Most species ovulate toward the end of estrus. However, cattle ovulate after estrus, and cats only ovulate following coitus.

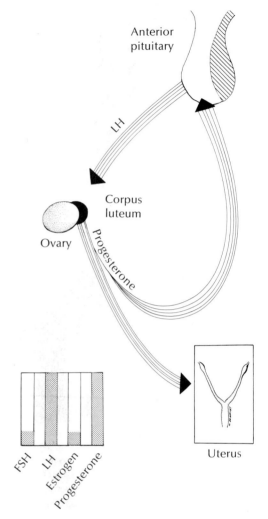

Fig. 16-4. Metestrus. Continued secretion of LH by anterior pituitary causes development of corpus luteum in ovary. Corpus luteum produces progesterone, which causes uterus to prepare for implantation of fertilized ova. Progesterone also inhibits FSH release by anterior pituitary.

Just prior to ovulation the pituitary secretes high levels of LH. The LH probably stimulates ovulation.

3. *Metestrus* (Fig. 16-4). During metestrus the pituitary secretes LH, which stimulates formation of the corpus luteum in the ovary. As the corpus luteum develops, it secretes progesterone. Progesterone inhibits the pro-

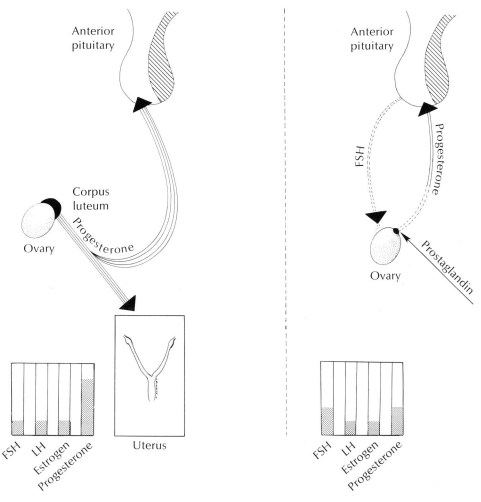

Fig. 16-5. Diestrus. In early diestrus *(left)*, pituitary activity is low. Corpus luteum continues to secrete progesterone, which inhibits secretion of either FSH or LH. Uterus is ready to accept fertilized ova. In late diestrus *(right)* in some species, prostaglandins cause corpus luteum to shrink and progesterone levels to drop. As progesterone secretion drops, FSH is secreted by anterior pituitary and animal is about to enter proestrus of new cycle.

duction of FSH by the pituitary and therefore prevents the development of more Graafian follicles. During metestrus, estrogen levels are low. The uterus adapts to prepare for the implantation of fertilized ova.

4. *Diestrus* (Fig. 16-5). During diestrus pituitary activity is low. The ovary contains a mature corpus luteum, which continues to secrete progesterone. The high concentration of progesterone in the blood continues

to inhibit the secretion of either FSH or LH by the pituitary and the development of Graafian follicles in the ovary. Estrogen levels are low. In some species, toward the end of diestrus, a chemical is released, probably by the uterus, that causes the corpus luteum to regress. This compound is probably prostaglandin. When the chemical is released and the corpus luteum regresses, blood concentrations of progesterone drop. This stimu-

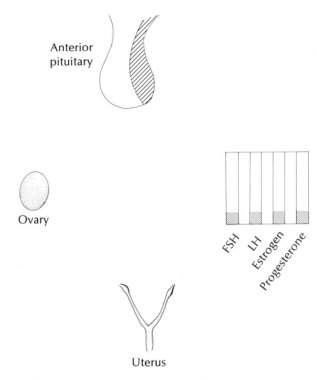

Fig. 16-6. Anestrus. During anestrus, there is virtually no production of gonadotropins in anterior pituitary, and ovary and uterus are inactive.

lates the anterior pituitary to secrete FSH and a new cycle begins. However, this does not occur in all species. In the dog and the cat, no compound has been demonstrated that will cause the corpus luteum to regress.[17] If pregnancy occurs, progesterone continues to be secreted by the corpus luteum to maintain a uterine environment hospitable for the fetus.

5. *Anestrus* (Fig. 16-6). In species in which anestrus does not occur, the female always goes from diestrus to proestrus. However, in other species, anestrus occurs under two sets of circumstances. For certain species such as the canine it occurs as part of their normal cycle. The canine estrus cycle is very long compared to most animals discussed in this text. After diestrus in the canine there is a long period of time when the reproductive tract is quiet. That period is referred to as "anestrus."

Some species of animals, for example, horses and sheep, only have sexual cycles during certain periods of the year. During those times when they are not cycling, they are said to be in a state of anestrus. However, when they are cycling, the cycle is typical as just described, consisting of proestrus, estrus, metestrus, and diestrus.

In either of these cases, animals during anestrus show little activity in the secretion of gonadotropins or in the ovaries and reproductive tract. Levels of progesterone and estrogen are low in such animals.

Bovine estrus cycle. The total cycle in the cow lasts on an average of 21 days, with a range of approximately 18 to 24 days. Proestrus lasts from 1.5 to 3 days and estrus from 1 to 2 days. Ovulation occurs about 10 hours after cows enter metestrus. Bovine metestrus lasts from 14 to 16 days. Diestrus occurs from 1.5 to 3 days. Ovulation is spontaneous. The fact that it occurs about 10 hours after cows leave estrus aids in the practice of artificial insemination. Cows show obvious signs of estrus, and when they are observed, the rancher can arrange to have the cow bred. Even if the cow comes out of estrus prior to the time the inseminator arrives, there is a good chance she will be inseminated prior to ovulation.

Ovine estrus cycle. Among the animals discussed in this text, only the ewe and mare have periods of the year during which they do not sexually cycle. It is likely that the period of anestrus developed in the species to help assure that they would give birth during the time when climatic conditions were most favorable for survival of the offspring. Ewes tend to cycle in the fall of the year. A major factor influencing their fertile periods is the shortening of daylight. Because they lamb 150 days after breeding, most births occur in the spring. The estrus cycle in the ewe lasts approximately 17 days. Estrus lasts approximately 30 to 40 hours. Ewes ovulate near the end of estrus.

Equine estrus cycle. In the northern hemisphere most mares come into heat from approximately February to August. Generally, mares are in anestrus between October and February. The gestation in horses is approximately 355 days. Estrus in the mare lasts about 5 days. They ovulate approximately 24 hours before the end of heat. Mares are usually bred on the second or third day of heat and, if estrus is prolonged, may be bred a second time.

Canine estrus cycle. In the dog each phase of the estrus cycle is approximately ten times longer than the same phase in the cow. The cycle is an average 217 days long. Unlike other domestic animals and humans, the normal cycle of the dog contains adequate periods of time for pregnancy and lactation. Pregnancy usually lasts approximately 63 days and lactation approximately 40 days. Proestrus is recognized by the vulva swelling and exuding a reddish discharge. Ovulation usually occurs on the first day of estrus as opposed to the last day in the cow. Various figures are given for the length of proestrus and estrus in the bitch. Jochle[18] states that proestrus lasts 5 to 12 days and estrus lasts 8 to 14 days. On about the ninth day after the first appearance of a vaginal discharge, the discharge shows a lightening or yellowing. Forty-eight hours after the light discharge appears, mating should be attempted. It should be repeated again in 48 hours.[23] If animals are not to be bred, they must be isolated during the entire proestrus and estrus periods.

During the first 4 days of estrus, estrogens increase to peak levels. After estrus, metestrus lasts for approximately 140 days and anestrus for 30 to 90 days.

There are numerous differences between the human sexual cycle and that of the bitch which are commonly misunderstood by dog owners. The primary differences are as follows:

1. Bitches commonly discharge from the vulva for a 21-day period, as opposed to a 4- to 5-day period in the human.

2. The vaginal discharge of the bitch signifies proliferation of tissues in the uterus for reception of the fertilized ova. In the human it signifies degeneration of uterine tissue following lack of implantation of a fertilized ova.

3. The sexual interest in the bitch is at a maximum approximately 9 to 12 days after heat is manifested. The chance for fertilization at this time is also optimal.[24]

Bitches should not be bred until they are full grown but under 7 years of age.

In addition to a unique estrus cycle, the bitch responds in a unique way to the sex hormones. The uterus of the dog may respond to certain androgenic, estrogenic, and progestrogenic hormones by extreme proliferation (glandular cystic hyperplasia). This can predispose the uterus to disease states such as pyometra, a condition in which the uterus becomes distended with pus.

Long-term administration of progesterone and its derivatives can cause a type of mammary tumor that commonly disappears when the administration of progesterone is discontinued.

The bitch's bone marrow is uniquely sensitive to natural and synthetic estrogens. When these are administered, uncontrollable bleeding due to a reduction in thrombocytes (which play an important role in the clotting process) can result.

Feline estrus cycle. The estrus cycle of the queen (female cat) is different from either the bitch or cow. Ovulation only results from coitus or mechanical stimulation of the cervix. If mating does not occur, the ripe follicles degenerate and shrink and willingness to mate vanishes temporarily. However, in about 7 to 10 days a new set of follicles begin to ripen. After parturition, cats have a fertile heat within 18 to 30 hours.

Antifertility compounds

Because of a large surplus of dogs and cats in the United States, some form of pet population control is necessary to prevent the destruction of approximately 15 million dogs and cats per year in American pounds. While surgical sterilization of males and females is a highly successful form of population control, it is too expensive for some owners and considered undesirable by others. Some reliable and easily administered chemicals that would prevent conception would be a highly desirable form of population control in pets.

Medroxyprogesterone acetate (MAP). Medroxyprogesterone acetate (MAP) is derived from progesterone. The drug has been used to delay estrus in the bitch for 6 months or more. The long-term effect of a single administration of the drug by subcutaneous or intramuscular injection probably results from its low solubility in body fluids and the resulting slow absorption from the injection site.

Effectiveness. The drug is highly effective. For example, in one trial MAP was used to delay estrus in beagle and mongrel bitches weighing approximately 10 kg each. When administered subcutaneously at the rate of 50 mg/kg, estrus was delayed an average of 12.5 months with a range from 6 to 26.5 months.[5]

Toxicity. In the 1960s MAP was removed from the American market as an antifertility drug in bitches because of numerous problems associated with its use. Among the reported problems are the following[5,29,30]:

1. Thinning of the hair over the subcutaneous injection site
2. A vaginal discharge that has a creamy appearance 30 days after treatment
3. Changes in the lining of the uterus that may predispose to pyometra, which necessitates surgical removal of the uterus

By far the most important side effects of MAP are the uterine changes referred to as "endometrial cystic hyperplasia." It has been observed that when bitches are treated with MAP in late metestrus or during anestrus, little change in uterine size results. However, those treated in proestrus have substantial increases in uterine size.[29]

It has been hypothesized that the uterine problems associated with the use of MAP occur if the drug is given when natural high levels of estrogen or progesterone exist. When estrogen is given alone to intact bitches, there is some uterine stimulation but no cystic hyperplasia. Estrogen stimulation followed by progesterone does produce cystic hyperplasia. In fact, large doses of progesterone given alone will cause cystic hyperplasia. However, when only 50 mg of MAP are injected subcutaneously, it does not cause proliferation of the endometrium in bitches with no ovaries. These dogs of course have low levels of estrogens and progesterones.[30] Therefore one may conclude that a 50 mg dose of MAP is safe in bitches with low estrogen levels.

Dose and administration. Although MAP is not currently available in the United States for use as an antifertility agent in the bitch, it has been reintroduced in Great Britain. Currently the recommended dose is 50 mg for dogs weighing less than 40 kg and 50 to 75 mg for those weighing more than 40 kg.[31]

To minimize side effects of the drug, the recommended dosage should be carefully followed. In addition, MAP should not be administered to animals with signs of genital disease. MAP must not be administered during estrus or proestrus because of the high levels of natural estrogens at that time. To administer MAP at the stage of the estrus cycle when damage to the endometrium is least likely to occur, it is suggested that bitches be allowed to experience their first heat prior to administration to establish without doubt the phase of the estrus cycle at the time of administration. The treatment should then be given 5 months after the start of proestrus as determined by vaginal discharge. Five months after the start of proestrus, estrogen and progesterone blood levels are low.

Megestrol acetate. Megestrol acetate is a potent synthetic progesterone that is orally effective. In the dog the drug is primarily excreted by the liver, with only 10% being excreted by the kidney. The half-life of megestrol in dogs is 8 days, which is ten times that found in women.[6,25] Megestrol acetate is used in dogs as an oral contraceptive.

Effectiveness. In an experimental trial it has been shown that when megestrol is given orally to bitches in proestrus at the rate of 2.2 mg/kg for 8 days, estrus is suppressed in 92% of bitches. Of animals on which follow-up data were obtained, 89% experienced estrus within 4 to 28 weeks after treatment was discontinued. When bitches in anestrus are administered megestrol, 0.55 mg/kg, for 32 days, signs of proestrus or estrus do not occur during the treatment period in 97% of animals. Follow-up reports on a limited number of these experimental animals indicate that normal estrus occurred in about 93% from 1 to 7 months after treatment was discontinued.[6]

Toxicity. Occasional adverse effects were reported in the bitches treated during anestrus in the trials just cited. These include mammary enlargement, listlessness, lactation, changes in temperament such as nervousness or irritability, increased or decreased appetite, exceptional weight gain, or intestinal disturbances. However, all such effects disappeared within a week after ceasing treatment. Even for animals treated during the proestrus stage, when estrogen levels were high, the adverse effects were mild and ceased within a week after the megestrol acetate was discontinued. Why is megestrol almost free of side effects, even when given to dogs in proestrus, when MAP would be expected to cause serious problems? The relative lack of serious side effects reported so far may be due to the relatively short time megestrol is present in the animal after administration, as compared to MAP. Megestrol is contraindicated in first heat bitches because there is substantial variability in the signs of the first heat and the animal may be sexually immature.

Megestrol acetate should not be used in bitches with disease or any reproductive disorders. It should not be used in pregnant dogs or in dogs with mammary tumors. Some mammary tumors may be stimulated by exogenous progesterones.

Dose and administration. Megestrol acetate is administered to the bitch for three purposes (Table 16-1):

1. During proestrus to postpone estrus
2. During anestrus to postpone estrus
3. For the treatment of false pregnancies

When used during proestrus for postponement of estrus, administration must be started during the first 3 days of proestrus. If

Table 16-1. Use of megestrol acetate in the bitch

Purpose	Remarks	Oral dose
During proestrus to postpone estrus	Start treatment during first 3 days of proestrus	2.2 mg/kg for 8 consecutive days
During anestrus to postpone proestrus and estrus	Start administration 7 days prior to date on which effect is desired	0.55 mg/kg for 32 days
Treatment of false pregnancies	Make sure condition is not a true pregnancy	2.2 mg/kg for 8 consecutive days

given later, the drug will be less effective. If started before or after the third day of proestrus, the bitch may proceed into estrus, or if estrus is postponed, she will return to estrus at a very early date, possibly as soon as 2 to 3 weeks. During proestrus megestrol acetate is administered orally at the rate of 2.2 mg/kg of body weight daily for 8 consecutive days.

When used during anestrus to postpone a pending estrus, the daily oral dose must be started 7 days prior to the desired onset of effect. Bitches will normally cycle 2 to 6 months after anestrus administration of megestrol acetate. During anestrus for postponement of estrus megestrol acetate is given orally at the rate of 0.55 mg/kg of body weight daily for 32 days.

Megestrol acetate can be used to treat false pregnancies when the bitch is free of uterine disease or disease of other reproductive organs. Care must be taken to be sure the condition is false pregnancy and not true pregnancy. For treating false pregnancies it is given orally at the rate of 2.2 mg/kg of body weight for 8 consecutive days. Improvement should occur in 3 to 4 days.

Other antifertility drugs. In addition to synthetic progesterones, other methods of contraception in the bitch have been proposed. The subcutaneous implantation of testosterone in a slow-release form has been suggested as one possible way to obtain reversible long-term contraception in the bitch.[27] Prior to its use clinically, however, further investigation is necessary.

It has also been suggested that population control could be achieved in dogs if males were immunized against bovine LH. Experimentally, such immunization has resulted in circulating antibodies that are associated with atrophy of the testes, epididymis, and prostate gland. There are preliminary indications that animals will eventually return to normal as the levels of antibodies drop.[12] This approach needs further investigation.

Drugs to produce abortion

Diethylstilbestrol (DES). DES is commonly administered to prevent pregnancy following the unwanted mating of a bitch.

Effectiveness. Best results are obtained if treatment is begun as soon after the mating as possible. However, successful treatments using DES have been reported up to 10 days after the mismating.

Toxicity. It should be recognized that administration of DES entails a risk of endometrial disturbances leading to pyometra. In addition, administration of natural and synthetic estrogens to bitches can cause uncontrollable bleeding due to a decrease in thrombocytes. Thrombocytes, which are essential to the clotting process, are produced in the bone marrow, which in the bitch is uniquely sensitive to estrogens.

Dose and administration. Recommended doses vary. They generally fall in the range of 1 to 20 mg per dog orally immediately followed by 1 mg orally daily for 5 days.

Malucidin. Malucidin, a yeast fraction isolated from spent brewers yeast, has been given intravenously to cause abortion in dogs. When given prior to the forty-fourth day of pregnancy, the fetuses will absorb within 48 to 60 hours. However, if the drug is administered after the forty-sixth day of pregnancy, fetuses will be aborted within 24 hours. This occurs with no apparent harm to the bitch.[34]

A serious side effect that can occur when administering malucidin is a severe drop in blood pressure. Some individuals recommend the use of epinephrine to counteract this drop in blood pressure. However, others contend that epinephrine may prevent the drug from causing abortion.

A total dose of 22 mg/kg of body weight is recommended. It should be given as follows: 2.2 mg/kg are initially given intravenously, followed in 10 minutes by the balance to avoid a severe drop in blood pressure.[25]

N-Desacetyl thiocolchicine (DCT). It has been reported that the administration of 2 mg/kg of body weight of DCT given once intravenously during the second half of gestation will induce death and abortion in a high percentage of canine litters within 2 days. Abortion closely imitates natural birth at term. The drug does not appear to affect subsequent fertility or quantity of litters.

Generally, after 24 to 48 hours, expulsion

of dead but intact fetuses and fetal membranes begins. It appears that the action of the drug is direct or indirect stimulation of smooth muscles. This is evidenced by vomiting, diarrhea, and contraction of the pregnant uterus. It appears that the pregnant uterus is highly sensitive to DCT and that other organ systems are less sensitive to it.

Toxic reactions include one or two evacuations of loose stools within 1 to 3 hours after administration of the drug and slight retching and vomiting. Other than that, discomfort should be minimal.[32] Further clinical investigation is necessary before recommending the drug for routine usage in small-animal practice.

Corticosteroids. It has been mentioned earlier in this chapter that certain corticosteroids produce abortion or early calving in cattle. Because it is imperative that both dairy and beef cows produce one calf annually, the clinical use of corticosteroids to produce abortion is limited. However, care must be exercised in the use of these drugs for other therapeutic purposes so that abortion is not caused inadvertently. If corticosteroids are used to produce either abortion or early calving, a high percentage of fetal membrane retention may result.

Drugs to synchronize estrus in cows

If methods could be developed to reliably synchronize fertile estrus periods in both dairy and beef herds, there would be great economic benefit. We have previously mentioned that substantial differences exist in the manner by which dairy and beef cattle are managed. One difference is the way cows are bred.

Dairy cattle are primarily bred by artificial insemination. Because dairy cows are handled twice daily, having them available for the artificial inseminator is little problem.

The advantages of artificial insemination in dairy cattle follow:

1. The rancher is able to breed his cows to higher quality bulls than he would be able to afford if he had to purchase his own. Many heifers born on dairy ranches are raised to replace retiring cows from the milking string.

The amount of milk they will be capable of producing over a lifetime is as dependent on the genes of the sire as those of the dam.

2. The rancher is saved the expense of maintaining his own bulls.

3. The rancher is spared the problems of maintaining dangerous dairy bulls.

4. Fertility of semen used in artificial insemination is proven. However, fertility of a bull standing in natural service is always in question.

Although theoretically artificial insemination would be useful in beef breeds, the management of beef animals usually makes artificial insemination impractical. As opposed to being handled twice a day, beef cattle roam on large pastures or range areas. It is therefore difficult to detect heat and to restrain the animals for artificial insemination. Because beef bulls are usually not as aggressive as those used in dairy practice, they are not as difficult to maintain on a ranch. However, if all cows on a ranch could be brought into heat at the same time, there would be several advantages to using artificial insemination in beef cattle. One is the proven fertility of the semen used. The other is that semen of higher genetic quality would be available for the average rancher to use.

Synchronization of fertile estrus in both beef and dairy cattle would be an effective management tool to increase production. For beef cattle it would also permit the use of artificial insemination on a practical basis. Synchronization would facilitate the detection of heat and allow a large group to be artificially inseminated at one time. In addition, a more uniform calf crop with a potentially higher value would be produced. In dairy breeds the synchronization of fertile heat periods would allow greater numbers of cattle to be inseminated at the time the inseminator visits the ranch.

For years attempts have been made to bring many cows into heat at the same time. It was recognized that when estrogens were administered to animals, the signs of heat were produced. However, the administration of estrogens produce a sterile heat because the animal is responding to the high levels of blood estrogen even though no Graafian follicle is present. Fertile estrus occurs only after a Graafian follicle develops and ovulation takes place. Only by understanding the endocrine interrelationships, can one understand the rationale behind the attempts to synchronize fertile estrus in cattle.

The drugs that have been used effectively to synchronize heat in cattle are the progesterones and prostaglandins.

Progesterones. Various progesterones have been used to synchronize heat in cattle. Progesterones are effective in synchronizing heat. However, most tests indicate that there is a high rate of infertility at the first synchronized heat period.[22] At the second heat period, fertility may be normal. The administration of progesterones to cattle probably synchronizes heat by preventing development of a new Graafian follicle after the lysis of the cow's corpus luteum. If the progesterone is given for a long enough period of time, all cows, regardless of the stage of their cycle at the initiation of therapy, would be at the same stage, that is, diestrus with no corpus luteum. When the progesterone is discontinued, the plasma levels of progesterone drop, FSH is then released by the anterior pituitary, allowing for the development of follicles and a relatively simultaneous appearance of estrus.

Melengestrol acetate (MGA). Melengestrol acetate (MGA) is an orally active progesterone with the ability to prevent estrus and ovulation. Chemically it is related to both MAP and megestrol. MGA, however, has been reported to be more than 300 times more potent than MAP in synchronizing estrus.[28]

Effectiveness. After giving MGA orally to cows for 14 days, heat could be expected in 3 to 11 days after discontinuance of the MGA.[8,28]

Comparing the total fertility rates resulting from breeding during the first and second heat periods after MGA administration, it appears that animals given MGA have a conception rate similar to that of animals not re-

ceiving MGA. If MGA is to be used to synchronize animals, it would, perhaps, be wise to administer 1500 IU of human chorionic gonadotropin, which is high in LH, to stimulate ovulation at the time of insemination. There are indications that this procedure will increase fertility rates of nonsynchronized heifers and heifers synchronized with progesterones.[4]

Toxicity. MGA seems to be relatively free of side effects. After administration, abnormally large amounts of vaginal mucous secretion have been reported in a few cows. There are some indications that MGA may prolong the estrus period in the first heat after discontinuance of the medication. If inseminated early in estrus and if ovulation does not occur until late during estrus, this effect could reduce fertility because the spermatozoa only remain alive in the cow for a short time.

Dose and administration. When used to synchronize heat, MGA is generally administered at the rate of 1 mg/24 hr per cow orally for 14 days.

Prostaglandins. Prostaglandins are naturally occurring fatty acids found in the tissues of many animal species. They are responsible for a variety of physiological activities in the body, one being a marked effect on the reproductive system. Prostaglandin $F_{2\alpha}$ ($PGF_{2\alpha}$) in cattle and sheep is produced by the uterus and causes destruction of the corpus luteum when the animal does not become pregnant. This usually results in estrus and ovulation 2 to 4 days later.

Generally, prostaglandins of the E and A types produce dilation in most vascular beds. However, those of the F type constrict vascular beds in most species. Prostaglandins are currently being studied for their potential in inducing abortion and parturition. In addition to their use in the reproductive system, prostaglandins are being investigated as inhibitors of gastric acid secretions, as bronchodilators, in the prevention of platelet aggregation in blood clotting, in inflammatory conditions, and in circulatory disturbances.

Effectiveness. $PGF_{2\alpha}$, given at the rate

of 30 mg subcutaneously to cows, has been successful in producing estrus in 2 to 4 days in heifers treated between the sixth and sixteenth days of their cycles. This probably occurs because prostaglandins cause regression of the corpus luteum, therefore allowing development of a Graafian follicle. Cows with functional corpus luteas show a marked decrease in the progesterone level within 24 hours after administration of prostaglandins. $PGF_{2\alpha}$ is not effective in producing estrus when given to cows on the first to fourth days of their cycles.[9,22] Probably prostaglandins are ineffective during the first 4 days of the cycle because no functional corpus luteum is present. An attempt to synchronize cattle randomly therefore will result in less than 80% of the animals in a normal population being in the proper stage for synchronization.

The use of progesterone followed by $PGF_{2\alpha}$ may be effective in eliminating the approximately 20% of animals that would not respond to $PGF_{2\alpha}$ because they are in the first 4 days of the cycle. Progesterone can be given for 7 days followed by $PGF_{2\alpha}$. This should prevent cows from entering proestrus until prostaglandins are administered. Such a regimen has been effective in producing fertile heat.[9]

It should be noted that a high percentage of cows treated with prostaglandins will develop mature follicles and ovulate even though they do not show external signs of heat. Therefore all animals receiving the drug should be inseminated whether they exhibit signs of heat. Although it can be expected that animals receiving $PGF_{2\alpha}$ will come into estrus 2 to 4 days after treatment, the period of time may range from 1 to 7 days. Seventy-two hours after treatment may be a good average time in which to inseminate the animals.

Toxicity. Toxic side effects in cattle from the use of prostaglandins have not been reported.

Dose and administration. Even though many experiments have been reported in which prostaglandins were administered di-rectly into the uterus, practical use requires that they be given by the intramuscular route. In cattle, therapeutic doses are approximately 30 mg given intramuscularly. In ewes the intramuscular dose used is 6 mg.[9]

Treatment of ovarian cysts in cows

Cows with cystic ovaries do not develop fertile heat. Depending on the type of cysts, signs in the cow may vary from nymphomania (showing continuous signs of heat) to anestrus (an absence of heat). While the cysts remain, the cow will not conceive. Various treatments have been advocated over the years. One is manual rupture of the ovarian cyst. Although the manual rupture of cysts is effective in some cases, complications such as severe hemorrhages have resulted. Two types of ovarian cysts occur in cows. One is a cystic Graafian follicle, the other is a cystic corpus luteum.

Cystic Graafian follicle. Cows with cystic Graafian follicles commonly exhibit nymphomania. To treat this condition medically, veterinarians use LH or gonadotropin-releasing hormone, which stimulates the pituitary to secrete LH.

Luteinizing hormone (LH). In cows the injection of LH has resulted in a 65% to 80% remission rate.[11] Clinically, LH can be administered in one of two forms:

1. Pituitary LH is available. It is usually administered to cattle at the rate of 25 mg intravenously.[25]

2. Human chorionic gonadotropin (HCG) is obtained from the urine of pregnant women. Although it contains fractions that mimic both LH and FSH activities, the predominant activity is similar to that of LH. For the treatment of ovarian cysts in cows 5000 to 10,000 units of HCG are recommended intramuscularly or 2500 to 5000 units intravenously. However, up to 10,000 units have been used intravenously in cattle.[11]

Gonadotropin-releasing hormone (GNRH). Studies have shown that administration of 50, 100, and 250 μg of GNRH intramuscularly to cows with cystic ovaries results in a favorable response in 64% to 82% of cows.[3,11] There appears to be no difference between the results from the use of LH or GNRH.

Cystic corpus luteum. Cows with cystic corpus luteum are in a perpetual state of early diestrus. They have relatively high levels of blood progesterone and will not come into heat.

Because prostaglandins cause disintegration of the corpus luteum in normal cows, they have been used in the treatment of cystic corpus luteum. For prostaglandins to be effective, the veterinarian must be sure the failure of the cow to come into heat is due to a cystic corpus luteum as opposed to some other condition or the failure of the rancher to observe estrus in a cow that is cycling normally.

Good results in the treatment of cystic corpus luteum have been reported using cloprostenol, an analog of prostaglandin.[10] Cloprostenol is administered at a dose of 500 μg by deep intramuscular injection.

Miscellaneous use of sex hormones

Pregnant mare serum (PMS). One source available for the therapeutic administration of gonadotropic hormones is pregnant mares' serum (PMS). PMS is obtained from pregnant mares between the fortieth and one-hundred fortieth day of pregnancy.

Primarily PMS activity is like pituitary FSH. Although it also has some action similar to pituitary LH, PMS is used primarily for its FSH activity. Because it does not pass the renal filter and remains in the circulation of an injected animal, it has a long duration of activity. Apparently the gonadotropin's function in the pregnant mare is to cause follicular development and finally multiple ovulations even though the mare is already pregnant. This results in multiple formation of corpora lutea, which helps to sustain the pregnancy.

In veterinary medicine PMS is used to induce follicular growth in anestrus ovaries of mature animals. In addition, the LH-like

activity in PMS may induce ovulation. Because PMS can result in superovulation, that is, formation of multiple follicles resulting in production of abnormally high numbers of ova, it is advisable not to breed animals on the first induced estrus following PMS administration. The next estrus is recommended for breeding.

Estrogens. The principle estrogens naturally found in animals are estradiol, estrone, and estriol.

Estrogens are sometimes used in spayed bitches to treat conditions related to the lack of ovarian production of estrogen. These include skin conditions and inability of some bitches to retain a normal amount of urine in the bladder (urinary incontinence). For these conditions 0.1 to 1 mg of estrogens are administered daily in increasing dose levels until success is observed. This is repeated within 2 weeks at the lowest possible dose. When using estrogens in the bitch, it must be kept in mind that they can cause serious side effects such as uterine disorders or generalized hemorrhages.

Diethylstilbestrol (DES). DES is a synthetic estrogen that has been widely used in veterinary medicine. Because of its potential for inducing cancer in humans, DES has come under intense fire from various sources. It is currently prohibited for use in food-producing animals, and injectable forms are not available in the United States.

Estradiol 17B-cypionate. Another commonly used estrogen in veterinary medicine is estradiol 17B-cypionate (ECP). It is only used intramuscularly. The appropriate dose will depend on the species on which it is used and the condition that is being treated. Ranges have been suggested as follows[25]:

Cattle	3 to 5 mg
Mares	5 to 10 mg
Ewes and sows	0.5 to 1 mg
Cats	0.2 to 0.5 mg
Dogs	0.2 to 2 mg

Other salts of estradiol are also available for clinical use.

Table 16-2. Use of progesterones in bitches

Progesterone compound	Route of administration
Progesterone	Injection
Hydroxyprogesterone	Oral
Hydroxyprogesterone	Injection
Medroxyprogesterone acetate (MAP)	Oral, injection solution, injection suspension
Megesterol acetate	Oral
Delmadinone acetate (DMA)	Oral, injection

Progesterones. Progesterones are available in many forms and for various routes of administration in the bitch. Table 16-2 shows the various types and possible routes of administration. Doses vary widely, depending on the reason the hormone is administered. Progesterone and progesterone-like compounds have many uses in dogs and cats. The progesterone and progesterone-like compounds inhibit release of the gonadotropic hormones. They prolong the normal anestrus stage of the female cycle.

Use. Progesterones inhibit the effects of estrogen in the female and androgens in the male. This may result in an inhibition of typical male or female behavior. For example, intact queens often have intense and prolonged or frequently repeated heat periods. One method of correcting this, without the use of drugs, is by the vigorous mechanical stimulation of the vagina and cervix with a blunt instrument such as a thermometer. In cases not associated with ovarian cysts, this usually causes ovulation and corpus luteum formation. If chemical therapy is desired, the use of progesterone may help. In either case, the results should be seen within hours. The animal will become quiet, and a pseudopregnancy condition will be established. It will last from 30 to 60 days. As blood concentrations of progesterone drop, normal cycle function is expected in most queens.

Estrus control. Various progesterones have been used for estrus control in the queen. Beginning treatment at any time seems to carry a lower risk of creating uterine disturbances in the queen than in the bitch. However, MAP and megestrol acetate have been implicated in the occurrence of uterine cystic hyperplasia and pyometra in queens. Delmadinone acetate (DMA) is currently being investigated for the control of reproduction in the queen. DMA is proposed to be administered as a pellet for subcutaneous implantation. This pellet should prevent heat for more than 6 months. In experimental trials safety has been claimed when DMA is used in this manner.[18]

Dermatitis. The use of megestrol acetate has been advocated as a replacement for corticosteroid therapy in certain dermatitis conditions of cats. There is clinical evidence that megestrol acetate is effective in treating some types of dermatitis due to hormonal imbalance. Doses of 2.5 to 5 mg given twice weekly until signs regress and then once weekly produce remission in a high percentage of clinical cases.[15]

Androgens. The male sex hormones are referred to as "androgens." Testosterone is the primary naturally produced androgen in most mammalian species. Under the influence of interstitial cell–stimulating hormone (ICSH), which is secreted by the pituitary, testosterone is produced by the interstitial cells of the testicle. The androgens in conjunction with FSH promote the development of sperm in the male. Androgens affect the development of the primary sex organs and secondary sex characteristics, such as male body conformation, voice patterns, hair growth, and sex drive.

Use. Androgens exert an anabolic effect, that is, they influence cellular metabolism to increase nitrogen retention, protein building, and an increase in muscle mass. Administration of testosterone parenterally has been reported to increase weight gain and nitrogen retention. This effect has resulted in the marketing of a group of compounds related to testosterone, commonly referred to as the "anabolic steroids." It should be kept in mind, however, that even though the ratio of androgenic to anabolic effects has been reduced in these compounds, some androgenic effect remains.

Effectiveness. Anabolic steroids promote positive nitrogen balance in animals, and increased weight gain can be achieved with the use of these compounds. In addition, red blood cell synthesis is stimulated. Indications for the use of anabolic steroids are not always clear. Although they promote an increase in muscle mass, a corresponding increase in strength has not been demonstrated. These drugs may be indicated in severely debilitated animals to help improve protein synthesis and appetite. Anabolic steroids are also of value in the treatment of some anemias.

Toxicity. The use of anabolic steroids is not without risk. Although the androgenic effects of these drugs have been reduced, the masculinizing effects are still present to some degree. Their use then can result in unwanted masculinizing effects and overaggressive behavior. The secretion of naturally occurring androgens increases with sexual maturity. Application of these compounds in immature animals can produce a false signal to the body, resulting in a premature slowing of long bone growth. Such a situation can result in a reduction of final stature. Toxicities have also been associated with the use of these drugs. These toxic effects, which follow, occur rarely at clinical doses but should nonetheless be kept in mind:

1. *Edema.* Anabolic steroids can cause retention of sodium and water. Water and salt retention is undesirable in animals with congestive heart disease or edematous conditions.

2. *Liver damage.* Anabolic and androgenic steroids that are substituted in the 17α position (Table 16-3) have been associated with cholestatic jaundice, in which the flow of bile is obstructed and pools in the biliary capillaries of the liver. It is recommended that the 17α-substituted compounds be given for no more than 3 to 4 weeks, then withheld for similar periods of time.

Dose and administration. For dose and administration of the anabolic steroids see Table 16-3.

Use of prostaglandins in mares. In mares that fail to conceive or even cycle due to persistent corpus luteum, analogs of prostaglandin have been successfully used to return the animals to normal fertile estrus cycles. Conditions in mares for which prostaglandins appear to be particularly well suited include failure of mares to cycle after early fetal death and resorption, mares in persistent diestrus (pseudopregnant mares), and noncycling lactating mares.

Toxicity. The early use of PGF$_{2\alpha}$ caused many toxic effects in horses. These included profuse sweating, spasms of the gastrointestinal tract, and increased rates of pulse and respiration. These effects were probably due to the activity of the prostaglandin on the smooth muscle. Newer analogs of prostaglandins have little or no smooth muscle activity at doses that cause regression of the corpus luteum. In limited trials they have been free of side effects in horses at therapeutic doses.

Dose and administration. For the treatment of persistent corpus luteum in mares, fluprostenol has been administered as a single intramuscular dose of 250 μg.[7] Prostalene has been administered at the rate of 5 μg/kg or 2 mg for the average-sized mare.[2] Both fluprostenol and prostalene are analogs of prostaglandins.

Oxytocin

The posterior portion of the pituitary secretes two closely related but different hormones: oxytocin and vasopressin (antidiuretic hormone). Since oxytocin and vasopressin have entirely different pharmacologic properties, there would rarely, if ever, be a condition in which both drugs should be administered simultaneously. It is important to recognize this because extracts of posterior pituitary glands containing both hormones are still available for veterinary use. It is strongly recommended that when oxytocin therapy is indicated, either oxytocin (USP)

Table 16-3. Androgenic and anabolic steroids

Compound	Primary activity	17α Substitution*	Dose†
Boldenone undecylenate	Anabolic	No	Horse: 250-500 mg IM every 2-4 weeks
Nandrolone decanoate	Anabolic	No	Dogs: 5 mg/kg IM every 3-4 weeks
Nandrolone phenpropionate	Anabolic	No	Horse: 200-400 mg Cat: 10-25 mg Dog: 10-50 mg SC or IM every 7-30 days
Stanozolol	Anabolic	Yes (CH₃)	Cats: 0.5-2 mg oral twice a day; 10-25 mg IM every 7 days Dogs: 0.5-4 mg oral twice a day; 10-50 mg IM every 7 days
Methyltestosterone	Androgenic	Yes (CH₃)	Dogs: 0.5-1 mg/kg Cats: 0.5-2 mg daily
Testosterone	Androgenic	No	Cattle: 100-300 mg SC or IM Cats and dogs: 2.2 mg/kg IM or SC

*17α substitution relates to potential hepatotoxicity (see text).
†Rossoff, I. S.: Handbook of veterinary drugs, New York, 1974, Springer Publishing Co.

or purified oxytocic principal (USP) be used rather than posterior pituitary extracts.

Oxytocin has two main effects on the body. It causes marked uterine contractions, particularly when the uterus has been sensitized by estrogen, and it causes contraction of the muscles surrounding the epithelium in the mammary glands, forcing milk into the collecting ducts and facilitating its passage to the exterior. This is referred to as "milk let-down."

The primary use of oxytocin is in veterinary obstetrics. When using purified oxytocin, administration by means of a slow intravenous drip is preferable to a large intramuscular injection. One must be assured, however, that when administering oxytocin to facilitate parturition that the cervix has been dilated prior to commencing the administration. The drug has particular value in assisting delivery in small animals such as the dog and cat when the uterus fails to contract. By stimulating uterine motility in the dog or cat, the use of oxytocin may force the fetus into the pelvic canal

where instruments can be used to help with delivery. However, the decision of an experienced clinician regarding the use of oxytocin is necessary because the cause of the inactive uterus will determine the treatment of choice. For example, when a bitch has a low level of blood calcium, the administration of calcium ion slowly may be more effective than the administration of oxytocin to stimulate uterine activity.

Because manual manipulation is possible in the cow, mare, and ewe, oxytocin is rarely used to assist with delivery in these species. However, in all species, oxytocin is of value in inducing contractions of the uterus after cesarean section to aid the expulsion of the placenta and the evacuation of uterine debris and to stimulate involution of the uterus (returning the uterus to its normal nonpregnant state). One of the primary actions of oxytocin is to cause uterine involution so that the animal can once again start to have normal estrus cycles.

If given right after a cow gives birth, oxytocin can be of use for preventing retained placenta in the cow. Doses of 60 units are administered intravenously to an adult cow.

It is also useful for treating retained placenta in the mare. Various figures have been quoted for the normal expulsion of fetal membranes in the mare. These figures vary from 2 to 12 hours. Generally, there is a concern when the time between parturition and failure to expel the fetal membranes exceeds 2 hours. Severe toxic reactions can result from retained fetal membranes, endangering the life or fertility of mares.

Clinically it has been observed that single intramuscular or intravenous injection of large doses of oxytocin results in intense and only sporadic uterine contractions. Separate, although multiple, administrations of oxytocin therefore are of little value for the treatment of retained fetal membranes in the mare. Prolonged effects of oxytocin are necessary to assist in the delivery of the fetal membranes. Slow intravenous infusion over a period of 30 to 60 minutes has therefore been recommended in treating mares with retained fetal membranes. During the administration period, 30 to 60 IU of oxytocin in 1 to 2 liters of normal saline are administered. Probably the best regimen is to give 60 units of oxytocin over a 60-minute period in 2 liters of normal saline.[33]

Vasopressin (antidiuretic hormone)

The primary pharmacological effect for which vasopressin is used in veterinary medicine is its action on the kidney to increase water resorption. Deficiencies of vasopressin hormone result in diabetes insipidus. Diabetes insipidus results in a lack of water resorption in the kidneys, causing excessive urine formation and increased consumption of water.

Although high doses of vasopressin raise blood pressure, its use for this purpose is limited because of its potentially serious side effects. Doses hundreds of times larger than those required for the antidiuretic effect are necessary to obtain pronounced vasopressor activity.

Vasopressin also possesses some activities in common with oxytocin. It slightly stimulates milk let-down and contraction of the uterus. However, oxytocin does not share the antidiuretic properties of vasopressin.

Vasopressin is available as vasopressin (USP). This form is preferred over posterior pituitary (USP). In the treatment of diabetes insipidus in dogs, various doses have been recommended in the range of 25 to 500 mg orally or parenterally. In cats the dose has ranged from 25 to 50 mg orally or parenterally. In horses 1 gm is administered orally daily.[25]

The hydrochlorothiazide group of diuretics have an antidiuretic effect in dogs with diabetes insipidus.[16] This effect has also been noted in humans with diabetes insipidus. The mechanism that results in diuretics having an antidiuretic effect in this disease is not known.

Thyroid hormone

As a result of stimulation by thyroid-stimulating hormone (TSH), the thyroid produces thyroxine and other chemicals with similar structure and activities. The thyroid active hormones contain iodine. Even with adequate levels of TSH, these thyroid hormones can only be produced if adequate iodine is present in the diet. Thyroxine and similar chemicals are stored in the thyroid gland and released into the blood.

Unlike most other hormones of a protein nature, thyroid hormone is active when given by the oral route. TSH from the anterior pituitary stimulates the formation, storage, and release of thyroxin in the thyroid gland. In the absence of TSH the thyroid gland will function at a minimal level. However, that level is inadequate to maintain animals in a normal physiological state.

Among the effects of thyroxine on the body are the following:

1. Oxygen utilization of every cell of the body is stimulated.

2. Carbohydrate utilization is increased.

3. Protein metabolism is increased.

4. Fats are more readily utilized.

The primary function ascribed to thyroxine is an increase in cellular metabolism. Although other drugs can increase the metabolic rate, only thyroxine provides relief from the clinical symptoms of thyroid deficiency. Thyroxine also produces an increase in the heart rate. It does this by lowering the threshold of response to the sympathetic nervous system.

If animals are presented to a veterinarian demonstrating signs of thyroid deficiency, various alternatives of therapy are available. In certain geographical areas the veterinarian must consider the possibility that the signs result from iodine deficiency. Adequate dietary intake of iodine is necessary for the thyroid gland to function properly. In certain parts of the country, iodine deficiencies are common so that iodine must be added to the diet.

Assuming adequate levels of dietary iodine, thyroid deficiencies can be treated with TSH, desiccated thyroid, thyroxine, or one of the chemical analogs.

Desiccated thyroid is administered to cats at the rate of 1 to 2 mg/kg daily as an initial dose, increasing to 10 to 20 mg/kg one to three times a day as the response indicates. In dogs, dessicated thyroid is given at the rate of 1 to 6 mg/kg daily as an initial dose, increasing if indicated to 10 to 20 mg/kg one to three times a day.[25]

Thyroxine can be administered to dogs at the rate of 0.001 to 0.01 mg/kg initially daily. If signs indicate, the dose can be increased to 0.02 to 0.03 mg/kg one to three times a day.[25]

Thyroid-stimulating hormone

TSH will only be effective in the treatment of thyroid deficiencies if a functional thyroid gland is present and the animal has adequate iodine reserves. The administration of TSH is based on units that are generally based on milligrams of purified glandular substance from bovine anterior pituitary glands.

As with the thyroid hormones, TSH should not be administered in animals with hyper-thyroidism (animals that produce too much thyroid hormone) or in animals with insufficient output of adrenocortical hormone.

For therapeutic purposes, TSH can be administered to dogs at the rate of 0.5-3 units daily for 5 days.

Thyrotropin-releasing hormone

The hypothalamus produces a chemical that stimulates the release of TSH. This chemical is referred to as thyrotropin-releasing hormone (TRH).

Acanthosis nigricans, a skin disease of dogs, has been traditionally treated with either thyroid hormone or TSH. Synthetic TRH has also been used in a series of clinical trials.[1] However, the efficacy of this method of treatment is disputed. Many clinicians now think that acanthosis nigricans is basically an inflammatory disease and is better treated with anti-inflammatory drugs.

Toxicity. In patients treated with TRH, adverse side effects attributed to TRH have not been observed. Because TRH directly affects TSH secretion by the pituitary, no thyroid preparation should be given concurrently with TRH.

Dose and administration. In a clinical trial, TRH was given at an initial dose of $100/\mu g$ intravenously twice weekly for 4 weeks and then once weekly for 4 weeks. After this therapy, the dose was reduced to 100 μg every other week for a month. Medicated baths were also given. Following this 3-month treatment regimen, 200 μg of TRH were administered subcutaneously once a week. The animal so treated weighed 22.27 kg.[1]

References

1. Austin, V. H.: New treatment for acanthosis nigricans, Mod. Vet. Pract. **55**:202, 1974.
2. Averkin, G., and Schlitz, R.: Summary of the effect of prostalene, a new synthetic prostaglandin, on the breeding efficiency of mares, Vet. Med. Small Anim. Clin. **71**:1616, 1976.
3. Bierschwall, C. J., Garverick, H. A., Martin, C. E., Youngquist, R. S., Cantley, T. C., and Brown, M. D.: Clinical response of dairy cows with ovarian cysts to GnRH[1,2,3,4], J. Anim. Sci. **41**:1660, 1975.
4. Brown, H., Wagner, J. F., Rathmacher, R. P.,

McAskill, J. W., Elliston, N. G., and Bing, R. F.: Effect of human chorionic gonadotropin on pregnancy rate of heifers, when used under field conditions, J. Am. Vet. Med. Assoc. **162:**456, 1973.

5. Bryan, H. S.: Parenteral use of medroxyprogesterone acetate as an antifertility agent in the bitch, Am. J. Vet. Res. **34:**653, 1973.
6. Burke, T. J., and Reynolds, H. A. Jr.: Megestrol acetate for estrus postponement in the bitch, J. Am. Vet. Med. Assoc. **167:**285, 1975.
7. Cooper, M. J.: Fluprostenol in mares: clinical trials for the treatment of infertility, Vet. Rec. **98:**523, 1976.
8. DeBois, C. H. W., and Bierschwal, C. J.: Estrus cycle synchronization in dairy cattle, given a fourteen day treatment of melengestrol acetate, Am. J. Vet. Res. **31:**1545, 1970.
9. Downey, B. R.: Control of the estrus cycle with protaglandins, Vet. Med. Small Anim. Clin. **69:**880, 1974.
10. Eddy, R. G.: Cloprostenol as a treatment for no visible oestrus and cystic ovarian disease in dairy cows, Vet. Rec. **100:**62, 1977.
11. Elmore, R. G., Bierschwal, C. J., Youngquist, R. S., Cantley, T. C., Kesler, D. J., and Garverick, H. A.: Clinical responses of dairy cows with ovarian cysts after treatment with 10,000 IU HCG or 100 mcg GNRH, Vet. Med. Small Anim. Clin. **70:**1346, 1975.
12. Faulkner, L. C.: An immunologic approach to population control in dogs, J. Am. Vet. Med. Assoc. **166:**479, 1975.
13. Hagg, D. D., and Schiltz, R. A.: The effect of intramammary corticosteroid administration during late gestation in cattle, Mod. Vet. Pract. **54:**29, Dec. 1973.
14. Herrick, J. B.: The proper use of corticosteroids, Vet. Med. Small Anim. Clin. **70:**921, 1975.
15. Houdeshell, J. W., Hennessey, P. W., and Bigbee, H. B.: Treatment of feline miliary dermatitis with megestrol acetate, Vet. Med. Small Anim. Clin. **72:**573, 1977.
16. Jackson, W. F.: Which diuretic? Small Anim. Clin. **2:**341, 1962.
17. Jochle, W.: Pet population control: chemical methods, Canine Pract. **1:**8, Sept. 1974.
18. Jochle, W.: Progress in small animal reproductive physiology, therapy of reproductive disorders, and pet population control, Folia Vet. Lat. **4:**706, 1974.
19. Kunesh, J. P.: Clinical use of glucocorticoids in large animals, Vet. Med. Small Anim. Clin. **72:**611, 1977.
20. Lauderdale, J. W.: Effect of corticoid administration on bovine pregnancy, J. Am. Vet. Med. Assoc. **160:**867, 1972.
21. Lavelle, R. B.: The treatment of Cushing's disease in the dog, Vet. Rec. **98:**406, 1976.
22. Mickelsen, D. W., and Degrofit, D.: Prostaglandin as an estrus-synchronizing agent in range cattle, Mod. Vet. Pract. **55:**289, 1974.

23. Nixon, G. F.: Watch and wait, Mod. Vet. Pract. **48:**64, Nov. 1967.
24. Pailet, A., and Smith, M. W., Jr.: Physical examination and reproductive physiology, Mod. Vet. Pract. **48:**64, Nov. 1967.
25. Rossoff, I. S.: Handbook of veterinary drugs, New York, 1974, Springer Publishing Co.
26. Schechter, R. D., Stabenfeldt, G. H., Gribble, D. H., and Ling, G. V.: Treatment of Cushing's syndrome in the dog with an adrenocorticolytic agent (*o,p*-DDD), J. Am. Vet. Med. Assoc. **162:**629, 1973.
27. Simmons, J. G., and Hamner, C. E.: Inhibition of estrus in the dog with testosterone implants, Am. J. Vet. Res. **34:**1409, 1973.
28. Simpson, M. J., Wilson, L. L., Rugh, M. T., Stout, J. M., and Varela-Alvarez, H.: Synchronization of estrus and fertility in beef cows fed melengestrol acetate, Vet. Med. Small Anim. Clin. **65:**491, 1970.
29. Sokolowski, J. H., and Zimbelman, R. G.: Effects of a single injection of medroxyprogesterone acetate on the reproductive organs of the bitch, Am. J. Vet. Res. **34:**1493, 1973.
30. Sokolowski, J. H., and Zimbelman, R. G.: Canine reproduction: effects of a single injection of medroxyprogesterone acetate on the reproductive organs of intact and ovariectomized bitches, Am. J. Vet. Res. **34:**1501, 1973.
31. Stabenfeldt, G. H.: Physiologic, pathologic and therapeutic roles of progestins in domestic animals, J. Am. Vet. Med. Assoc. **164:**311, 1974.
32. Thiersch, J. B.: Abortion of the bitch with *N*-desacetyl thiocolchicine, J. Am. Vet. Med. Assoc. **151:**1470, 1967.
33. Vandeplassche, M. J., and Spincemaille, R. B.: Aetiology, pathogenesis and treatment of retained placenta in the mare, Equine Vet. J. **3:**144, Oct. 1971.
34. Williams, R. H.: Malucidin for advanced cases, Mod. Vet. Pract. **46:**57, June 1965.

Additional readings

Anderson, R. K., Gilmore, C. E., and Schnelle, G. B.: Utero-ovarian disorders associated with use of medroxyprogesterone in dogs, J. Am. Vet. Med. Assoc. **146:**1311, 1965.

Arbeiter, K.: The use of progestins in the treatment of persistent uterine hemorrhage in the postpartum bitch and cow: a clinical report, Theriogenology **4:**11, July 1975.

Cantley, T. C., Garverick, C. J., Bierschwal, C. J., Martin, C. E., and Youngquist, R. S.: Hormonal responses of dairy cows with ovarian cysts to GnRH [1,2,3,4,5,6], J. Anim. Sci. **41:**1666, 1975.

Chesney, C. J.: The response to progestogen treatment of some diseases of cats, J. Small Anim. Pract. **17:**35, Jan. 1976.

Dermody, W. C., Sakowski, R., Vaitkus, J. W., and Beck, C. C.: Pituitary LH responses of lactating anestrous ewes to varying doses of luteinizing hormone-releasing hormone administered by different routes and vehicles, Vet. Med. Small Anim. Clin. **71**:687, 1976.

Edquist, L. E., Edman, L., Gustafsson, B., and Lindell, J.: The clinical and hormonal effect of luteinizing hormone (LH-RH) in cows with cystic ovaries, Nord. Vet. Med. **26**:556, 1974.

Keye, W. R., Young, J. R., and Jaffe, R. B.: Hypothalmic gonadotropin releasing hormone: physiologic and clinical considerations, Obstet. Gynecol. Surv. **31**:635, 1976.

King, G. J., and Macpherson, J. W.: Fertility of beef cows treated during estrus with human chorionic gonadotropin, Can. Vet. J. **14**:221, Sept. 1973.

Kirk, M. D.: Field diagnosis and treatment of secondary adrenocortical insufficiency in the horse, Vet. Med. Small Anim. Clin. **69**:1383, 1974.

Kittock, R. J., Britt, J. H., and Edgerton, L. A.: Serum steroids after gonadotropin treatment in cows with ovarian follicular cysts, Am. J. Vet. Res. **35**:1575, 1974.

Liptrap, R. M., and McNally, P. J.: Steroid concentrations in cows with corticotropin-induced cystic ovarian follicles and the effect of prostaglandin $F_{2\alpha}$ and in-

domethacin given by intrauterine injection, Am. J. Vet. Res. **37**:369, 1976.

McKenzie, B. E., and Kenney, R. M.: Histologic features of ovarian follicles of gonadotropin-injected heifers, Am. J. Vet. Res. **34**:1033, 1973.

O'Connor, J. J., Stillions, M. C., Reynolds, W. A., Linkenheimer, W. H., and Maplesden, D. C.: Evaluation of boldenone undecylenate as an anabolic agent in horses, Can. Vet. J. **14**:154, July 1973.

Seguin, B. E., Convey, E. M., and Oxender, W. D.: Effect of gonadotropin-releasing hormone and human chorionic gonadotropin on cows with ovarian follicular cysts, Am. J. Vet. Res. **37**:153, 1976.

Studer, E., and Holtan, A.: Luteinizing hormone-releasing hormone evaluation in anestrous beef cows with suckling calf, Vet. Med. Small Anim. Clin. **70**:1047, 1975.

Sullivan, J. J., Parker, W. G., and Larson, L. L.: Duration of estrus and ovulation time in nonlactating mares given human chorionic gonadotropin during three successvie estrous periods, J. Am. Vet. Med. Assoc. **162**:895, 1973.

Wagner, W. C., Willham, R. L., and Evans, L. E.: Controlled parturition in cattle, J. Anim. Sci. **38**:485, 1974.

17

Fluid, electrolyte, metabolic, and vitamin imbalances

FLUID AND ELECTROLYTE IMBALANCE

Water accounts for approximately 70% of the body weight of animals. Body water is essential to all life processes. It is the vehicle in which metabolism is carried out; it is the medium by which ions, nutrients, and wastes are transported, and it is essential to the secretion of enzymes and hormones. Body water also plays important roles in the maintenance of body temperature, blood volume and pressure, and the lubrication of body surfaces.

Body water is classified as intracellular and extracellular (Fig. 17-1). Approximately 50% of body weight consists of intracellular water. The intracellular water provides a diffusion medium for ions, molecules, and enzyme systems within the cells. Extracellular body water consists of plasma (5% of body weight) and interstitial fluid (15% of body weight). The interstitial fluid is located between the cells of the body. Extracellular water transports nutritive and waste substances to and from cells.

In the normal animal the amount of water taken in by ingestion plus the water formed by chemical reactions oxidizing hydrogen (metabolic water) is equal to the amount of water lost by way of the urine, feces, sweat, and respiration. In many disease conditions, however, the intake of water is reduced or the excretion is increased so that a net loss of body water results (Fig. 17-2). Such disease conditions can rapidly result in dehydration.

Although a starving animal can lose nearly all its glycogen and fat, half of its protein, and two fifths of its body weight without dying, a loss of 10% of body water results in serious metabolic disturbances and losses of 20% are nearly always fatal.

70% of body weight is water

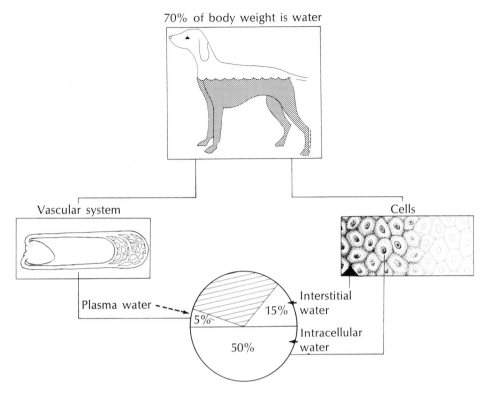

Vascular system

Cells

Plasma water - - - →   5%   15%   Interstitial water

Intracellular water

50%

Fig. 17-1. Distribution of body water. Approximately 70% of body weight is water. Intracellular water equals about 50% of body weight. Extracellular water consists of interstitial water (15% of body weight) and plasma water (5% of body weight).

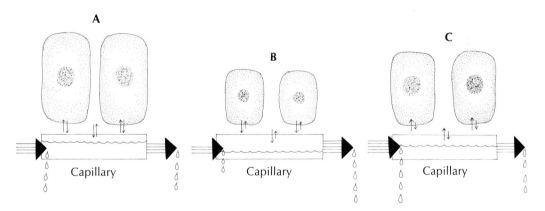

A

B

C

Capillary   Capillary   Capillary

Fig. 17-2. Dehydration. **A,** Normally intake of water and electrolytes is in balance so that there is proper distribution of water and electrolytes in blood, interstitial space, and intracellular space. **B,** When loss of water and electrolytes is greater than intake, there is reduction of blood volume shift of water and electrolytes from cells and interstitial space to blood. **C,** To correct dehydration, water and electrolytes are given, and they restore blood volume and also move from blood to interstitial and intracellular spaces.

In dehydration, blood volume decreases. This is referred to as "hemoconcentration." Eventually all compartments, that is, intracellular and interstitial, share the water deficit. Electrolytes are lost with the water, and acid-base balance is often compromised. In order for fluid therapy to be effective in the treatment of dehydration, water must reach both the interstitial and intracellular compartments by way of the blood. Proper electrolytes must be available to transport the water through cellular membranes.

Sodium, potassium, chloride, bicarbonate, calcium, magnesium, and other ions are present at different concentrations in the intracellular and extracellular fluid. Intracellular fluid tends to be high in potassium and magnesium and low in sodium, chloride, bicarbonate, and calcium ions. On the other hand, extracellular fluid contains relatively high amounts of sodium, chloride, bicarbonate, and calcium ions.

Herbivorous animals take in large amounts of potassium in their normal diets. Because they take in more potassium than they require, large quantities of potassium are excreted in the urine, feces, and sweat. However, herbivorous animals generally will take in minimal levels of sodium in their normal diet. There is a comparatively low and unavoidable loss of sodium ions in sweat, feces, and urine. In general, the horse is able to conserve sodium well. However, its ability to conserve potassium is less efficient. Therefore, when intake of potassium is reduced as, for example, when an animal quits eating, severe potassium depletion may result.

In animals, the correct acid-base balance must be maintained. If the pH drops beyond certain limits, many enzymatic processes fail. For example, in horses the pH should range between 7.35 and 7.45; a pH in the range of 7 to 6.8 is incompatible with life.

When there is a drop in the normal pH, a state of acidosis exists. Acidosis is generally classified as metabolic or respiratory. Metabolic acidosis results from increased production and retention of acid compounds or from an abnormal deficit of bicarbonate ions. For example, diarrhea results in considerable losses of bicarbonate, sodium, and potassium ions. In kidney failure, hydrogen ions may be retained. In conditions such as shock, inadequate perfusion of tissues by the blood reduces the available tissue oxygen and leads to the increased production of acid metabolites. Respiratory acidosis is caused by inadequate alveolar exchange of oxygen and carbon dioxide in the lungs. As a result, there is a retention of carbon dioxide and a drop in the pH of body fluids as carbonic acid (H_2CO_3) levels increase.

Treatment. Metabolic acidosis is treated by administering bicarbonate ion or lactate ion, which is converted rapidly to bicarbonate ion in the liver. To treat respiratory acidosis, effective respiration must be established to get rid of the retained carbon dioxide.

The treatment of fluid and electrolyte imbalances can be accomplished by the oral or parenteral administration of appropriate electrolyte solutions. Before initiating fluid therapy, three questions need to be answered:

1. What is the existing water and electrolyte deficit?

2. What are the continuing abnormal losses?

3. What is the amount of fluid required for normal maintenance?

Fluid and electrolyte solutions can be administered orally, intravenously, subcutaneously, or intraperitoneally (Fig. 17-3). Oral administration is preferred whenever administration by this route is practical and adequate. In animals that are vomiting, comatose, anesthetized, or have diseases of the gastrointestinal tract, which interfere with absorption of ions and sugars, the oral route should generally be avoided. The preferred parenteral routes of administration are the intravenous and subcutaneous routes. Intraperitoneal injection of fluids presents considerable risk of infection. In order not to overload the heart with an excessive intravenous fluid volume, intravenous administration of fluids must be done slowly.

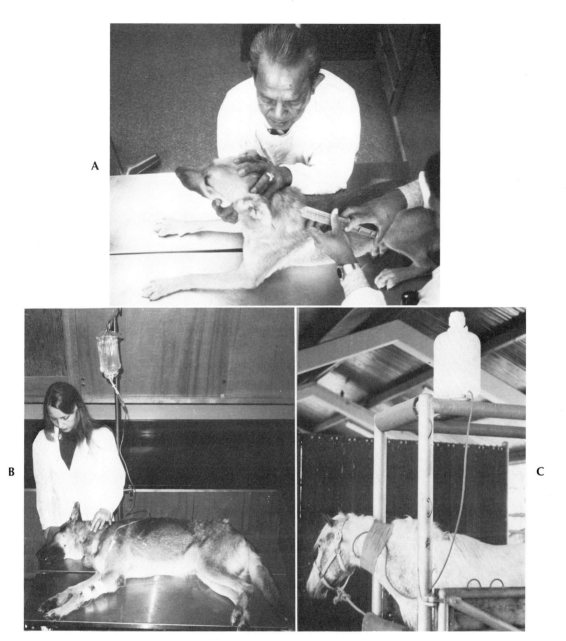

Fig. 17-3. Parenteral water and electrolyte administration to a dog subcutaneously **(A)**, to a dog intravenously **(B)**, and to a horse intravenously **(C)**.

Fluids administered by the subcutaneous route should be isotonic, that is, they must have the same osmotic tension as serum. If the solutions are hypertonic prior to their absorption from the site, they will draw fluid from the vascular system. In a severely de- hydrated animal, this could be fatal. In addition to being isotonic, fluids administered by the subcutaneous route should closely approximate the normal ion composition of extracellular fluid, so that ions will not diffuse into the site of administration, further com-

Table 17-1. Composition of commonly used fluids

Fluid	Tonicity	Calories/liter	Ions mEq/liter				
			NA+	K+	CA+	Cl-	HCO₃ equivalent*
5% Dextrose in water	Isotonic	170					
10% Dextrose in water	Hypertonic	340					
50% Dextrose in water	Hypertonic	1700					
2.5% Dextrose in 0.45% saline	Isotonic	85	77			77	
5% Dextrose in 0.45% saline	Hypertonic	170	77			77	
5% Dextrose in normal saline	Hypertonic	170	155			155	
Lactated Ringer's solution	Isotonic	9	131	4	3	110	28
Normal saline	Isotonic		155			155	
Ringer's solution	Isotonic		147	4	4.5	155.5	
⅙ M Sodium lactate	Isotonic	55	167				171
7.5% Sodium bicarbonate	Hypertonic		890				890

*Assuming complete metabolism of lactate.

promising an animal in severe electrolyte imbalance. Ringer's solution is isotonic and contains electrolytes in proportions similar to normal canine plasma.

A description of the commonly used fluids in veterinary medicine and the concentration of ions in each appears in Table 17-1.

Small animals. Commercially available fluids are usually employed in parenteral fluid therapy of small animals. These fluids are sterile. They are also pyrogen-free, that is, they are free of substances that are likely to cause a fever after administration. The electrolyte solutions are available in 250 ml, 500 ml, and 1000 ml containers. It is important to remember that such solutions do not contain antibacterial preservatives. When the seal is broken on the container, the fluids become contaminated with organisms from the air. This contamination is minimal and generally presents no problem to the patient if the total contents are used at one time. However, if the container is partially used and then kept for reuse, the organisms may multiply, resulting in a grossly contaminated solution that if administered to a patient could endanger its life. Therefore any unused portion of these solutions must be discarded.

Generally, when administering electrolyte solutions to animals, the exact electrolyte excesses and deficiencies are not determined. Rather solutions such as isotonic sodium chloride or Ringer's solution are administered. The animal's kidneys are relied on to eliminate excess electrolytes and conserve those that are deficient. In an animal with good kidney function and an ability to conserve electrolytes, this will probably occur. However, kidney disease in the dog is common, particularly in older animals, and in these animals one cannot assume that proper electrolyte balance will develop after administration of an electrolyte solution containing excess or deficient amounts of electrolytes. The most rational approach is to supply the deficient electrolytes in an isotonic solution.

Dose and administration. When using fluid therapy in small puppies or kittens with diarrhea, a dosage of 22 to 33 ml/kg of body weight is usually adequate. Administration of fluid subcutaneously in dogs and cats is often more practical than the intravenous route. Intravenous administration requires much closer monitoring over extended periods of time.

Large animals. Fluid therapy in large animals presents several unique problems, since extremely large volumes of fluid may be required. Volumes in excess of 40 liters daily are commonly employed in the therapy of water and electrolyte–wasting diseases in the horse.

In horses, the route of administration of fluid therapy is an important consideration. When the intestinal tract is normal, water, electrolytes, and food substances may be given by stomach tube. A dose of up to 5 liters of fluid every 3 hours is recommended. Frequent administration allows the body some control over the absorption of water and selective excretion of electrolytes. When the gut is not normal, fluids must be administered intravenously.

The economics and logistics of supplying commercially available sterile fluids in the amounts required for horses often become overwhelming. For this reason it is common for the large-animal practitioner to devise an alternate method of supplying fluid and electrolyte solutions to his patients. Several balanced electrolyte powders are available in the veterinary market that can be mixed with appropriate volumes of distilled water to yield concentrations compatible with parenteral administration. Although the fluids prepared in this manner are not proved to be either pyrogen free or sterile, if they are made with distilled water and are not stored after mixing, the risk of serious contamination is minimal.[18]

KIDNEY DISEASE

Kidney disease is an important geriatric problem in dogs. When functioning normally, the kidneys filter water, electrolytes, and urea from the blood. Normally more than 99% of the water filtered by the glomeruli is reabsorbed in the kidney tubules (Fig. 17-4). In addition, those electrolytes needed by the body are reabsorbed and those in excess are passed in the urine. Upon reaching certain levels of concentration in the blood, various chemicals pass into the urine. This is a common disposal route for drugs. Therefore in kidney disease the blood level of drugs may be substantially increased because the kidneys are not excreting them at a normal rate.

When kidneys first start to malfunction, the only clinical sign that may be apparent is that the amount of water an animal drinks and the amount of urine it produces increase. The urine will also be of lower specific gravity than normal. These signs indicate that the animal has a reduced capacity for reabsorbing water in the tubules. The animal therefore is not able to concentrate its urine and conserve water. As long as enough water is available to the animal and the kidneys clear the blood of waste products, the animal can be maintained in good health.

As kidney disease becomes more severe, an animal on a normal diet may not be able to get rid of all the urea produced by normal protein metabolism. As blood levels of urea increase, the animal is said to be uremic. Because of its toxicity, high levels of blood urea are eventually fatal. If the kidneys are not too severely damaged, uremia can be controlled by feeding the animal a diet that is relatively low in protein but high enough to meet the animal's daily protein need and that consists of protein of high biological value. Proteins of high biological value are those that are effectively used by the body with a resultant low urea production. Commercial diets containing relatively low amounts of protein of high biological value are available for use in dogs. Veterinarians can also recommend formulas for creating appropriate diets at home. No drugs are available to help the kidney become more efficient in excreting waste products. Although diuretics give the appearance of increasing kidney function by increasing the amount of urine volume and electrolyte excretion, they may actually impair kidney function by preventing selective reabsorption of certain electrolytes and water. Therefore they are not appropriate drugs to be used to increase kidney activity. Rather they are used to selectively increase the excretion of water and electrolytes in animals suffering from other organ problems such as cardiac disease or mammary edema.

Peritoneal dialysis

In animals suffering from acute uremia that have a chance of returning to relatively normal kidney function, one means of removing metabolic waste products is peritoneal dialy-

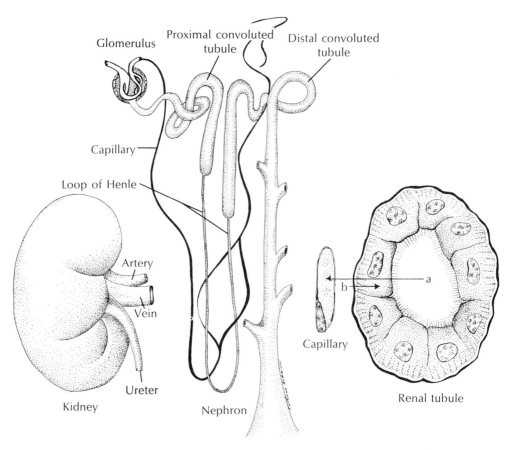

Fig. 17-4. The functional unit of the kidney is the nephron. In the nephron, blood is filtered in the glomerulus, producing glomerular filtrate. In the proximal convoluted tubule, loop of Henle, and the distal convoluted tubule, there is selective reabsorption into blood of electrolytes and water. There is also a small amount of secretion of water and electrolytes from blood to the renal tubule. This process results in 99% of glomerular filtrate being reabsorbed, and 1% becomes urine. *a,* Reabsorption of water and electrolytes; *b,* secretion of water and electrolytes.

sis. It is relatively easy to perform and can be done repeatedly until clinical improvement is seen.

Peritoneal dialysis is performed as follows: A mixed electrolyte solution is warmed to 37 to 40° C. It is administered in a dose equal to approximately 5% of the patient's body weight. Because it is given intraperitoneally, strict aseptic techniques such as shaving, washing, and disinfecting the site of injection and using absolutely sterile equipment and fluids are necessary. After an hour, fluid is drained from the peritoneum. When continuous dialysis is required, the fluid is drained every hour and replaced with an equal volume of warm electrolyte solution. The procedure can be continued for 12 hours or longer. While the solution is in the peritoneal cavity, electrolytes and waste products diffuse through the various membranes in the peritoneal cavity from the circulation into the fluid. These waste products are eliminated from the body when the fluid is removed.

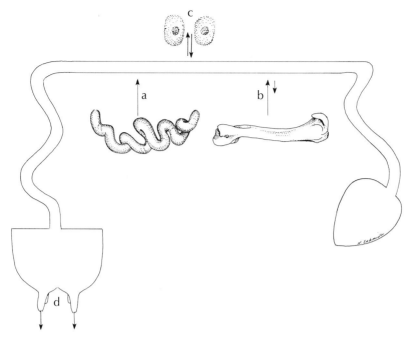

Fig. 17-5. Calcium metabolism. *a,* Calcium is absorbed from the gut. *b,* It is deposited and, in times of need, reabsorbed from the bone. *c,* It is used by various body cells and, *d,* excreted in milk.

CALCIUM, PHOSPHORUS, AND MAGNESIUM METABOLISM

The metabolism of calcium and phosphorus is largely influenced by parathyroid hormone, which is secreted by the parathyroid glands. The parathyroid glands are located next to the thyroid gland in the neck. Parathyroid hormone raises the blood concentration of calcium and decreases the blood concentration of phosphorus. The parathyroid glands produce parathyroid hormone in response to calcium and phosphorus blood levels. If the calcium level drops or the phosphorus level increases, parathyroid hormone is released. For example, in dogs with severe kidney disease, blood levels of phosphorus increase. This results in increased production of parathyroid hormone and absorption of calcium from the bone and in severe cases causes generalized demineralization of bones. In the jawbone this occurs to such an extent that it becomes pliable. This condition is known as "rubber jaw."

Calcium and phosphorus metabolism refers to the total chemical processes involving these minerals (Fig. 17-5). Among these processes are their absorption from the gastrointestinal tract, maintenance of adequate blood levels, deposition in and reabsorption from bones, and utilization by various cells. Bones are important in calcium and phosphorus metabolism. They are composed of a protein matrix impregnated with calcium and phosphorus salts, which when needed by the body can be mobilized from the bone into the blood. In addition to the relationship of calcium and phosphorus to bone, these minerals affect the function of the nervous system and heart and are also involved in the coagulation of blood. Abnormally low calcium blood levels in most species cause tetanic muscle spasms and can result in death.

To maintain good health, adequate dietary intake of calcium and phosphorus is necessary. Growing animals and pregnant or lactating animals require the greatest amounts of calcium, phosphorus, and vitamin D. In addition to the need for adequate dietary intake, it is equally important that the calcium and phosphorus be ingested in a proper ratio. For dogs and cats that ratio is approximately 1.2 parts of calcium to 1 part phosphorus. At that ratio there is optimum utilization of these minerals. When the intake of either mineral is too high or too low, some insoluble phosphates are formed, and absorption of both calcium and phosphorus from the intestine is reduced.

Vitamin D exerts great influence on calcium and phosphorus metabolism. Adequate levels of vitamin D will allow greater intestinal absorption and utilization of calcium and phosphorus even when an imbalance of these minerals is present. However, when there is a serious imbalance of calcium and phosphorus and/or a vitamin D deficiency, rickets can result. Rickets is a condition in which there is a failure to deposit proper amounts of tricalcium phosphate in the bones.

Large breeds of dogs are predisposed to rickets during their rapid growth phase. If fed properly, the condition will be self-corrective when they obtain full growth. Currently, high-quality commercial pet foods are available for growing puppies and pregnant and lactating bitches. Such products contain optimal amounts of calcium and phosphorus. Supplementation of these minerals to dogs fed such diets should not be necessary. If supplementation is attempted, products containing calcium and phosphorus at a 1.2:1 ratio should be used.

Parturient paresis (milk fever)

Milk fever is a metabolic disease primarily of dairy cattle occurring about the time of parturition. It is characterized by hypocalcemia, general muscular weakness, a flaccid paralysis, and depression of consciousness. It primarily occurs in high milk-producing cows. If untreated, it usually terminates in death.

Although many ranchers treat this condition unaided by a veterinarian, it is important for them to realize that other conditions in dairy cattle, such as overwhelming mastitis or severe uterine infection may mimic milk fever. Diagnosis by a veterinarian is necessary to distinguish milk fever from other conditions.

In cows with milk fever, lowered blood calcium and phosphorus are constant findings. The concentration of magnesium in the serum may vary. In normal parturient cows the serum magnesium concentration is elevated relative to that of the cow before parturition.[1] In those with milk fever this elevation seems to become a little more pronounced. Cows with milk fever are often hyperglycemic (they have increased blood levels of glucose). Hyperglycemia may in fact play an important role in milk fever, and there may be a correlation between recovery and the return to normal blood sugar levels. It has been shown that after calcium borogluconate is given intravenously, a significant decrease in plasma glucose concentration occurs.[2]

Prevention. To prevent milk fever, the oral or parenteral use of vitamins D_2 and D_3 during the last days of pregnancy and the first days after parturition have been recommended. However, further study is needed to evaluate the effectiveness of vitamin D in preventing milk fever.

The oral use of calcium chloride gel prophylactically may be of value in preventing parturient paresis. Two regimens have been proposed. In one study 150 gm of calcium chloride was administered during a period 1 day before to 1 day after calving. In another, 100 gm of calcium chloride was given daily 5 to 7 days before the estimated calving date to 2 days after parturition. Further investigation into the value of calcium chloride gel in the prevention of parturient paresis is necessary.[11]

Treatment. Milk fever is normally treated by the administration of intravenous calcium solutions. Five hundred milliliters of 20% calcium borogluconate or calcium gluconate sterile solution is administered intravenously. Twenty percent calcium borogluconate solution contains 8.3% calcium, and 20%

calcium gluconate contains 9.3% calcium. However, calcium borogluconate is less likely to precipitate the calcium gluconate. Either solution must be administered slowly to prevent heart block from sudden high blood calcium levels. The animal's pulse rate should be monitored during administration of calcium solutions. If cardiac irregularities develop, administration should be stopped immediately.

Commercially available preparations of 20% calcium gluconate or calcium borogluconate solutions combined with various electrolytes are available. The other electrolytes may include potassium, magnesium, and phosphorus. Some preparations also contain glucose.

If done under strict aseptic conditions, inflation of the udder with air gives a more sustained elevation of plasma calcium than does the administration of calcium intravenously.[15] However, if performed carelessly, udder inflation can result in a severe mastitis. It has therefore not been used as a common form of therapy. When producing milk, cows absorb minerals from their bones into their blood. These minerals may then be secreted into the milk. When the udder is inflated with air, milk secretion is reduced and the concentration of blood calcium increases. Udder inflation may also have a beneficial effect on the blood levels of other minerals such as magnesium, phosphorus, and potassium.

Because of the hyperglycemia that commonly accompanies milk fever, cows that remain down following calcium therapy might be candidates for insulin therapy. A dose of protamine zinc insulin at the rate of 0.5 to 1 unit/kg has been recommended. The effectiveness of this dose, however, has not been reported in clinical trials.[15]

Eclampsia

One to 3 weeks after parturition, eclampsia, or hypocalcemia, sometimes occurs in bitches. As opposed to the flaccid paralysis of cows with milk fever, dogs with eclampsia are in a state of tetany. To treat the condi-

tion, 5 to 10 ml of a 10% calcium gluconate solution is administered intravenously. The solution must be injected slowly to prevent cardiac fibrillation.[16]

Grass tetany

Grass tetany is a disease characterized by low blood concentrations of calcium and magnesium (hypocalcemia and hypomagnesemia). The disease tends to occur in adult cattle and sheep that are pastured on rapidly growing young grass in the spring and in calves fed entirely on milk. Milk has a low-magnesium content. Adult cows contracting the disease are usually of the beef breeds.

Prevention. Many methods have been advocated for the prevention of grass tetany. One method is to administer 60 gm of magnesium oxide orally daily to individual cows and 15 gm daily to calves. Another method is to add magnesium oxide to feed so the cows receive at least 60 gm daily. Because an adult cow cannot build up usable stores of magnesium in the body, the chemical must be given within a few hours before cattle are turned on to lush, green pasture.

Magnesium oxide can also be applied to the pasture. The amounts required will vary with different soil conditions. However, a rule of thumb is that 450 kg of the material to an acre can give protection for six grazing seasons. It is best to apply the chemical during the winter and spring so the magnesium can be taken up by the spring grasses.

Another method is to feed a commercial mineral mixture with 20% magnesium oxide added. The mixture can be fed free choice. If it is not readily consumed, sodium chloride can be added in up to equal parts to increase the palatability.[22]

The following formula for a ton of supplement has been developed to prevent grass tetany in cattle: 1000 pounds of old process cottonseed meal, 370 pounds of sodium chloride, 150 pounds of magnesium oxide, 200 pounds of dicalcium phosphate, 200 pounds of calcium carbonate, and 80 pounds of a vitamin premix. The supplement is kept under cover and offered free choice in the winter and spring months.[2]

Under no circumstances should magnesium sulfate be fed to cattle to prevent grass tetany. Microorganisms in the rumen react with the sulfate ion to produce toxic substances.

Treatment. Five hundred milliliters of calcium gluconate or calcium borogluconate with magnesium added are administered intravenously. As in the treatment of milk fever, the calcium must be administered slowly to prevent heart block. In general, cows with grass tetany do not respond as well to therapy as those with milk fever.

MAMMARY EDEMA

Mammary edema commonly occurs in dairy cattle and is associated with parturition. The condition causes concern because edematous udders are prone to trauma, mastitis, and injuries to the end of the teat. Other problems include difficulty in applying the milking machine, difficulty in removing normal amounts of milk, infiltration of the udder with fibrous connective tissue, and damage to the suspensory apparatus of the udder. Even though the condition normally resolves itself in a few days without treatment, diuretics, with or without corticosteroids, are often administered to reduce mammary edema. The efficacy of this treatment is in question.[21]

Treatment. Among those drugs which are used to treat mammary edema are diuretics. The action of diuretics is discussed in Chapter 18. Chlorothiazide is administered orally at the rate of 2 gm once to twice a day for 3 to 4 days. Hydrochlorothiazide can be given intramuscularly at the rate of 100 to 250 mg, by slow intravenous administration at the rate of 100 to 150 mg, or orally at the rate of 100 to 250 mg once or twice a day. It is claimed that in cattle the drug is two to four times as effective as chlorothiazide. Another diuretic, furosemide, can be given either intramuscularly or intravenously at 6- to 12-hour intervals at the rate of 0.5 to 1 mg/kg, or orally once a day at the rate of 5 mg/kg. A diuretic, trichlormethiazide can be

used in combination with dexamethasone in a ratio of forty parts trichloromethiazide to one part dexamethasone. It is administered at the rate of 200 to 400 mg as an initial dose, followed by 100 to 200 mg daily for 2 additional days if needed.[24]

UROLITHIASIS IN CATS

Urolithiasis, the obstruction of the urethra with a urinary stone (calculus), commonly occurs in male cats. Urolithiasis results from the formation of crystals in the urine. These crystals increase in number when the urine is alkaline and disappear when the acidity drops below a pH of 6.8. The incidence in male cats may be as high as 10%. In affected cats, the mortality rate may approach 50%.

Obstruction of the urethra causes urine to accumulate within the bladder. Other urinary problems, perhaps related to urethral obstruction, also occur in cats. Hematuria (blood in the urine) occurs in male cats without resulting obstruction. Hematuria is also common in female cats. Generally associated with hematuria is an increased frequency of urination with passage of small volumes of urine.

Twelve to 24 hours after a complete urethral obstruction occurs, the symptoms of acute uremia will be evident in the cat. In addition to the accumulation of urea and other toxic products in the blood, potassium moves from within the cell to the extracellular fluid. Because a uremic animal does not eat, there is an increased breakdown of glycogen and protein, which releases additional amounts of potassium into the extracellular fluid. As a result, the most frequent cause of death in uremic cats is elevated blood potassium levels (hyperkalemia) due to the inability of the kidneys to excrete potassium and return blood and extracellular fluid values to normal.

Prevention. The addition of 1% sodium chloride to the feed of cats has been recommended to increase urine output with the hopes of preventing the formation of struvite crystals.[23] However, the value of sodium chloride in the prevention of phosphate uroliths in cats is a question. The addition of 4% sodium chloride to the diet has been shown to be ineffective in controlling the formation of diet-induced phosphate uroliths in cats.[4] The sodium chloride was effective in causing the cats to drink more water but was not effective in preventing calculi formation. Whether the addition of sodium chloride to the diet of cats will help prevent naturally occurring calculi is open to question.

Treatment. Acidification of urine is recommended in the therapy of urinary calculi and other related urinary disorders in cats. The following methods of acidification can be tried:

1. Ammonium chloride, in addition to acidifying urine, acts as a diuretic. However, its effectiveness is limited to 5 or 6 days. It is given at the rate of 25 mg/kg.[24]

2. Ascorbic acid can be administered in large doses to acidify urine without causing systemic acidosis.

3. Methionine can be given at a dose of 100 to 400 mg one to three times a day.[24]

4. Sodium phosphate, monobasic, is commonly used to prevent formation of urinary calculi composed of calcium salts. It is given orally at the rate of 30 mg/kg two to three times a day.[24]

In the presence of kidney or hepatic failure, urinary acidifiers should not be used. In hepatic failure, the use of urinary acidifiers may induce coma. Other potential contraindications include diabetes mellitus, prolonged diarrhea, vomiting large quantities of intestinal juices, and starvation.

To medically treat struvite urethral obstructions in cats, the use of Walpole's acetate buffer solution, pH 4.5, has been suggested. The solution is prepared by combining 57 ml of 0.2 molar acetic acid and 43 ml of 0.2 molar sodium acetate. The solution should be sterilized by filtering it through a Millipore filter prior to use. By flushing the solution into the urethra, the obstruction can be dissolved. (For details on the use of the solution, see Jackson.[9])

In cats with hyperkalemia as a result of urethral obstruction, intravenous fluid therapy should be performed once the urethral obstruction is cleared. The intent of the fluid therapy is to restore blood volume, correct dehydration, provide maintenance fluid requirements, and replace fluids and ions lost during the diuresis that follows relief of the urethral obstruction.

The fluid therapy must be aimed at correcting the hyperkalemia. Addition of sodium bicarbonate will cause a rapid influx of potassium from the intravascular space to the intracellular space. Caution must be used, however, because massive doses of sodium bicarbonate can interfere with cardiac activity.[26]

Another approach is to administer intravenously a multiple electrolyte solution to cats at the time the urethral obstruction is cleared. By anticipating the dehydration as a percent of body weight, the losses can be corrected by intravenous administration of fluids in a 1-hour period. Subsequent maintenance of fluids can be given by subcutaneous injections.[3]

Peritoneal dialysis offers an effective approach to the management of hyperkalemia. The use of regular insulin has also been suggested in the treatment of hyperkalemic uremic cats. Regular insulin is suggested because it acts rapidly, has a relatively short duration, and can be given intravenously. Insulin facilitates the transfer of glucose from the intravascular space to the intracellular compartment in many tissues. This transfer of glucose is accompanied by a shift in serum potassium in a similar direction. Cats are extremely sensitive to insulin. The dose for this use still needs to be established.[3,26]

UROLITHIASIS IN CATTLE AND SHEEP

Urinary calculi occur frequently in feedlot cattle and sheep. Generally, they are treated surgically. However, even when treated, the affected animals may be so uremic that they die. Up to 5% sodium chloride may be included in the ration as an aid in the prevention of urinary calculi. Whereas adding sodium chloride to cat rations produces no results, the addition of sodium chloride in the ration of sheep and cattle appears to be effective in preventing urinary calculi. Two explanations have been suggested. One is that the addition of sodium chloride increases the consumption of water, thereby decreasing the concentration of minerals and organic substances that make up the urinary calculi. Another suggestion is that the chloride ion displaces phosphate from the less soluble magnesium phosphate to the more soluble magnesium chloride.

KETOSIS

Etiology. Ketosis is primarily a disease of dairy cattle and sheep. It is characterized by increased levels of ketone bodies in the blood. In cattle and sheep the condition can occur secondarily to other illnesses when the animals stop eating. Primary ketosis, which is associated with pregnancy in ewes and early lactation in dairy cattle, can have serious economic consequences. In ewes the condition frequently occurs during the last month of pregnancy; ewes carrying multiple fetuses are most susceptible. Because sheep develop ketosis prior to parturition, the economic losses may be compounded by loss of lambs as well as ewes. In dairy cattle the economic losses primarily result from a decrease in milk production.

In the development of both primary and secondary ketosis, the level of substances necessary for the formation of glucose in the liver is no longer sufficient to meet the demands of the body. Because of this, the following occur:

1. Concentration of glucose in the blood is decreased (hypoglycemia).

2. Adequate glucose for synthesis and energy is not available.

3. The fat reserve is utilized for energy production.

4. Free fatty acids are transported to the liver and are oxidized, resulting in a higher than normal production of ketone bodies.

Prevention. Of primary importance in the prevention of ketosis is an adequately balanced diet. The formulations for adequate diets are beyond the scope of this text; the student is referred to Kronfeld.[14]

Treatment. Cows with ketosis may recover spontaneously. It is therefore difficult to attribute improvements in a given animal to the therapy employed. To minimize the frequency of relapses, treatments such as propylene glycol with glucose or insulin with glucocorticoids are sometimes used, but the efficacy of such treatments is not well established.

Glucose. Because glucose is fermented in the rumen, it is administered parenterally to ruminants. When treating ketosis in cows, 500 ml of a 50% glucose solution is given intravenously over a period of 5 to 10 minutes. This usually produces a peak glucose concentration of 300 mg/100 ml, which returns to the preinjection levels in about 2 hours. If an infusion is given over a 90-minute period, the blood glucose level will be sustained for about 4 hours after the injection. With such a treatment, blood ketones drop but rise again to preinjection levels within 16½ hours. High blood glucose levels may be achieved by giving a continuous glucose intravenous drip. Under most circumstances, however, this is impractical.

When glucose is administered, the cows usually improve and increase milk production for at least one milking period. However, the improvements are generally temporary, with nervous signs returning in 12 to 24 hours followed by a decline in the milk production on the second or third day. Repeat treatments are therefore needed. To increase the possibility that glucose therapy will benefit cows, the following procedures are recommended:

1. Repeat the administration of glucose as often as necessary. (Treatments may be required from two or three times a day to once every 2 or 3 days.)

2. Administer the glucose continuously for as long as required.

3. Supplement the glucose therapy with long-acting glucocorticoids, or supplement the glucose by feeding a glucose precursor for several days.[13]

Glucose precursors. The oral administration of sodium propionate, lactates, glycerol, or propylene glycol (which are glucose precursors) is followed by a less dramatic and less consistent improvement than is expected from administration of glucose parenterally. Therefore glucose precursors are only recommended as the sole therapy in mild cases or in combination with glucose therapy in severe cases.

Glucose precursors are used as a drench or mixed with the feed for preventing ketosis.

The glucose precursors have some disadvantages. Sodium propionate may cause digestive disturbances and depress the intake of feed and the butterfat content of milk. Ammonium and sodium lactates may have a laxative action. Calcium lactate is unpalatable and poorly accepted. Mixed lactate salts (calcium-sodium lactate) are the most palatable and do not have undesirable side effects. Sodium lactate masks the unfavorable flavor characteristics of calcium lactate.[28] In trials, when fed at the rate of 6% to 10% of the concentrate mixture, mixed lactate salts were acceptable and effective. Under farm conditions, prolonged feeding at this rate did not produce any adverse side effects during a 3-month period. The rations were accepted by 95% of the cows after the third feeding.[28]

Unlike glycerol, propylene glycol resists fermentation in the rumen and becomes available for conversion to glucose in the liver. Cows tolerate about 1500 gm before developing incoordination and diarrhea. Generally, the recommended dose of 125 to 250 gm administered twice a day causes no ill effects. When administered this way, propylene glycol generally causes no problems, diminishes the incidence of clinical ketosis, and increases the milk production from 0.5 to 1 kg/day. However, the drug will not be universally effective in all herds.

Glucocorticoids. Glucocorticoids are commonly used in the treatment of ketosis. Dexamethasone and betamethasone are popular because they result in the most prolonged hyperglycemic effect. Regardless of which glucocorticoid is used, the dose recommended by the manufacturer for the treatment of ketosis must be closely followed. Overdosing can result in many prob-

lems, including reduction in appetite, which will further complicate the disease.

Unfortunately not all cows with ketosis respond favorably to glucocorticoids. Some become worse. Such a response, however, may indicate a concurrent complication.

Insulin. Because insulin facilitates transport of glucose into cells where it is needed, when cows do not respond to glucocorticoid therapy, the use of insulin may be beneficial. A low dose of long-acting insulin has been used. For example, 200 units of protamine zinc insulin appears to reduce fat mobilization and formation of ketone bodies in the liver.[12,13]

Insulin and glucocorticoids. Insulin and glucocorticoids can be used in combination. Doses of the combination consist of 200 units of protamine zinc insulin together with either 10 mg of dexamethasone or 2.5 mg of flumethasone. Because this combination acts for about 48 hours, it should be readministered only every 2 days if necessary.

Lipotropic drugs. Some success has been claimed for the use of various lipotropic drugs in the treatment of ketosis. Lipotropic drugs decrease deposition of fat in the liver and also increase utilization of fat from the liver. Among the lipotropic drugs advocated for the treatment of ketosis are choline, cysteamine, and l-methionine. Because they are unstable, lipotropic agents must be kept dry before use.

Vitamins. Vitamins will only be effective in the treatment of ketosis caused by a vitamin deficiency.

Anabolic steroids. It appears that the anabolic steroid, trienboline acetate, may have some use in the treatment of primary ketosis in cattle.[5] Doses of 60 to 120 mg are administered. Although no hyperglycemic effect is observed in the cows after the steroid therapy, blood concentrations of ketone bodies are decreased 24 and 48 hours after treatment. An immediate improvement of appetite after therapy is also noted. This in itself might initiate a chain of metabolic events reversing the effects of ketosis. Further investigation on the use of anabolic steroids in the treatment of ketosis is in order.

Summary. In summary, for the treatment of primary ketosis, it is recommended that glucose be given initially by intravenous injection and supplemented by propylene glycol orally. An alternative would be to use a long-acting glucocorticoid in conjunction with a long-acting insulin.

If the ketosis is secondary to another condition, the primary condition must be determined and treated to bring about successful resolution of the ketotic condition.

DIABETES MELLITUS

Diabetes mellitus is a disease in which there is insufficient insulin to regulate carbohydrate metabolism. The insulin is produced by an important endocrine tissue, the islets of Langerhans, which is located throughout the pancreas. The α cells in the islets of Langerhans secrete the polypeptide hormone glucagon. The β cells produce the protein hormone insulin. Both these hormones have important functions in the regulation of glucose metabolism.

In domestic animals, diabetes mellitus is primarily seen in dogs and cats. The disease is characterized by an increase in the volume of urine, increased consumption of water, weight loss despite an increased appetite, hyperglycemia (increase blood levels of glucose), glucose in the urine, ketosis, and acidosis. The condition can eventually lead to coma and death. As a result of the decreased insulin production, many biochemical abnormalities take place. Most of these can be traced to a reduced entry of glucose into the cells of various tissues and an increased liberation of glucose from the liver into the circulation. The decreased production of insulin results in reduced glucose uptake by skeletal muscle, cardiac muscle, smooth muscles, fatty tissue, and other organs. Internally then the cells of these tissues are starved for their primary source of energy, glucose. Their metabolism is grossly disturbed.

The hyperglycemia that occurs in diabetes mellitus by itself is relatively harmless. However, increased levels of sugar in the urine (glycosuria), a result of the hyperglycemia, causes an increased urine output and water intake. In addition, there is an appreciable urinary loss of sodium and potassium as well. As glucose is lost through urine, substantial calories are lost to the body, resulting in starvation. If possible, the animal will compensate by increasing its oral caloric intake, which raises the blood glucose and further increases the glycosuria. It is therefore unavoidable in uncontrolled diabetes mellitus that mobilization of fat stores and weight loss follow. Because the cells can no longer effectively utilize glucose, energy is provided by the metabolism of fat and protein. When fat is broken down, ketone bodies are formed. Because the metabolism of fat in severe insulin deficiencies takes place faster than the body's ability to dispose of the ketone bodies, blood ketone levels rise. As ketones are excreted in the urine, there is a resultant loss of sodium, potassium, and calcium. A severe metabolic acidosis results. During the state of metabolic acidosis, potassium ions leave the cells in exchange for hydrogen ions. Even though an overall potassium deficiency results, plasma levels are higher than normal. As the blood becomes more concentrated from dehydration, the potassium levels appear even greater.

Treatment

Insulin. In dogs and cats with diabetes mellitus, the primary treatment consists of the administration of insulin.

Types. Three general categories of insulin exist: rapid, intermediate, and long-acting. Among the rapid-acting insulins are soluble insulins, which are solutions of regular or zinc insulin crystals. For intravenous administration, only soluble insulin should be used.

NPH insulin is an intermediate acting insulin. Protamine zinc insulin is a long-acting insulin.

Dose and administration. For animals in a diabetic coma, a rapid, short-acting insulin is required. Regular insulin has a maximum effect in 2 hours, and the total effect is gone in 6 hours. An initial dose of 2.2 units/kg is administered by intravenous injection. If in 2 hours the blood ketone or glucose level has not dropped, 4.4 units/kg should be administered intravenously. Once the blood glucose level falls, repeated doses should not be given until the full effect of the last dose is known. If the animal is acidotic but not in shock, then 1.1 units/kg of regular insulin can be given intravenously and 1.1 units/kg subcutaneously.[16]

In addition to insulin therapy, the diet of diabetic animals must be controlled.

Toxicity. Some practices have noted that previously well-regulated diabetic dogs and cats that have been receiving intermediate-acting insulin may develop hypoglycemic reactions 6 to 8 hours after daily insulin injections. However, 18 to 24 hours after the insulin treatment, they become hyperglycemic. This is manifested clinically by the appearance of glucose in the urine. This syndrome can result from an individual reaction to intermediate insulin, which causes an earlier peak and shorter duration of action in the particular patient. The problem can be overcome by dividing the total daily dose of insulin into two equal doses, each to be administered 30 minutes before the morning and evening meals at 8 to 12-hour intervals. Urine should be monitored twice daily to establish the correct dose of insulin. The evening dose should be increased until the morning glycosuria ranges between ⅛% and ¼%. Similarly, the morning insulin dose should be increased until the evening urine is minimally glycosuric at ⅛% to ¼%.[27]

It is important to remember that in addition to animals being presented with hypoglycemia secondary to insulin therapy, the condition can result from other causes. In the dog, glucose values of less than 50 mg/100 ml of blood are considered hypoglycemic. The primary condition must be determined by the veterinarian and treated.

Fluid therapy. Fluid therapy may be necessary to correct the dehydration, provide daily water needs, correct the acidosis, pro-

vide potassium replacement, and perhaps provide glucose if the administration of insulin results in severe hypoglycemia. Hypoglycemia is the primary toxic reaction of insulin overdosage and, if severe, can result in coma and death. It can be corrected by the intravenous injection of glucose.

IRON DEFICIENCIES

If animals receive balanced diets, iron deficiencies generally do not occur. When they do, various oral and parenteral preparations can be administered by the veterinarian. It is important that proper doses are used because overdosing with iron preparations can be toxic.

Baby pig anemia

Baby pigs commonly suffer from iron deficiency anemia. In baby pig anemia there is a reduction of the hemoglobin content of the blood. Hemoglobin is the oxygen-carrying chemical in the blood. The anemia results from an inadequate assimilation from the placenta of iron for future hemoglobin formation. The piglet is born without adequate reserves of iron to support increased hemoglobin formation during its rapid growth.

To supplement hemoglobin formation, the baby pig needs 7 mg of iron daily. In nature it obtains this iron by rooting in the soil. However, in most farrowing operations, cement floors are used, and the baby pig cannot pick up iron by rooting. The piglet must rely entirely on the mother's milk for iron during the first few weeks of life. However, the sow's milk does not contain enough to meet the needs of the baby pig, and without iron supplementation, a high percent of piglets develop anemia in about the third week of life.

Treatment. Various techniques have been used to administer supplemental iron to baby pigs. Oral preparations can be given as long as the doses recommended by the manufacturer are followed. Doses that are too high result in diarrhea and further limit the ability of the gut to absorb iron. Because of the time consumed in the administration of oral doses, parenteral preparations have become more popular. Iron salts have been complexed to relatively large molecular weight organic molecules like dextran, dextrin, and other polysaccharides to reduce their toxicity so that therapeutic doses can be given parenterally. Some injectable iron compounds also contain vitamin B_{12}, cobalt, and zinc.

Intramuscular injections of 100 to 200 mg of complexed iron, such as iron-dextran, are probably the most popular therapy for the treatment of baby pig anemia. This treatment is highly effective in preventing anemia and allowing the animal to gain weight rapidly.

These products, if used at the proper dose and in baby pigs, are generally safe. No objectionable staining of the muscle results at slaughter (if pigs are slaughtered at normal weight) in pigs given injections on or before 4 weeks of age. However, when injected into the ham at 2 months of age or older, some noticeable discoloration and a significant increase in muscular iron will result.[19,20]

SELENIUM AND VITAMIN E

Use. In recent years selenium and vitamin E have been recommended to prevent and treat various conditions in animals. Although there is evidence that selenium and vitamin E have value in preventing or treating certain conditions, such as white muscle disease in sheep and cattle and "tying up" in horses, their use in other conditions such as lameness and arthritic conditions in dogs is based on little hard evidence. In those conditions for which they are effective, response to treatment is greater with combinations of vitamin E and selenium than to either used alone.

Action. About 85% of administered selenium salts are absorbed from the small intestine in monogastric animals. However, ruminants only absorb about 35%, perhaps because ruminal microorganisms reduce the selenite to an insoluble form.

It appears that one biological role of selenium is its incorporation in a blood protein that acts as a carrier of vitamin E. This carrier may prolong blood levels of the vitamin and increase its absorption.

Wheat germ contains vitamin E. When isolated from wheat germ, vitamin E consists of a mixture of three tocopherols: α, β, and γ. α-Tocopherol, which possesses the greatest biological activity, occurs both as a levo and dextro form. The dextro form is approximately 30% more active than the levo form.[6]

Perhaps the basic action of vitamin E is antioxidation of lipids. It may prevent either the oxidation of essential cellular constituents or prevent the formation of toxic products from unsaturated fatty acids. Apparently there is no efficient storage mechanism for vitamin E in the body. Therefore a constant intake is necessary. It appears that selenium protects the body to some degree from vitamin E deficiencies.

Effectiveness. Combinations of vitamin E and selenium have been effective in treating and preventing white muscle disease in sheep and cattle. This condition, which can cause severe pathology in both the skeletal and cardiac muscles, can result in decreased weight gain, stiffness, abortion, and cardiac arrest.

Various other conditions also seem to respond favorably to treatment with vitamin E and selenium. For example, in cows on an apparently selenium-deficient diet, a combined injection of vitamin E and potassium selenite 3 weeks before the estimated calving date reduced the incidence of retained placenta.[29] It has also been reported that the administration of sodium selenite at the rate of 0.1 mg/kg to underweight lambs in areas deficient in natural selenium increased the mean body weight at weaning and at 1 year of age over control groups receiving no selenium. In addition, the weight of the fleece in selenium-treated lambs was greater than in lambs that received no selenium.[17]

A condition referred to as "tying up"

DOSES OF SELENIUM-d-α-TOCOPHEROL COMBINATIONS*

BO-SE

Contains per milliliter: sodium selenite, 2.19 mg (equivalent to 1 mg selenium), plus vitamin E, (as d-α-tocopherol acetate) 50 mg (68 IU).
Inject subcutaneously or intramuscularly:

Calves	2.5 to 3.75 ml/45 kg
Lambs	1 ml/18 kg (minimum 1 ml) in lambs 2 weeks and older
Ewes	2.5 ml/45 kg

E-SE

Contains per milliliter: sodium selenite, 5.48 mg (equivalent to 2.5 mg selenium), plus vitamin E (as d-α-tocopherol acetate), 58 mg (68 IU).
Inject intravenously or by deep intramuscular injection in divided doses in two or more sites:

Horses	1 ml/45 kg, may be repeated at 5- to 10-day intervals

MU-SE

Contains per milliliter: sodium selenite, 10.95 mg (equivalent to 5 mg selenium), plus vitamin E (as d-α-tocopherol acetate), 58 mg (68 IU).
Inject subcutaneously or intramuscularly:

Weanling cattle	1 ml/90 kg, may be repeated in 5 to 10 days
Breeding beef cattle	1 ml/90 kg during the middle third of pregnancy; repeat 30 days before calving

SELETOC

Injection =	per milliliter: sodium selenite, 2.19 mg (equivalent to 1 mg selenium) plus vitamin E (as d-α-tocopherol acetate), 56.2 mg (68 IU)
Capsule =	each capsule contains sodium selenite, 2.19 mg (equivalent to 1 mg selenium), plus vitamin E (as d-α-tocopherol acid succinate), 56.2 mg (68 IU)
Minicaps =	each capsule contains sodium selenite, 0.548 mg (equivalent to 0.25 mg selenium) plus vitamin E (as d-α-tocopherol acid succinate), 14 mg (17 IU).
Dogs	Initial therapy: Injection subcutaneously or intramuscularly in divided doses in two or more sites: 1 ml/9 kg (minimum 0.25 ml and maximum 5 ml), repeated every 3 days until a satisfactory response is obtained, then shifting to a maintenance dose; if no response after 14 days, the therapy should be reevaluated by a veterinarian
	Maintenance: Capsules for dog 9 kg and over: 1 capsule/18 kg (minimum 1 capsule) every 3 to 7 days or longer as required; minicaps for dogs under 9 kg: 1 minicap/4.5 kg (minimum 1 minicap) every 3 to 7 days or longer as required

*These are products of Burns-Biotec.

in horses results from inflammation of the muscles as demonstrated by severe muscle cramping. It commonly occurs in race horses. A large percentage of the cases occur on the first day or so upon returning to training and after 1 or 2 days of rest from a rigid training schedule. Good results have been reported using a selenium-vitamin E combination to prevent recurrence of muscle typing up in horses.[7]

It has been postulated that selenium and vitamin E have some benefit in the treatment of lamenesses and arthritic-like conditions in dogs, but further clinical evaluation is in order before a recommendation can be made.

Toxicity. Selenium is a highly toxic trace element. For medical use, however, it has an adequate margin of safety. Single parenteral doses of 0.875 to 3.5 mg/kg are fatal in rats, rabbits, and dogs. Oral doses of 2.2 to 11 mg/kg will kill lambs, horses, and cows.[6] Selenium can be irritating to tissues when given intramuscularly, so when large doses must be administered, multiple sites are recommended.

Dose and administration. According to the manufacturer of a selenium-vitamin E preparation, doses as shown in the boxed material on p. 279 can be given.

VITAMINS

Vitamins are organic substances that must be present in the body in small amounts for normal metabolism to take place. When clinical deficiencies of one or more vitamins exist, serious disease and even death may result. When diets are deficient in one or more vitamins, supplementing those diets with products containing the missing vitamins will have a profound beneficial effect on the health and well-being of the animals. Probably because of the profound differences in weight gain, general appearance, and health of animals on vitamin-deficient diets and those receiving adequate nutrition, therapeutic value has been ascribed to vitamins over and above their ability to prevent deficiency syndromes.

For example, despite the lack of experimental evidence, many people consume doses of vitamins many times larger than those required to prevent deficiency syndromes in the hopes that their general health will be improved. Large quantities of vitamin C are taken to prevent colds, large doses of various B vitamins are ingested to prevent and treat neurological diseases, and large quantities of vitamin E are ingested for a variety of reasons from the prevention of atherosclerosis to increasing the libido. The question as to whether such uses of vitamins in humans are beneficial will probably not be answered in our lifetime.

Just as humans in our culture administer vitamins to themselves in massive doses on the chance that they may be beneficial, so, too, do many people administer massive doses to their pets and farm animals. Even though most commercial pet foods have adequate levels of all known vitamins needed for the nutrition of dogs and cats, large quantities of pet vitamins are sold by veterinarians and pharmacists and in the lay markets. Frequently, veterinarians administer vitamin B complex parenterally to dogs and cats that have stopped eating secondary to an illness. Even though no evidence exists that such animals suffer from vitamin B deficiency as a result of their self-imposed short-term fast, such vitamins are administered on the hope that they will increase the appetite and provide a biochemical basis for returning the animal to a more normal metabolic state. Only well-controlled experiments, which at best are difficult to perform, will determine whether such veterinary uses of vitamins are well-founded.

Although there is little indication that quantities of most vitamins over and above those needed to prevent deficiencies contribute to animal or human health, there is also little evidence that large quantities of most vitamins are harmful. However, severe toxic reactions from overdosing with vitamins A and D can result. The toxicity of vitamins A and D is described later.

Animals either obtain vitamins from within their own body or from external sources in their natural diet. In addition, vitamins can be artificially administered to animals by supplementing their diet or by parenteral administration. The production of vitamins within animals is an important source of some vitamins for species discussed in this text. With the exception of guinea pigs and primates, animals do not have to receive external sources of ascorbic acid (vitamin C). The animals discussed in this text synthesize sufficient quantities of vitamin C to meet their metabolic needs. Vitamin D is synthesized in the skin of animals exposed to sunlight. Various factors, to be discussed later determine whether adequate levels of vitamin D are produced or whether dietary intakes are necessary to meet an animal's requirement. Different amounts of the various vitamin Bs are produced in the gastrointestinal tract of animals. Large amounts of vitamin B complex are synthesized by ruminal microorganisms. Therefore naturally occurring vitamin B deficiencies in ruminants are rare.

Well-balanced diets will provide vitamins needed to prevent deficiencies. In formulating diets for any animal, one must be cognizant of the minimum vitamin needs and be sure to include those nutrients containing adequate sources of the vitamins.

Although the metabolic requirements of various species of animals for vitamins are similar, the amount of vitamins that need to be included in the diet varies greatly between the species. This difference primarily results from the variability between species in synthesizing their own vitamins.

Traditionally, vitamins are classified as fat or water soluble. The fat-soluble vitamins include vitamins A, D, E, and K. The water-soluble vitamins are the vitamin B complex and vitamin C.

Vitamin A

Animals synthesize vitamin A from carotenes, which are naturally contained in various plants. The synthesis occurs in the intestinal wall and liver. Vitamin A is stored in large quantities in the liver.

Generally, carotenes are found in young growing green plants. Good quality, rapidly growing pasture is usually a good source of vitamin A. However, as plants mature, levels of carotene drop. In addition to plant sources, various animal products are good sources of vitamin A. The primary commercial source of vitamin A is the liver oil of various fish.

One of the primary problems in attempting to supplement the dietary intake of vitamin A is that both carotenes and vitamin A are easily destroyed by oxidation. Even newly cut hay, which has substantial amounts of carotene when growing, rapidly loses its carotene content through the oxidation process. Mature pastures and those that have been bleached out due to long summer droughts experienced in the western United States commonly have little if any vitamin A content. Therefore animals maintained on such pasture or animals totally maintained on cut hay can develop vitamin A deficiencies. How effectively feed supplements prevent these deficiencies depends on how fresh the supplements are, the conditions of storage, and what measures were taken by the manufacturers to prevent oxidation of either carotene or vitamin A in the supplements. It is imperative that supplements be stored in such a way as to protect them from air and heat. Although heat has no direct deleterious effect on the vitamin A, it will speed up the oxidation process in the presence of air. It is important to obtain feed supplements that have been produced in such a way as to minimize oxidation. This is primarily accomplished by coating the vitamin A with a gelatinous material and/or adding antioxidants such as vitamin E to the mixture. Another method of assuring that feed supplements have adequate levels of vitamin A is to use only those which have been freshly prepared. Generally, feed supplements should be used within 3 months of manufacture.

Vitamin A deficiency. Animals suffering

from severe deficiencies of vitamin A show the classical signs, which include impaired vision in dim light, reproductive failures, increased keratinization of the skin and mucous membranes, slow growth rate, skeletal deformities, and cranial and spinal nerve damage. Livestock with marginal deficiencies of vitamin A may not exhibit the classical signs but will not be as "healthy" as animals with adequate vitamin A reserves. They may not grow as quickly and may have reproductive disorders and reductions in milk production. If fed high-quality commercial diets, dogs and cats are unlikely to suffer from vitamin A deficiencies.

Toxicity. There is a wide margin of safety in the administration of vitamin A, but doses forty to a hundred times normal intake can result in toxic reactions. Toxic doses result in skeletal abnormalities, hemorrhage, and high concentrations of fats in the blood.

Administration of vitamin A. When livestock or horses are subjected to conditions in which vitamin A deficiency is likely, they should receive supplements to provide minimum daily requirements as recommended in current textbooks on nutrition. When vitamin A is to be administered parenterally before animals are placed on ranges deficient in vitamin A, a dose should be given that will provide their minimum requirements during the time that they are to be on the range. Following are sample doses for injectable vitamin A:

Calves	1,000,000 to 1,500,000 IU
Adult cattle	250,000 to 2,500,000 IU
Lambs	125,000 to 250,000 IU
Sheep	250,000 to 500,000 IU
Growing swine	125,000 to 250,000 IU
Breeding swine	500,000 IU

These doses may be repeated in 30 to 60 days.

Because of the inclusion of antioxidants in most parenteral vitamin A preparations, their destruction by oxidation is unlikely. The parenteral administration of vitamin A therefore is more likely to prevent vitamin A deficiencies than the use of feed supplements, which may have been oxidized.

Vitamin D

The function of vitamin D has already been discussed on p. 270. The primary source of vitamin D in animals is the formation of vitamin D_3 under the influence of ultraviolet radiation from sunlight. Vitamin D_3 is formed from 7-dehydrocholesterol (provitamin D_3). Provitamin D_3 is formed in the intestinal mucosa from cholesterol. The rate of synthesis of vitamin D_3 from cholesterol is generally adequate in adult animals exposed to sunlight. However, in young growing animals or adults with limited exposure to sunlight, total reliance on natural vitamin D_3 may result in rickets. Diets of such animals should be supplemented with some form of vitamin D. Vitamin D supplements are obtained primarily from two sources. One is from an animal source (such as livers), which provides vitamin D_3. The other, ergosterol, is from plant sources and can be converted by irradiation into calciferol (vitamin D_2). These compounds are widely distributed in plants.

In most animals, vitamins D_2 and D_3 are equally effective. However, in some animals, vitamin D_3 is the only effective vitamin D. For example, chickens and New World nonhuman primates can only utilize vitamin D_3.

Excessive doses of vitamin D can be toxic. In dogs, doses of approximately 528,000 units/kg of body weight can result in fatalities. Toxic effects of massive doses of vitamin D include calcified deposits in the soft tissues, malformed teeth, and decalcification of bones.[10]

In feed supplements, vitamin D is more stable under most conditions than vitamin A. However, oxidation of vitamin D in supplements can occur.

As with other vitamins and minerals, dogs and cats fed quality commercial diets usually receive adequate levels of vitamin D. However, during lactation, pregnancy, or periods of rapid growth, some supplementation of the diet with vitamin D may be helpful. This is especially true if the animals receive an unbalanced calcium or phosphorus supplement, which, as mentioned earlier in the section on calcium, phosphorus, and magnesium metabolism, increases the demands for vitamin D.

Doses of injectable vitamin D_2 for livestock follow:

Calves	150,000 to 225,000 IU
Cattle	37,500 to 375,000 IU
Lambs	18,750 to 37,500 IU
Sheep	37,500 to 75,000 IU
Growing pigs	18,750 to 37,500 IU
Breeding swine	75,000 IU

These doses may be repeated in 30 to 60 days. Dogs' feed should be supplemented at the rate of 22 to 275 IU/kg on a daily basis.

Vitamin E

The use of vitamin E was discussed on pp. 278 to 280. In addition to its physiological activity, vitamin E is often added to vitamin preparations to reduce the oxidation of vitamin A and D.

Vitamin K

Because of its abundance in plants and bacteria, clinical deficiencies of vitamin K rarely occur. The normal population of intestinal bacteria synthesize adequate amounts of vitamin K. Generally, vitamin K deficiency occurs only from the prolonged administration of oral antibacterial drugs, which interfere with the normal gut flora, or from conditions such as obstruction of the bile duct or chronic diarrhea that reduce the absorption of fat-soluble materials such as vitamin K from the intestinal tract.

Vitamin K is necessary for the proper clotting of blood. It is used clinically to treat dicumarol poisoning, which interferes with vitamin K's activity in the formation of prothrombin, resulting in spontaneous hemorrhages. The effects of dicumarol can be reversed by increasing the available amount of vitamin K.

Doses of vitamin K injectable, in the form of menadione (a fat-soluble synthetic vitamin K), are as follows: dogs and cats, 5 to 10 mg; cattle and horses, 80 to 250 mg intramuscularly every 12 hours for 2 days.

Vitamin C

Because the animals discussed in this text are able to synthesize adequate levels of vitamin C, ascorbic acid is not used to prevent vitamin C deficiencies. However, as mentioned on p. 273, ascorbic acid can be used to acidify the urine of cats.

B vitamins

Each vitamin in the vitamin B complex is distinct chemically and produces a unique set of signs when deficient. However, our discussion of the group will be limited because animals receiving adequate nutrition should not suffer vitamin B deficiencies. That is, to prevent any of the vitamin B deficiencies adequate nutrition alone is sufficient rather than vitamin B supplementation. When it is impossible to provide a diet containing adequate amounts of the B vitamins and/or when adequate levels are not produced in the intestinal tract, such as during oral antibacterial therapy, then either parenteral or oral administration of the B vitamins is in order.

Unlike the fat-soluble vitamins, the B vitamins are not stored for prolonged periods in the liver. Therefore a single parenteral injection does not provide the long-term benefits that are obtained with single injections of the fat-soluble vitamins. In chronic deficiencies, therefore, daily supplementation of the diet is necessary. This is best accomplished by the oral administration of vitamin B complex according to the directions of the manufacturer. Vitamin B complex consists of the following: thiamine (vitamin B_1), riboflavin (vitamin B_2), niacin, pantothenic acid, biotin, the folic acid group, and cyanocobalamin (vitamin B_{12}).

With the exception of vitamin B_{12}, vitamin B deficiencies in adult ruminants are unlikely. The rumen microflora produce adequate levels of the B vitamins. However, in cobalt deficient areas, deficiencies of vitamin B_{12} in ruminants do occur. Cobalt is contained in vitamin B_{12} and needed by the ruminal microflora to synthesize the vitamin. Such deficiencies can be treated by either the oral or parenteral administration of cobalt or by parenterally administering vita-min B_{12}.[8,25] Cobalt can be given in the feed at the rate of 5 mg/24 hr for calves; 10 mg/24 hr for cattle; and 0.1 mg/24 hr for sheep.[24]

References

1. Blum, J. W., Ramberg, C. F., Johnson, K. G., and Kronfeld, D. S.: Calcium (ionized and total), magnesium, phosphorus, and glucose in plasma from parturient cows, Am. J. Vet. Res. 33:51, 1972.
2. Crouch, J. Quoted in J. Am. Vet. Med. Assoc. 160:725, 1972.
3. Finco, D. R.: Induced feline urethral obstruction: response of hyperkalemia to relief of obstruction and administration of parenteral electrolyte solution, J. Am. Anim. Hosp. Assoc. 12:198, 1976.
4. Hamar, D., Chow, F. C. H., Dysart, M. I., and Rich, L. J.: Effect of sodium chloride in prevention of experimentally produced phosphate uroliths in male cats, J. Am. Anim. Hosp. Assoc. 12:514, 1976.
5. Heitzman, R. J., and Walker, M. S.: The antiketogenic action of an anabolic steroid administered to ketotic cows, Res. Vet. Sci. 15:70, 1973.
6. Herrick, J. B.:Selenium-tocopherol in veterinary medicine, Vet. Med. Small Anim. Clin. 70:1455, 1975.
7. Hill, H. E.: Selenium-vitamin E treatment of tying up in horses, Mod. Vet. Pract. 43:66, 1962.
8. Hogan, K. G., Lorentz, P. P., and Gibb, F. M.: The diagnosis and treatment of vitamin B_{12} deficiency in young lambs, N. Z. Vet. J. 21:234, Nov. 1973.
9. Jackson, O. F.: The treatment of struvite urethral obstruction in cats using Walpole's acetate buffer solution pH 4.5, Feline Pract. 6:52, May 1976.
10. Jones, L. M.: Veterinary pharmacology and therapeutics, ed. 3, Ames, Iowa, 1965, Iowa State Press.
11. Jonsson, G., and Simesen, M. G.: Parturient paresis: a review, Aust. Vet. J. 49:252, 1973.
12. Kronfeld, D. S.: Insulin therapy in bovine ketosis, Mod. Vet. Pract. 49:26, Feb. 1968.
13. Kronfeld, D. S.: Bovine ketosis: the problems of treatment, Mod. Vet. Pract. 50:47, Feb. 1969.
14. Kronfeld, D. S.: Nutritional management and bovine ketosis, Mod. Vet. Pract. 50:45, April 1969.
15. Kronfeld, D. S.: Management of downer cows, Mod. Vet. Pract. 57:599, 1976.
16. Lorenz, M. D.: Metabolic emergencies, Vet. Clin. North Am. 2:331, 1972.
17. McDonald, J. W.: Selenium-responsive unthriftiness of young merino sheep in Central Victoria, Aust. Vet. J., 51:433, 1973.
18. Miller, R. M.: Uses of commercially-bottled water in emergency intravenous fluid therapy for large animals, Vet. Med. Small Anim. Clin. 71:442, 1976.
19. Miller, E. R., Ullrey, D. E., Brent, B. E., Merkel, R. A., Bradley, B. L., and Hoefer, J. A.: Effects of age of pig and form of parenteral iron upon tissue

20. Miller, E. R., Ullrey, D. E., Brent, B. E., Merkel, R. A., Laidlaw, V. A., and Hoefer, J. A.: Iron retention and ham discoloration: a comparison of five injectable iron preparations, J. Am. Vet. Med. Assoc. 146:331, 1965.
21. Mitchell, R. G., Mather, R. E., Swallow, W. H., and Randy, H. A.: Effects of a corticosteroid and diuretic agent on udder edema and milk yield in dairy cows, J. Dairy Sci. 59:109, 1976.
22. Morgan, W. D.: Magnesium oxide prophylaxis for grass tetany in beef cattle, Mod. Vet. Pract. 48:60, March 1967.
23. Rich, L. J.: Current concepts and feline urethral obtruction, Vet. Clin. North Am. 1:245, 1971.
24. Rossoff, I. S.: Handbook of veterinary drugs, New York, 1974, Springer Publishing Co.
25. Russel, A. J. F., Whitelaw, A., Moberly, P., and Fawcett, A. R.: Investigation into diagnosis and treatment of cobalt deficiency in lambs, Vet. Rec. 96:194, 1975.
26. Schaer, M.: The use of regular insulin in the treatment of hyperkalemia in cats with urethral obstruction, J. Am. Anim. Hosp. Assoc. 11:106, 1975.
27. Schaer, M.: Transient insulin response in dogs and cats with diabetes mellitus, J. Am. Vet. Med. Assoc. 168:417, 1976.
28. Shaw, J. C.: Oral glucogenic compounds for bovine ketosis, Vet. Med. 56:357, 1961.
29. Trinder, N., Hall, R. J., and Renton, C. P.: The relationship between the intake of selenium and vitamin E on the incidence of retained placentae in dairy cows, Vet. Rec. 92:641, 1973.

Additional readings

Baird, G. D., Heitzman, R. J., Hibbitt, K. G., and Hunter, G. D.: Bovine ketosis; a review with recommendations for control and treatment, part II, Br. Vet. J. 130:318, 1974.
Bild, C. E.: An outline of the clinical uses of fluid-electrolytes in canines, Anim. Hosp. 3:40, 1967.
Burtis, C. A., Troutt, H. R., Goetsch, G. D., and Jackson, H. D.: Effects of glucagon, glycerol and insulin on phlorizin-induced ketosis in fasted, nonpregnant ewes, Am. J. Vet. Res. 29:647, 1968.
Chaney, C. H., and Barnhart, C. E.: The effect of iron supplementation on the prevention of anemia in baby pigs, Am. J. Vet. Res. 25:420, 1964.
Edwards, A. J., and Williams, L. L.: Fluid therapy in treating dehydration from calf scours (a practical approach), Vet. Med. Small Anim. Clin. 67:273, 1972.
Giesecke, D.: Metabolic kinetics of the anti-ketotic compound 1,2-propanediol in the rumen, Arch. Int. Physiol. Biochem. 82:645, 1974.
Hall, R. F., and Reynolds, R. A.: Concentrations of magnesium and calcium in plasma of Hereford cows during and after hypomagnesemic tetany, Am. J. Vet. Res. 33:1711, 1972.

Hall, R. F., Sanders, W. L., Bell, M. C., and Reynolds, R. A.: Effects of season and grass tetany on mineral composition of Hereford cattle hair, Am. J. Vet. Res. 32:1613, 1971.

Herigstad, R. R., and Whitehair, C. K.: Local and systemic effects of parenteral injections of sodium selenite in cattle and swine, Vet. Med. Small Anim. Clin. 69:1035, 1974.

Herin, R. A.: Toxicologic, hematologic, and growth studies on pigs given hydrogenated iron-dextran intramuscularly, J. Am. Vet. Med. Assoc. 141:1062, 1962.

Herrick, J. B.: Vitamin E and selenium in animal nutrition, Vet. Med. Small Anim. Clin. 67:568, 1972.

Kirkham, W. W., Guttridge, H., Bowden, J., and Edds, G. T.: Hematopoietic response to hematinics in horses, J. Am. Vet. Med. Assoc. 159:1316, 1971.

Littledike, E. T., Glazier, D., and Cook, H. M.: Electrocardiographic changes after induced hypercalcemia and hypocalcemia in cattle: reversal of the induced arrhythmia with atropine, Am. J. Vet. Res. 37:383, 1976.

Mason, T. A.: A practical approach to fluid therapy in the horse, Aust. Vet. J. 48:671, 1972.

Naga, M. A., Harmeyer, J. H., Holler, H., and Schaller, K.: Suspected "B"-vitamin deficiency of sheep fed a protein-free urea containing purified diet, J. Anim. Sci. 40:1192, 1975.

Nurmio, P., and Alanko, M.: A clinical study of the compound Astra 2045 in the treatment of bovine hypocalcemia with special reference to dosage levels, Nord. Vet. Med. 25:104, 1973.

Nurmio, P., Roine, K., Juokslahti, T., and Loman, A.: A study of the effects of nicotinic acid in cattle, with special reference to ketosis therapy, Nord. Vet. Med. 26:370, 1974.

Odegaard, S. A.: Parturient paresis in dairy cows, Nord. Vet. Med. 25:634, 1973.

Osbaldiston, G. W., and Lowrey, J. L.: SAC allopurinol in the prevention of hyperuricemia in Dalmatian dogs, Vet. Med. Small Anim. Clin. 66:711, 1971.

Owen, C. A.: The discoveries of vitamin K and dicumarol and their impact on our concepts of blood coagulation, Mayo Clin. Proc. 49:912, 1974.

Scheel, E. H., and Patton, I. M.: Urinary calculi in feedlot cattle—report on treatment with amino promazine, J. Am. Vet. Med. Assoc. 137:665, 1960.

Stockman, V.: Treatment of urolithiasis in the male cat, Vet. Rec. 93:602, 1973.

Van Vleet, J. F.: Experimentally induced vitamin E-selenium deficiency in the growing dog, J. Am. Vet. Med. Assoc. 166:769, 1975.

Zuschek, F., Gillingham, J., and Clark, F.: Clinical studies of a parenteral polysaccharide-iron complex, Vet. Med. 55:63, Dec. 1960.

18

DRUGS FOR TREATMENT OF

Cardiovascular disorders

CARDIAC FUNCTION

The heart is a pump responsible for the movement of blood through the circulatory system (Fig. 18-1). Most of the heart is a strong muscle referred to as the "myocardium." The myocardium and valves direct the flow of blood in one direction. Although the heart is regarded as a single organ, it functions as two pumps, the right and left heart. The right heart receives blood from the general circulation and pumps it to the lungs where the blood gives up carbon dioxide and receives oxygen. The oxygenated blood then returns through the pulmonary vein to the left heart, which pumps it throughout the body.

The two main events of cardiac function are relaxation of the organ (diastole) and contraction (systole) (Fig. 18-2). Both the right heart and left heart have two chambers each, an atrium and a ventricle. The right atrium receives blood from the major vein in the body, the vena cava. The left atrium receives blood from the pulmonary vein. The atria empty into the ventricles, the primary pumping chambers of the heart. The right ventricle pumps blood into the pulmonary artery and the left into the aorta. The atria and ventricles are separated by valves that prevent the regurgitation of blood from the ventricles into the atria during systole. Valves in the pulmonary artery and aorta prevent the back flow of blood into the ventricles during diastole.

Oxygenated blood is pumped by the left heart throughout the general circulation (Fig. 18-3). It exits the left heart by way of the aorta, which branches into the major arteries of the body, which in turn branch into arterioles and finally into capillaries. The capillaries have very thin walls only one cell thick. They are so small that blood cells must line up in single file to pass through them. In the capillaries, oxygen and carbon dioxide are exchanged between the blood and the cells. Also in the capillaries, water and electrolytes pass into the interstitial space. These are returned to the general circulation by making their way into dead-end lymph capillaries, which direct the lymph toward the thoracic cavity where the major lymph vessel, the thoracic duct, joins the vena cava prior to its entering the heart. Blood is returned to the heart from capillaries through a network of venules that sup-

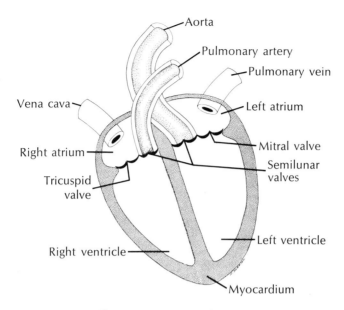

Fig. 18-1. Anatomy of heart.

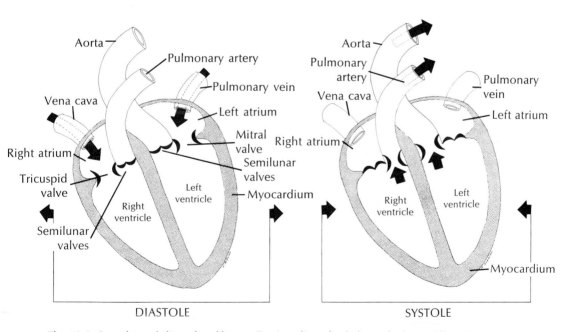

Fig. 18-2. Systole and diastole of heart. During diastole *(left)*, right heart fills with blood with high carbon dioxide content returning from general circulation, and left heart fills with blood rich in oxygen returning from lungs. During systole *(right)*, heart contracts and forces blood into aorta and pulmonary artery.

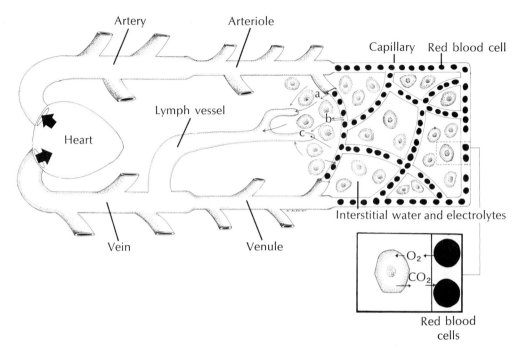

Fig. 18-3. General circulation. Left heart pumps blood into arteries, which branch into arterioles, which branch into capillaries. In capillaries, red blood cells exchange oxygen (O_2) for carbon dioxide (CO_2). *a,* Water and electrolytes leave capillaries to space between cells (interstitial fluid). Interstitial fluid is either reabsorbed in capillaries *(b)* or moves into lymph vessels *(c),* which eventually empty into venous system. As blood moves toward heart, capillaries merge to form venules, and venules merge to form veins.

ply veins, which eventually merge into the vena cava.

One factor that strongly influences cardiac function is the rhythm of systole and diastole. A series of events must take place in a coordinated step-by-step fashion or the heart will not pump blood efficiently. There must be an adequate diastolic phase allowing the atria and ventricles to fill. Systole must occur initially in the atria to maximize ventricular filling. Then the ventricles contract, forcing blood into the arteries.

Cardiac output is the amount of blood pumped by the heart in a given period of time. It is usually expressed in liters per minute. This is determined by the amount of blood ejected during each systole multiplied by the pulse rate. Cardiac output can be increased by maximizing the amount pumped with each beat and/or by increasing the pulse rate up to a point that does not prevent adequate cardiac filling during diastole. In many cases, cardiac output is increased when the pulse rate is lowered from a rate that does not permit proper cardiac filling during diastole.

CARDIAC FAILURE

Even though the heart may not function perfectly, various compensating mechanisms may provide an animal with adequate circulation. One compensatory mechanism of the heart is slight enlargement, thereby increasing the volume of blood pumped during each systole. (Severe enlargement may actually reduce cardiac output by weakening the myocardium.) Another mechanism is an increase in the rate of heart beat.

When the circulation becomes compromised as a result of cardiac malfunction, then a degree of cardiac failure is said to exist. If the failure is complete, blood pressure drops to zero, and death will ensue in a matter of minutes unless cardiac function is restored. In less severe cardiac failure various signs related to the compromised circulation result. The signs vary from relatively mild ones such as shortness of breath upon exercise to severe chronic disability that eventually leads to death.

Various conditions can adversely affect cardiac function. Generally, problems fall into one of the following categories:

1. *Disease of the myocardium (the heart muscle).* When a substantial portion of the myocardium is diseased, less forceful systole results. In humans, myocardial damage frequently results from blockage of the coronary arteries, which supply the myocardium. When the coronary arteries are blocked, a portion of the myocardium is deprived of oxygen and dies. If the patient survives, the damaged myocardium is replaced with scar tissue. Such a process does not commonly occur in domestic animals.

2. *Valvular defects.* Any malfunction of the valves will allow misdirection of a portion of the blood to be pumped during systole. The severity of the problem is proportional to the amount of blood that is misdirected. If valvular malfunctions are to be treated, they must be treated surgically. The surgical treatment of such conditions is beyond the scope of this text.

3. *Shunts.* Certain defects can cause blood to bypass the normal circulatory path, resulting in inadequate cardiac function and inadequate oxygenation of the blood. One of the most common sites for such bypasses between the right and left heart are defects in the ventricular wall (ventricular septum) separating the right and left ventricles. Defects in the ventricular septum must be treated surgically and from a practical standpoint are usually not treated in veterinary practice. Another cause of bypass between the right and left heart is patent ductus arteriosus. The ductus arteriosus is a vessel that exists in the fetus to shunt blood from the pulmonary artery to the aorta. The pulmonary circulation can essentially be bypassed in a fetus because blood is oxygenated by an exchange of gases with the mother's blood in the placenta. At birth the ductus arteriosus normally closes. When it does not, cardiac function is seriously compromised. Traditionally, patent ductus arteriosus has been treated surgically. There are indications that prostaglandins (Chapter 16) keep the ductus open in the fetus. The administration of a prostaglandin inhibitor, such as indomethacin, has been effective in causing the patent ductus to close in the human newborn.

4. *Unusual cardiac rates and rhythm (arrhythmias).* If the cycle of cardiac diastole and systole, a coordinated event initiating with contraction in the atria and gradually extending through the ventricles, occurs out of sequence, cardiac arrhythmia exists. There are numerous types of arrhythmias. For example, the atria and ventricles may beat independently of one another, substantially reducing cardiac effectiveness. Heart rates that are too slow or too fast can decrease cardiac output substantially.

5. *Strictures and obstructions.* A decrease in the internal size of any of the heart chambers or the lumen of the major vessels will restrict the flow of blood. In Chapter 11 we discussed the effect on circulation caused by adult heartworms located in the pulmonary artery. Although strictures or obstructions of the major vessels are not technically cardiac defects, they can result in impaired circulation.

Edema

One of the most important aspects of cardiac failure is the accumulation of fluid in various parts of the body. Left-sided failure causes an increase in venous pressure in the pulmonary vein and the lung. Right-sided failure causes an increase in pressure in the vena cava and the veins and capillaries in the general circulation.

Associated with these increased pressures

is the accumulation of abnormally high amounts of interstitial fluid. This is associated with retention of sodium ions. Such tissues are termed "edematous." The edema commonly occurs in the lungs and liver. When fluid accumulates in the lungs, animals may cough and give the appearance of suffering from respiratory disease. In humans the lower extremities such as the ankles often become edematous; however, this sign is not normally seen in domestic animals. As right-sided failure progresses, fluid will collect in the peritoneal cavity. This is referred to as "ascites."

The exact mechanism for the sodium and water retention associated with cardiac disease is not known. However, it has been well demonstrated clinically that if total body sodium levels can be decreased, edema and ascites can be controlled. With the resolution of the edema, organ systems such as the lung and liver can return to normal function.

Treatment

The medical treatment of cardiac failure is a complicated process requiring the efforts of a skilled clinician who can evaluate various laboratory and clinical findings, initiate therapy, and adjust that therapy as needed to meet the needs of an individual patient. Although the evaluation of cardiac disease and the specifics that determine the choice of therapy are beyond the scope of this text, the basic principles of the management of cardiac disease will be discussed. For greater detail students are referred to Ettinger[4] and Ettinger and Suter.[5]

The medical treatment of cardiac conditions is aimed at three areas:
- Strengthening of the myocardial contraction
- Elimination of edema
- Correction of abnormal cardiac rates and rhythm

Cardiac glycosides

Cardiac glycosides are derived from various plants and have the effect of increasing the force of cardiac contraction and slowing the heart rate, thus increasing cardiac output.

Types. Frequently used cardiac glycosides include the following[5]:

1. Powdered digitalis (USP), which is available as tablets for oral administration. It has a relatively long action.

2. Digitalis tincture (NF), which is produced in a strength so that 1 ml is equivalent to 100 mg of powdered digitalis. It is given orally and has a relatively long action.

3. Ouabain injection (USP), a rapid-acting preparation for intravenous use.

4. Digitoxin (USP), which is available for oral administration and in an injectable form. It has a relatively long action.

5. Digoxin (USP), which is available as a tablet and elixir for oral administration and in an injectable form. It has a moderate duration of activity.

6. Lanatoside C (NF), which is available in tablet form for oral use. It has a moderate duration of action.

7. Deslanoside (NF), which is produced from the alkaline hydrolysis of lanatoside C. It is for injectable use. Its action is of moderate duration.

In addition to these, other cardiac glycosides are available.

Use. Because of the potential toxic effects of cardiac glycosides, during a course of therapy the patient must continually be evaluated by a skilled veterinary clinician. In general, these drugs are used to treat congestive heart failure and certain arrhythmias, in particular atrial fibrillation.

The elimination of cardiac glycosides is delayed by severe liver or kidney damage. Therefore doses are lower in animals with hepatic or renal damage than those with normal liver and kidney function.

Effectiveness. One problem of clinical evaluation of drugs is that clinicians often are biased significantly to report erroneous opinions on the effectiveness of drugs. For example, it has been reported that 16 of 18 veterinarians given placebos, described as a digitalis diuretic compound effective in a university setting, stated that they and their clients observed that the placebo was at least as good, if not better, than the best available cardiac therapy. However, of 6 veterinarians who had been told that the drug was ineffective in a university setting, all agreed that the same placebo was ineffective. Prior to using the drug, both groups were told that the placebo had the potential for causing drowsiness and diarrhea. Fifty percent reporting on the use of the placebo noticed either drowsiness or diarrhea.[8]

Because cardiac glycosides are almost always used in conjunction with either diuretics, a low-sodium diet, or both, the primary factor responsible for the alleviation of signs such as coughing, difficulty in breathing, edema, and ascites is difficult to assess.

Although the use of cardiac glycosides to treat a wide variety of heart conditions will undoubtedly continue for many years, there is not universal agreement that the drugs actually prolong the life of canine cardiac patients. Most clinicians believe that, when used properly, cardiac glycosides are an important part of the total therapeutic regimen for cardiac disorders. There is virtually universal agreement that cardiac glycosides are responsible for clinical improvement in dogs with heart failure resulting from atrial fibrillation. This probably results from the cardiac glycosides' slowing of the rapid ventricular rate that occurs in this condition.

In one study[9] 131 dogs with congestive heart failure treated as outpatients were separated into three categories. One group received digoxin, another digitoxin, and the other no digitalis glycoside. In those receiving cardiac glycosides, doses were adjusted to meet the individual needs of patients. All three groups were fed low-sodium diets and were given diuretic therapy.

Cardiac glycosides were shown to be effective in 13 dogs with atrial fibrillation. In dogs receiving digoxin there was a decrease in heart rate of about 80 beats/min. The decrease in dogs receiving digitoxin was about 47 beats/min. In dogs receiving neither glycoside, a decrease in the heart rate of about 31 beats/min was noted. These were statis-

tically significant differences that indicated digitalis glycosides caused reduction in ventricular rates. Digoxin was more effective in slowing the ventricular rate than digitoxin. There was no difference in the duration of survival between the dogs receiving digoxin and digitoxin. However, both groups survived an average of 4 months longer than the group not given digitalis glycosides.

Of the dogs with cardiac diseases other than atrial fibrillation, those given no glycoside lived longer than those maintained on digitalis-like compounds. However, there was no significant difference in the survival rate of dogs receiving digitoxin as compared to those receiving digoxin.

A significantly greater number of dogs given digoxin exhibited toxic reactions than those given digitoxin or no glycoside.

This study questions the effectiveness in cardiac conditions other than atrial fibrillation of one of the oldest group of drugs used by man. It has therefore been hypothesized that for many cardiac conditions the use of diuretics and restriction of sodium in the diet is a much safer and equally efficacious treatment of cardiac disorders than the use of digitalis glycosides. Reducing pulmonary edema through the use of diuretics may allow better oxygenation of pulmonary capillary blood. This would benefit all organs including the heart.

The validity of the conclusions drawn from this study have been questioned.[14] Certainly further study of a large sample of clinical cases treated with and without cardiac glycosides is necessary to determine the effectiveness of the drugs relative to survival time of patients. We cite this study to make the following points:

1. There is not total agreement that cardiac glycosides benefit patients afflicted with many cardiac conditions for which they are commonly used.

2. It is necessary for controlled experiments to be designed to continue to evaluate a wide variety of accepted therapeutic regimens.

3. Clinicians can be fooled into thinking

improvements are due to drug therapy even when they are not.

Toxicity. The digitalis glycosides can be difficult drugs to use because of their toxicity. They may have varying rates of excretion because dogs in which they are used may have various stages of liver and/or kidney disease. Different manufacturers' preparations may appear to have varying potencies because of the physical nature of the preparation, which affects its absorption from the gastrointestinal tract. The signs of digitalis toxicity in dogs include the following: changes in pulse rate, cardiac arrhythmias, vomiting, diarrhea, loss of appetite, and depression. To reverse toxic effects of cardiac glycosides, administration should be discontinued. Toxicity of digitalis glycosides is enhanced by hypokalemia (a low serum potassium level). Therefore, in most conditions, serum potassium levels should be determined and potassium supplementation or potassium-sparing diuretics used if arrhythmias tend to persist beyond 24 hours after digitalis has been stopped. If arrhythmias are severe and persistent, antiarrhythmic agents should be used. If heart block occurs rather than an arrhythmia, usually only the withdrawal of digitalis is necessary. A heart block is either a partial or complete blockage of impulses conducted from the atria to the ventricles. In the treatment of heart block, potassium therapy and antiarrhythmic therapy are contraindicated.[2]

Digitalis can be resumed at a lower dose level after all toxic signs have regressed.

The evaluation of the toxic effects of digitalization can be difficult because signs referrable to the gastrointestinal tract such as loss of appetite, salivation, vomiting, and diarrhea may result from gastrointestinal irritation by the drug. This can be particularly suspected if such signs are evident after the first oral dose. Changes in the electrocardiograph give a good indication as to the level of toxicity produced by cardiac glycosides.

The treatment for cardiac glycoside intoxication is to discontinue therapy until the dog regains appetite and acts normal and electrocardiographic abnormalities disappear.

Selection. Given the choice of various cardiac glycosides, one is faced with the decision to select the most effective. Probably the most effective cardiac glycoside in a given circumstance is as much a function of the experience of the clinician as the basic pharmacological properties of the compound.

The most commonly used cardiac glycosides in veterinary medicine are digoxin and digitoxin. Each have their own supporters. For example, Ettinger[3] contends and cites references to show that digoxin is more effective than digitoxin or whole leaf digitalis in controlling heart failure in dogs. Hamlin et al.,[7] on the other hand, state that digitoxin as an alcoholic solution given orally or digitoxin given intravenously is the preferred drug for treating heart failure of dogs because of its effectiveness, low incidence of toxic reactions, wide margin of safety, and rapid excretion.

In dogs with right heart failure caused by dirofilariasis, the force of right ventricular contractions increased after intravenous administration of digoxin and digitoxin at the rate of 1 mg/10 kg of body weight. The mean contractility produced by digitoxin (54%) was significantly greater than that produced by the same dose of digoxin (27%).[7] Hamlin's preference for digitoxin is based on the following:

1. Alcoholic solutions of digitoxin are absorbed rapidly and completely from the gastrointestinal tract of the dog. (NOTE: Other forms may not be so well absorbed.)

2. Both parenteral digitoxin and oral tincture of digitoxin are given in identical amounts.

3. When compared to digoxin, digitoxin is at least as effective and probably more so for increasing the strength of ventricular contraction.

4. In dogs at therapeutic doses of 0.5 mg/10 kg of body weight from one to three times a day, digitoxin rarely produces vomiting, diarrhea, or central nervous sytem de-

pression. However, equivalent doses of digoxin frequently produce toxic signs. This forces a reduction in the dose of digoxin and the amount of drug available to stimulate heart action.

5. The reputation that digoxin has for being safer than digitoxin was observed in humans and does not necessarily hold true for dogs. In dogs these drugs are absorbed from the gastrointestinal tract and cleared from the blood at different rates than in humans.

If dissolved in alcohol, solutions of digitoxin must be kept hermetically sealed in brown glass bottles if its activity is to be maintained. Tinctures of digitoxin can be administered to canine patients orally by placing the material into freshly made gelatin capsules or a bolus of dog food.

Dose and administration. For the various cardiac glycosides no single digitalization dose will be appropriate for all animals. In presenting doses on a milligram per kilogram basis a clinician will have to exercise judgment as to whether the dose should be raised or lowered. One factor that must be considered relative to the weight of the animal is that animals with cardiac failure often have severe edema. That edema can substan-

tially increase body weight and result in higher doses than appropriate for the animal. During the first 10 days of cardiac glycoside therapy, animals should be weighed daily to keep track of their body weight as they get rid of retained body fluids.

It is best to hospitalize animals during intial digitalization. This will give the veterinarian a chance to see the effects of the drug, determine if toxicity is occurring, and provide enforced cage rest for the patient.

When using cardiac glycosides, one of three methods of initiating therapy is used: loading dose method, initial maintenance therapy (Table 18-1), and rapid parenteral digitalization.

Loading dose method. The idea behind giving a loading dose of cardiac glycosides is to establish therapeutic blood levels early in the course of therapy and then drop to a maintenance dose that replaces the cardiac glycosides at a rate similar to their rate of removal from the body.

The animal is hospitalized, and an approximate loading dose is calculated and divided into 5 equal doses to be given over a 48-hour period 12 hours apart. For example, if it was calculated that 1 mg was the total loading dose to be given over a 48-hour

Table 18-1. Administration of cardiac glycosides

	Loading dose		Maintenance dose
	Calculated loading dose	Administered	
Digoxin for dogs	0.11-0.22 mg/kg	0.02-0.04 mg/kg every 12 hours for 48 hours or until appearance of toxic signs	Approximately 0.011 mg/kg every 12 hours
Digitoxin for dogs	0.022-0.044 mg/kg	0.004-0.009 mg/kg every 12 hours for 48 hours or until appearance of toxic signs	Approximately 0.002-0.004 mg/kg every 12 hours
Digoxin for cats	—	—	Approximately 0.004 mg/kg every 12 hours; if no clinical improvement after 2 weeks, increase dose no more than 0.002 mg/kg at weekly intervals until clinical improvement or appearance of toxic signs

period, then 0.2 mg would be given every 12 hours until either toxic signs occurred or the 48 hours passed, whichever comes first. The cardiac glycoside is withheld for 24 hours, and if toxic signs regress, a maintenance dose is then administered daily. If toxic signs continue, no additional cardiac glycosides are given until the animal has returned to normal for at least 24 hours.

For digoxin when a loading dose schedule is employed, a total calculated dose of 0.11 to 0.22 mg/kg is administered in five divided doses (0.02 to 0.04 mg/kg per dose) until either signs of toxicity occur or 48 hours elapse. After toxic signs appear, the drug is withheld until no toxic signs have been present for 12 to 24 hours. A maintenance dose is then administered at the rate of 0.022 mg/kg daily divided into two doses at 12-hour intervals.[3]

Because it is questionable how much digitoxin is absorbed from the gastrointestinal system of dogs when tablets or powder are given, only the alcoholic elixir is recommended. A preparation is available that supplies 0.10 mg of digitoxin per milliliter. There is evidence that elixirs of digitoxin are absorbed well from the gastrointestinal tract of dogs. The manufacturer recommends a loading dose of approximately 0.022 to 0.044 mg/kg of body weight divided into doses over a 48-hour period. This amounts to 0.004 to 0.009 mg/kg per dose. The daily maintenance dose should approximate one sixth of the total loading dose. It should be divided into two equal portions administered approximately 12 hours apart for patients with normal renal function. Thus the maintenance dose would be about 0.002 to 0.004 mg/kg every 12 hours.

Regardless of the cardiac glycosides used, animals should remain under hospital observation for 3 to 5 days after initiation of the maintenance dose.

Initial maintenance dose. Therapeutic blood levels can be obtained in about 5 days when initial maintenance doses are administered to animals as opposed to a loading dose. Various problems are associated with

initiating therapy with the maintenance dose, however. It is possible to underdose an animal without realizing it for a long period of time. Also, the signs of toxicity with this regimen generally do not occur until the fifth to seventh day. If the animals are in the hospital, adequate monitoring is possible. However, if the animals are at home, the owner may fail to observe and report the toxicity to the veterinarian so that the dose can be readjusted. Digoxin 0.022 mg/kg divided into two doses every 12 hours, can be given. Less is required proportionately for larger breeds of dogs. It will require from 6 to 10 days for digitalization to occur.[3]

Digitoxin elixir can be given to dogs at the rate of 0.004 to 0.008 mg/kg divided into two doses given 12 hours apart.

Little is known about the clinical use of digitalis glycosides in cats. Cats appear to be more susceptible to the toxic effects of these drugs than dogs. The mean lethal dose of digitalis for the dog is approximately 1.7 times that of the cat. (This is probably not due to an inherent toxicity of the compound in cats but rather a blood level effect resulting from slower metabolism of cardiac glycosides in the cat than in the dog.) Digoxin in an elixir form can be administered to cats at an average rate of 0.004 mg/kg twice daily orally. No loading dose is used. Two weeks should pass prior to increasing the initial dose. If there is no clinical improvement or toxic signs after 2 weeks, the daily dose can be increased no more than 0.002 mg/kg at weekly intervals. After development of toxic signs the next two doses should be withheld. Reduced doses are then administered.[1]

Rapid parenteral digitalization. Rapid parenteral administration of cardiac glycosides is only performed in crisis situations. For cases not in imminent danger of death the oral route is preferred. Because of long residual effects, parenteral administration is not given if animals have received cardiac glycosides within 14 days.

Even though many textbooks advocate intramuscular administration, that route should be used only in fractious dogs because cardiac glycosides when injected intramuscularly are irritating. Therefore the intravenous route is generally preferred.

Both ouabain and digoxin can be used parenterally. Because each have different durations of activity, they are administered differently. A total dose of ouabain is estimated at approximately 0.044 mg/kg. Before the initial administration and continuously until administration is complete, there should be continued electrocardiographic monitoring. Following the initial intravenous administration of 25% to 50% of the total calculated dose, 25% of the total calculated dose is given intravenously every 30 minutes until either digitalization is complete or electrocardiographic disturbances develop. Because ouabain has a short duration of activity, it is not used for maintenance therapy. Maintenance therapy is provided with either parenteral digoxin or orally administered cardiac glycosides.[5]

The total calculated dose for the intravenous administration of digoxin is the same as for ouabain and is 0.044 mg/kg. Generally, 25% to 50% of the total calculated dose is administered initially. Twenty-five percent more is then given every hour to every 6 hours until digitalization occurs. Once digitalization occurs, maintenance doses of injectable digoxin can be given once daily at approximately 25% of the total digitalization dose required. As an alternative, oral maintenance therapy with digoxin may be utilized. The same oral maintenance dose normally calculated for a dog of a particular size is administered.[5]

Diuretics

In heart failure, kidney function changes and sodium and water tend to be retained

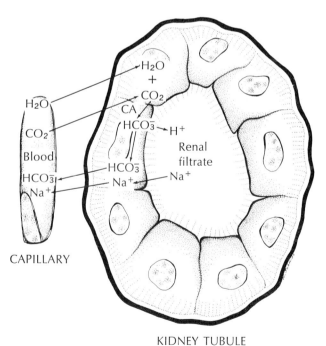

KIDNEY TUBULE

Fig. 18-4. Function of carbonic anhydrase to conserve sodium. In kidney tubule cells, carbonic anhydrase *(CA)* stimulates formation of carbonic acid *(H_2CO_3)*. Carbonic acid ionizes to hydrogen *(H^+)* and bicarbonate *(HCO_3^-)*. H^+ is exchanged with either sodium *(Na^+)* or potassium *(K^+)* (not shown) in renal filtrate. Sodium or potassium then shifts to blood and is retained by body.

in the body. When this occurs, diuretic drugs may be used to restore normal water and sodium balance. To fully appreciate the benefits derived from the use of diuretics, some understanding of kidney function is necessary.

Urine is produced in the kidney nephron. The nephron consists of the glomeruli, proximal convoluted tubule, loop of Henle, and distal convoluted tubule. (See Fig. 17-4.) The kidney maintains water and electrolyte balance by filtering waste products, electrolytes, and water from the blood as it passes through the glomeruli. The fluid that results is the glomerular filtrate. In the normal kidney, protein and fats do not diffuse across the glomerular membrane. In the kidney tubules a large percentage of water and electrolytes that make up the glomerular filtrate are reabsorbed into the blood. Some excretion of water and electrolytes also occurs in the kidney tubules.

Sodium is reabsorbed from the glomerular filtrate in exchange for hydrogen ion (H^+) due to the action of the enzyme carbonic anhydrase. Carbonic anhydrase stimulates the formation of carbonic acid from carbon dioxide and water. Carbonic acid then breaks down to hydrogen ion and bicarbonate ion (HCO_3^-). Some hydrogen ions replace sodium ions in the filtrate. This mechanism helps to maintain proper acid-base balance and conserves body sodium (Fig. 18-4).

When diuretics are used to treat the generalized edema that is associated with cardiac disease, they do not improve the excretory function of a failing kidney. Rather they give the appearance of increased kidney function by reducing the ability of the kidney to reabsorb sodium. This results in increased urine output.

Upsets in electrolyte and acid-base balance can occur when diuretics are used (Table 18-2). Toxicities from diuretics result both from such imbalances and the specific toxicities of the drugs. For example, in humans, chlorothiazide and furosemide tend to increase potassium excretion, organic mercurials increase chloride excretion, and the thiazides and furosemide may induce a diabetic reaction or cause uric acid retention, producing gouty symptoms.[11]

To maximize the clinical benefit and reduce the risk of toxic effects, the dose and frequency of administration of diuretics must be tailored to the individual needs of the patient.

Mercurials. The mercurial diuretics are seldom used, since they have been virtually replaced by newer types. However, they may be useful in dogs that are unresponsive to other diuretics.

Table 18-2. Effects of diuretics

Class of diuretic	Action	Effect on electrolytes
Mercurials	Depress tubular reabsorption of Na^+ and Cl^-	Cl^- deficiency resulting in possible metabolic alkalosis
Thiazides	Inhibit carbonic anhydrase	K^+ deficiency
		Retain Cl^- and lose HCO_3^- ⟵ Tend to cancel each other
	Mercurial-like action	Lose Cl^- and retain HCO_3^- ⟵
Carbonic anhydrase inhibitors	Inhibit carbonic anhydrase	Metabolic acidosis
		Retain Cl^-
		Lose HCO_3^- and K^+
Furosemide	Inhibits reabsorption of Na^+ and Cl^-	K^+ deficiency may cause metabolic alkalosis when Cl^- loss is excessive
Aldosterone-inhibiting agents	Inhibits Na^+ reabsorption	

Action. Mercurials are organic compounds containing mercury, which is liberated in the kidney. In the kidney the ionic mercury inhibits the specific enzyme systems responsible for reabsorption of sodium and chloride in the tubules.

Toxicity. Because of the danger of accumulation of mercury, mercurials are contraindicated in acute renal failure or in other conditions in which urinary output is decreased.

Dose and administration. Mercurials are only partially absorbed from the gastrointestinal tract and are therefore given only by the parenteral route. This generally limits their use to either hospitalized animals or those seen on a daily outpatient basis. After parenteral administration, the absorption of the mercurials is rapid. Diuresis starts in 1 or 2 hours and reaches a peak in 6 hours. Within a day mercurials are completely eliminated through the kidneys.

An example of a mercurial diuretic is meralluride, a mercurial-theophylline complex. It is available in 1 or 2 ml vials containing 30 mg of mercury per milliliter. It can be administered by either the subcutaneous or intramuscular route at the rate of 1 ml/ 13.5 kg. No more than 2 ml should be administered to any one animal. The drug should not be given by the intravenous route because it may be lethal when administered by that route. Two regimens have been suggested for dogs. In one, meralluride is administered once daily for the first 2 or 3 days and then is discontinued and followed by oral diuretics. Another method is to administer the drug no more than once or twice weekly.[5]

Thiazides. The thiazide diuretics include chlorothiazide, hydrochlorothiazide, and bendroflumethiazide and are popular for treating edema associated with cardiac disease. They are highly effective, are well ab-

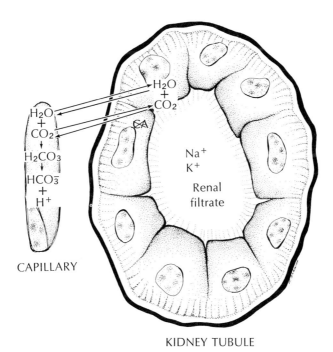

Fig. 18-5. Action of carbonic anhydrase inhibitor diuretics. By blocking action of carbonic anhydrase *(CA)* in cells of kidney tubule, hydrogen ion *(H⁺)* is not available to replace sodium *(Na⁺)* or potassium *(K⁺)* in renal filtrate. This results in excessive urinary excretion of Na^+ and K^+ and excessive retention in blood of H^+.

sorbed, and rarely cause gastric irritation after oral administration. Unlike other categories of diuretics, no tolerance appears to develop as a result of regular and continued use of thiazides.

Action. The thiazides act on the renal tubule to inhibit the reabsorption of sodium, potassium, and chloride. They cause diuresis by two mechanisms. One is the inhibition of carbonic anhydrase, which produces diuresis by inhibiting the formation of carbonic acid in the renal tubules. This prevents the exchange of hydrogen for sodium or potassium. As sodium and potassium remain in the tubules, water is carried with them (Fig. 18-5). In addition, like mercurials, thiazides act directly on the renal tubule to depress sodium reabsorption. This combination of actions is advantageous. The carbonic anhydrase activity favors body retention of chloride and a loss of bicarbonate, leading to acidosis, which is cancelled by the mercurial-like action favoring a loss of chloride, leading to alkalosis.

Toxicity. The primary disadvantage of thiazides is that with continued use, potassium deficiencies in the blood (hypokalemia) may result. Hypokalemia can be serious in cardiac patients because it can induce digitalis intoxication. To prevent hypokalemia, potassium supplements or foods rich in potassium should be administered simultaneously with the thiazide.

There is concern that in humans the thiazides can cause an increase in blood sugar in latent diabetics and an upset of the sugar balance in controlled diabetics.[11]

Dose and administration. After oral administration, thiazide diuretics are well-absorbed, resulting in diuresis within an hour, which persists for 12 to 24 hours. Initially thiazides are usually given twice daily. When the animal has improved clinically, the frequency may be reduced to once a day, and half the original dose may be administered. Occasionally the drug may be skipped for a day to assure maintenance of normal potassium levels.

Doses recommended are as follows[15]: chlorothiazide (for dogs), 10 to 25 mg/kg of body weight given from one to three times per day; hydrochlorothiazide (for dogs), 11 to 33 mg/kg of body weight intramuscularly or orally twice a day, and bendroflumethiazide (for dogs), 5 mg orally twice a day.

Carbonic anhydrase inhibitors. The carbonic anhydrase–inhibiting diuretics result in a substantial diuresis.

Toxicity. Because of undesirable side effects, these drugs are rarely indicated in treating congestive heart failure. They result in the development of metabolic acidosis by preventing the exchange of hydrogen for sodium and potassium (Fig. 18-5). In addition, the degree of diuresis achieved is no better and possibly less than can be achieved using safer drugs such as the thiazides. In addition to edema, they are used to treat glaucoma (Chapter 15).

Dose and administration. Acetazolamide, the classical carbonic anhydrase inhibitor diuretic, can be administered to dogs at the rate of 5 to 15 mg/kg of body weight once or twice a day.[15]

Furosemide. Furosemide is used for treating edema resulting from cardiac, lung, liver, or kidney disease. Because it is rapidly effective, it is especially useful in edema of the lungs.

Action. Furosemide reduces the reabsorption of sodium in the proximal and distal convoluted tubules and in the loop of Henle. Furosemide does not interfere with aldosterone or carbonic anhydrase inhibitors. Therefore it may be used concurrently with those diuretics. Even if glomerular filtration is reduced, furosemide is effective.

Toxicity. Results of furosemide overdosage include marked dehydration and sodium, hydrogen, and chloride depletion. Hypokalemia may also result. Even though the development of hypokalemia resulting from the use of furosemide is reported to be minimal, frequent blood electrolyte determinations and electrocardiograms are recommended when the drug is used on a long-term basis. When used intramuscularly, it may cause tissue sloughing.

Dose and administration. Furosemide works quickly. Within 5 minutes after intravenous administration, diuresis begins. The evening dose should be given to dogs early so that they may urinate before the time that the owner retires for the day. Furosemide can be given to cats and dogs at the rate of 1 to 2 mg/kg intravenously and orally at 12- to 24-hour intervals at the rate of 3 to 5 mg/kg. In horses it can be given intramuscularly or intravenously at the rate of 250 to 300 mg. Intravenous use is usually reserved for emergency therapy.[15]

Aldosterone-inhibiting agents

Action. Spironolactone is a synthetic steroid compound. In the distal renal tubule it is an effective antagonist to the adrenal steroid, aldosterone. In the distal tubule, spironolactone exerts a diuretic effect by inhibiting sodium reabsorption. In addition, spironolactone prevents potassium loss from the distal renal tubules. It is therefore indicated for the treatment of edema caused by uncomplicated excessive aldosterone secretion and for congestive heart failure accompanied by excessive aldosterone secretion.

Spironolactone results in a relatively limited diuresis and requires 3 to 5 days to achieve the diuretic effect. Therefore it is not used as the primary diuretic in treating congestive heart failure. However, because of its potassium-sparing effect, it may be used to offset the potassium loss that occurs when thiazides are administered alone. Spironolactone is expensive, and its use in veterinary medicine is not widespread.

Toxicity. When using spironolactone, one should check for hyperkalemia by periodic electrocardiograms and blood electrolyte determinations.

Dose and administration. A tablet containing 25 mg of spironolactone and 25 mg of hydrochlorothiazide is available. It is generally administered at the recommended rate for hydrochlorothiazide. It should be administered frequently and, if possible, divided into four equal daily doses.[5]

Low-sodium diets

For some patients, low-sodium diets can be used instead of diuretics. In cases of moderate heart disease a low-sodium diet and limited physical activity may reverse signs of cardiac insufficiency. When the use of digitalis glycosides is indicated, restriction of dietary sodium can be a valuable addition to drug therapy.

In addition to the diet, however, water is an important source of sodium. When the water table is low, concentrations of sodium can increase severalfold in municipal water supplies. When restricting dietary sodium, the amount of sodium that will be ingested with drinking water must be considered. If tap water contains more than 150 parts per million of sodium, distilled water should be furnished to animals on sodium-restricted diets. One can determine the level of sodium in drinking water by calling the local water utility. Dogs with congestive heart failure should not be given water that has been chemically softened. Water softeners add sodium to the water.

Restricted intake of sodium for the treatment of congestive heart failure in humans consists of diets at three levels: 7 mg of sodium per kilogram daily, 13 mg/kg daily, and 35 mg/kg daily. Depending on the degree of congestive heart failure, a similar approach may be effective in dogs.

When treating congestive heart failure in dogs by limiting their sodium intake, it is probably best to start with the most restrictive regimen. Such a strict reduction would require a diet that would contain no more than 50 mg of sodium per 100 gm of dry diet, resulting in a sodium intake of approximately 7 mg/kg. Some dogs with only mild cardiac problems respond favorably when fed diets containing about 250 mg of sodium per 100 gm of dry diet, resulting in an intake of approximately 40 mg/kg per day. Such restrictions raise the question of the possibility of producing sodium deficiency in the patient. However, there are indications that dogs have an excellent ability to conserve sodium. It appears that minimum dietary sodium requirement of the dog is less than 4.4 mg/kg and that animals could be maintained at this rate when attempting to treat congestive heart failure without causing sodium depletion.[12]

Diets produced commercially for the management of canine cardiac disease are low in sodium and modest in potassium content when compared to commonly used canine feeds. They do contain sufficient levels of calcium, phosphorus, and magnesium to adequately nourish dogs.

Antiarrhythmic drugs

The clinician must take into account various factors in deciding the choice of drugs for treating cardiac arrhythmias. Arrhythmias fall into various categories: (1) those that do not threaten cardiac function or that are likely to resolve spontaneously before they threaten cardiac function, (2) those that limit cardiac function but do not require immediate treatment, and (3) those that are an immediate threat to life and require prompt treatment. Depending on the category, cardiac arrhythmias can be left untreated, be subjected to a well-thought out and well-planned treatment, or be treated with the therapy most likely to resolve the arrhythmia in the shortest possible time.

There is always the possibility that drugs used in the treatment of cardiac arrhythmias may make matters worse. This is particularly a danger if the cardiac arrhythmia is not limiting cardiac function. The use of drugs can produce an arrhythmia that either seriously limits cardiac function or even causes death. Therefore the use of antiarrhythmic drugs must be determined by a clinician experienced in the management of cardiac arrhythmias.

Quinidine

Action. Quinidine is chemically related to quinine. It has various effects on the heart as follows:

1. It decreases spontaneous discharge of the pacemaker tissue.

2. It reduces conduction of the impulses that cause contraction of the heart.

3. It prolongs the period of time that both the conduction fibers and cardiac muscles are refractory to impulses.

4. It reduces contractility of the cardiac muscles.

While these effects tend to depress cardiac activity, quinidine in therapeutic doses is likely to result in an increased heart rate. Quinidine counteracts the activity of the vagus nerve, which supplies parasympathetic innervation to the heart. In addition, quinidine, to some extent, counteracts the effects of acetylcholine. The decreased arterial blood pressure that results from quinidine administration may also be partially responsible for the increased heart rate. Quinidine may lose its effectiveness after it is used for several months.

Toxicity. Quinidine must be used with great caution in congestive heart failure. If there is already decreased cardiac contractility, quinidine will decrease it even further. Although it can be safely administered with digitalis when there are no signs of digitalis intoxication, it should not be used to treat arrhythmias caused by intoxication from the cardiac glycosides.

Signs of intoxication of quinidine therapy include vomiting, diarrhea, depression, incoordination, and convulsions. Certain changes in the electrocardiogram will also be noted. When signs of overdosage occur, the drug should be discontinued. To increase the safety of administration, quinidine at low doses may be used in combination with other antiarrhythmic drugs such as procainamide.

Dose and administration. Quinidine is available as tablets and capsules, as long-acting tablets composed of quinidine polygalacturonate, and as an injectable product, quinidine gluconate.

When quinidine is given orally, it is completely absorbed from the gastrointestinal tract. To obtain a cumulative effect, it must be administered every 2 to 4 hours because it has a maximum effect in 1 to 3 hours and persists for 6 to 8 hours. When given intramuscularly, the peak effect is reached in 30 to 90 minutes.

There is no fixed dose for quinidine preparations. Doses are adjusted to meet the individual needs of patients. However, if results are to be favorable, high doses are necessary. Substantially higher doses are given on a body weight basis to dogs than are given to humans. Doses of approximately 7 to 22 mg/kg of body weight orally or intramuscularly have been suggested.[5] When given orally, the initial dose is followed by a second dose 2 to 8 hours later, depending on the severity of the condition. In acute situations, doses following the initial dose are given every 2 hours for four or five doses. This regimen is continued until the arrhythmia ceases or toxic levels of the drug are reached. Once the arrhythmia has been abolished and there is less urgency, maintenance doses are administered every 6 to 8 hours.

When given intramuscularly, the dose of quinidine is followed by similar doses every 2 to 4 hours until either the arrhythmia is resolved or signs of intoxication develop. Once the arrhythmia ceases, maintenance therapy with either oral or intramuscular administration is initiated. Maintenance therapy involves levels of drugs between approximately 7 and 22 mg/kg of body weight every 6 to 8 hours. Long-acting quinidine preparations may be administered every 12 hours to reduce the frequency of administration.

Procainamide

Action. Procainamide is closely related chemically to procaine, a local anesthetic. Like procaine it reduces the sensitivity of the ventricles to electrical stimulation. Its effects on the cardiovascular system are similar to those of quinidine. Procainamide slows conduction and depresses excitability in the atria and ventricles. At normal doses the contractility of the heart is depressed to a lesser extent than with quinidine. The heart rate of dogs receiving procainamide may increase due to its antivagal and anticholinergic effects. Unlike quinidine, procainamide usually has little effect on blood pressure when administered orally or intramuscularly. However, it causes a decrease in blood pressure due to vasodilation when given intravenously.

Toxicity. If a dog receiving procainamide stops eating, becomes nauseated, vomits, or develops certain electrocardiographic abnormalities, the drug must be discontinued.

When the drug is used intravenously a severe drop in blood pressure is the major toxic reaction. Procainamide should not be given intravenously to dogs with preexisting low blood pressure. If the drug is to be given intravenously, blood pressure should be monitored. It must be used cautiously in dogs with decreased kidney function because it is primarily excreted by the kidneys. Toxic reactions are treated by discontinuing administration of the drug.

Dose and administration. Procainamide is available in both oral and parenteral forms. When given orally, it is completely and rapidly absorbed from the gastrointestinal tract, resulting in maximum plasma concentrations in 1 hour. When given intramuscularly, maximum plasma levels are obtained within 15 minutes to 1 hour. Intravenous administration results in effective blood level within minutes. The drug must be administered every 4 to 6 hours because plasma levels diminish rapidly.[5] As a guideline only, oral doses for dogs have been recommended at the level of 50 mg/kg initially, followed by 25 to 50 mg/kg. Procainamide can be given by slow intravenous administration at 10 to 15 mg/kg of body weight.[15]

Lidocaine

Action. Although it is primarily a local anesthetic, lidocaine has also been used for the management of ventricular arrhythmis. Lidocaine decreased ventricular excitability and conductivity. Unlike quinidine, in therapeutic doses lidocaine does not greatly affect myocardial contractility, systemic arteriole blood pressure, or the refractory period.

Toxicity. When lidocaine is used, continuous electrocardiographic monitoring is essential. Certain electrocardiographic changes are indications that lidocaine therapy should be discontinued.

High doses of lidocaine can cause convulsions. These convulsions usually subside shortly if lidocaine administration is stopped. If necessary, the administration of ultra–short-acting barbiturates intravenously will control convulsions.

When used as a local anesthetic, lidocaine is commonly combined with epinephrine to prolong the removal of lidocaine from the site of injection. When used for the treatment of cardiac arrhythmias, an intravenous form of lidocaine in 2% solution *without* epinephrine should be used.

Dose and administration. Lidocaine is cleared from the blood within 20 minutes and therefore has a short duration of activity. It is metabolized approximately 90% by the liver; the metabolites are excreted in the urine. Approximately 10% of lidocaine is excreted by the kidney in an unchanged form. Because of its short activity, it is best used in conjunction with other antiarrhythmic drugs such as quinidine, which are given either orally or intramuscularly. Lidocaine will then control the acute problem until the other antiarrhythmic drug has a chance to take effect.

Lidocaine is administered intravenously at the rate of 4.4 to 8.8 mg/kg over a 1- to 2-minute period. Its effect lasts from 10 to 20 minutes. It may be administered in intermittent doses intravenously every 10 to 20 minutes or as a continuous intravenous drip.[5]

SHOCK

Shock is defined as a decrease in the effective circulatory blood volume. In shock, cardiac output and blood pressure are low. It can be caused by a condition such as trauma where blood may pool in the intestinal viscera and be lost for effective circulation. Shock may also result from the loss of blood volume from hemorrhage. When shock is caused by extreme blood loss, there is a deficiency of red cells and plasma proteins, in addition to a relative deficiency of blood volume.

Shock, regardless of the cause, stimulates a reflex constriction in the vascular bed. This vasoconstriction is apparently an effort by the body to restore blood pressure and to divert the flow of blood to vital organs such as the heart, brain, and lungs. However, vasoconstriction can result in insufficient blood flow to other organs, especially the kidneys, liver, and intestines. Reduced blood supply to these organs can cause severe disruption

in cellular function and eventual cellular death. If there is extensive cellular damage in these organs, the animal will die, even if normal blood pressure is eventually restored. This is referred to as "irreversible shock."

Vasopressor shock therapy

Vasopressor drugs act to increase blood pressure by vasoconstriction and by increasing cardiac contractility. They are used with the hope that perfusion to vital organs will improve. However, studies of shock show that intensive vasoconstriction is already present in shock. Further vasoconstriction can seriously impair already reduced blood flow to organs such as the kidney and liver.

Vasopressor drugs may be useful as an emergency measure in the treatment of hemorrhagic shock until other therapy such as blood replacement can be instituted. However, there is the danger that vasopressor drugs can increase the risk of further circulatory collapse by obscuring the extent of blood loss and causing loss of fluid from the vascular compartment.

The pros and cons of the various vasopressor drugs in the treatment of shock are beyond the scope of this text. The student is referred to Ogburn.[13]

Vasodilator shock therapy

If circulation to the brain, heart, and lungs can be maintained in the treatment of shock, the use of vasodilators, such as chlorpromazine, may be warranted. However, such use should only be made by clinicians highly experienced in the treatment of shock and able to use various mechanical, surgical, and pharmacological means for maintaining the animal in a proper physiological state. In the hands of inexperienced persons, vasodilators are contraindicated in the treatment of shock.

Corticosteroid shock therapy

Although there is no conclusive proof that corticosteroids benefit the patient in shock, many veterinary clinicians believe that corticosteroids may help prevent the serious consequences of shock. On the other hand, some veterinarians believe the use of corticosteroids in the treatment of shock may be harmful.

Various mechanisms have been suggested to explain the value of the use of corticosteroids in treating the shock patient. These include the following[6,10]:

1. Increasing cardiac output and raising the blood pressure.

2. Inhibiting the action of various vasoconstrictor substances that are released during the early stages of shock, thus preventing intensive vasoconstriction in peripheral organs such as the liver and kidney, increasing the return of blood to the venous circulation, increasing cardiac output, and preventing irreparable damage to vital organs.

3. Preventing the buildup of lactic acid, serum fatty acids, and amino acids, which contribute to the development of acidosis in shock patients. Corticosteroids probably prevent acidosis by increasing oxygenation of the tissues through the maintenance of adequate blood circulation and by inducing enzymes that improve maintenance of normal metabolic processes.

4. Stabilizing the cellular membranes, thus preventing the release of enzymes that aid in the formation of myocardial depressant factor. Once those enzymes are released, their action cannot be blocked by corticosteroids. This may explain why large doses must be administered early in shock for corticosteroids to be effective. Also, by stabilizing cellular membranes, the shift of water from the extracellular spaces to the intracellular spaces is prevented, contributing to a reduction in blood volume.

5. Helping to maintain adequate microcirculation by preventing adhesiveness of platelets, decreasing platelet and white blood cell viscosity, and perhaps returning platelets trapped in the pulmonary vessels to systemic circulation.

Corticosteroids may prevent shock produced by bacterial endotoxins by neutralizing the effects of the endotoxins. It has been hypothesized that when endotoxin is released on the death of bacteria, it combines with complement and antibody to form anaphylatoxin. Anaphylatoxin may stimulate release of hormones that cause vasoconstriction.

It is important to remember that massive doses are employed when using corticosteroids in the treatment of shock and that their administration must be started as soon as possible. Perhaps one reason massive doses are needed is because corticosteroids are readily bound to many serum proteins. For example, in the treatment of shock in the dog, prednisolone sodium succinate at the rate of 11 mg/kg has been recommended administered intravenously over a 2- to 3-minute period. Three hours after the initial dose, administration of prednisolone sodium succinate may be repeated. Dexamethasone is generally given at the rate of 4.4 to 11 mg/kg.[10] For hemorrhagic shock the following doses of any one of the following drugs have been recommended[6]: prednisolone, 30 mg/kg; dexamethasone, 5 mg/kg; and hydrocortisone, 50 mg/kg.

The use of corticosteroids in hemorrhagic shock enjoys less support than their use in endotoxin-caused shock. Generally, massive doses of corticosteroids for shock are terminated within 24 to 48 hours after the first treatment.

In general, corticosteroids alone will not be sufficient to treat shock. Other therapy must be initiated, depending on the cause. For example, in shock due to hemorrhage, blood volume replacement is the most important consideration. In addition, appropriate electrolytes should be administered to animals in shock to maintain the proper acid-base balance.

Blood transfusions

Physiologically the most desirable method of treating hemorrhagic shock is to replace lost blood by whole blood transfusion. Hemorrhagic shock is rarely a problem in large animal species such as cattle and horses because of their large blood volumes. However, hemorrhagic shock can be serious in dogs and cats and is commonly treated by the administration of whole blood.

Blood consists of a liquid in which various types of cells are suspended. The liquid phase of blood is plasma. When plasma is allowed to coagulate, the remaining liquid fraction is serum, which has essentially the same components as interstitial water. The three types of blood cells are the red cells, which are primarily involved with the transportation of oxygen to the tissues and carbon dioxide to the lungs; the white cells, which have a multitude of functions, including the destruction of invading organisms; and the platelets, which in conjunction with the plasma proteins are involved in the clotting process.

Depending on the condition to be treated, fractions of blood or whole blood can be transfused. For example, in severe hemorrhages the transfusion of whole blood may be life-saving. However, in certain anemic conditions the animal has an adequate blood volume but suffers a deficiency of red cells. In treating such conditions it is best to transfuse red cells rather than whole blood. This can be accomplished by storing the blood containers upside down in the refrigerator, allowing the red cells to settle by gravity. By transfusing only the portion of the container with red cells, approximtely 70% cells are administered to the animal. In burn cases in which there is a substantial loss of plasma without the loss of cells or in certain cases of shock in which there is a pooling of blood and a reduced effective circulating blood volume, the administration of plasma may restore circulatory function to normal.

Whether transfusing whole blood or blood fractions, the veterinarian should first be certain that transfusion is really necessary. Because of problems that can be encountered when blood is transfused, transfusion should never be performed for frivolous reasons. When the decision is made to transfuse blood, enough of it must be administerd to correct the deficiency that is being treated. The dose will be dependent on the deficiency which is determined on the basis of various clinical pathological examinations conducted by the veterinarian.

Blood collection. Sterile containers must be used when collecting blood from a donor. Commercially, containers are available that already contain premeasured amounts of anticoagulants. The anticoagulants are usually either acid citrate dextrose (ACD) or citrate phosphate dextrose (CPD). The containers must be filled with donor blood to the level recommended by the manufacturer to prevent the presence of excess anticoagulant. Such an excess decreases the clotting ability of the recipient's blood, posing sever problems for an animal in need of transfusion. Dextrose is present in the anticoagulant solutions to help preserve the red cells. When blood is properly collected and stored in either ACD or CPD solutions at 1° to 6° C (34° to 43° F), the red blood cells will remain usable for up to 21 days.

As an alternative to the anticoagulants, heparin can be used. However, because heparin contains no dextrose preservative and because heparin is neutralized by thromboplastic and antiheparin materials in the blood, heparinized blood must be used immediately or stored at 1° to 6° C for no longer than 48 hours.

Heparin is commonly used as an anticoagulant for feline blood because the small volume removed from the donor is not enough to fill standard commercial ACD or CPD containers. When using heparin, it is important that no more than necessary be utilized as an anticoagulant. An appropriate dose for cats would be 250 USP units of heparin in 3 ml of saline per 15 ml of blood.

Blood typing. Blood is a tissue, and as with any tissue transplantation from one animal to another, there is the possibility of the donated tissue being rejected by the recipient. Blood in various species is assigned to group designations according to the antigens contained in the sample. Although the groups usually refer to antigens of the red blood cells, plasma incompatabilities are also possible. When blood of a particular type is injected into an animal that has been previously sensitized with that same type, a reaction may take place that causes destruction of the red blood cells or anaphylaxis.

Various blood types are recognized in dogs. The most important red cell antigen is the A type, which occurs in approximately 60% of the random dog population. The Tr type, which is present in about 50% of the random dog population, may also be capable of causing transfusion reactions. The ideal donor dog would be both A and Tr negative. Because the other blood types can cause problems if transfused, cross matching of donor and recipient should be performed prior to initiating a transfusion.

Cats have at least three blood groups. Cross matching of donor and recipient should also be practiced in that species. Except in lifesaving emergencies, one must be assured that the cells of the donor are compatible with the recipient. Under no circumstances should transfusions be performed from one species to another.

References

1. Beck, A. M.: Digitalis for cats? Mod. Vet. Pract. **50:**22, Aug. 1969.
2. Bolton, G.: The management of digitalis-induced arrhythmias, Am. Anim. Hosp. Assoc. **7:**72, 1971.
3. Ettinger, S. J.: A new controlled digoxin elixir for use in small animals, Vet. Med. Small Anim. Clin. **67:**972, 1972.
4. Ettinger, S. J.: Textbook of veterinary internal medicine: diseases of the dog and cat, Philadelphia, 1975, W. B. Saunders Co.
5. Ettinger, S. J., and Suter, P. F.: Canine cardiology, Philadelphia, 1970, W. B. Saunders Co.
6. Grinstein-Nadler, E., and Bottoms, G. D.: Dexamethasone treatment during hemorrhagic shock: changes in extra cellular fluid volume and cell membrane transport, Am. J. Vet. Res. **37:**1337, 1976.
7. Hamlin, R. L., Dutta, S., and Smith, C. R.: Effects of digoxin and digitoxin on ventricular function in normal dogs and dogs with heart failure, Am. J. Vet. Res. **32:**1391, 1971.
8. Hamlin, R. L., Pipers, F. S., and Carter, K. L.: Preferences of veterinarians for drugs used to treat heart failure in dogs, J. Am. Vet. Med. Assoc. **161:**504, 1972.
9. Hamlin, R. L., Pipers, F. S., Carter, K. L., and Lederer, H.: Treatment of heart failure in dogs without use of digitalis glycosides, Vet. Med. Small Anim. Clin. **68:**349, 1973.
10. Hankes, G. H.: Therapy of shock: the corticosteroid question, Vet. Clin. North Am. **6:**277, 1976.
11. Modell, W.: Drugs of choice, ed. 8, St. Louis, 1972, The C. V. Mosby Co.
12. Morris, M. L. Jr., Patton, R. L., and Teeter, S. M.: Low sodium diet in heart disease: how low is low? Vet. Med. Small Anim. Clin. **71:**1225, 1976.
13. Ogburn, P.: The role of vasoactive agents in shock therapy, Vet. Clin. North Am. **1:**245, 1971.
14. Patterson, D. F., Abt, D. A., Detweiler, D. K., Buchanan, J. W., Knight, D. H., and Pyle, R. L.: On digitalis glycosides in treatment of heart failure: criticism and reply, Vet. Med. Small Anim. Clin. **68:**708, 1973.
15. Rossoff, I. S.: Handbook of veterinary drugs, New York, 1974, Springer Publishing Co.

Additional readings

Breznock, E. M.: Application of canine plasma kinetics of digoxin and digitoxin to therapeutic digitalization in the dog, Am. J. Vet. Res. **34:**993, 1973.
Hamlin, R. L., Smith, R. C., Powers, T. E., and Haschen, T.: Efficacy of various diuretics in normal dogs, J. Am. Vet. Med. Assoc. **146:**1417, 1965.
Linnell, M. R.: Liothyronine in treatment of canine ischemic heart disease, Vet. Med. Small Anim. Clin. **62:**972, 1967.
Phillips, L. R., and Ruebush, E. E.: Dietetic management of canine cardiac disease, J. Am. Vet. Med. Assoc. **148:**254, 1966.

19

DRUGS FOR TREATMENT OF

Gastrointestinal disorders

ANATOMY AND PHYSIOLOGY

Although the anatomy and physiology of the gastrointestinal tract is somewhat unique for each species discussed in this text, the functional purpose of the system is the same. Regardless of the species, the primary functions of the gastrointestinal tract are as follows:

- To break down fats, carbohydrates, and proteins into basic structures that can be absorbed into the blood and utilized by the body for energy and/or tissue growth and repair
- To absorb into the bloodstream water, minerals, and vitamins
- To pass from the body portions of ingested material that were not utilized by the body and other waste products
- To conserve water by reabsorbing it into the general circulation
- To provide a suitable environment for microorganisms that assist in the digestion processes
- To prevent absorption into the systemic circulation of microorganisms from the gastrointestinal tract

When one or more of these functions is incompletely achieved, gastrointestinal disease results. Drugs used in the treatment of gastrointestinal disorders should help to restore the functions listed.

Although the functions of the gastrointestinal tract are common among the animals discussed in this text, the means by which those functions are accomplished may vary significantly. Some understanding of the anatomy and physiology of the digestive tract for each species is necessary if one is to appreciate how drugs are used to correct gastrointestinal disorders.

As the term "digestive system" implies, the primary function of the gastrointestinal tract is to break down complex structures into those that can be absorbed and utilized

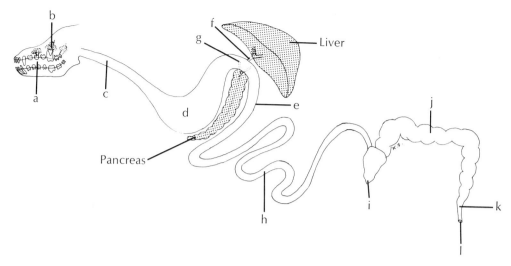

Fig. 19-1. Typical digestive tract. *a,* Mouth; *b,* salivary glands; *c,* esophagus; *d,* stomach; *e,* duodenum; *f,* bile ducts; *g,* pancreatic ducts; *h,* small intestine; *i,* cecum; *j,* colon; *k,* rectum; and *l,* anus.

by the body. Carbohydrates are broken down to sugars, proteins are broken down to amino acids, and fats are broken down to fatty acids and triglycerides. Fats, carbohydrates, and proteins are broken down to basic structures by the actions of enzymes that are formed in the salivary glands, the stomach, the pancreas, and the mucosa of the small intestine.

The basic structures of the digestive system include the mouth, including the teeth, tongue, and salivary glands; esophagus; stomach; duodenum; pancreas; liver, gallbladder in some species; bile ducts; small intestine (jejunum and ileum); cecum; colon; rectum; and anus (Fig. 19-1).

The salivary glands produce enzymes that break down starch into smaller carbohydrates. In the stomach, two major types of enzymes are formed. One type acts to digest proteins, and the other begins the breakdown of fats. Pancreatic enzymes are delivered to the duodenum by the pancreatic ducts. Various pancreatic enzymes act on carbohydrates, fats, and proteins. In addition, intestinal glands produce enzymes that act on all three major categories of nutrients.

Of primary importance in the digestion of fats are the bile salts that are produced in the liver and delivered to the duodenum by the bile duct. In some animals, bile is stored in the gallbladder; however, horses do not have gallbladders. Bile salts help to emulsify fats in the small intestine.

In simple stomach animals, the stomach primarily serves to store newly ingested material and to initiate some enzymatic digestion. The anatomy and physiology of the rumen were previously discussed in Chapter 12. As a result of the action of rumen microorganisms, complex carbohydrates that cannot be broken down by simple stomach animals can be digested by ruminants.

The cecum tends to be larger in herbivores than in carnivores. Some digestion of complex carbohydrates by microorganisms and possibly some absorption resulting from that digestion takes place in the cecum.

In all species, the primary function of the colon is to absorb water, certain minerals, and perhaps vitamins formed by activity of microorganisms in the posterior part of the digestive tract. As the intestinal contents become more solid in the colon, they pass to the rectum for expulsion through the anus.

ANTACIDS

Although antacids are commonly used in human medicine, they are rarely used in veterinary medicine. For the most part, animals do not suffer gastric and duodenal ulcers, which in humans are the most significant lesions caused by hyperacidity. Humans use antacids to obtain relief from indigestion associated with hyperacidity. If animals do suffer from hyperacidity indigestion, they are unable to communicate their discomfort and therefore do not receive antacids for relief.

Probably the most common use for antacids in veterinary medicine is for the treatment of indigestion resulting from overeating in ruminants. In this condition, carbohydrates are rapidly fermented, resulting in extreme acidity in the rumen. This condition is described in greater detail on p. 315.

Antacid preparations generally contain one or more of the following: aluminum hydroxide, magnesium oxide, magnesium hydroxide, or sodium bicarbonate.

Aluminum hydroxide. Aluminum hydroxide reacts with excess stomach acid. The formula for this reaction is $AL(OH)_3 + 3HCl \rightarrow AlCl_3 + 3H_2O$. The aluminum chloride resulting from the combination of the aluminum hydroxide and hydrochloric acid is an acid salt producing a mildly acidic stomach content. This result is desirable because if the stomach contents become alkaline, the stomach reacts to produce more hydrochloric acid. This phenomenon is referred to as "acid rebound."

Besides its use for neutralizing stomach and intestinal acids, aluminum hydroxide has an astringent action and is capable of adsorbing bacteria and toxins.

In addition to its use in the gastrointestinal tract, aluminum hydroxide is used for other purposes as well. For example, it reduces or prevents acidosis and the formation of phosphate calculi in the urinary tract because it decreases absorption of acidic phosphate ion. It should not be given with tetracycline because it may prevent adequate absorption of the antibiotic from the intestinal tract. Prolonged use can cause

phosphorus deficiency. Aluminum hydroxide can be constipating.

Magnesium oxide and magnesium hydroxide. Probably the most commonly used antacids in veterinary medicine are magnesium oxide and magnesium hydroxide. They are used both for their antacid and laxative effects. In addition, as discussed in Chapter 17, magnesium oxide can be used to supplement magnesium-deficient diets.

Both magnesium oxide and magnesium hydroxide have a laxative effect. Only a small amount of the magnesium ion is absorbed from the intestinal tract. The unabsorbed magnesium ion causes the intestinal contents to become hypertonic. To make the gastrointestinal contents isotonic, water is drawn into the intestinal tract from the circulation. The resulting large volume stimulates contraction of the intestine, reducing the amount of time for its contents to pass through the tract and resulting in watery feces.

If either magnesium oxide or magnesium hydroxide are given to animals with intestinal blockage and/or reduced kidney function, blood concentrations of magnesium can increase and depress central nervous system function.

When supplied as a powder, magnesium oxide or magnesium hydroxide can be administered to cattle at a dose of approximately 100 to 500 gm mixed in 4 liters of water. Commercially available milk of magnesia preparations, which contain approximately 8% of magnesium hydroxide in a water suspension, can be given in the following doses[9]:

Adult cattle	1 to 4 liters
Foals	30 to 60 ml
Sheep	250 ml
Cats	1 to 5 ml
Dogs	1 to 20 ml

Sodium bicarbonate. Sodium bicarbonate can be used as an antacid, but generally it is not employed for this purpose because, unlike the poorly absorbed compounds just discussed, it can cause a systemic alkalosis. However, in conditions in which there is a need for an intestinal antacid and to reverse systemic acidosis, the use of sodium bicarbonate can be considered.

ANTI-DIARRHEAL DRUGS
Protectives and adsorbents

Protectives and adsorbents are drugs that form a protective coat on inflamed mucosal surfaces and adsorb toxic substances, facilitating their excretion. They are contained in many commercial antidiarrheal products. Among the drugs commonly classified as protectives and adsorbents are the following: insoluble bismuth salts such as bismuth subnitrate, subcarbonate, and salicylate; various hydrated colloidal aluminum silicates, including bentonite, kaolin, and fuller's earth; and pectin, which is a carbohydrate obtained from the inner rind of apples and other fruits. Activated charcoal is, in our opinion, the adsorbent of choice for use in both large and small animals.

Anti-infective drugs

As discussed in the chapters on infectious diseases, various microorganisms—viruses, bacteria, protozoa, and fungi—can cause digestive problems. The anti-infective drug and the dose chosen depends on the species and the type of infecting organism (Chapters 3 to 7).

Salicylazosulfapyridine. Salicylazosulfapyridine (Azulfidine) is worthy of special mention. It has been used in the treatment of one specific intestinal disorder of dogs—ulcerative colitis. Its effectiveness in treating other diarrheal diseases has not been demonstrated.

The drug is contraindicated in cats because it can cause anemias in that species. In addition, keratoconjunctivitis sicca has been associated with the use of this drug in dogs.

When used to treat ulcerative colitis, it is administered at the rate of 44 to 55 mg/kg three times a day. No more than 6 gm is given to any individual in a day.[6] Some clinicians now believe that better control of ulcerative colitis can be achieved without the risk of side effects by manipulation of the animal's diet.

Antispasmodics

Opium derivatives. Opium contains various substances that act directly on the smooth muscle of the gastrointestinal tract to reduce spasms. Although various opiate preparations can be used to treat diarrhea, probably the most common is camphorated opium tincture (paregoric). It contains approximately 0.4% opium and 0.04% morphine. It can be administered to calves and foals at the rate of 15 to 30 ml two to three times a day and to dogs at the rate of 2 to 5 ml two to four times a day.

Because the opium derivatives are narcotics and subjected to strict federal regulation, they are generally not as popular for the treatment of diarrhea as other nonnarcotic antispasmodic drugs.

Parasympatholytics (cholinergic blocking drugs). The parasympathetic nerves stimulate activity of the gastrointestinal system. By employing drugs that counter the muscarinic effects of acetylcoline (parasympatholytics), the gastrointestinal secretions and movement of the intestinal tract are reduced. For a review of the parasympathetic nervous system, see Chapter 8.

Belladonna alkaloids. The prototype of the cholinergic blocking drugs is atropine, which is obtained from the root and leaf of the belladonna plant *Atropa belladonna* (deadly nightshade). The belladonna plant contains various alkaloids with anticholinergic action, of which atropine and scopolamine are the most significant. Belladonna alkaloids are commonly contained in antidiarrheal drugs. Whenever belladonna alkaloid–containing products are administered to animals, the dose used should be that recommended by the manufacturer. Overdoses can result in serious toxicity.

Isopropamide. Isopropamide, a cholinergic blocking drug, is included in a popular veterinary preparation with the phenothiazine tranquilizer-antiemetic prochlorperazine (Darbazine). The formulation is recommended by the manufacturer for use in dogs with nonspecific gastroenteritis, vomiting, or motion sickness and for infectious or drug-induced diarrhea. The combination product should be given according to the manufacturer's recommendation.

When used alone, isopropamide can be given orally to dogs twice a day at the rate of 0.22 to 1.32 mg/kg.

Diphenoxylate. A commercial product (Lomotil) developed for humans is popular with some veterinarians for the treatment of diarrhea in dogs. It is manufactured as a tablet or liquid. Each tablet and each 5 ml of the liquid contains 2.5 mg diphenoxylate hydrochloride and 0.025 mg atropine sulfate. Diphenoxylate is a derivative of meperidine (Chapter 14). It reduces spasms of the gastrointestinal tract smooth muscles.

When dispensing this drug, clients must be warned that diphenoxylate is a potent compound and must be kept out of the reach of children. If ingestion by children occurs, immediate medical attention is necessary. The toxic effects can be reversed with the narcotic antagonist, naloxone. However, patients must be observed for a long period of time because the effects of naloxone may wear off before the diphenoxylate is cleared from the body.

The dose of diphenoxylate in dogs that weigh 9 kg or greater is one tablet or 5 ml as needed for diarrhea. This dose may be repeated in 2 to 6 hours.[6]

CATHARTICS

Cathartics are drugs that promote evacuation of the bowels. They work primarily by one or more of the following mechanisms:
- Irritation of the intestine, which causes hypermotility of the intestinal tract
- Increase in the bulk in the intestinal tract, causing a reflex stimulation that produces hypermotility of the intestinal tract

- Lubrication and/or softening of the intestinal contents
- Stimulation of the parasympathetic innervation of the gastrointestinal system

In the United States there exists a cultural fixation on bowel habits that has led to widespread use and abuse of cathartic drugs. Those persons dispensing veterinary products should attempt to discourage a similar abuse of cathartics in animals.

There are few clinical reasons for using cathartics in dogs and cats. Although constipation can occur, particularly in older animals, it generally results from the failure to evacuate hard dry stools in the colon. These can often be removed by means of an enema. As in humans, the long-term use of cathartics in dogs and cats can make the animal dependent on them.

Certain clinical conditions in cattle and horses require the use of cathartics. The choice of cathartics to treat the specific condition is made by a veterinarian. Cathartics can be lifesaving when used to treat cattle and horses suffering from overeating concentrated carbohydrates, as well as horses suffering from certain types of intestinal impactions. Such uses will be described later in the chapter.

Irritant cathartics

Irritant cathartics work by irritating the mucosa of the gastrointestinal tract, producing hypermotility. Clincally they are not used as often as bulk or lubricant cathartics because they irritate an already malfunctioning intestinal tract. Irritant cathartics can also cause discomfort to the animal patient.

Two irritant cathartics that have been used in veterinary medicine, castor oil and croton oil, are, in our opinion, obsolete drugs that should be totally replaced with cathartics that are safer to use.

Cascara sagrada. Cascara sagrada is a commonly used cathartic in veterinary medicine, derived from the shrub, *Rhamnus purshiana*, the California buckthorn. The active ingredient in cascara sagrada is emodin. Cascara sagrada is administered orally. Compared to other irritant cathartics it is mild in action. After oral administration, 6 to 8 hours are required for it to take effect.

There are claims that no tolerance develops even when it is administered regularly to a patient.

Dose and administration. Cascara sagrada fluid extract can be administered to dogs orally at the rate of 1 to 4 ml and to cats at the rate of 0.5 to 1.5 ml. The dry extract can be administered orally to dogs at the rate of 0.1 to 0.5 gm and to cats at the rate of 30 to 150 mg.[9]

Raw linseed oil. Although it is not as popular as other cathartics, raw linseed oil has been used for years, especially in horses, as a cathartic. When purchasing linseed oil, one must be sure that it is *raw* because boiled linseed oil contains large amounts of lead, which will cause lead poisoning. In addition, other linseed oil products sometimes have added chemicals that are toxic to animals but improve the utilization of the material in paint products.

Although linseed oil is generally considered as a lubricant cathartic, it is included here as an irritant cathartic because intestinal secretions partially saponify the linseed oil, forming soap and glycerin, both of which are mildly irritating to the intestinal tract. Raw linseed oil is not used in dogs and cats because in those species it produces severe nausea.

Dose and administration. The dose in cattle and horses is 500 ml per adult animal given by way of a stomach tube. This assures delivery of the linseed oil to the stomach and prevents accidental inhalation by the animal in the struggle that results when an attempt is made to administer the medication with a dosing syringe. Only those persons highly skilled in the placement of stomach tubes should administer linseed oil or other preparations using this method, since it is easy to misplace the tube in the trachea (windpipe). Delivering oily products to the lung can result in a fatal inhalation pneumonia.

Bulk cathartics

Saline cathartics. Various salts that are not readily absorbed from the intestinal tract increase the bulk of intestinal contents by holding or drawing water into the intestine. This bulk stimulates an intestinal reflex that propels the intestinal contents through the gastrointestinal tract more rapidly than normal. Therefore, if hypertonic solutions of saline cathartics are given, water will be drawn into the intestinal tract. For this reason, hypertonic solutions should be avoided in the administration of cathartics to severely sick animals because the solution tends to further dehydrate the patient. If isotonic solutions of saline cathartic are given, the administered volume will pass through the intestinal tract without absorption of water from the gastrointestinal tract into the general circulation. If hypotonic solutions are given, there will be some absorption of water from the gastrointestinal tract until isotonicity within the gastrointestinal tract is achieved.

Magnesium salts. Magnesium sulfate, magnesium oxide, and magnesium hydroxide are among the magnesium salts used as cathartics. We have already mentioned that magnesium oxide and magnesium hydroxide are also used as antacids. In addition, magnesium oxide is used as a magnesium feed supplement for the prevention of grass tetany in cattle (Chapter 17).

Dose and administration. When magnesium sulfate is used as a cathartic, it can be administered orally at the following doses[9]:

Cattle	500 gm
Calves and foals	30 to 60 gm
Sheep and large hogs	30 to 120 gm
Cats	2 to 5 gm
Dogs	2 to 60 gm

Since dogs commonly vomit after being given capsules containing magnesium sulfate, it is best administered to them in solution form.

The dose of magnesium oxide and magnesium hydroxide for cathartic action is the same as for antacid action.

Sulfates. Certain salts containing sulfate ion produce cathartic action. Sodium sulfate and magnesium sulfate can be used as cathartics. Sodium sulfate may be more effective in horses than magnesium sulfate.

Dose and administration. The dose of magnesium sulfate was given previously.

For a mild laxative action the following oral doses of sodium sulfate have been recommended[9]: horses, 30 to 60 gm, and sheep, 10 to 15 gm. For stronger cathartic action, the following oral doses are recommended[9]: horses, 250 to 375 gm, and sheep, 60 gm.

Sodium phosphate dibasic. Sodium phosphate dibasic is more pleasant tasting than other saline cathartics. Its action is also milder than magnesium or sodium sulfate. As a laxative the following oral doses are used[9]:

Cattle	500 to 1000 gm
Horses	250 to 500 gm
Calves, foals, sheep, and swine	30 gm
Cats	2 to 5 gm
Dogs	5 to 50 gm

One to 2 gm of sodium phosphate dibasic mixed with 2.5 to 5 gm of sodium phosphate monobasic in 30 ml of water can be used as an enema in small dogs and adult cats. Three times this amount is used in large dogs.[9]

Solid nonabsorbable bulk cathartics. Various solid undigestable materials, particularly those that have an affinity for water, act as bulk cathartics by swelling as they absorb water after they have been ingested. Their bulk action provides a stimulus for increased movement within the intestinal tract. For example, hemicellulose, a lumber industry by-product, can be used for this purpose. Traditionally, wheat bran has been fed to horses as a mild laxative because it contains a large portion of fibrous material that cannot be digested.

Plantago seed also provides bulk by absorbing water and swelling up to fifteen to twenty times its size in the intestinal tract. It is administered to cats at the rate of 2 to 4 gm once or twice a day and to dogs at the rate of 2 to 10 gm once or twice a day in moist or liquid food.

Lubricants

Mineral oil (liquid petrolatum). Mineral oil is probably the most popular lubricant cathartic used in animals. Because the oil is indigestable and not absorbed, it passes through the intestinal tract unchanged.

Dose and administration. Mineral oil should only be administered to cattle and horses by means of a stomach tube. Care must be taken to see that none of the mineral oil is introduced into the respiratory tract because this will cause a fatal foreign body pneumonia. It is administered to cattle and horses at the dose of 0.5 to 4 liters as needed.

Mineral oil is tasteless. Therefore, when given to dogs and cats orally, a flavoring agent such as cod-liver oil should be added so that they will taste the oil and swallow it. It is administered orally to cats at the dose of 2 to 10 ml and to dogs at the rate of 2 to 60 ml as needed.

Petrolatum (petroleum). Petrolatum is often dispensed as a lubricant laxative for cats. The formulations used for this purpose generally also contain a flavoring substance such as yeast or malt to encourage the cat to readily swallow the material. The formulation is used especially to prevent and treat intestinal impactions—especially from "hairballs." Because at body temperature the petrolatum liquifies in the intestine, the formulation is an effective lubricant laxative. Because it is semisolid when administered, there is no danger of the cat inhaling the drug. It is therefore much safer than mineral oil. In chronic oral use, fat-soluble vitamin deficiencies can be created.

When administered petrolatum is usually smeared on the gums, lips, or nose of cats. Generally, cats readily accept the product. It is given orally at the rate of 2 to 5 gm daily or every other day as needed to prevent or remove intestinal impactions.

Fecal softeners

Dioctyl sodium sulfosuccinate. Dioctyl sodium sulfosuccinate (DSS) can be administered orally or by enema as a fecal softener. (It is also used in the treatment of cattle bloat to reduce surface tension as discussed later in this chapter.)

Dose and administration. When used as a fecal softener in cattle and horses, DSS is administered at the rate of 5 to 15 gm orally as needed. The dose in dogs is 15 to 120 mg orally and in cats, 15 to 30 mg orally.

As an enema it can be administered as a 0.5% aqueous solution at the rate of 1 to 3 liters for horses, 40 ml for cats, and 40 to 160 ml for dogs.[9]

Parasympathomimetics (cholinergics)

Parasympathomimetics—autonomic drugs that mimic the muscarinic effects of acetylcholine—act by one of two mechanisms. One is to function like acetylcholine and the other is to block the ability of cholinesterase to break down acetylcholine.

In many respects these drugs are not properly listed as cathartic drugs because they are not routinely employed for that purpose. In mild cases of constipation they would be totally inappropriate. Far less toxic drugs, such as those discussed previously, should be used. In serious impactions, parasympathomimetics are contraindicated because the violent intestinal activity that results from their use may rupture the intestinal tract.

Independent of the gastrointestinal tract, cholinergics have other uses, for example, as miotics in ophthalmology. For such uses they are described under appropriate sections of this text.

None of the cholinergic drugs mentioned here should be used in pregnant animals. They should not be used in old animals or those with intestinal obstructions. They may produce a severe drop in blood pressure and bronchoconstriction.

Ruminatorics. The primary use of cholinergic drugs in the treatment of gastrointestinal disorders is as a ruminatoric, a drug that stimulates contraction of the rumen. The bulk, irritant, and lubricating cathartics are not effective ruminatoric drugs. The primary indications for ruminatorics are overeating, indigestion, and rumen bloat.

Carbachol (carbamylcholine, Lentin, Caride). Carbachol functions like acetylcholine—it stimulates those structures stimulated by acetylcholine. Like actycholine its effects are blocked by atropine. It can be administered to cattle as a ruminatoric at the rate of 4 mg subcutaneously.[9] Higher doses should not be used because they sometimes inhibit ruminal activity by a still unknown mechanism.

Pilocarpine. Pilocarpine is a naturally occurring alkaloid. Like carbachol it stimulates parasympathetic activity. It is rarely used as a ruminatoric. However, when it is used this way, it is administered subcutaneously at the rate of 65 mg to adult cattle. Its primary veterinary use is as a miotic, as discussed in Chapter 15. Besides these uses, the only other likely clinical application is as an antidote for atropine poisoning.

Physostigmine and neostigmine. Physostigmine and neostigmine are ruminatorics that act by inhibiting cholinesterase. Their ruminatoric effect lasts for about 1 hour. They cannot be used in animals that have been recently exposed to cholinesterase-inhibiting pesticide drugs. In cattle, physostigmine salicylate can be given as a ruminatoric at the rate of 30 to 50 mg subcutaneously. Neostigmine is given subcutaneously at the rate of 1 mg/45 kg to cattle. It can be repeated every 2 hours as needed.[9]

ANTIFLATULENTS

Flatulence is the presence of gas in the stomach or intestines. Although some gas can come from the swallowing of air, the primary source is the fermentation of stomach or intestinal contents by microorganisms. Other than antibiotics, which may decrease the population of gas-producing organisms, drugs will not prevent the formation of gas.

The primary action of antiflatulents then is to assist in the removal of gas from the gastrointestinal tract.

Powdered ginger root and oil of turpentine have been widely used as antiflatulents. We are unaware of any controlled experiment that demonstrates the effectiveness of these drugs for this purpose.

Simethicone and poloxalene may act as antiflatulents by breaking down air bubbles. This permits larger pockets of gas that can be expelled from the gastrointestinal tract.

Simethicone. Simethicone is a polymerized methylsilicone preparation that may break down foam in the gastrointestinal tract. It is said to reduce the surface tension of the gastrointestinal contents. Variable results have been reported with simethicone because apparently some commercial products are not properly activated to achieve the desired antifoaming effect. Recommended doses for the use of Simethicone in treating bloat in cattle may also be too low. Oral doses in excess of 200 ml of a 2.5% weight/volume (w/v) emulsion have been recommended for bloat in cattle, and 60 ml of a 2.5% w/v emulsion have been recommended for bloat in goats and sheep.[9] As will be discussed later, the use of antiflatulents only constitutes one part of antibloat therapy.

Poloxalene. Poloxalene, which is a nonionic surfactant (a substance that reduces surface tension), has been shown to be effective when administered orally at the rate of 25 to 50 gm to cattle with alfalfa bloat.[1]

DIGESTANTS

The only true digestants administered to animals are bile salts and pancreatic enzymes. Bile acids and bile salts are used to stimulate the flow of bile. In addition, they can be of benefit in treating pancreatitis in dogs when the production of pancreatic enzymes is reduced. Use of bile salts in these conditions helps to form more readily absorbable fatty acid complexes, activates lipase, and aids in the absorption of fat-soluble vitamins. Bile acids are administered to dogs after eating at a dose of 100 to 300 mg.[9]

Pancreatin is a source of pancreatic enzymes. The dose usually employed in dogs is 500 mg to 6 gm daily. The dose in cats is 500 mg to 2 gm daily. A powdered pancreatin (NF) is available and provides a palatable and convenient dose form that can be sprinkled on the animal's food.

If pancreatin does not provide clinical relief as evidenced by the disappearance of fatty, foul-smelling stools, the administration of raw uncooked pancreas should be considered. It can be administered to cats at the rate of 5 to 15 gm with each meal and to dogs at the rate of 5 to 60 gm with each meal. Prior to use, raw uncooked pancreas should be stored in the freezer to prevent deterioration of the enzymes.

EMETICS

Emetics are drugs that cause vomiting. They are used to expel ingested poisons from the stomach.

Apomorphine. Perhaps the most widely used emetic in veterinary medicine is apomorphine. Although it is listed as a schedule II narcotic (Appendix G), the primary use of apomorphine is to induce vomiting. The dosage range of apomorphine is 1.5 to 8 mg subcutaneously. The average dose in dogs is 3 mg. In cats a total dose of 1 to 2 mg given subcutaneously is generally recommended. However, doses as high as 25 mg/kg subcutaneously have been suggested.[9]

Syrup of ipecac. Another emetic used in veterinary medicine is syrup of ipecac. It is a 7% solution of ipecac in glycerin. It also contains 2% alcohol. It should not be confused with the more potent fluid extract. The emetic activity of ipecac is due to the alkaloids emetine and cephaline, both of which cause gastric irritation and stimulation of the vomit center in the brain. In dogs, syrup of ipecac can be administered at the rate of 4 to 30 ml orally.[9] Previously recommended doses for cats are probably too low. In experimental trials it has been shown that by administering 6.6 ml/kg, a mean latent period of 11.5 minutes elapses between the time the drug is administered and vomiting.

This latent time is satisfactory for its use in treating the ingestion of poisons. However, when administered at the rate of 2.2 ml/kg, the mean latent time is 52 minutes, which is not satisfactory for treating the ingestion of poisons.[11] In cats doses of 6.6 ml/kg of body weight are therefore recommended.

SPECIAL CONDITIONS OF CATTLE
Indigestion (rumen overload)

When ruminants ingest excessive amounts of concentrated carbohydrate substances such as grain, a rapid buildup of lactic acid within the rumen occurs. Under such conditions, carbohydrates are fermented to lactic acid faster than lactic acid can be removed from the rumen and metabolized in the liver. This results in increased osmotic pressure in the rumen. As a result, excessive fluid moves into the rumen, and the animal becomes severely dehydrated. Because of the buildup of lactic acid, the pH of the rumen falls, killing beneficial microflora. Rumen motility also decreases. As the normal microflora of the rumen die, conditions are set up that encourage the growth of pathogenic organisms. The lowered pH causes severe inflammation to the mucosa in the rumen and can result in ulceration. Pathogenic microorganisms can invade these ulcerated areas and by way of the bloodstream may infect other organs such as the liver.

The most effective method of preventing rumen overload is to keep concentrated carbohydrates, primarily grains, in locked rooms to which cattle have no access.

Treatment. If animals are discovered within the first few hours, surgery can be performed to remove the feed from the rumen. If surgery is not practical, chemical means must be used to neutralize the effects of the ingested carbohydrates. Commonly, a 500 gm dose of magnesium hydroxide is given to neutralize the buildup of lactic acid and to facilitate the passage of the ingested grain through the gastrointestinal tract as quickly as possible.

To reestablish rumen motility, ruminatorics can be used. Ruminatorics that are most effective in cattle include physostigmine, 30 to 50 mg subcutaneously; neostigmine, 1 mg/45 kg subcutaneously; and carbachol, 4 mg subcutaneously.

In previous times, strychnine or the plant from which it is extracted, *Nux vomica*, have been used as ruminatorics. Most authorities believe that they have no value as ruminatorics and their use should be discontinued.

Antimony and potassium tartrate (tartar emetic) is traditionally included in commercial preparations as a ruminatoric. Experiments have shown that it has little or no effect in stimulating the activity of a normal rumen. Whether it stimulates an atonic rumen is an open question. Because it is known that physostigmine, neostigmine, and carbachol are effective ruminatorics, there appears to be no reason to use tarter emetic.

Because of rapid dehydration, cattle suffering from overeating indigestion are appropriate candidates for intravenous fluid administration. Although it is unlikely that such administration is practical in range cattle, it can be feasible in dairy cattle if administered by the same methods as recommended for the horse in Chapter 17.

Traumatic reticuloperitonitis (hardware disease)

Traumatic reticuloperitonitis is a condition that is truly unique to veterinary medicine with an unusual preventive and therapeutic regimen. Cattle often accidentally ingest wire or nails. Such heavy materials fall into the reticulum and can perforate that structure, resulting in a variety of signs. When the foreign body first punctures the reticulum, an acute local peritonitis is established. That reaction may be walled off with no further complications. On the other hand, a chronic local peritonitis or an acute diffuse peritonitis can result. Either of these conditions may result in chronic illness or death. If the foreign body migrates toward the head, it can puncture the diaphragm, the pericardium, and even the heart itself.

The diagnosis of hardware disease must be made by a veterinarian. It is made on the

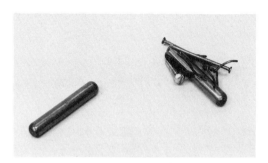

Fig. 19-2. Bar magnets. When given orally to cattle, bar magnet will attract wire or nails in reticulum, preventing their migration.

basis of clinical signs and sometimes by using specially designed metal detectors.

Prevention. To prevent hardware disease, many ranchers administer bar magnets to their animals prophylactically (Fig. 19-2). If one questions whether an animal has received a magnet, a simple direction compass held close to the animal can determine whether a magnet is present.

In addition to prophylactically administering bar magnets to livestock, on some ranches, all chopped hay to be fed to cattle is run under strong magnets so that pieces of wire and nails will be removed.

Treatment. Once a diagnosis of hardware disease is made, a veterinarian must decide on either surgical or medical therapy. If surgery is decided on, he will make an incision

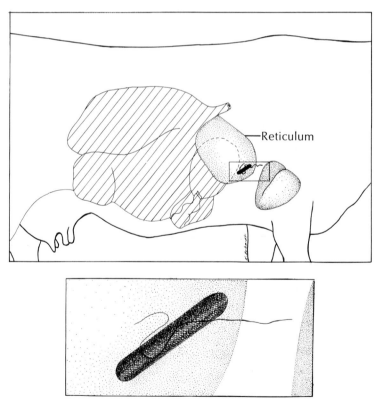

Fig. 19-3. Bar magnet holding wire in reticulum. By attracting wire or nails in reticulum, bar magnet can prevent migration of object and allow body's defenses to "wall off" object.

in the rumen and attempt to locate and remove the foreign body. To treat this condition medically, the cattle is confined (preferably with the anterior portion of the cow elevated) and a bar magnet is administered orally.

The magnet drops into the reticulum and hopefully will attract the foreign body, preventing its migation and allowing the cattle's own defense system to wall off the foreign body (Fig. 19-3), resulting in clinical improvement.

Ruminal bloat

Ruminal bloat is the accumulation of unusually large amounts of gas in the rumen. In the rumen the fermentation process causes a large production of various gases. Bloat results from the inability of the animal to get rid of that gas. Primary bloat results from the development of foam in the rumen, which prevents the eructation (burping) of gases.

Secondary bloat results from an obstruction of the esophagus, often with a foreign body such as an apple or potato. Secondary bloat can be relieved by removing the obstruction.

Because primary bloat responds to medical treatment, our discussion shall be limited to that condition.

Etiology. Various mechanisms for the development of bloat have been suggested as follows:

- Certain microorganisms in the rumen that may cause rapid gas production, resulting in a frothing of the ingesta
- Other ruminal microorganisms breaking down natural plant antifoaming substances
- Ingestion of young plants
- Lack of roughage in the diet
- Genetic factors that may result in lowered salivary flow and a decrease of antifoaming substances
- Ingestion of plants that have been subjected to frost, ingestion of green legumes (such as alfalfa or clover), or gestion of large amounts of easily digestable carbohydrates

When there is frothing of the ingesta, large gas pockets do not form at the cardia (that portion of the rumen where the esophagus enters). Because of the lack of these large gas pockets, eructation does not occur. Toxic substances in plants can also interfere with eructation.

Distention of the posterior digestive tract, rapid feeding, and various genetic factors can also interfere with eructation. The eructation reflex is also depressed when rumen motility decreases, favoring gas accumulation. As bloat develops, rumen motility decreases or stops entirely (ruminal atony).

Prevention. Because acute primary bloat can affect the majority or even all animals in a herd and because mortality among affected animals is so high, the prevention of bloat is an essential component of managing a herd of cattle.

If pastures are maintained with less than 50% legumes and hay is fed prior to pasturing animals, the incidence of bloating will be materially reduced. Pasturing animals on nonlegumes overnight has prevented animals from developing bloat when moved to an alfalfa pasture the next day.

The feeding of antifoaming agents at times when bloat is most likely to develop is another means of preventing bloat. Various mineral and vegetable oils are effective, within limits, as antifoaming agents. Detergents and silicones are less reliable. Bloat can be prevented for 3 to 4 hours in animals feeding on legumes when animals ingest 50 to 100 gm of fat that has been sprayed on the feed. However, the ingestion of fat does not prevent feedlot bloat, which develops when animals ingest high levels of easily digestible carbohydrates.

Because of individual variability in drinking patterns, adding antifoaming agents to drinking water has been unreliable. In some cases, effective and practical prevention of bloat has been accomplished by the spraying of pastures with emulsified peanut oil or tallow.

The oral administration of low levels of antibiotics has been suggested as a means of preventing bloat. The intent is to kill bacteria that may contribute to the frothing. Although low level feeding of antibiotics may be practical in beef cattle and dry dairy cows, it has limited application in lactating dairy cows. The low level use of antibiotics in lactating dairy cows can result in contamination of the milk.

The practice of feeding low levels of antibiotics to herds of animals is a controversial one. We believe that in the near future such use will be prohibited or at least severely limited by the FDA.

In summary, the most practical means of preventing bloat include the following:

1. Pasturing animals on pastures consisting of a combination of legume and grass, with grasses predominating (palatability is maintained by clipping)
2. Supplementing with good quality grass hay when legumes predominate
3. Supplementing legume soilage with grass hay
4. When practical, the use of antifoaming agents either by feeding fats or spraying herbage

Treatment. The primary aim in the treatment of bloat is to relieve the distention of the rumen caused by the trapped gas. Because of the high rate of mortality associated with bloat, the condition should always be treated by a veterinarian.

The treatment of secondary bloat is uncomplicated. The veterinarian can pass a stomach tube, thereby relieving the obstruction and allowing the accumulated free gas to escape.

The treatment of primary bloat requires greater skill. The most important aspect of the treatment is to pass a stomach tube and administer a medication that will reduce the surface tension of the rumen contents. This will break down the foam and allow free gas to accumulate, which can then either pass through the stomach tube or be naturally eructated.

Poloxalene, a nonionic surfactant, is used to reduce the surface tension of ruminal contents. When administered at the rate of 25 to 50 gm by either stomach tube or drench, poloxalene is effective in treating bloat.[1]

Poloxalene is diluted with a large volume of water when administered with a stomach tube. This results in a rapid dispersal of the poloxalene throughout the rumen, breaking down the froth over a large area.

Traditionally drugs have been injected through the left flank area directly into the rumen (intraruminal injection). Such injections deliver medication to the posterior part of the rumen in an area removed from the cardia (Fig. 19-4, A). Because ruminants only eructate in response to free gas at the cardia, injecting poloxalene or other surfactants intraruminally will do little to relieve bloat. When administered orally or by means of a stomach tube, poloxalene acts in the region of the cardia, allowing formation of a gas pocket and eructation (Fig. 19-4, B).

Vegetable or mineral oils can be given by stomach tube to animals with bloat to break down the foamy ruminal contents. For cattle 500 ml to 1 liter are administered.

Silicones such as simethicone can be given as a drench or by way of a stomach tube. A 2.5% w/v emulsion of simethicone is given at the rate of 200 ml to cattle and 60 ml to sheep.[9]

DSS is used in veterinary medicine primarily as a fecal softener and for cleaning earwax from the external ear canal. It is also used as a surfactant for the treatment of rumen bloat. Fifteen grams are given to cattle as a drench and by stomach tube.[9]

Once the foam starts to break up, ruminatorics can be administered to stimulate ruminal activity. Any one of the following can be used: carbachol, 4 mg injected subcutaneously; neostigmine, 1 mg/45 kg injected subcutaneously; pilocarpine, 65 mg injected subcutaneously; and physostigmine, 30 to 50 mg injected subcutaneously.

At the discretion of the attending veterinarian, oral antibiotics are often administered in an attempt to reduce the number of bacteria in the rumen that are contributing to the production of frothy bloat. Since the

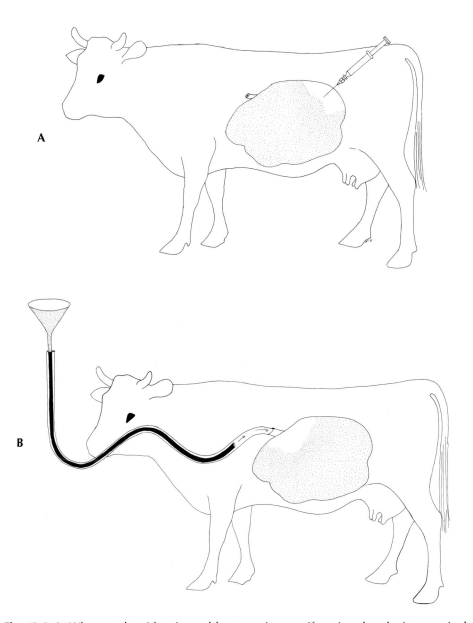

Fig. 19-4. A, When cattle with primary bloat are given antifoaming drug by intraruminal injection, they are unable to belch resulting free gas pocket. **B,** When cattle with primary bloat are given antifoaming drug by oral administration, gas pocket is produced near terminal end of esophagus, facilitating belching.

offending organisms are generally unidentified, the value of this practice is questionable at best.

SPECIAL CONDITIONS OF HORSES
Equine digestive tract

The horse is not a ruminant. Because it does not have the built-in advantages of the ruminant digestive system, the horse evolved with a completely different type of gastrointestinal tract to allow it to efficiently digest plant material. The large intestine is a more important digestive organ in the horse and is many times larger than it is in other domestic animals. Horses have an enormous cecum. Various digestive processes take place in the cecum and ventral colon. Among these are cellulose digestion and absorption. Water reabsorption is the primary function of the dorsal and small or transverse colon. To fit into the abdominal cavity, the voluminous colon is folded with the formation of the sternal, pelvic, and diaphragmatic flexures (Fig. 19-5). There are numerous places in the large intestine where the movement of ingesta may be potentially impeded. These include the cecum; the flexures, particularly the pelvic flexure; and the origin of the small colon. The anatomy of the large intestine therefore predisposes the horse to impactions of the cecum and colon.

Colic

When horses suffer from abdominal distress and show signs of pain, owners usually refer to the condition as "colic." However, colic is not a specific disease, and there is no single drug or treatment regimen that can be effectively used for its treatment. Because many conditions that result in abdominal distress are potentially fatal, all horses showing abdominal distress should be treated by a veterinarian as soon as possible. Among those conditions likely to predispose a horse to abdominal pain are poor physical condition, improper management, abnormal ex-

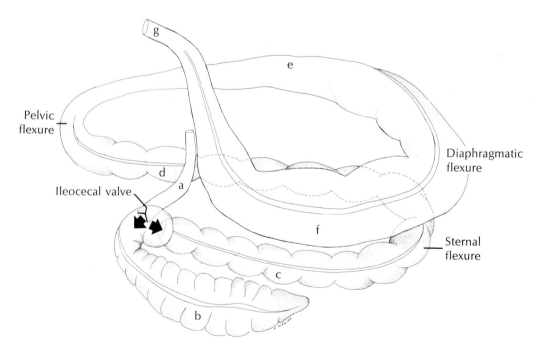

Fig. 19-5. Equine large intestine. *a,* Terminal end of ileum; *b,* cecum; *c,* right ventral colon; *d,* left ventral colon; *e,* left dorsal colon; *f,* right dorsal colon; and *g,* origin of small colon.

ercise, bacterial and viral infections, and parasitism.

Anytime a horse shows colicky signs, there are alterations in intestinal motility. In most instances there will be a cessation of motility in at least one segment of the gut. However, hyperactivity of the gut also results in colicky signs.

Colic can be related to the blood and nerve supply of the intestines. Essentially all the blood to the small intestine and large intestine is supplied by the cranial mesenteric artery. Disruption in the flow of blood to the cranial mesenteric artery can decrease the blood supply to part of the intestine. Intimately associated with the cranial mesenteric artery is a plexus of nerves that innervate the large and small intestines. If the plexus is disrupted, pain or malfunction of the intestines can result.

Treatment. Because it is possible to surgically treat many conditions causing colic in the horse, early selection of surgical cases is important. If abdominal surgery is performed on the horse, fluid and electrolyte balance must be maintained. The treatment of acute abdominal diseases should be based on the likely physiologic changes occurring in the patient. Of primary concern is the control of pain, prevention of shock, and relief of the primary condition.

Analgesics. Numerous analgesic drugs are used in the treatment of colic. Among these are dipyrone, meperidine, and pentazocine (Chapter 14). However, because of the possibility of shock in horses suffering from abdominal distress, analgesics that reduce blood pressure should not be administered if there is any evidence of hemoconcentration or toxemia.

Pentazocine. On the basis of clinical trials, pentazocine appears to be an effective analgesic for the management of abdominal pain from a variety of causes.[5] In humans, it is a strong analgesic that is effective against both visceral pain and pain of musculoskeletal origin. It appears to have a minimal depressant effect on either gut motility or arterial blood pressure.[4] For the treatment of

colic, a combination of the intravenous and intramuscular routes appears to be the best method of administration.

Analgesic effects are obtained after an initial intravenous dose of 0.33 to 0.44 mg/kg, followed 10 minutes later by a similar dose intramuscularly.[5]

Flunixin. In clinical trials the administration of flunixin at a 1.1 mg/kg of body weight intravenously produced a rapid favorable effect in the remission of signs of equine colics of varying causes. In horses that required more than one injection, the drug had a duration of activity that averaged 6 to 8 hours. Generally, excellent results in the relief of pain were noted.[10]

Preventing shock. The prevention of shock is complicated. The control of pain by the use of analgesics will help to prevent shock. As explained in Chapter 18, if the animal is in the initial stages of shock, there will be substantial peripheral vasoconstriction that may shut off blood supply to vital organs. Phenothiazine-derivative tranquilizers (Chapter 14) can be used to prevent peripheral vasoconstriction prior to the outright evidence of shock. However, such drugs should not be administered if there is evidence (such as increased pulse or pale mucous membranes) of a decreased blood volume due to lack of fluid intake or because of fluid pooling in the gastrointestinal tract.[3]

Fluid and electrolyte therapy. Previous studies indicate that horses in acute abdominal crisis usually have a slight elevation of plasma sodium, a slight to moderate decrease in plasma potassium, a slight to moderate and on occasion marked decrease in plasma chloride, normal plasma proteins, increased blood lactate, and high plasma glucose concentration.[4] This primarily is due to a hypovolemia caused by a loss of water, electrolytes, and protein into the lumen of the gastrointestinal tract and the peritoneal cavity. To correct this fluid and electrolyte imbalance, vigorous fluid therapy, as discussed in Chapter 17, is necessary.

In an animal that is not eating or drinking, parenteral administration of balanced electrolyte solutions can help to prevent the development of shock. The acid-base status of the horse must be evaluated prior to initiating treatment for that condition. The incidence of acidosis will be high. However, in horses with obstruction of the large bowel, metabolic alkalosis can occur. In the presence of acidosis or if the acid-base status of a horse cannot be determined, therapy should be aimed at correcting acidosis. The administration of 50 gm of sodium bicarbonate in one liter of sterile, distilled water will temporarily buffer a moderate acidosis and will not injure a horse in alkalosis.[4]

Parasitic colic

Among the most important causes of colic are parasites. *Strongylus vulgaris* is the most significant parasite causing altered intestinal motility in the horse. As larvae of the parasite migrate and develop in the mesenteric artery, they cause two types of lesions. One lesion is a true aneurysm with enlargement of the lumen of the artery and sacculation of the wall. It is relatively uncommon. More often, a verminous arteritis with roughening of the lining of the vessel and thrombosis results from the parasites. The thrombosis may result in emboli blocking small branches of the mesenteric arteries, which supply the intestines. Both aneurysms and verminous arteritis may lead to alterations in intestinal motility.

Strongyle parasites in the arteries may result in colicky symptoms in several ways:

1. A thrombosis may completely block the lumen of a major intestinal artery, resulting in an acute rapidly fatal colic. Fortunately this condition is relatively rare.

2. Major branches of an artery may become blocked by thrombosis or embolism. This leads to stasis of large segments of the intestine, impaction, intussuception, or torsion.

3. More commonly, mild thromboembolic lesions may occur. These lesions are present in more than 90% of all horses. Because of the presence of thrombi in the arteries, small emboli occasionally pass into and block

smaller branches, temporarily stopping motility of the gastrointestinal tract. Such occurrences may be chronic and recurring. Thrombi can also predispose a horse to colic from other gastrointestinal insults such as overeating grain or deprivation of water.

4. The nerve supply to the gut can be interfered with when aneurysms cause an enlargement of the cranial mesenteric artery and its major branches, resulting in pressure on adjacent nerves.

Treatment. Because foals commonly eat their mother's feces, it is highly recommended that mares be treated for gastrointestinal parasites during the last 2 weeks of gestation and again within 24 hours after foaling. A relatively nontoxic anthelminic such as one of the benzimidazoles should be used. Doses are given in Chapter 13. Although it is difficult to eliminate *Strongylus vulgaris* from horses, it is possible to do so by improved sanitation alone. Five days are required for strongyle eggs to develop into infective larvae. It has been demonstrated that if mares and foals are kept in isolation from all other horses and all fecal material is removed every 24 hours, it is possible to raise foals that are free of strongyles.[2]

Intestinal obstructions

Horses are highly susceptible to intestinal obstructions. The skill of an experienced equine practitioner is necessary to diagnose the location of the impaction and the best form of therapy.

Impactions of the colon often respond to the administration of a mild lubricant cathartic, like mineral oil, and if necessary, administration of pain-relieving drugs.

Impaction of the ileocecal valve is often fatal and frequently requires surgical intervention and aggressive postsurgical fluid therapy. In addition, conditions such as torsion of the intestine or intussusception in which there is a telescoping of the intestine upon itself will result in death unless immediate surgical intervention by a veterinarian is provided. In addition to the surgery, intensive fluid therapy, as discussed in Chapter 17, must be employed.

Because obstruction of the gastrointestinal tract causes secretion of water, sodium, and potassium into the intestine, drugs such as saline laxatives, which cause fluid to pool in the intestine, should not be administered. Magnesium sulfate therefore is contraindicated in such conditions. Mineral oil should *not* be used if surgery is anticipated. If during surgery it is necessary to excise the gut, the presence of mineral oil in the intestine increases the probability of the peritoneal cavity becoming contaminated. In other cases, mineral oil is probably the laxative of choice. It does not result in potential hemoconcentration as do the saline laxatives.

Stomach distention must be relieved early in the treatment of abdominal conditions. It has been shown that an obstructed bowel begins to secrete rather than absorb water and electrolytes within 12 hours of the onset of intestinal obstruction. The rate of secretion increases with time. By passing a stomach tube to remove the accumulated fluid, the passage of extracellular water and electrolytes into the gut lumen may be slowed, relieving gastric and intestinal distention, reducing pain, and minimizing the risk of stomach rupture.

Gastrointestinal stimulants such as neostigmine may aggravate the pain that commonly occurs with intestinal obstruction and have the potential of causing rupture of the distended, devitalized gastrointestinal tract. Despite that, the use of such drugs is recommended by some veterinary clinicians. After animals have been treated with lubricant to soften and lubricate the intestinal impaction, the use of 10 to 12 mg of neostigmine intramuscularly has been recommended.[8] Neostigmine generally causes the animal to defecate within 20 to 30 minutes. Sometimes animals show intestinal discomfort 10 to 15 minutes after the injection. If evidence of severe pain is present, atropine at a dose of from 15 to 30 mg subcutaneously can be used to block the action of neostigmine.

Sand colic. So-called sand colic is an intestinal impaction with sand, which is sometimes ingested by horses maintained on pasture. When mineral oil is used to treat sand colic, it often passes around firm sand impactions and therefore does not aid in correcting the problem. Some practitioners use a hemicellulose obtained from plantago seed to treat sand impactions.[7] Plantago seed is used as a bulk-forming laxative. It absorbs water and swells to fifteen to twenty times its size into a jellylike mass in the intestinal tract.

For a 450 kg horse, 0.23 to 0.45 kg of plantago seed are added to 8 to 12 liters of warm water and administered to the horse by way of a stomach tube. After the initial treatment, the owner is instructed to mix 0.11 to 0.15 kg of the plantago seed flakes with the horse's feed for 5 to 7 days. The plantago seed is mixed with either chopped alfalfa and molasses or other sweet feed.

When an extremely hard sand impaction is present 5 to 15 gm of DSS can be added to the plantago seed mixture and given initially by way of a stomach tube.

Spasmodic colic

A condition that produces the most severe signs of abdominal distress but generally results in little permanent damage to horses is a spastic (hyperactive) gut. Among the causes of spasmodic colic are gastrointestinal parasites, change in diet, spoiled feed, overeating, or nervousness. Animals demonstrate extreme abdominal pain and often there is increased gas production. Treatment by the veterinarian is usually designed to relieve the pain and reduce peristaltic activity.

Treatment. Dipyrone is used in colic for its analgesic effect. It is administered to horses at a dose of 2.5 to 10 gm intramuscularly or subcutaneously. Frequently, to provide immediate relief it is administered intravenously at a dose of approximately 5 to 10 gm. The manufacturer states that the drug may be repeated once or twice daily at 8-hour intervals. Dipyrone should not be administered to animals with a history of blood dyscrasia or in conjunction with phenylbutazone or barbiturates.

Meperidine provides analgesic and antispasmodic relief. It is a class II narcotic. It can be administered to horses at a dose of 150 to 200 mg/45 kg of body weight as needed to relieve pain.

Atropine also has an antispasmodic effect that will help to reduce colicky pains. Horses should receive approximately 15 to 30 mg subcutaneously as needed to reduce gut spasms.

The offending material that stimulated the gut to hyperactivity should be removed by giving the patient a mild cathartic such as mineral oil.

References

1. Bartley, E. E., Stiles, D. A., Meyer, R. M., Scheidy, S. F., Clark, J. G., and Boren, F. W.: Poloxalene for treatment of cattle with alfalfa bloat, J. Am. Vet. Med. Assoc. **151:**339, 1967.
2. Bennett, D. G.: Predisposition to abdominal crisis in the horse, J. Am. Vet. Med. Assoc. **161:**1189, 1972.
3. Coffman, J. R., and Garner, H. E.: Acute abdominal disease of the horse, J. Am. Vet. Med. Assoc. **161:**1195, 1972.
4. Donawick, W. J.: Metabolic management of the horse with an acute abdominal crisis, J. Afr. Vet. Assoc. **46:**107, March 1975.
5. Dresher, K., Kind, R. E., and Miller, R. M.: Clinical assessment of pentozocine in treatment of equine colic, Vet. Med. Small Anim. Clin. **67:**683, 1972.
6. Enos, L. R.: Formulary, Veterinary Medical Teaching Hospital, 1976, University of California.
7. Ferraro, G. L.: Diagnosis and treatment of sand colic in the horse, Vet. Med. Small Anim. Clin. **68:**736, 1973.
8. Gertsen, K. E., Dawson, H. A., and Wales, L.: The use of cholinergic drugs in treating intestinal impaction in the horse, Vet. Med. Small Anim. Clin. **67:**760, 1972.
9. Rossoff, I. S.: Handbook of veterinary drugs, New York, 1974, Springer Publishing Co.
10. Vernimb, G. D., and Hennesseey, P. W.: Clinical studies on flunixin meglumine in the treatment of equine colic, J. Equine Med. Surg. **1:**111, March 1977.
11. Yeary, R. A.: Syrup of ipecac as an emetic in the cat, J. Am. Vet. Med. Assoc. **161:**1677, 1972.

Additional readings

Edds, G. T., Kirkham, W. W., Wang, Y., and Holden, C. A.: Viability of bovine rumen bacteria, Vet. Med. Small Anim. Clin. **68:**50, 1968.
Editors: The mechanism and mangement of bovine bloat, Mod. Vet. Pract. **46:**47, Feb. 1965.
Mullenax, C. H.: Clinical observations of an effective ruminatoric, Vet. Med. Small Anim. Clin. **62:**794, 1967.
Nichols, R. E.: The control of experimental legume bloat with an enzyme inhibitor, alkyl aryl sulfonate sodium, J. Am. Vet. Med. Assoc. **143:**998, 1963.
Tennant, B., Evans, C. D., Schwartz, L. W., Gribble, D. H., and Kaneko, J. J.: Equine heptic insufficiency, Vet. Clin. North Am. **3:**279, 1973.

20

Musculoskeletal disorders

As used in this text, musculoskeletal disorders are those conditions resulting in abnormal locomotion due to lesions located in areas other than the brain or spinal cord. Musculoskeletal disorders primarily result from lesions in one or more of the following structures:

- Sensitive structures in the feet such as the digital pads in dogs and cats or the sensitive laminae in hooved animals
- Bone
- Cartilage
- Joints
- Ligaments
- Tendons
- Skeletal muscles
- Blood vessels
- Peripheral nerves

There are many causes of musculoskeletal disorders, including thrombi, infection, trauma, and autoimmune diseases (those diseases resulting in the production of antibodies that destroy certain tissues within the animal's own body). The causes of many musculoskeletal disorders have not been determined.

The primary sign of muscular disorders is lameness. Because they are maintained primarily for their locomotor ability, lamenesses are a particular problem in horses. Although many of the products and philosophies of therapy discussed in this chapter are applicable to all domestic species, our primary focus is on the therapy of equine lamenesses.

One of the primary problems in the therapy of equine lameness is that laypersons tend to think of lameness as a specific condition rather than a wide variety of conditions affecting different structures and resulting from various causes but showing similar signs. This lumping of all lamenesses into one category by laypersons tends to be reinforced by the presence of many OTC preparations for "curing" lamenesses. There are many problems associated with the use of these common remedies. Most have never been shown to hasten recovery from musculoskeletal disorders. Others are actually harmful. Many musculoskeletal disorders cannot be treated medically. Some must be

325

treated surgically, and for others, neither surgical nor medical treatment will result in a cure.

COUNTERIRRITANTS

Counterirritants are drugs that, by irritating the intact skin, relieve pain originating in underlying tissue. Many counterirritant formulations are available for application to the skin of horses to prevent or treat lamenesses. The effectiveness of these compounds is highly questionable. Those that are mild probably cause no harm. However, strong counterirritants can severely inflame and even blister the skin.

Counterirritants break down into three major categories:

1. Rubefacient drugs result in dilation of the blood vessels, increasing the circulation and reddening the area of the skin to which they are applied.

2. Blisters increase capillary dilation and the permeability of capillaries. This results in plasma escaping into the tissues and fluid collecting under the epidermis to form blisters.

3. Caustics cause corrosive effects on the skin, resulting in necrosis. Because such necrosis results in the formation of scars and permanent blemishes, caustics have no place in a therapeutic regimen.[2]

Rubefacient drugs

Rubefacient drugs are commonly contained in liniments and braces.

Liniments

Liniments have a water or alcohol base in which an oil or fatty substance is emulsified or suspended. Liniments are designed to be rubbed or massaged into the affected area. Massage in combination with liniments is used in subacute and chronic swellings. Probably the primary benefit is from massage, with the lubrication quality of liniments aiding the massage. To be of value massage must be performed several times a day. The benefits of massage are reduction of tissue edema and some freeing of adhesions of the skin to underlying structures. If used under a bandage and/or if not thoroughly rubbed in, liniments may blister the skin. An example of a liniment is white liniment, which consists of strong ammonia solution, turpentine, gum camphor, ammonium chloride, and oleic acid in a water base. Other examples of liniments include a formulation of camphor and cottonseed oil; a formulation of hard soap, camphor, rosemary oil, and alcohol; and a formulation of chloroform, camphor, and soap.

Brace

A brace is generally less irritating than a liniment and is used routinely after workouts. A typical formulation may include oil of chenopodium, thymol, chloroxylenol, menthol, and acetone. Isopropyl alcohol (70%) also serves as a satisfactory brace.

Blisters

Blisters are drugs that produce blistering of the skin. The most common blisters contain red iodide of mercury or cantharides (Spanish fly).

When applying a blister, the area to which it will be applied should be clipped. Because blisters are as irritating to human as to animal skin, they should only be applied with a piece of cork, a stick, or a brush rather than with bare hands. Blisters should be rubbed into the animal's skin for about 5 minutes. Before applying, petroleum jelly should be applied around the perimeter so that the formulation will not disturb adjacent tissues. The animal should be cross-tied so that it is unable to lick or chew the area to which the blister is being applied. After the appropriate period, the blister should be removed according to the directions on the formulation.

Because of the danger of the blistered area becoming infected, horses that are blistered should receive either preexposure or postexposure tetanus immunization (Chapter 7).

The effectiveness of blistering horses is questionable at best. It is a painful and probably ineffective form of therapy. Positive results probably are due to the enforced rest of the animal rather than from the chemical burn produced by the drug. In our opinion, blisters are inappropriate for the treatment of equine lameness with one exception. The only proved therapeutic use of blisters is to increase the rate of hoof growth in the equine when the wall of the hoof is cracking. In such instances, blisters are applied at the coronary band (the area where the skin joins the hoof) (Fig. 20-2). Because infections accelerate hoof growth, blisters are never needed when the hoof is infected.

Cantharides. Cantharides consists of ground, dried insects, *Cantharis vesicatoria*, which contain a highly irritating substance called "cantharidin." Cantharadin causes blisters when applied to the skin.

When cantharides is used as a blister, it is usually present in a concentration of 10% to 35% in waxes or ointments for external application. It generally results in a blister in 3 to 10 hours, depending on the concentration. Once the blister forms, the irritant should be removed to prevent further blistering, which might lead to necrosis and a permanent blemish.

Cantharidin must not be ingested orally by either man or animals. It produces an intense irritation of mucous membranes, resulting in vomiting, diarrhea, colic, and collapse in severe cases. The drug is excreted by way of the urinary tract which becomes extensively irritated. As it is excreted from the urethra in the male, this irritant action may result in penile erection. This has led to the myth that cantharides is an aphrodisiac. However, rather than increasing libido, its toxic effect tends to reduce the appetite for sexual activities.

Cantharides should not be used in animals with nephritis, on large areas of the skin, or in young animals.

Red iodide of mercury (mercuric iodide). Red iodide of mercury is generally applied as an ointment in a concentration of 6% to 25%. Because it is highly irritating, it should not be used in young animals.

CORTICOSTEROIDS

When administered systemically or injected into the affected area, corticosteroids reduce inflammation in many musculoskeletal disorders. When properly used, they are valuable in treating acute laminitis, osteitis, tendonitis, arthritis, periostitis, tenosynovitis, myositis, and musculoskeletal trauma. When corticosteroids are used for the treatment of musculoskeletal disorders, animals must receive sufficient rest to allow healing. If healing is not complete prior to the animal returning to normal activity, permanent tissue damage may result. The use of corticosteroids often eliminates signs of lameness even though the affected tissues have not healed. Because horse owners often want to put a horse into service as soon as clinical signs subside rather than wait for nature to completely heal the lesion, many clinicians have curtailed their use of corticosteroids for lamenesses in horses.

Acute conditions respond most favorably to corticosteroid therapy.

Systemic administration

When given systemically for the treatment of musculoskeletal disorders, the excessive use of corticosteroids can result in toxicity as discussed in Chapter 16. Among problems encountered with excessive corticosteroid use are electrolyte imbalances, excessive protein breakdown, suppression of the immune system with increased susceptibility to infectious disease, and a retardation of bone and wound healing.

Table 20-1 shows the dose and route of administration for commonly used veterinary corticosteroids used to treat equine lamenesses.

Intraarticular administration

To deliver active corticosteroid preparations directly to the site of injured joints, certain corticosteroids can be injected directly into the joint. A joint is encapsulated, with the joint capsule lined by the synovial membrane (Fig. 20-1). Ligaments that attach from bone to bone and tendons that attach from

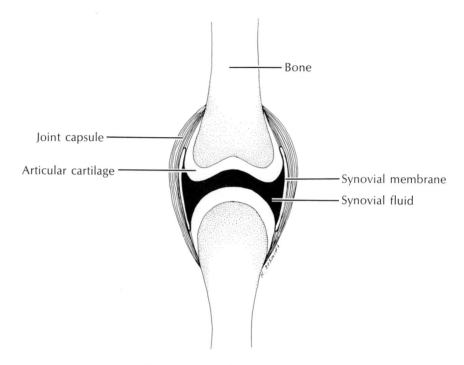

Fig. 20-1. Diagram of major joint structures.

Table 20-1. Use of corticosteroids for equine musculoskeletal disorders

Drug	Systemic	Intraarticular	Reference
Betamethasone (sodium phosphate 3.9 mg/ml; acetate 12 mg/ml)	No dose given	2.5-5 ml	4
Dexamethasone	2.5-5 mg IV or IM; 5-10 mg orally; 20 mg	Not used by this route	4
Flumethasone	1.25-2.5 mg IM, IV	Up to 10 mg	5
9-Fluoroprednisolone	20-60 mg orally; 20 mg IM	5-20 mg	5
Methylprednisolone acetate	200 mg IM	120 mg	5
Prednisolone	50-250 mg IM	50-100 mg	5
Prednisone	100-300 mg IM	50-250 mg	4
Triamcinolone	10-20 mg IM	6-18 mg	5

muscles to bone often pass over joints. The space within the joint contains synovial fluid, which acts as a lubricant. The ends of the bone in the joint are covered with cartilage.

The primary sign of joint disease in the horse is lameness. Mere distention of the joint by excessive synovial fluid is not considered a sure indication of joint disease.

The articular cartilage does not contain pain-sensing nerves. Therefore pain associated with joint disease in the horse does not originate with the cartilage. Rather the signs of pain are referrable from pain-sensitive soft tissues in the region of the joint and possibly bone that lies under the cartilage. The lubrication of joints is aided by the synthesis of polymerized hyaluronic acid, which is contained in the synovial fluid. Pain on motion may result from a loss of lubrication of the synovial membrane due to the low viscosity of the synovial fluid from either reduced polymerization of hyaluronic acid or from dilution of the polymerized hyaluronic acid by excessive synovial fluid production. Other factors that contribute to joint pain are alterations in tensions on tendons and ligaments, distention of blood vessels by inflammation, and muscle spasms.[6]

It appears that the site of action of corticosteroids when injected intraarticularly is the synovial membrane. Following successful administration of an intraarticular corticosteroid there is a reduced volume and increased viscosity of synovial fluid.

When administering corticosteroids by the intraarticular route, the area in which the injection is to be made must be prepared as for surgery. It should be clipped, shaved, washed, and rinsed. A disinfectant such as tincture of iodine should be applied to the site and allowed to dry prior to the introduction of the hypodermic needle. As much synovial fluid as possible should be withdrawn before injecting the corticosteroid preparation. No more corticosteroids should be administered than can be absorbed into the synovial membrane because excess amounts diffuse into the systemic circulation or are hydrolyzed in the synovial fluid to a biologically inactive residue that is eventually removed from the joint cavity.[6] Corticosteroids must never be injected into joints that are infected.

Only certain corticosteroid formulations may be injected into joints. The more common ones are shown in Table 20-1. Corticosteroid preparations that are not specifically recommended for use in joints must not be injected intraarticularly.

Betamethasone is claimed to be long acting when injected into the joint.[6] The commercial product (Betavet) contains betamethasone sodium phosphate, which is relatively soluble, resulting in rapid anti-inflammatory action, and betamethasone acetate, which is less soluble and has the advantages of being less easily hydrolyzed in the joint and of persisting for long periods of time in the synovial tissues.

Intraarticular injection of corticosteroids results in decreased swelling and tenderness on palpation of the joint. The animal's gait will improve or return to normal as the pain is reduced or alleviated. Generally, these changes will take place within the first 24 hours after intraarticular injection. However, maximum reduction in signs may take up to 3 days to achieve. Additonal injections into the joint should only be made as the need arises. Intraarticular use of corticosteroids eliminates the toxic effects commonly associated with systemic administration.

Intraarticular injection of corticosteroids is particularly effective when combined with rest and protection of the joint from continued trauma. When using corticosteroids, it is important to remember that relief of pain and inflammation does not indicate the complete or even partial healing of the affected joint. Rest is an important element of healing.

Because they can interfere with healing, the use of corticosteroids systemically or by intraarticular injection is contraindicated in severe forms of traumatic arthritis with internal damage of the affected joint and marked hemorrhage.

MISCELLANEOUS DRUGS TO TREAT MUSCULOSKELETAL DISORDERS
Dimethyl sulfoxide (DMSO)

DMSO is an oxidation product of dimethyl sulfide. It is an exceptionally potent solvent for many organic and inorganic compounds. DMSO can absorb more than 70% of its weight in water from air at 20° C and 65% relative humidity. Therefore, when not in use, any container of DMSO must be tightly closed to avoid dilution.

Physiologically the most important characteristic of DMSO is its percutaneous absorption (the passage from the outside through the entire thickness of skin). When applied topically, DMSO reaches the systemic circulation.

DMSO has been approved by the FDA for clinical use in dogs and horses. It is used for a wide variety of clinical conditions in strengths usually ranging from 50% to 90%. However, it has not been approved for horses intended for human consumption nor for horses or dogs intended for breeding purposes.

Even though not approved by the FDA, veterinarians and/or animal owners commonly add drugs to DMSO. Most frequently corticosteroids are added, and occasionally antibiotics or other drug preparations are added, depending on the condition being treated. DMSO increases the permeability of the skin to a wide variety of drugs. The ability of DMSO to increase the penetrability of other drugs depends on the nature of the second drug, the concentration of it and of DMSO, and the site of application. In certain instances normal penetrability can be increased up to a hundred times. Among the drugs that have increased absorption when applied with DMSO are glucocorticoids, local anesthetics, antifungal drugs, antibacterial drugs, and anticholinesterase compounds.

In addition to increasing the penetrability of hydrocortisone, however, there is also an increased risk of systemic toxicity when such drugs are topically applied with DMSO.[3] Until good research studies determine the benefits and liabilities of combining drugs with DMSO, the practice cannot be recommended.

Effectiveness. When used alone, the most common use of DMSO is to reduce soft tissue inflammation resulting from acute trauma. When used for this purpose, response to treatment is considered excellent. In experiments and clinical studies, DMSO appears to reduce acute inflammation related to the musculoskeletal system in horses.[1,3] Clinical studies indicate that the sooner the drug is applied following trauma the more dramatic the results.

Toxicity. DMSO was recalled from clinical evaluation in the United States in 1965 following a report of a change in the refractive index of the lenses in the eyes of dogs and other animals being treated with topical or oral DMSO. There appears to be a difference in species' susceptibility to this effect and in the ability of the lens to return to normal after discontinuance of the drug. For example, toxicology studies revealed no clinically significant effects were present in the eyes of horses that had been treated topically each day with 100 to 300 ml of medical grade DMSO for a period of 90 days, even though much smaller amounts produced eye changes in other species.

DMSO should be used with caution in the presence of drugs that affect the cardiac and central nervous systems. Work in experimental animals indicate that there may be some potentiation of the effects of such drugs in the animal.[1]

The parenteral administration of DMSO should not be performed. It has resulted in fetal abnormalities and death in hamsters.

Clinical studies with horses show that the presence of iodine liniments and strong irritants on DMSO-treated skin produces a marked temporary local reaction. If other topical agents are used, they should not be applied to the skin until DMSO is thoroughly dry.

An occasional transient irritation and/or blistering follows the use of DMSO in horses. These effects appear to be self-limiting and reversible and do not necessarily indicate that the drug needs to be discontinued. These signs usually disappear even with continued use of the drug.

Dose and administration. To assure that contaminants are not contained in DMSO, only the medical grade should be used.

The site to be treated with DMSO should be thoroughly washed, rinsed, and dried before application because DMSO has the ability to penetrate the skin barrier and carry with it certain other chemicals that may be present on the skin.

Because it is rapidly absorbed by the skin, DMSO should not be applied with the bare hands. Either rubber gloves, cotton swabs, glass rods, dabbers, or brushes should be used. The amount of DMSO to be applied should be transferred to a suitable container and the original bottle recapped to prevent the absorption of water. Brushes of synthetic material should not be used for application because DMSO is a highly potent organic solvent.

The maximum recommended daily dosage for horses is 100 ml divided equally among two or three applications, not to exceed 30 days. For dogs the maximum dose is 20 ml/24 hr divided equally among two or three applications, not to exceed 14 days.[5]

Flunixin meglumine

Flunixin meglumine is a nonnarcotic, nonsteroidal drug with analgesic anti-inflammatory and antipyretic activity in the horse. It is discussed in Chapter 14.

Meclofenamic acid

Meclofenamic acid has been recently marketed as an anti-inflammatory analgesic and antipyretic drug for use in the horse. Its use is discussed in Chapter 14.

Methocarbamol

Another name for methocarbamol is glyceryl guaiacol ether carbamate. It is used to produce skeletal muscle relaxation without seriously altering respiration. The manufacturer recommends it as an adjunct to therapy of acute inflammatory and traumatic conditions of the skeletal muscles to reduce muscular spasms and relax skeletal muscles in a variety of conditions. The conditions for which it is recommended in dogs include spinal cord trauma, sprain and strain of muscles and ligaments, inflammation of muscles and joints, muscular spasms, strychnine poisoning, and tetanus. In the horse it is recommended for traumatic strain and sprain of muscles and ligaments; inflammation of muscles, bursae, and joints; the tying-up syndrome (Chapter 17); and tetanus.

Effectiveness. Because the drug is relatively new in the veterinary field, adequate evaluation of its effectiveness has not been made.

Toxicity. In both dogs and cats the administration of large doses and/or a rapid injection rate may result in excessive salivation, vomiting, muscular weakness, or incoordination.

The drug is not approved for use in horses intended for food.

It should not be used during pregnancy unless in the judgment of the clinician the possible hazards are outweighed by the potential benefits of the medication. Injectable methocarbamol should not be administered to animals with known or suspected kidney disease or known hypersensitivity to the drug.

Dose and administration. Methocarbamol is available as an injectable solution for use in horses, dogs, and cats and as 500 mg tablets for use in dogs and cats.

The dose and frequency of administration of methocarbamol is based on the severity of the condition and response noted. For acute conditions a therapeutic dose should be administered by intravenous injection. When satisfactory muscular relaxation is achieved in dogs and cats, the effective blood concentration can be maintained with tablets.

For dogs and cats with moderate conditions, the injectable solution can be administered intravenously at the rate of 45 mg/kg and for severe conditions at the rate of 55 to 220 mg/kg. When giving intravenous injections to dogs and cats, the rate of injection should not exceed 2 ml/min of the 100 mg/ml intravenous solution. Because the drug is hypertonic it must not be administered paravascularly. By placing dogs and cats in a recumbent position during the injection, the possibility of toxic reactions is reduced.

When using tablets in dogs, the first day's loading dose should be 45 mg/kg three times a day. That is followed on subsequent days by doses of 22 to 45 mg/kg. For horses, only the intravenous route is used. For moderate conditions, 4.4 to 22 mg/kg are administered. In severe conditions such as tetanus, 22 to 55 mg/kg are administered. In contrast to the dog and cat, the rapid intravenous injection with a 15 or 17 gauge needle gives the most effective response in the horse.

Naproxen

Naproxen is a new anti-inflammatory, analgesic, and antipyretic drug intended for use in horses. It is discussed in Chapter 14.

Phenylbutazone

Phenylbutazone has been used for many years in veterinary medicine as an anti-inflammatory, analgesic, and antipyretic drug in horses, dogs, and cats. Its use is discussed in Chapter 14.

Orgotein

Orgotein is used as an anti-inflammatory in horses. It is produced from the liver of cattle and is a water-soluble protein of low molecular weight chelated with magnesium, copper, and zinc. Orgotein is used in horses for the treatment of soft tissue inflammation associated with the musculoskeletal system. The manufacturer recommends a dose in horses of 5 mg given intramuscularly every day for 2 weeks, then twice a week for 2 to 4 weeks. In severe cases, daily injections are given initially.

Adequate data are not yet available on the effectiveness of orgotein.

Sodium oleate

Sodium oleate is recommended by the manufacturer to accelerate healing of conditions such as bucked shins and splints, particularly in race horses. Bucked shins is an inflammatory condition of the periosteum

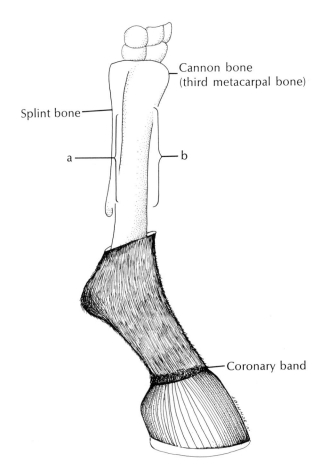

Fig. 20-2. Equine lower leg. Splints occur at site *a*, and bucked shins occur at site *b*.

(the membrane covering bones) primarily of the lower front legs of horses. Splints is an inflammatory condition involving the ligament between the splint and cannon bones on the front legs of horses (Fig. 20-2). Both of these conditions commonly occur in young race horses. Previously, the primary therapy for alleviation of these conditions was rest for periods of about 30 days. The manufacturer contends that sodium oleate stimulates the production of fibrous and fibrocartilagenous tissue, hastening the recovery from these inflammatory conditions.

In our opinion, further controlled clinical evaluations are necessary before one could recommend shortening the convalescent period for horses suffering from either buck shins or splints, even when sodium oleate is used.

Toxicity. The safety of using sodium oleate in pregnant animals has not been established. The drug has not been cleared for use in horses intended for food. There is a possibility that excessive tissue reaction will occur if sodium oleate is administered following or concurrent with the administration of corticosteroids.

Dose and administration. The commercial product contains 50 mg sodium oleate per milliliter. The amount to be injected depends on the area to be treated. One milliliter is used to produce a response in an area approximately 15 cm², and 2 ml is used to produce a response in an area approximately 30 cm². For areas larger than 30 cm² a second injection site adjacent to the first is necessary. Volumes greater than 2 ml per injection site will not produce proportionately larger areas of response. However, regardless of the number of injection sites, the total volume administered per animal should not exceed 10 ml. Massage to the area is recommended to distribute the solution after it has been injected.

Selenium and vitamin E

The primary use of selenium and vitamin E in animals—to prevent white muscle disease in cattle and sheep and the tying-up syndrome in horses—is discussed in Chapter 17.

References

1. Editors: Dimethyl sulfoxide (DMSO), Vet. Med. Small Anim. Clin. **65:**1051, 1970.
2. Jones, L. M.: Veterinary pharmacology and therapeutics, ed. 3, Ames, Iowa, 1965, Iowa State Press.
3. Koller, L. D.: Clinical application of DMSO by veterinarians in Oregon and Washington, Vet. Med. Small Anim. Clin. **71:**591, 1976.
4. McDonald, L. E.: Endocrine pharmacology. In Jones, L. M., Booth, N. H., and McDonald, L. E., editors: Veterinary pharmacology and therapeutics, ed. 4, Ames, Iowa, 1977, Iowa State Press.
5. Rossoff, I. S.: Handbook of veterinary drugs, New York, 1974, Springer Publishing Co.
6. Van Pelt, R. W., Tillotson, P. J., and Gertsen, K. E.: Intra-articular injection of betamethasone in arthritis in horses, J. Am. Vet. Med. Assoc. **156:**1589, 1970.

Additional readings

Asheim, A., and Lindblad, G.: Intra-articular treatment of arthritis in racehorses with sodium hyaluronate, Acta Vet. Scand. **17:**379, 1976.
Averkin, E., Killian, J., O'Brien, T., and Sickles, J.: Experimental design of clinical trials testing the efficacy of 90% DMSO solution in injuries to the musculoskeletal system in the dog, Vet. Med. Small Anim. Clin. **70:**177, 1975.
Decker, W. E., Edmondson, A. H., Hill, H. E., Holmes, R. A., Padmore, C. L., Warren, H. H., and Wood, W. D.: Local administration of orgotein in horses, **55:**773, 1974.
Jacob, S. W., and Wood, D. C.: Dimethyl sulfoxide (DMSO)—a status report, 1971, Department of Surgery, University of Oregon Medical School.
Mendenhall, H. V., Litwak, P., Yturraspe, D. J., Ingram, J. T., and Lumb, W. V.: Aggressive pharmacologic and surgical treatment of spinal cord injuries in dogs and cats, J. Am. Vet. Med. Assoc. **168:**1026, 1976.
Van Pelt, R. W., Tillotson, P. J., Gertsen, K. E., and Gallagher, K. F.: Effects of intraarticular flumethasone suspension on synovial effusion enzyme activity of arthritic horses, J. Am. Vet. Med. Assoc. **160:**186, 1972.
Vernimb, G. D., Van Hoose, L. M., and Hennessey, P. W.: Onset and duration of corticosteroid effect after injection of Betasone for treating equine arthropathies, Vet. Med. Small Anim. Clin. **72:**241, 1977.
Wisner, A. B.: Clinical use of Osteum in the horse, Vet. Med. Small Anim. Clin. **71:**1181, 1976.

How to organize a pharmacy inventory in a veterinary hospital

I. Drugs should be placed on the shelf in some sort of systematic manner.
  A. Drugs can be placed on the shelf by the dosage form of the drug and container size. These will usually be further subdivided, perhaps by alphabetical order by generic or brand names. For example; solutions in 1 quart containers could all be kept on one shelf in alphabetical order.
    1. Classification of drugs by dosage form
      a. Topical preparations
        (1) Solutions
        (2) Tinctures
        (3) Lotions
        (4) Liniments
        (5) Powders
        (6) Ointments and creams
      b. Oral preparations
        (1) Solid preparations
          (a) Powders
          (b) Capsules
          (c) Tablets
          (d) Boluses (very large tablets)
        (2) Liquid preparations
          (a) Syrups
          (b) Elixirs
          (c) Solutions
          (d) Suspensions
        (3) Semisolid preparations
          (a) Electuary (paste)
      c. Parenteral preparations
        (1) Solutions
          (a) Aqueous
          (b) Nonaqueous
        (2) Suspensions
          (a) Aqueous
          (b) Nonaqueous
        (3) Multiple dose injectables
        (4) Single dose injectables
  B. Drugs can be placed on the shelf by drug action. These may be subdivided alphabetically by generic or brand names or by dosage form. For example; one section of shelves could contain all anthelmintics in alphabetical order by brand name.
    1. Classification of drugs by action
      a. Antibacterials
        (1) Sulfas
        (2) Antibiotics
        (3) Nitrofurans
      b. Anesthetics
        (1) General
        (2) Local
      c. Topical skin products
      d. External pesticides
      e. Fungicides
      f. Anthelmintics
      g. Anticonvulsants
      h. Tranquilizers
      i. Ophthalmic preparations
      j. Hormones
      k. Corticosteroids
      l. Parenteral fluids
      m. Vitamin and mineral supplements
      n. Cardiac drugs
      o. Diuretics
      p. Gastrointestinal preparations
      q. Prescription diets
      r. Cancer chemotherapeutic drugs
II. Certain drugs and biologics must be kept refrigerated as indicated on the container.
III. Controlled drugs in schedule II, III, IV, and V (Appendix G) usually need to be kept under lock and key.
IV. Inventory and ordering.
  1. Determine generics and brands that will be kept in stock.
    a. Determine container size.
  2. Determine minimum number to be kept on hand before reordering.

Dispensing and prescribing drugs

I. Dispensing drugs
  A. Establish a routine
    1. Never deviate from that routine
    2. Have built-in safety checks
    3. Consider dosage errors in orders and *question any irregular requests*
    4. Double-check
    5. Do not decipher—if you cannot read or hear the order clearly, ask for clarification
  B. Sample system
    1. Read or hear the order
    2. Select the drug *(read the label)*
    3. Consider the dose and quantity
    4. *Read the label,* count, or pour into the container
    5. Prepare and affix dispensing labels one at a time
    6. Check the final preparation
    7. Return stock drugs to the shelf—*read the label*
    8. Dispense medication to the client; check the label and explain it to the client
  C. Dosage calculations
    1. Preferably prepare dosages in milligrams per kilogram
    2. Always convert everything to one system (e.g., metric) for calculations
    3. Proceed with caution and great care; double-check all calculations

II. Prescribing drugs
  A. A prescription should contain the following (see sample prescription below):
    1. The date it was written
    2. The name and address of the animal owner
    3. The name and species of the patient

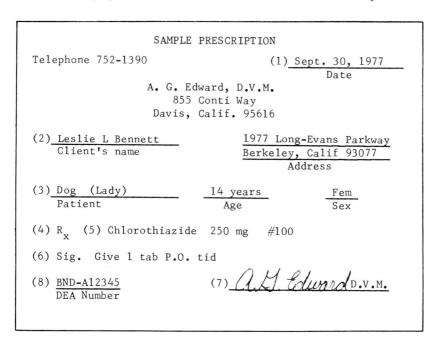

```
                    SAMPLE PRESCRIPTION
Telephone 752-1390              (1) Sept. 30, 1977
                                        Date

              A. G. Edward, D.V.M.
                  855 Conti Way
              Davis, Calif. 95616

    (2) Leslie L Bennett        1977 Long-Evans Parkway
         Client's name          Berkeley, Calif 93077
                                        Address

    (3) Dog  (Lady)            14 years            Fem
         Patient                  Age              Sex

    (4) R   (5) Chlorothiazide  250 mg   #100
         x

    (6) Sig.  Give 1 tab P.O. tid

    (8) BND-A12345        (7) A.G. Edward D.V.M.
         DEA Number
```

```
┌────────────────────────────────────────────────────────────────┐
│                    SAMPLE PHARMACY LABEL                         │
│                                                                  │
│                 (1) The Corner Pharmacy                          │
│                     Medical Center Way                           │
│                 Cow Hollow, Calif. 94930                         │
│                 Telephone (415) 285-7447                         │
│                                                                  │
│   (2) No. 123-456                    (3) Dr. A. G. Edward        │
│                                                                  │
│   (4) Give one tablet orally three times a day                   │
│                                                                  │
│   (5) Chlorothiazide 250 mg #100  (M.S.D.)                       │
│                                                                  │
│   (6) Bennett.  Dog "Lady"                                       │
│                                                                  │
│   (7) Filled Aug. 6, 1977            (8) Expires July 1982       │
│                                                                  │
└────────────────────────────────────────────────────────────────┘
```

```
┌────────────────────────────────────────────────────────────────┐
│                                                                  │
│                    SAMPLE VETERINARY LABEL                       │
│                                                                  │
│                 (1) City Veterinary Clinic                       │
│                     855 Conti Way                                │
│                     Davis, Calif., 95616                         │
│                     916-752-1390                                 │
│                                                                  │
│   (2) Give one tablet orally three times a day.                  │
│                                                                  │
│   (3) Leslie L. Bennett, Canine "Lady"                           │
│                                                                  │
│   (4) 8/6/77                                                     │
│                                                                  │
│   (5) Chlorothiazide 250 mg.  #100 (M.S.D.)                      │
│                                                                  │
│                   (6) Expires July, 1982                         │
│                                                                  │
│                   (7) A. G. Edward, D.V.M.                       │
│                                                                  │
└────────────────────────────────────────────────────────────────┘
```

4. The superscription "℞," an abbreviation of the Latin word for recipe or "take thou"
5. The inscription, which lists the names and amounts of drugs to be included in the prescription; the drug names should be written in English rather than Latin and the amounts in the metric system (see Appendix C for prescription abbreviations)
6. The transcription, preceded by the Latin abbreviation "Sig" ("write thou"), which gives the instruction to be written on the label
7. The signature of the prescriber

8. For controlled substances, the prescriber's Drug Enforcement Administration (DEA) number

B. The following information should be included on labels prepared by a pharmacy (see sample label above):
   1. The name and address of the pharmacy
   2. The prescription number
   3. The prescriber's name
   4. Directions for use
   5. Drug name, strength, quantity (trade name of manufacturer)
   6. Name of client and description of patient
   7. Date filled

8. Expiration date
C. The following information should be included on the label prepared by a veterinary hospital (see sample label on p. 336):
   1. The name and address of the hospital
   2. Directions for use
   3. Name of client and description of patient
   4. Date filled
   5. Drug name, strength, quantity (trade name of manufacturer)
   6. Expiration date of the drug
   7. Name of veterinarian dispensing the drug

Common drug abbreviations

TYPE OF MEDICATION

amp	Ampule
Aq, H_2O	Water
cap	Capsule
el, elix	Elixir
ext	Extract
haust	Drench
pil	Pill
pv	Powder
sol	Solution
Sp	Spirit
Supp	Suppository
Syr	Syrup
tab	Tablet
tr, tinct	Tincture
ung	Ointment

MEDICATION DOSE (AMOUNT)

aa	Of each
cc	Cubic centimeter
fl	Fluid
gal, C	Gallon
Gm	Gram
gr	Grain
mg	Milligram
min	Minim
no	Number
oz	Ounce
pt, O	Pint
qt	Quart
$\overline{ss}$, ss	One-half
T, tbls	Tablespoon
t, tsp	Teaspoon

MANNER OF ADMINISTRATION (METHOD)

$\overline{c}$	With
H, hypo	Hypodermically
IM	Intramuscular
IV	Intravenous

OD	Right eye
oral, PO	By mouth
OS	Left eye
OU	Both eyes
PR	By rectum
$\overline{s}$, s	Without
SC, Subq	Subcutaneous

TYPE OF ADMINISTRATION (WHEN TO GIVE MEDICINE)

$\overline{a}$	Before
ac	Before meals
ad lib	As freely or as often as is desired
am or AM	Morning
bid	Twice a day
h	Hour
hs	Bedtime, hour of sleep
non rep, nr	Do not repeat
p	After
pc	After meals
PM	Afternoon
prn	When required, as necessary
q, qq	Every
qd, qqd	Once daily
qh, qqh	Every hour
q2h	Every 2 hours
qid	Four times a day
qod	Every other day
sos	If necessary, or one time
stat	Immediately
tid	Three times a day

OTHER

eq pts	Equal parts
et	And
ft	Make
M	Mix
S, Sig	Write (on the label)

Weights

METRIC WEIGHT

Micrograms	Milligrams	Grams	Kilograms
1	0.001	10^{-6}	10^{-9}
1000	1	0.001	10^{-6}
10^6	1000	1	0.001
10^9	10^6	1000	1

APOTHECARY WEIGHT

Grains	Scruples	Drams	Ounces	Pound
1	0.05	0.02	0.002	0.00017
20	1	0.33	0.04	0.003
60	3	1	0.13	0.01
480	24	8	1	0.08
5760	288	96	12	1

AVOIRDUPOIS WEIGHT

Grains	Ounces	Pound
1	0.0023	0.00014
437.5	1	0.0625
7000	16	1

CONVERSION OF MILLIGRAMS TO GRAINS

Milligram	Grain
1	0.0154
2	0.0308
3	0.0462
4	0.0616
5	0.0770
6	0.0924
7	0.1078
8	0.1232
9	0.1386
10	0.1540
15	0.231
20	0.308
30	0.462
40	0.616
50	0.770
60	0.924
70	1.078
80	1.232
90	1.386
100	1.54
200	3.08
300	4.62
400	6.16
500	7.70
600	9.24
700	10.78
800	12.32
900	13.86
1000	15.40

CONVERSION OF GRAINS TO METRIC VALUES (MILLIGRAMS OR GRAMS)

Grains	Milligrams or grams		Grains	Milligrams or grams	
$1/600$	0.1	mg	10	648	mg
$1/400$	0.16	mg	15	972	mg
$1/300$	0.2	mg	20	1.3	gm
$1/200$	0.3	mg	30	1.94	gm
$1/100$	0.6	mg	40	2.59	gm
$1/60$	1	mg	50	3.24	gm
$1/30$	2	mg	60	3.89	gm
$1/15$	4	mg	70	4.54	gm
$1/10$	6	mg	80	5.18	gm
$1/8$	8	mg	90	5.83	gm
$1/4$	16	mg	100	6.48	gm
$1/2$	32	mg	200	13	gm
$3/4$	49	mg	300	19.4	gm
1	64.8	mg	400	25.9	gm
2	130	mg	500	32.4	gm
3	194	mg	600	38.9	gm
4	259	mg	700	45.4	gm
5	324	mg	800	51.8	gm
6	389	mg	900	58.3	gm
7	454	mg	1000	64.8	gm
8	518	mg	1 oz (Ap)	31.1	gm
9	583	mg	1 oz (Av)	28.35	gm

CONVERSIONS OF KILOGRAMS TO POUNDS

Kilograms	Pounds	Kilograms	Pounds
1	2.2	23	50.7
2	4.4	24	52.9
3	6.6	25	55.1
4	8.8	35	77.1
5	11.0	40	88.2
6	13.2	45	99.2
7	15.4	50	110.2
8	17.6	55	121.2
9	19.8	60	132.2
10	22.0	65	143.3
11	24.2	70	154.3
12	26.4	75	165.3
13	28.7	80	176.3
14	30.9	85	187.3
15	33.1	90	198.4
16	35.3	95	209.4
17	37.5	100	220.4
18	39.7	200	440.8
19	41.9	300	661.2
20	44.1	400	881.6
21	46.3	500	1102
22	48.5		

CONVERSION OF POUNDS TO KILOGRAMS

Pounds	Kilograms	Pounds	Kilograms
1	0.45	37	16.78
2	0.91	38	17.24
3	1.36	39	17.70
4	1.81	40	18.15
5	2.27	41	18.60
6	2.72	42	19.06
7	3.18	43	19.51
8	3.63	44	19.96
9	4.08	45	20.42
10	4.54	46	20.87
11	4.99	47	21.32
12	5.44	48	21.78
13	5.90	49	22.23
14	6.35	50	22.68
15	6.80	51	23.14
16	7.26	52	23.59
17	7.71	53	24.05
18	8.17	54	24.50
19	8.62	55	24.95
20	9.07	56	25.41
21	9.53	57	25.86
22	9.98	58	26.32
23	10.44	59	26.77
24	10.89	60	27.22
25	11.34	70	31.76
26	11.80	80	36.30
27	12.25	90	40.83
28	12.70	100	45.37
29	13.16	200	90.74
30	13.61	300	136.12
31	14.07	400	181.49
32	14.52	500	226.68
33	14.97	600	272.23
34	15.43	700	317.59
35	15.88	800	362.98
36	16.33	900	408.35
		1000	453.72

Fluid measure

METRIC MEASURE

Milliliters	Cubic centimeters	Liter
1	1	0.001
500	500	0.5
1000	1000	1

UNITED STATES FLUID MEASURE

Minims	Ounces	Pints	Quarts	Gallons
480	1	0.0625	0.001	0.0003
7680	16	1	0.5	0.125
15360	32	2	1	0.25
61440	128	8	4	1

CONVERSIONS

Milliliters*	Liter	Ounces	Pints
1	0.001	0.034	0.002
29.57	0.030	1	0.0625
473.12	0.473	16	1
1000	1	34	2.13

*1 teaspoon = 5 ml; 1 tablespoon = 15 ml.

Other units of measure

1. Milliequivalent (mEq) = an amount of a substance with an equivalent reaction potentional of one millimole of hydrogen ion. It is determined by dividing the atomic weight by the ionic valence and expressing the answer in milligrams.

$$mEq = \frac{\text{Atomic weight}}{\text{Ionic valance}}$$

EXAMPLE: Sodium (Na^+) has an atomic weight of 23 and valence of 1. Calcium (Ca^{++}) has an atomic weight of 40 and a valence of 2. Therefore for sodium

$$1 \text{ mEq} = \frac{23}{1} = 23 \text{ mg}$$

For calcium

$$1 \text{ mEq} = \frac{40}{2} = 20 \text{ mg}$$

To determine the milliequivalent per liter the following formula is used:

$$mEq/liter = \frac{\text{mg/liter} \times \text{Ionic valance}}{\text{Atomic weight}}$$

EXAMPLE: In Ringer's solution there are 2369 mg of sodium per liter. To find the milliequivalents per liter, we use the following formula:

$$mEq/liter = \frac{2369 \times 1}{23} = 103$$

2. Percent (%) = "per hundred," that is, grams per 100 gm (gm/100 gm); pounds/100 pounds, or handfuls per 100 handfuls.

Percent (%) in pharmaceutical systems may be indicated as follows:

% w/w = % weight/weight (6% = 6 gm/100 gm, 6 mg/100 mg, or 60 mg/gm)

% w/v = % weight/volume (6% = 6 gm/100 ml or 60 mg/ml)*

% v/v = % volume/volume (6% = 6 ml/100 ml or 60 ml/liter)

*Unless otherwise indicated, percent in pharmaceutical systems is % w/v.

Controlled substances*: inventory requirements

The Controlled Substances Act (P.L. 91-513) requires each registrant to make a complete and accurate record of all stocks of controlled substances on hand every two years. The biennial inventory date of May 1, may be changed by the registrant to fit his regular general physical inventory date, if any, so long as the date is not more than six (6) months from the biennial date that would otherwise apply. The actual taking of the inventory should not vary more than four (4) days from the biennial inventory date.

Whether or not you use this inventory format, the inventory record must:

1. List the name, address, and DEA registration number of the registrant
2. Indicate the date and the time the inventory is taken, i.e., opening or close of business
3. Be signed by the person or persons responsible for taking the inventory
4. Be maintained at the location appearing on the registration certificate for at least two years
5. Keep records of Schedule II drugs separate from all other controlled substances

When taking the inventory of Schedule II controlled substances, an exact count or measure must be made. When taking the inventory of Schedule III, IV, and V controlled substances, an estimated count may be made unless the container holds more than 1000 dosage units, in which case an exact count must be made if the container has been opened.

SCHEDULES OF CONTROLLED SUBSTANCES

The drugs that come under jurisdiction of the Controlled Substances Act are divided into five schedules. They are as follows:

*From the Drug Enforcement Administration (DEA), Washington, D.C., revised January 1977. Subject to the Controlled Substance Act of 1970 (Public Law 91-513).

Schedule I substances

Drugs in this schedule are those that have no accepted medical use in the United States and have a high abuse potential. Some examples are heroin, marihuana, LSD, peyote, mescaline, psilocybin, tetrahydrocannabinols, ketobemidone, levomoramide, racemoramide, benzylmorphine, dihydromorphine, morphine, methysulfonate, nicocodeine, micomorphine, etorphine, and others.

Schedule II substances

The drugs in this schedule have a high abuse potential with severe psychic or physical dependence liability. Examples of Schedule II controlled substances are certain narcotic drugs, and drugs containing amphetamines or methamphetamines as the single active ingredient, or in combination with each other. Additional examples of Schedule II controlled substances are opium, morphine, codeine, hydromorphone (Dilaudid), methadone (Dolophine), pantopon, meperidine (Demerol), cocaine, oxycodone (Percodan), anileridine (Leritine), oxymorphone (Numorphan), and amphetamine (Benzedrine, Dexedrine) and methamphetamine (Desoxyn). Also in Schedule II are phenmetrazine (Preludin), methylphenidate (Ritalin), amobarbital, pentobarbital, secobarbital, methaqualone, etorphine HCl, and dyphenoxylate.

Schedule III substances

The drugs in this schedule have an abuse potential less than those in Schedules I and II and include compounds containing limited quantities of certain narcotic drugs, and nonnarcotic drugs such as derivatives of barbituric acid except those that are listed in another schedule, glutethimide (Doriden), methyprylon (Noludar), chlorhexadol, phencyclidine, sulfondiethylmethane, sulfonmethane, nalorphine, benzphetamine, chlorphentermine, clortermine, mazindol, phendimetrazine. Paregoric is in this schedule.

343

Schedule IV substances

The drugs in this schedule have an abuse potential less than those listed in Schedule III and include such drugs as barbital, phenobarbital, methylphenobarbital, chloral betaine (Beta Chlor), chloral hydrate, ethchlorvynol (Placidyl), ethinamate (Valmid), meprobamate (Equanil, Miltown), paraldehyde, methodexital, fenfluramine, diethylpropion, phentermine, chlordiazepoxide (Librium), diazepam (Valium), oxazepam (Serax), clorazepate (Tranxene), flurazepam (Dalmane), clanazepam, and mebutamate.

Schedule V substances

The drugs in this schedule have an abuse potential less than those listed in Schedule IV and consist of preparations containing limited quantities of certain narcotic drugs generally for antitussive and antidiarrheal purposes.

SYMBOLS AND LABELING

Each commercial container of controlled substances is required to have on its label a symbol designating to which schedule it belongs. The symbol for Schedules I through V controlled substances is as follows: C or C-I; C^{II} or C-II; C^{III} or C-III; C^{IV} or C-IV; and C or C-V. These symbols are not required on prescription containers dispensed by a pharmacist to a patient in the course of his professional practice.

ORDER FORMS

A triplicate order form is necessary for the transfer of controlled substances in Schedules I and II. Under the Controlled Substances Act, the use of the order forms will be for Schedules I and II drugs only. A registrant desiring DEA order forms can obtain them by using the requisition form (DEA-222D). Once a registrant has obtained DEA order forms, they will then utilize Form DEA-222B which is in each order form book. No charge is made for order forms.

When a registrant issues an order form for Schedule II controlled substances and when he receives the items ordered, he must record on his retained copy the number of packages and the date such packages were received. A space is provided for this on the DEA order form.

DEA order form books consist of six sets of order forms. Each registrant is allowed a maximum of three books at one time unless it can show that its needs exceed this limit. In such case, the registrant should contact the Regional Office of DEA in its area and explain its needs.

LOST OR STOLEN ORDER FORMS

Lost or stolen order forms should not be reported to the Registration Section of DEA. Instead, direct your information to: Drug Enforcement Administration, Compliance Division, Investigations Section, 1405 I Street, N.W., Washington, D.C. 20537.

DRUG SECURITY AND CONTROL

The following methods of drug security and control are required by the Drug Enforcement Administration:

Security—Schedules II, III, IV, and V controlled substances must be kept in a locked cabinet or dispersed throughout the noncontrolled stock in such a manner to obstruct theft.

Disposal—Those wishing to dispose of any excess or undesired stocks of controlled substances must contact the nearest DEA Regional or District Office and request the necessary forms (DEA-41). Three copies of Form DEA-41 will be forwarded to the Regional Office that serves the area in which the registrant is situated. (*A cover letter from the registrant must be attached to the reports stating that the controlled substances are not desired and the registrant wishes to dispose of them.*)

Regional office action upon receipt of request to destroy controlled substances. Upon receipt of the required DEA-41 forms and the letter from the registrant, one of four courses of action will be utilized. The course of action chosen by the Regional Director or his designee will be stated in letter form, attached to the original copy of the DEA-41 form, and returned to the registrant.

The four courses of action in disposing of excess or undesired stock of controlled substances are:

1. The return letter to the registrant will advise that the drugs may be destroyed by two responsible parties employed or acting on behalf of the registrant. This course of action will be used when there are factors which preclude an on-the-site destruction witnessed by DEA personnel, such as the firm's history of compliance and the abuse potential of the drugs involved.

2. The return letter to the registrant will advise to forward the excess or undesired stocks or controlled substances to the appropriate state

agency for destruction. In lieu of actual surrender to the state agency, destructions witnessed by state personnel are acceptable.

3. The return letter will advise to hold the substances until DEA personnel arrive at a mutually convenient time to witness the destruction of the substances. DEA personnel will date and sign the reports or forms after witnessing the destruction.

4. The return letter will advise to forward the substances to the Regional Office of DEA which serves the area in which the registrant is located. Upon receipt of the substances, the Regional Director or his designee will verify the actual substance submitted. If errors are found, a corrected form must be prepared and the registrant duly notified. The original form will be returned to the registrant.

Drug theft — Any registrant involved in loss of controlled substances must notify the DEA Regional Office in its region of the theft or significant loss upon discovery. The registrant must make a report regarding the loss or theft by completing DEA Form 106.

Such report shall contain the following information:

1) Name and address of firm
2) DEA Registration Number
3) Date of theft
4) Local police department notified
5) Type of theft (night break-in, armed robbery, etc.)
6) Listing of symbols or cost code used by registrant in marking containers (if any)
7) Listing of controlled substances missing through theft

The above report should be made in triplicate. The registrant should keep the original copy for its records and forward the remaining two copies to the nearest DEA Regional or District Office.

Biologicals—types and brand names

This list contains the biologicals discussed in the text and examples of available brands. Abbreviations used in this appendix are as follows:

MLV = Modified live virus
TCO = Tissue culture origin
IBR = Infectious bovine rhinotracheitis
ICH = Infectious canine hepatitis
PI3   = Parainfluenza 3

Anaplasmosis vaccine

Anaplaz (Fort Dodge)	Anaplasmosis vaccine, killed, bovine origin

Anthrax vaccine—Sterne's South African strain

Anvax (Jen-Sal)	Anthrax spore vaccine—Sterne's nonencapsulated strain
Sternvac (Haver-Lockhart)	Anthrax spore vaccine, avirulent

Autogenous bacterins

Autogenous bacterins (Fort Dodge)

Bacillary hemoglobinuria (red water) vaccine

(*See Clostridium haemolyticum* bacterin)

Blackleg vaccine

(*See Clostridium chauvoei* bacterin)

Blue tongue vaccine

Blue tongue vaccine (Colorado Serum)

Bovine mixed antisera

Virobactin (Fort Dodge)	*Escherichia coli, Pasteurella multocida, Salmonella typhimurium* antiserum, bovine isolates, and origin
E.P.S. serum (Bio-Ceutic)	*Escherichia coli, Pasteurella multocida, Salmonella typhimurium* antiserum, bovine isolates, and origin

Bovine viral diarrhea vaccine

(*See also* bovine viral diarrhea–parainfluenza 3 vaccine; bovine viral diarrhea–parainfluenza 3 vaccine–*Pasteurella haemolytica-multocida* bacterin; infectious bovine rhinotracheitis–viral diarrhea vaccine; infectious bovine rhinotracheitis–viral diarrhea vaccine–*Leptospira* bacterin; infectious bovine rhinotracheitis–viral diarrhea–parainfluenza 3 vaccine; infectious bovine rhinotracheitis–bovine viral diarrhea–parainfluenza 3 vaccine–*Leptospira* bacterin; infectious bovine rhinotracheitis–viral diarrhea–parainfluenza 3 vaccine–*Pasteurella haemolytica-multocida* bacterin)

Bovine Virus Diarrhea Vaccine (Abbott)	MLV, porcine TCO
Bovine Virus Diarrhea Vaccine (Fort Dodge)	MLV, porcine TCO
Bovine Virus Diarrhea Vaccine (BVD) (Bio-Ceutic)	MLV, embryonic bovine TCO
BVD Vac (Diamond)	Bovine virus diarrhea vaccine
BVD Vaccine (Bio-Ceutic)	Bovine virus diarrhea vaccine, MLV, embryonic bovine TCO
Jensine B (Jen-Sal)	Bovine virus diarrhea, MLV, porcine TCO
Mucovax (Pitman-Moore)	Bovine virus diarrhea vaccine, MLV, bovine TCO
Resbo BVD (Norden)	Bovine virus diarrhea vaccine, MLV, bovine TCO

Bovine viral diarrhea–infectious bovine rhinotracheitis vaccine

(*See* infectious bovine rhinotracheitis–viral diarrhea vaccine)

Bovine viral diarrhea–parainfluenza 3 vaccine

Mucovax 3 (Pitman-Moore)	Bovine virus diarrhea vaccine, MLV, bovine TCO; PI3 vaccine

Bovine viral diarrhea–parainfluenza 3 vaccine–*P. haemolytica–multocida* bacterin

Mucovax plus *Pasteurella* (Pitman-Moore)	Bovine virus diarrhea vaccine, MLV, bovine TCO; PI3 vaccine–*Pasteurella haemolytica-multocida* bacterin

Bovine wart vaccine

Wart Vaccine (Abbott)	Killed virus, bovine origin
Wart vaccine (Diamond)	Killed virus, bovine origin
Wart vaccine (Fort Dodge)	Killed virus, bovine origin
Wart vaccine (Haver-Lockhart)	Bovine, inactivated
Wart Vaccine (Norden)	Killed virus, bovine origin

Brucella abortus vaccine

Brucella abortus Vaccine (Colorado Serum)	
Brucella abortus Vaccine (Fort Dodge)	Live culture
Brucella abortus Vaccine (Jen-Sal)	Strain 19, live culture

Brucellosis vaccine

(*See Brucella abortus* vaccine)

BVD vaccine

(*See* bovine viral diarrhea vaccine)

Calf scours vaccine

(*See* reovirus vaccine)

Canine distemper vaccines

(*See also* canine distemper–hepatitis vaccine; canine distemper–hepatitis–*Leptospira* antisera; canine distemper–hepatitis vaccine–*Leptospira* bacterin; canine distemper–hepatitis–parainfluenza vaccine; canine distemper–hepatitis–parainfluenza vaccine–*Leptospira* bacterin; canine distemper vaccine–*Leptospira* bacterin; canine distemper–measles vaccine)

A.B.D. (Affiliated)	Canine distemper virus, MLV, canine TCO
Cytogen (Jen-Sal)	Canine distemper vaccine, MLV, canine TCO

Biocine D. (Burns-Biotec)	Canine distemper vaccine, MLV, canine TCO
Delcine (Dellen)	Canine distemper vaccine, MLV, canine cell line origin
Distemperoid (Fromm)	Canine distemper vaccine, MLV, ferret TCO
Enduracell D (Norden)	Canine distemper vaccine, MLV, canine cell line origin
Fromm D (Fromm)	Canine distemper vaccine, MLV, chick embryo TCO
Tissuvax (Pitman-Moore)	Canine distemper vaccine, MLV, canine cell line origin

Canine distemper–hepatitis vaccines

A.B.D.H. (Affiliated)	Canine distemper virus, live attenuated, canine cell TCO; infectious canine hepatitis virus, live attenuated, porcine cell TCO
Biocine DH (Burns-Biotec)	Canine distemper–hepatitis vaccine, MLV, canine TCO
Canine distemper–hepatitis vaccine (Abbott)	MLV, canine TCO
Canine distemper–hepatitis vaccine (Colorado Serum)	
Canovax (Fort Dodge)	Canine distemper vaccine, hepatitis vaccine, MLV, canine and bovine TCO
Certi-Vac dh (Diamond)	Canine distemper and hepatitis vaccine, MLV, canine TCO
Delcine-H (Dellen)	Canine distemper vaccine, MLV, canine cell line origin; infectious canine hepatitis vaccine, MLV, canine cell line origin
D-Vac-H Vaccine (Bio-Ceutic)	Canine distemper–hepatitis vaccine, MLV, nontransmissible, ICH fraction–porcine lung TCO
Enduracell D-H (Norden)	Canine distemper–hepatitis vaccine, MLV, canine cell line origin
Fromm-DH (Fromm)	Canine distemper–hepatitis vaccine, MLV, chick

embryo cell culture origin
and canine cell culture
origin, respectively

Havacine DH (Haver-Lock-hart) — Canine distemper vaccine, MLV, Cabasso strain, chick embryo culture origin; infectious canine hepatitis vaccine, porcine TCO

Tissuvax D-H (Pitman-Moore) — Canine distemper–hepatitis vaccine, MLV, canine cell line origin

Canine distemper–hepatitis–*Leptospira* antisera

Anti-DHL Serum (Fromm) — Canine distemper antiserum, canine infectious hepatitis antiserum, *Leptospira canicola* antiserum

Canine distemper–hepatitis vaccine–*Leptospira* bacterin

A.B.D.H. with Lepto (Affiliated) — Canine distemper virus, live attenuated, canine cell TCO; infectious canine hepatitis, live attenuated, porcine cell TCO; *Leptospira canicola* and *L. icterohaemorrhagiae* bacterin

Biocine DHL (Burns-Biotec) — Canine distemper–hepatitis vaccine, MLV, TCO (canine); *Leptospira* bacterin

Canine Distemper–Hepatitis Vaccine with *Leptospira* Bacterin (Abbott) — MLV, canine TCO

Canine Distemper–Hepatitis—*Leptospira* bacterin (Colorado Serum)

Can-O-Vax-L (Fort Dodge) — Canine distemper vaccine, MLV, canine kidney cell TCO; canine hepatitis vaccine, MLV, bovine kidney cell TCO; *Leptospira* bacterin

Certi-Vac dh-l (Diamond) — Canine distemper and hepatitis vaccine, MLV, ca-

nine TCO; concentrated *Leptospira canicola-icterohaemorrhagiae* bacterin

Delcine-HL (Dellen) — Canine distemper–hepatitis vaccine, MLV, canine cell line origin; *Leptospira canicola-icterohaemorrhagiae* bacterin

D-Vac-HL vaccine (Bio-Ceutic) — Canine distemper–hepatitis vaccine, MLV, nontransmissible TCO; *Leptospira canicola-icterohaemorrhagiae* bacterin

Enduracell D-H-L (Norden) — Canine distemper–hepatitis vaccine, MLV, canine cell line origin; *Leptospira canicola-icterohaemorrhagiae* bacterin

Fromm DHL (Fromm) — Canine distemper vaccine, MLV, chick cell culture origin; canine hepatitis vaccine, MLV, canine cell culture origin; *Leptospira canicola-icterohaemorrhagiae* bacterin

Havacine DHL (Haver-Lock-hart) — Canine distemper vaccine, MLV; canine hepatitis vaccine; *Leptospira* bacterin

Tissuvax 4 (Pitman-Moore) — Canine distemper–hepatitis vaccine, MLV, canine cell line origin, *Leptospira canicola-icterohaemorrhagiae* bacterin

Trioid Plus (Fromm) — Canine distemper–hepatitis vaccine, inactivated; *Leptospira canicola-icterohaemorrhagiae* bacterin

Canine distemper–hepatitis–parainfluenza vaccine

Tissuvax D-H-P (Pitman-Moore) — Canine distemper–hepatitis–parainfluenza vaccine, MLV, canine cell line origin

Canine distemper–hepatitis–parainfluenza vaccine–*Leptospira* bacterin

Tissuvax 5 (Pitman Moore) — Canine distemper–hepatitis–parainfluenza vaccine, MLV, canine cell line origin; *Leptospira canicola-icterohaemorrhagiae* bacterin

Canine distemper vaccine–*Leptospira* bacterin

Biocine DL (Burns Biotec)
: Canine distemper vaccine, MLV, canine TCO; *Leptospira* bacterin

Delcine-L (Dellen)
: Canine distemper vaccine, MLV, canine cell line origin; *Leptospira canicola-icterohaemorrhagiae* bacterin

Fromm-DL (Fromm)
: Canine distemper vaccine, MLV, chick embryo cell culture origin; *Leptospira canicola-icterohaemorrhagiae* bacterin

Canine distemper–measles vaccine

Enduracell-D-M (Norden)
: Canine distemper–measles vaccine, MLV, canine cell line origin

Canine hookworm vaccine

Canine Hookworm Vaccine (Jen-Sal)
: Attenuated live larvae

Canine infectious hepatitis vaccine

(*See* canine distemper–hepatitis vaccine; canine distemper–hepatitis–*Leptospira* antisera; canine distemper–hepatitis vaccine–*Leptospira* bacterin; canine distemper–hepatitis–parainfluenza vaccine; canine distemper–hepatitis–parainfluenza vaccine–*Leptospira* bacterin)

Canine infectious tracheobronchitis vaccine

(*See also* canine distemper–hepatitis–parainfluenza vaccine; canine distemper–hepatitis–parainfluenza vaccine–*Leptospira* bacterin)

Paramune-P (Dellen)
: Canine parainfluenza vaccine, MLV, canine perma-cell line origin

***Clostridium chauvoei* bacterin**

(*See* following mixed bacterins containing *Clostridium chauvoei*)

***Clostridium chauvoei-novyi-sordellii* bacterin**

Electrogen-CSNS (Jen-Sal)
: *Clostridium chauvoei-novyi-sodellii* bacterin

***Clostridium chauvoei-septicum* bacterin**

CCS (Bio-Ceutic)
: *Clostridium chauvoei-septicum* bacterin

C.C.S. (Dellen)
: *Clostridium chauvoei-septicum* bacterin

Clostri-Bac CS (Haver-Lockhart)
: *Clostridium chauvoei-septicum* bacterin

Clostridium chauvoei-septicum bacterin (Abbott)

Clostridium chauvoei-septicum bacterin (Affiliated)

Clostridium chauvoei-septicum bacterin (Colorado Serum)

Clostridium chauvoei-septicum bacterin (Dellen)

Clostroid CS (Fort Dodge)
: *Clostridium chauvoei-septicum* bacterin

Fermicon 2 (Bio-Ceutic)
: *Clostridium chauvoei-septicum* bacterin

D-Ferm CCS (Diamond)
: *Clostridium chauvoei-septicum* bacterin

Electrogen-CS (Jen-Sal)
: *Clostridium chauvoei-septicum* bacterin

***Clostridium chauvoei-septicum-novyi* bacterin**

Clostridium chauvoei-septicum-novyi bacterin (Colorado Serum)

Electrogen-CSN (Jen-Sal)
: *Clostridium chauvoei-septicum-novyi* bacterin

***Clostridium chauvoei-septicum-novyi-sordellii-perfringens* types C and D bacterin**

Electroid 7 (Jen-Sal)
: *Clostridium chauvoei-septicum-novyi-sordellii-perfringens* types C and D bacterin

***Clostridium chauvoei-septicum-novyi* bacterin-toxoid**

CCSN (Bio-Ceutic)
: *Clostridium chauvoei-septicum-novyi*-bacterin-toxoid

Clostroid CSN (Fort Dodge)
: *Clostridium chauvoei-septicum-novyi* bacterin-toxoid

***Clostridium chauvoei-septicum-novyi-sordellii* bacterin-toxoid**

C.C.S.N.S. (Dellen)
: *Clostridium chauvoei-septicum-novyi-sordellii* bacterin-toxoid

Clostri-Bac (Haver-Lockhart)
: *Clostridium chauvoei-septicum-novyi-sordellii*-bacterin-toxoid

Clostri-Bac 4 (Haver-Lock-hart)   *Clostridium chauvoei-sep-ticum-novyi sordellii* bacterin-toxoid

Clostroid CSNS (Fort Dodge)   *Clostridium chauvoei-sep-ticum-novyi sordellii* bac-terin-toxoid

Clostridium haemolyticum bacterin

Clostridium haemolyticum Bacterin (Bio-Ceutic)

Clostridium haemolyticum Bacterin (Dia-mond)

Electrogen H (Jen-Sal)   *Clostridium haemolyticum* bacterin

Redwol (Haver-Lockhart)   *Clostridium haemolyticum* bacterin

Clostridium novyi-sordellii bacterin-toxoid

Sardol (Haver-Lockhart)   *Clostridium novyi-sordellii* bacterin-toxoid

Clostridium novyi-sordellii-perfringens types C and D bacterin-toxoid

Electroid NSCD (Jen-Sal)   *Clostridium novyi-sordellii-perfringens* types C and D bacterin-toxoid

Clostridium perfringens antitoxin, types C and D

Clostridium per-fringens Anti-toxin Types C and D (Ab-bott)

Clostridium per-fringens Anti-toxin Types C and D (Colo-rado Serum)

Dybelon (Bio-Ceutic)   *Clostridium perfringens* types C and D antitoxin, equine origin

Clostridium perfringens type C bacterin-toxoid

Deltox-C (Del-len)   *Clostridium perfringens* type C bacterin-toxoid

Ultrabac C (Af-filiated)   *Clostridium perfringens* type C bacterin-toxoid

Clostridium perfringens type C toxoid

Clostridium per-fringens Type C toxoid (Bio-Ceutic)

Electroid C (Jen-Sal)   *Clostridium perfringens* type C toxoid

Fringol C-2 (Haver-Lock-hart)   *Clostridium perfringens* type C toxoid

Clostridium perfringens types C and D bacterin-toxoid

Clostroid-C-D (Fort Dodge)   *Clostridium perfringens* types C and D bacterin-toxoid

Deltox C-D (Dellen)   *Clostridium perfringens* types C and D bacterin-toxoid

Entrotox-CD (Haver-Lock-hart)   *Clostridium perfringens* types C and D bacterin-toxoid

Ultrabac CD (Affiliated)   *Clostridium perfringens* types C and D bacterin-toxoid

Clostridium perfringens types C and D toxoid

Clostridium per-fringens Types C and D Tox-oid (Bio-Ceu-tic)

Electroid CD (Jen-Sal)   *Clostridium perfringens* types C and D toxoid

Clostridium perfringens type D bacterin-toxoid

Deltox-D (Del-len)   *Clostridium perfringens* type D bacterin-toxoid

Entrobac-D-2 (Haver-Lock-hart)   *Clostridium perfringens* type D bacterin-toxoid

Entrobac-D (Haver-Lock-hart)   *Clostridium perfringens* type D bacterin-toxoid

Ultrabac D (Af-filiated)   *Clostridium perfringens* type D bacterin-toxoid

Clostridium perfringens type D toxoid

Clostridium per-fringens Type D Toxoid (Bio-Ceutic)

Clostroid D (Fort Dodge)   *Clostridium perfringens* type D toxoid

Electroid D (Jen-Sal)   *Clostridium perfringens* type D toxoid

Fringol D-2 (Haver-Lock-hart)   *Clostridium perfringens* type D toxoid

Clostridium perfringens type D toxoid plus tetanus toxoid

Clostroid D-T (Fort Dodge)   *Clostridium perfringens* type D toxoid–tetanus toxoid

Clostridium tetani antitoxin

Tetanus Anti-   Equine Origin
toxin (Ab-
bott)

Tetanus Anti-
toxin (Colo-
rado Serum)

Tetanus Anti-   Equine origin
toxin (Fort
Dodge)

Tetanus Anti-   Equine origin
toxin (Haver-
Lockhart)

Tetanus Anti-   Equine origin
toxin (Jen-
Sal)

Clostridium tetani toxoid

(*See* also *Clostridium perfringens* type D toxoid
plus tetanus toxoid)

Super-Tet   Tetanus toxoid
(Haver-Lock-
hart)

Tetanus Toxoid
(Colorado Se-
rum)

Tetanus Toxoid
(Fort Dodge)

Tetoid (Affili-   *Clostridium tetani* (cell free)
ated)   toxin (tetanus toxoid)

Unitox (Jen-Sal)   Tetanus toxoid

Colibacilosis vaccine

(*See* mixed bacterins-bovine)

Enterotoxemia vaccines

(*See Clostridium perfringens* antitoxin, types
C and D; *Clostridium perfringens* type C bacterin-toxoid; *Clostridium perfringens* type C
toxoid; *Clostridium perfringens* types C and
D bacterin-toxoid; *Clostridium perfringens*
types C and D toxoid; *Clostridium perfringens* type D bacterin-toxoid; *Clostridium perfringens* type D toxoid; *Clostridium perfringens* type D toxoid plus tetanus toxoid;
*Clostridium chauvoei-septicum-novyi-sordel-
lii-perfringens* types C and D bacterin; *Clostridium novyi-sordellii-perfringens* types C
and D bacterin-toxoid)

**Equine encephalomyelitis vaccine, eastern
and western**

Cephalovac-EW   Eastern and western en-
(Jen-Sal)   cephalomyelitis vaccine,
    killed, avian TCO

Encephaloid   Encephalomyelitis vaccine,
I.M. (Fort   eastern and western,
Dodge)   killed virus, chick TCO

Encephaloid   Encephalomyelitis vaccine,
(Fort Dodge)   killed virus, eastern and
    western, chick TCO

Encevac (Hav-   Eastern and western en-
er-Lockhart)   cephalomyelitis vaccine,
    TCO

Myelovac (Nor-   Encephalomyelitis vaccine,
den)   eastern and western,
    killed virus, chick TCO

**Equine encephalomyelitis vaccine,
Venezuelan**

Cephalovac-V   Venezuelan encephalomye-
(Jen-Sal)   litis vaccine, MLV,
    guinea pig TCO

VEE-Vac (Nor-   Encephalomyelitis vaccine,
den)   Venezuelan, MLV,
    guinea pig TCO

Equine influenza vaccine

Equicine (Hav-   Equine influenza vaccine,
er-Lockhart)   killed virus, chick embryo
    origin

Equi-Flu II   Equine influenza vaccine,
(Jen-Sal)   killed virus, chick embryo
    origin

Flumune (Nor-   Equine influenza vaccine,
den)   killed virus, chick embryo
    origin

Fluvac (Fort   Equine influenza vaccine,
Dodge)   killed virus, chick embryo
    origin

**Equine rhinopneumonitis (equine herpesvirus
I) vaccine**

Pneumabort   Equine rhinopneumonitis
(Fort Dodge)   virus, live virus, hamster
    origin

Rhinomune   Equine rhinopneumonitis
(Norden)   vaccine, MLV, equine
    cell line origin

Erysipelas vaccine

(*See Erysipelothrix rhusiopathiae* antiserum;
Erysipelothrix rhusiopathiae avirulent living
vaccine; *Erysipelothrix rhusiopathiae* bacterin)

Erysipelothrix rhusiopathiae antiserum

Secon-2x (Bio-   *Erysipelothrix rhusiopath-
Ceutic)   iae* antiserum, equine
    origin, concentrate

Swine Erysip-
elas Antise-
rum (Dia-
mond)

Swine Erysip-
elas Anti-Se-
rum (Jen-Sal)

***Erysipelothrix rhusiopathiae* avirulent living vaccine**

Alva (Haver-Lockhart)	Avirulent erysipelas vaccine
EVA (Norden)	*Erysipelothrix rhusiopathiae* vaccine, avirulent live culture

***Erysipelothrix rhusiopathiae* bacterin**

Alobac 2 (Haver-Lockhart)	Erysipelas bacterin
Eravac (Jen-Sal)	Erysipelas bacterin
Erocon (Dellen)	*Erysipelothrix rhusiopathiae* bacterin
Erogen (Burns-Biotec)	Erysipelas bacterin
Ersipelin (Fort Dodge)	*Erysipelothrix rhusiopathiae* bacterin
Ery-Jex bacterin (Bio-Ceutic)	Concentrated erysipelas bacterin, *Erysipelothrix rhusiopathiae*
Erysipelas Bacterin (Affiliated)	*Erysipelothrix rhusiopathiae* (insidiosa) bacterin
Erysipelas Bacterin (Diamond)	
Erysipelothrix rhusiopathiae Bacterin (Abbott)	
Erysipelothrix rhusiopathiae Bacterin (Diamond)	
Neo-Vac (Diamond)	*Erysipelothrix rhusiopathiae* bacterin
Rhusigen (Pitman-Moore)	Erysipelas bacterin

Feline calicivirus vaccine

(*See* feline rhinotracheitis–calcivirus vaccines; feline rhinotracheitis–calcivirus–panleukopenia vaccine)

Feline panleukopenia vaccine

(*See also* feline rhinotracheitis–calcivirus–panleukopenia vaccine; feline rhinotracheitis–panleukopenia vaccine)

Delpan (Dellen)	Feline panleukopenia vaccine, killed virus, feline cell line origin
Deltab (Dellen)	Feline panleukopenia vaccine, MLV, feline cell line origin
FDV-TC (Burns-Biotec)	Feline distemper vaccine, inactivated feline TCO
Feline Panleukopenia Vaccine (Burns-Biotec)	
Feline Panleukopenia Vaccine (Haver-Lockhart)	MLV, feline TCO
Felocell (Norden)	Feline panleukopenia vaccine, MLV, feline cell line origin
Felocine (Norden)	Feline panleukopenia vaccine, killed virus, feline cell line origin
Fel-O-Vax (Fort Dodge)	Feline panleukopenia vaccine, killed virus, feline origin
Fevac TC (Fromm)	Feline panleukopenia vaccine, killed virus, feline TCO
Leukogen-TC (Bio-Ceutic)	Feline distemper vaccine, MLV, first single dose, TCO
Leukoid TC (Fromm)	Feline panleukopenia vaccine, MLV, feline TCO
Panacine-L (Affiliated)	Feline panleukopenia vaccine, MLV, ferret TCO
Panagen (Pitman-Moore)	Feline panleukopenia vaccine, killed virus, feline TCO
Panavac (Affiliated)	Feline panleukopenia vaccine, feline tissue cell culture origin, inactivated
Panleukovac (Diamond)	Feline panleukopenia vaccine

Feline pneumonitis vaccine

Feline Pneumonitis Vaccine (Fromm)	Modified live *Chlamydia*, chick embryo origin
Feline Pneumonitis Vaccine (Haver-Lockhart)	

Feline rhinotracheitis vaccine

FVR (Pitman-Moore)	Feline rhinotracheitis vaccine, MLV, feline cell line origin
Rhinoid TC (Fromm)	Feline rhinotracheitis vaccine, MLV, feline TCO

Feline rhinotracheitis–calcivirus vaccine

Felomune CVR	Feline rhinotracheitis–

(Norden) — calici vaccine, MLV, feline cell line origin

FVR-C (Pitman-Moore) — Feline rhinotracheitis–calici vaccine, MLV, feline cell line origin

Feline rhinotracheitis–calcivirus–panleukopenia vaccine

FVR C-P (Pitman-Moore) — Feline rhinotracheitis–calici–panleukopenia vaccine, MLV, feline cell line and TCO

Feline rhinotracheitis–panleukopenia vaccine

FVR-P (Pitman-Moore) — Feline rhinotracheitis–panleukopenia vaccine, MLV, feline cell line and TCO

Hog cholera vaccine and antiserum

(Not available in United States)

Human rabies immune globulin

Hyperab (Cutter) — Rabies immune globulin–human; for use in humans

IBR vaccine

(*See* infectious bovine rhinotracheitis vaccine)

Infectious bovine rhinotracheitis vaccine

(*See also* infectious bovine rhinotracheitis vaccine–*Leptospira* bacterin; infectious bovine rhinotracheitis–parainfluenza 3 vaccine; infectious bovine rhinotracheitis–parainfluenza 3 vaccine–*Leptospira pomona* bacterin; infectious bovine rhinotracheitis–parainfluenza 3 vaccine–*Pasteurella haemolytica-multocida* bacterin; infectious bovine rhinotracheitis–viral diarrhea vaccine; infectious bovine rhinotracheitis–viral diarrhea vaccine–*Leptospira* bacterin; infectious bovine rhinotracheitis–viral diarrhea–parainfluenza 3 vaccine; infectious bovine rhinotracheitis–viral diarrhea–parainfluenza 3 vaccine–*Leptospira* bacterin; infectious bovine rhinotracheitis–viral diarrhea–parainfluenza 3 vaccine–*Pasteurella haemolytica-multocida* bacterin)

Bovine Rhinotracheitis Vaccine (Abbott) — MLV, bovine TCO

Bovine Rhinotracheitis Vaccine (Diamond) — MLV, bovine TCO

Delvine (Dellen) — Infectious bovine rhinotracheitis vaccine, MLV, bovine cell line origin

IBR Vaccine — Bovine rhinotracheitis vac-

(Bio-Ceutic) — cine, MLV, Lamb kidney TCO

IBR Vaccine (Colorado Serum)

Jencine I (Jen-Sal) — Bovine rhinotracheitis vaccine, MLV, bovine TCO

Nasamune-IP (Affiliated) — Infectious bovine rhinotracheitis vaccine, attenuated porcine tissue cell culture origin

Piggyback I (Burns-Biotec) — Bovine rhinotracheitis vaccine, MLV, TCO

Resbo IBR (Norden) — Bovine rhinotracheitis vaccine, MLV, bovine cell line origin

Rhinocine (Haver-Lockhart) — Bovine rhinotracheitis vaccine, MLV, guinea pig TCO

Rhivax (Pitman-Moore) — Bovine rhinotracheitis vaccine, MLV, bovine TCO

Infectious bovine rhinotracheitis vaccine–*Leptospira* bacterin

Bovine Rhinotracheitis Vaccine with *Leptospira pomona* bacterin (Abbott) — MLV, bovine TCO

Delvine-L (Dellen) — Infectious bovine rhinotracheitis vaccine, MLV, bovine cell line origin; *Leptospira pomona* bacterin

IBR-Lepto Vaccine (Bio-Ceutic) — Bovine rhinotracheitis vaccine, MLV, lamb kidney TCO; *Leptospira pomona* bacterin

IBR-Lepto (Colorado Serum)

IBR-Lepto (Fort Dodge) — Bovine rhinotracheitis vaccine, MLV, bovine TCO; *Leptospira pomona* bacterin

Jencine IL (Jen-Sal) — Bovine rhinotracheitis vaccine, MLV, bovine TCO, *Leptospira pomona* bacterin

Piggyback I + L (Burns-Biotec) — Bovine rhinotracheitis vaccine, MLV, TCO; *Leptospira pomona* bacterin

Resbo IBR-LP (Norden)

Bovine rhinotracheitis vaccine, MLV, bovine cell line origin; *Leptospira pomona* bacterin

Rhino-Lep (Diamond)

Bovine rhinotracheitis vaccine, *Leptospira pomona* bacterin

Rhino-Mona (Haver-Lockhart)

Bovine rhinotracheitis vaccine, MLV, guinea pig, TCO; *Leptospira pomona* bacterin

Rhivax L (Pitman-Moore)

Bovine rhinotracheitis vaccine, MLV, bovine TCO; *Leptospira pomona* bacterin

Infectious bovine rhinotracheitis–parainfluenza 3 vaccine

Bovine Rhinotracheitis–Parainfluenza 3 Vaccine (Abbott)

MLV, bovine and porcine TCO

Delvine-P (Dellen)

Bovine rhinotracheitis–parainfluenza 3 vaccine, MLV, bovine cell line origin

IBR-PI 3 (Bio-Ceutic)

Bovine rhinotracheitis–parainfluenza 3 vaccine, MLV, cell line origin

IBR-PI3 Vaccine (Colorado Serum)

Nasalgen IP (Jen-Sal)

Bovine rhinotracheitis, intranasal, MLV, lapine TCO; parainfluenza 3, intranasal, MLV culture, porcine TCO

Piggyback 2 (Burns-Biotec)

Bovine rhinotracheitis–parainfluenza 3, MLV, porcine TCO

Rea-Plex (Fort Dodge)

Bovine rhinotracheitis–parainfluenza 3 vaccine, MLV, bovine TCO

Resbo IBR-PI3 (Norden)

Bovine rhinotracheitis–parainfluenza 3 vaccine, MLV, bovine cell line origin

Respacin "2" (Diamond)

Bovine rhinotracheitis–parainfluenza 3 vaccine

Rhino-Paracine (Haver-Lockhart)

Bovine rhinotracheitis MLV, guinea pig and porcine tissue; parainfluenza 3 vaccine

Rhivax P (Pitman-Moore)

Bovine rhinotracheitis vaccine, MLV, bovine TCO; parainfluenza 3 vaccine, MLV, bovine TCO

Infectious bovine rhinotracheitis–parainfluenza 3 vaccine–*Leptospira pomona* bacterin

Delvine-PL (Dellen)

Infectious bovine rhinotracheitis–parainfluenza 3 vaccine, MLV, bovine perma-cell line origin; *Leptospira pomona* bacterin

IBR-PI 3-Lepto (Colorado Serum)

Rea-Plex-L (Fort Dodge)

Bovine rhinotracheitis–parainfluenza 3 vaccine, MLV, bovine TCO; *Leptospira pomona* bacterin

Respacine "2" L (Diamond)

Bovine rhinotracheitis–parainfluenza 3 vaccine–*Leptospira pomona* bacterin

Rhino-Para-Lept (Haver-Lockhart)

Bovine rhinotracheitis vaccine, MLV, guinea pig tissue culture and porcine cell line origin; parainfluenza 3 vaccine, MLV; *Leptospira pomona* bacterin

Infectious bovine rhinotracheitis–parainfluenza 3 vaccine–*Pasteurella haemolytica–multocida* bacterin

Bovine Rhinotracheitis–Parainfluenza 3 Vaccine with *Pasteurella haemolytica-multocida* Bacterium (Abbott)

MLV, bovine and porcine TCO

Piggyback 2 + P (Burns-Biotec)

Bovine rhinotracheitis–parainfluenza 3, MLV, porcine TCO; *Pasteurella* bacterin

Quadraplex (Bio-Ceutic)

Bovine rhinotracheitis–parainfluenza 3 vaccine, killed virus, bovine TCO; *Pasteurella haemolytica-multocida* bacterin

Rhivax P *Pasteurella* (Pitman-Moore)

Bovine rhinotracheitis–parainfluenza 3 vaccine, MLV, bovine TCO; *Pas-*

teurella haemolytica-mul-tocida bacterin

Infectious bovine rhinotracheitis–viral diarrhea vaccine

Bovine Rhino-tracheitis–Virus Diar-rhea (Abbott)	MLV, bovine and porcine TCO
IBR-BVD Vaccine (Colorado Serum)	
Jencine IB (Jen-Sal)	Bovine rhinotracheitis vaccine, MLV, bovine TCO; viral diarrhea vaccine, MLV, porcine TCO
Resbo IBR-BVD (Norden)	Bovine rhinotracheitis vaccine, MLV, bovine cell line origin; bovine viral diarrhea vaccine, MLV, bovine TCO
RVD (Diamond)	Bovine rhinotracheitis–viral diarrhea vaccine

Infectious bovine rhinotracheitis–viral diarrhea vaccine–*Leptospira* bacterin

IBR-BVD-Lep-to (Colorado Serum)	
Jencine (Jen-Sal)	Bovine rhinotracheitis vaccine, MLV, bovine TCO; viral diarrhea vaccine, MLV, porcine TCO; *Leptospira pomona* bacterin
Jencine IBL (Jen-Sal)	Bovine rhinotracheitis–viral diarrhea vaccine, MLV, bovine TCO and porcine cell line origin; *Leptospira pomona* bacterin
Resbo IBR-BVD-LP (Norden)	Bovine rhinotracheitis–viral diarrhea vaccine, MLV, bovine cell line and TCO; *Leptospira pomona* bacterin
RVD-L (Dia-mond)	Bovine rhinotracheitis–viral diarrhea vaccine–*Leptospira pomona* bacterin

Infectious bovine rhinotracheitis–viral diarrhea–parainfluenza 3 vaccine

Bovine rhino-tracheitis–virus diar-rhea–para-	MLV, bovine and porcine TCO

influenza 3 vaccine (Abbott)

IBR-BVD-PI3 Vaccine (Bio-Ceutic)	Bovine rhinotracheitis vaccine, MLV, bovine TCO; viral diarrhea–parainfluenza 3 vaccine, MLV, bovine TCO
IBR-BVD-PI3 Vaccine (Colorado Serum)	
Resbo-3 (IBR-BVD-PI3 (Norden)	Bovine rhinotracheitis–viral diarrhea–parainfluenza 3 vaccine, MLV, bovine cell line and TCO
Respacine "3" (Diamond)	Bovine rhinotracheitis virus, bovine TCO, MLV; viral diarrhea vaccine, bovine TCO; MLV; parainfluenza 3 vaccine, MLV, porcine TCO

Infectious bovine rhinotracheitis–viral diarrhea–parainfluenza 3 vaccine–*Leptospira* bacterin

IBR-BVD-PI3-Lepto (Colorado Serum)	
Resbo-4 (IBR-BVD-PI3-LP) (Norden)	Bovine rhinotracheitis–viral diarrhea–parainfluenza vaccine, MLV, bovine cell line and TCO; *Leptospira pomona* bacterin
Respacine "3" L (Diamond)	Bovine rhinotracheitis–viral diarrhea–parainfluenza vaccine–*Leptospira pomona* bacterin

Infectious bovine rhinotracheitis–viral diarrhea–parainfluenza 3 vaccine–*Pasteurella haemolytica-multocida* bacterin

Bovine Rhino-tracheitis–Viral Diar-rhea-Parain-fluenza 3 Vaccine with *Pasteurella haemolytica-multocida* Bacterin (Abbott)	Bovine and porcine TCO

Infectious necrotic hepatitis (black disease) vaccine

(*See Clostridium chauvoei-novyi-sordellii* bacterin; *Clostridium chauvoei-septicum-novyi* bacterin; *Clostridium chauvoei-septicum-novyi-sordellii-perfringens* types C and D bacterin; *Clostridium chauvoei-septicum-novyi* bacterin-toxoid; *Clostridium chauvoei-septicum-novyi-sordellii* bacterin-toxoid; *Clostridium novyi-sordellii-perfringens* types C and D bacterin-toxoid)

Influenza vaccine

(*See* equine influenza vaccine)

***Leptospira canicola-icterohaemorrhagiae* bacterin**

(*See also* canine distemper–hepatitis–*Leptospira* antisera; canine distemper–hepatitis vaccine–*Leptospira* bacterin; canine distemper–hepatitis–parainfluenza vaccine–*Leptospira* bacterin; canine distemper vaccine–*Leptospira* bacterin)

Bi-Lep (Burns-Biotec)	*Leptospira canicola-icterohaemorrhagiae* bacterin
Canictero-Bac (Bio-Ceutic)	*Leptospira canicola-icterohaemorrhagiae* bacterin
Canictogen (Pitman-Moore)	*Leptospira canicola-icterohaemorrhagiae* bacterin
Havo-Lep-2 (Haver-Lockhart)	*Leptospira canicola-icterohaemorrhagiae* bacterin
L.C.I. (Dellen)	*Leptospira canicola-icterohaemorrhagiae* bacterin
Leptobac (Fromm)	*Leptospira canicola-icterohaemorrhagiae* bacterin
Lepto C-I (Norden)	*Leptospira canicola-icterohaemorrhagiae* bacterin
Leptospira canicola (Fort Dodge)	*Leptospira canicola-icterohaemorrhagiae* bacterin
Leptospira canicola-icterohaemorrhagiae Bacterin (Affiliated)	
Leptospira canicola-icterohaemorrhagiae Bacterin (Colorado Serum)	
Leptospira canicola-icterohaemorrhag-	

iae Bacterin (Diamond)	
Leptospira canicola-icterohaemorrhagiae Bacterin (Fort Dodge)	
Leptospira canicola-icterohaemorrhagiae Bacterin (Jen-Sal)	

***Leptospira grippotyphosa-hardjo-pomona* bacterin**

Leptomune GHP (Affiliated)	*Leptospira grippotyphosa-hardjo-pomona* bacterin
Leptovac G-H-P (Norden)	*Leptospira grippotyphosa-hardjo-pomona* bacterin

***Leptospira pomona* bacterin**

(*See also* infectious bovine rhinotracheitis vaccine–*Leptospira* bacterin; infectious bovine rhinotracheitis–parainfluenza 3 vaccine–*Leptospira pomona* bacterin; infectious bovine rhinotracheitis–viral diarrhea vaccine–*Leptospira* bacterin; infectious bovine rhinotracheitis–viral diarrhea–parainfluenza 3 vaccine–*Leptospira* bacterin)

Leptin (Burns-Biotec)	*Leptospira pomona* bacterin
Leptocon (Dellen)	*Leptospira pomona* bacterin
Leptogen (Pitman-Moore)	*Leptospira pomona* bacterin
Leptomune (Affiliated)	*Leptospira pomona* bacterin
Lepto R.F. (Jen-Sal)	*Leptospira pomona* bacterin
Leptospira Pomona Bacterin (Abbott)	
Leptospira Pomona Bacterium (Colorado Serum)	
Lepto-SR (Bio-Ceutic)	*Leptospira pomona* S R bacterin
Leptovac-P (Norden)	*Leptospira pomona* bacterin
L.P.B.-2 (Haver-Lockhart)	*Leptospira pomona* bacterin
Neo-Lep (Diamond)	*Leptospira pomona* bacterin

Utilep (Fort Dodge)   *Leptospira pomona* bacterin

Leptospirosis vaccine (bovine and ovine)
(*See Leptospira grippotyphosa-hardjo-pomona* bacterin, *Leptospira pomona* bacterin)

Leptospirosis vaccine (canine)
(*See Leptospira canicola-icterohaemorrhagiae* bacterin; canine distemper vaccine–*Leptospira* bacterin; canine distemper–hepatitis vaccine–*Leptospira* bacterin; canine distemper–hepatitis–parainfluenza vaccine–*Leptospira* bacterin)

Malignant edema vaccine
(*See Clostridium chauvoei-septicum* bacterin; *Clostridium chauvoei-septicum-novyi* bacterin; *Clostridium chauvoei-septicum-novyi-sordellii* bacterin-toxoid; *Clostridium chauvoei-septicum-novyi-sordellii-perfringens* types C and D bacterin)

Measles vaccine
(*See also* canine distemper–measles vaccine)

D-Vac-M (Bio-Ceutic)   Measles vaccine, MLV

Heterovac (Diamond)   Measles vaccine, MLV, canine TCO

Measles Vaccine (Jen-Sal)   MLV, canine TCO

Mixed bacterins–bovine

Bovibac 3 (Fort Dodge)   *Escherichia coli, Salmonella typhimurium, Pasteurella multocida-haemolytica* bacterin

CCSP (Bio-Ceutic)   *Clostridium chauvoei-septicum* bacterin, *Pasteurella* bacterin

Bovibac I (Fort Dodge)   *Corynebacterium pyogenes* bacterin, *Pasteurella multocida-haemolytica* bacterin

Clostri-Bac SP-5 (Haver-Lockhart)   *Clostridium chauvoei-septicum* bacterin, *Pasteurella haemolytica-multocida* bacterin

Clostridium chauvoei-septicum-Pasteurella Bacterin (Abbott)

Clostridium chauvoei-septicum-Pasteurella Bacterin (Affiliated)

Clostridium chauvoei-septicum-Pasteurella Bacterin (Colorado Serum)

Clostroid CSP (Fort Dodge)   *Clostridium chauvoei-septicum* bacterin, *Pasteurella haemolytica-multocida* bacterin

Corynebacterium-Pasteurella Antiserum (Colorado Serum)

Corynebacterium pyogenes–Pasteurella haemolytica-multocida Bovine Isolates (Haver-Lockhart)

Electrogen-CSP (Jen-Sal)   *Clostridium chauvoei-septicum* bacterin, *Pasteurella* bacterin

Ultrabac-Bovine No. 1 (Affiliated)   *Corynebacterium pyogenes–Pasteurella haemolytica-multocida* bacterin, bovine isolates

Ultrabac-Bovine No. 3 (Affiliated)   *Escherichia coli–Pasteurella haemolytica-multocida–Salmonella typhimurium* bacterin, bovine isolates

Orf vaccine
(*See* ovine ecthyma vaccine)

Ovine ecthyma (sore mouth, orf) vaccine

Ovine-Ecthyma Live Vaccine (Cutter)

Parainfluenza 3 vaccine
(*See* Bovine viral diarrhea–parainfluenza 3 vaccine; infectious bovine rhinotracheitis–parainfluenza 3 vaccine; infectious bovine rhinotracheitis–parainfluenza 3 vaccine–*Leptospira pomona* bacterin; infectious bovine rhinotracheitis–parainfluenza 3 vaccine–*Pasteurella haemolytica-multocida* bacterin; infectious bovine rhinotracheitis–viral diarrhea–parainfluenza 3 vaccine; infectious bovine rhinotracheitis–viral diarrhea–parainfluenza 3 vaccine–*Leptospira* bacterin; infectious bovine rhinotracheitis–viral diarrhea–parainfluenza 3 vaccine–*Pasteurella haemolytica-multocida* bacterin)

***Pasteurella* antiserum**

Pasteurella Antiserum (Colorado Serum)

***Pasteurella haemolytica-multocida* bacterin**

(*See also* infectious bovine rhinotracheitis–parainfluenza 3 vaccine–*Pasteurella haemolytica-multocida* bacterin; infectious bovine rhinotracheitis–viral diarrhea–parainfluenza 3 vaccine–*Pasteurella haemolytica-multocida* bacterin)

Encon-P (Bio-Ceutic)	*Pasteurella haemolytica-multocida* bacterin (bovine isolates)
Hemseptol (Haver-Lockhart)	*Pasteurella haemolytica-multocida* bacterin
Pasteurella Bacterin (Colorado Serum)	
Pasteurella haemolytica-multocida Bacterin (Abbott)	
Pasteurella-mh (Diamond)	*Pasteurella haemolytica-multocida* bacterin
Pastin (Burns-Biotec)	*Pasteurella* bacterin
Pasturgen (Pitman-Moore)	*Pasteurella haemolytica-multocida* bacterin
Septobac (Fort Dodge)	*Pasteurella haemolytica-multocida* bacterin, bovine isolates
Ultrabac-P Bovine (Affiliated)	*Pasteurella multocida-haemolytica* bacterin

***Pasteurella multocida-haemolytica* bacterin**

(*See* *Pasteurella haemolytica-multocida* bacterin)

PI-3 vaccine

(*See* parainfluenza 3 vaccine)

Porcine virus diarrhea vaccine

Viocine (Burns-Biotec)	Virus diarrhea vaccine, porcine TCO

Rabies vaccine–inactivated

Rabies Vaccine (Bandy)	Inactivated caprine origin
Rabies Vaccine (Lilly)	Duck embryo, killed virus USP, for use in humans
Trimune (Fort Dodge)	Rabies vaccine, killed virus, murine origin

Rabies vaccine (MLV)

Endurall-R (Norden)	Rabies vaccine, MLV, canine cell line origin, high egg passage, Flury strain
ERA Strain Rabies Vaccine (Jen-Sal)	Porcine TCO, high cell passage, SAD strain
Neurogen-TC (Bio-Ceutic)	Rabies vaccine, SAD strain, MLV, canine TCO
Rabies Vaccine (Pitman-Moore)	Bovine kidney TCO, high cell passage, SAD strain
Rabies Vaccine (Haver-Lockhart)	MLV, Flury strain, chick embryo origin
Rabies Vaccine (Schering)	Chick embryo origin, low egg passage, Flury strain
Raboid (Fromm)	Rabies vaccine, MLV, chick embryo origin, Flury strain
Rabtec (Affiliated)	Rabies virus, attenuated, Kissling strain, hamster tissue culture cell line origin

Reovirus vaccine

Scourvax II (Norden)	Reo-corona viral calf diarrhea vaccine, MLV, bovine cell line origin
Scourvax-Reo (Norden)	Reoviral calf diarrhea vaccine, MLV, bovine cell line origin

Sore mouth vaccine

(*See* ovine ecthyma vaccine)

Strangles vaccine

(*See* *Streptococcus equi* bacterin)

Streptococcus equi bacterin

Equibac II (Fort Dodge)	*Streptococcus equi* bacterin

Tetanus vaccines

(*See* *Clostridium tetani* antitoxin; *Clostridium tetani* toxoid; *Clostridium perfringens* type D toxoid plus tetanus toxoid)

Transmissible gastroenteritis vaccine

TGE-Vac (Diamond)	Transmissible gastroenteritis vaccine, MLV, porcine TCO

Venezuelan equine encephalomyelitis vaccine

(*See* equine encephalomyelitis vaccine, Venezuelan)

Vibrio bacterin

Bo-Vibrio (Burns-Biotec)	*Vibrio fetus* bacterin

Tri-Vib (Fort Dodge)

Vibrio fetus bacterin (bovine isolates)

Vibo (Bio-Ceutic)

Vibrio fetus bacterin

Vibrio-Bac (Haver-Lockhart)

Vibrio fetus bacterin

Vibrio Fetus Bacterin-Bovine (Colorado Serum)

Vibrio Fetus Bacterin-Ovine (Colorado Serum)

Vibrio-Leptospira bacterin

Vibo-P (Bio-Ceutic)

Vibrio fetus–Leptospira pomona bacterin

Vibrio-Bac-L (Haver-Lockhart)

Vibrio fetus–Leptospira pomona bacterin, bovine isolates

Western and Eastern equine encephalomyelitis vaccines

(*See* equine encephalomyelitis vaccine, eastern and western)

Wart vaccine

(*See* bovine wart vaccine)

Pharmaceuticals—types and brand names

This list contains the pharmaceuticals discussed in the text and examples of available brands. Abbreviations used in this appendix are as follows:

gm = Gram
gr = Grain
IM = Intramuscular
IU = International unit
IV = Intravenous
LA = Long-acting
mEq = Milliequivalent
mg = Milligram
min = Minim
po = Oral
SC = Subcutaneous
tsp = Teaspoon
USP = United States Pharmacopeia

The term "various" in parentheses means the drug is available from numerous wholesalers under the generic rather than a brand name.

Acetylpromazine
Acepromazine Maleate (Ayerst)
Dosage form: Solution for IV, IM, or SC administration; 10 and 25 mg tablets for po administration

Acetazolamide
Diamox (Lederle) (manufactured for human use)
Dosage form: 125 mg and 250 mg tablets for po administration

Acetic acid
Cetaboro Otic (Summit Hill)
Dosage form: 2% solution for topical use

Adrenocorticotropic hormone (ACTH)
ACTH (Parke, Davis) (manufactured for human use)
Dosage form: Sterile lyophilized powder for reconstitution 25 and 40 USP units/vial for IM or SC administration

Acthar (Armour) (manufactured for human use)
Dosage form: Sterile lyophilized powder for reconstitution 25 and 40 USP units/vial for IM or SC administration

Adrenomone (Burns-Biotec)
Dosage form: 40 and 80 USP units/ml gel for IM or SC administration

Albendazole (experimental drug, not available commercially)

D-Alpha-tocopherol (*see* vitamin E; multiple vitamins; multiple vitamins with minerals; sodium selenite and vitamin E)

Alum
Methoform Dressing Powder (Haver-Lockhart) (also contains tannic acid, camphor, methylene blue, cresylic acid, and iodoform)
Dosage form: Powder for topical use

Aluminum hydroxide
AIU-Cap (Riker) (manufactured for human use)
Dosage form: 475 mg capsules for po administration

Amphojel (Wyeth) (manufactured for human use)
Dosage form: 320 mg/5 ml suspension and 300 mg tablets for po administration

Aminophylline
Aminophyllin (various) (manufactured for human use)
Dosage form: 100 and 200 mg tablets for po administration; 125 and 250 mg/ml solution for IM administration; 25 and 50 mg/ml solution for IV administration

Ammonium chloride
Ammonium chloride (various) (manufactured for human use)
Dosage form: 500 mg tablets for po administration

Anti-Tuss with Antihistamine (Med-Tech) (also contains glyceryl guaiacolate, 8 gr/30 ml; sodium citrate, 8 gr/30 ml; pyrilamine maleate, 50 mg/30 ml; and phenylephrine HCL, 50 mg/30 ml)

Dosage form: 8 gr/30 ml solution for po administration

Expectorant Compound (Bio-Ceutic) (also contains glyceryl guaiacolate, 36.29 gm/pound, and ethylenediamine dihydroiodide, 16.6 gm/pound)
Dosage form: Powder, 226.8 gm/pound, for po administration

Glycon (Bio-Ceutic) (also contains glyceryl guaiacolate, 36.29 gm/pound, and ethylenediamine dihydroiodide, 16.6 gm/pound)
Dosage form: Powder, 226.8 gm/pound, for po administration in drinking water

Glytussin with Iodides (Affiliated) (also contains glyceryl guaiacolate, 7%, and potassium iodide, 2%)
Dosage form: 75% powder for po administration in drinking water

Guiamol with Hi-Amine (Pitman-Moore) (also contains guaiacol and ethylenediamine dihydroiodide)
Dosage form: Powder for po administration

Vetussin (Parlam) (also contains glyceryl guaiacolate, 180 mg/30 ml; ascorbic acid; methapyrilene fumarate; ephedrine hydrochloride; sodium citrate; and citric acid)
Dosage form: 600 mg/30 ml for po administration

Respacell (Albion) (also contains glyceryl guaiacolate, vitamins A and D_3, potassium iodide, sodium chloride, phosphorus, zinc, and magnesium)
Dosage form: Bolus for po administration

Respacell "P" (Albion) (also contains glyceryl guaiacolate, potassium iodide, sodium chloride, magnesium chloride, and zinc chloride)
Dosage form: Powder for po administration in drinking water

Amoxicillin

Amoxi-Drop (Beecham)
Dosage form: Powder for reconstitution to 50 mg/ml suspension for po administration

Amoxil (Beecham) (manufactured for human use)
Dosage form: 250 and 500 mg capsules, 125 and 250 mg/5 ml suspension, and 50 mg/ml pediatric drops for po administration

Amoxi-Tabs (Beecham)
Dosage form: 50, 100, and 200 mg tablets for po administration

Larocin (Roche) (manufactured for human use)
Dosage form: 250 and 500 mg capsules, 125 mg/5 ml oral suspension, 250 mg/5 ml suspension, and 50 mg/ml pediatric drops for po administration

Polymox (Bristol) (manufactured for human use)
Dosage form: 250 and 500 mg capsules, 125 and 250 mg/5 ml oral suspension, and 50 mg/ml pediatric drops for po administration

Amphotericin B

Fungizone Intravenous for Infusion (Squibb) (manufactured for human use)
Dosage form: 50 mg/vial powder for reconstitution to solution for IV administration

Ampicillin

Ampi-Bol (Beecham)
Dosage form: 50 and 100 mg tablets and 400 mg bolus for po administration

Polycillin-N (Bristol) (manufactured for human use)
Dosage form: 125, 250, 500, 1000, and 2000 mg/vial for reconstitution to solution for IV administration; 125, 250, and 500 mg capsules for po administration

Polyflex (Bristol)
Dosage form: Sterile powder for reconstitution to solution for IM or SC administration

Princillin (Squibb), Ampicillin
Dosage form: 400 mg bolus; 10 gm/ounce soluble powder; 125, 250, and 500 mg capsules; 125 mg/ml powder for reconstitution to oral suspension for po administration; 200 mg/ml sterile suspension for IM or SC administration

Principen/N (Squibb) (manufactured for human use)
Dosage form: 125, 250, and 500 mg and 1 gm and 2 gm/vial for reconstitution to solution for IV administration; 250 and 500 mg capsules for po administration

Rea-Cil (Fort Dodge)
Dosage form: 125 and 250 mg capsules for po administration

Totacillin/N (Beecham) (manufactured for human use)
Dosage form: Powder, 250, 500, and 1000 mg/vial for reconstitution to solution for IV administration; 250 and 500 mg capsules for po administration

Amprolium

Corid (Merck)
Dosage form: 9.6% solution for po administration in drinking water or as drench

Apomorphine

Apomorphine Hydrochloride (Lilly) (manufactured for human use)
Dosage form: 6 mg hypodermic tablets for SC administration

Arecoline-acetarsol
Nemural (Winthrop)
 Dosage form: 18 and 54 mg tablets for po administration
Arecoline hydrobromide (*see also* arecoline-acetarsol)
Areco-Caine (Fort Dodge) (also contains procaine hydrochloride)
 Dosage form: 16.2 mg tablets for po administration
Aspirin (acetylsalicylic acid)
Aspirin (Haver-Lockhart)
 Dosage form: 50 gr tablets for po administration
Aspirin (Med-Tech)
 Dosage form: 250 gr bolus and 60 gr tablets for po administration
Aspirin (Parke, Davis)
 Dosage form: 5 gr tablets for po administration
Aspirin (various) (manufactured for human use)
 Dosage form: 1, 1.5, 2, 5, and 10 gr tablets for po administration
Ascorbic acid (*see* vitamin C; multiple vitamins; multiple vitamins with minerals)
Atropine
Atro-Dote (Hart-Delta)
 Dosage form: 2 mg/ml LA solution; 0.5 mg/ml short-acting solution for IV administration
Atro-Ject (Hart-Delta)
 Dosage form: 0.5 mg/ml solution for IV administration
Atropectate (Burns-Biotec) (also contains kaolin, pectin, bismuth subcarbonate)
 Dosage form: Suspension for po administration
Atropine (Fort Dodge)
 Dosage form: 2 mg/ml LA solution; 0.5 mg/ml short-acting solution for IV, IM, or SC administration
Atropine 1% (Maurry)
 Dosage form: Solution for topical use
Atropine Sulfate (Burns-Biotec)
Atropine Sulfate (Med-Tech)
 Dosage form: 0.5 and 15 mg/ml solutions for IM, IV, or SC administration
Atropine sulfate (various) (manufactured for human use)
 Dosage form: 0.3, 0.4, 0.5, 0.6, 1, 1.3, and 2 mg/ml solutions for IV administration
Atropine Sulfate Ophthalmic Ointment (Burns-Biotec)
 Dosage form: 0.5% ophthalmic ointment for topical use
Atropo (North American Pharm.)
 Dosage form: Powder, 32 mg/level tsp for po administration

Atrosol (Burns-Biotec)
 Dosage form: Solution for SC, IM, or IV administration
Atro-Sol (Haver-Lockhart)
 Dosage form: 2 mg/ml solution for IM, SC, or IV administration
Butropine (Burns-Biotec)
 Dosage form: Solution for IV, IM, or SC administration
Metropine (Pennwalt) (manufactured for human use)
 Dosage form: 1 mg tablets for po administration
P/M Atropine Sulfate (Pitman-Moore)
 Dosage form: 0.5 mg/ml solution for IM or SC administration
Bacitracin (*see also* neomycin-bacitracin–polymyxin B)
Baciferm (IMC Chemical Group) (contains zinc bacitracin)
 Dosage form: Soluble powder for po administration
Bacitracin USP (Upjohn) (manufactured for human use)
 Dosage form: Sterile powder for reconstitution to suspension for IM administration
Entromycin (Pitman-Moore) (also contains streptomycin, 15 mg)
 Dosage form: 150 unit tablets for po administration
Bar magnet
Bar magnet (various)
 Dosage form: Bolus shape for po administration to cattle
Belladonna tincture
Belladonna Tincture USP (Purepac) (manufactured for human use)
 Dosage form: Solution for po administration
Bendroflumethiazide
Naturetin-2.5, -5, -10 (Squibb) (manufactured for human use)
 Dosage form: 2.5, 5, and 10 mg tablets for po administration
Benoxinate
Benoxinate Ophthalmic Solution (Barnes-Hind) (manufactured for human use)
 Dosage form: 0.4% ophthalmic solution for topical use
Dorsacaine Hydrochloride (Dorsey) (manufactured for human use)
 Dosage form: 0.4% ophthalmic solution for topical use
Benzathine cloxacillin
Boviclox (Squibb)

Dosage form: 500 mg/ml suspension for intra-mammary administration

Dry-Clox (Bristol)

Dosage form: 50 mg/ml oil-gel in 10 ml syringe for intramammary administration

Orbenin-DC (Beecham)

Dosage form: 500 mg suspension in syringe for intramammary administration

Benzathine penicillin G

Benza-Pen (Beecham) (also contains procaine penicillin G)

Dosage form: Sterile suspension

Bicillin Fortified Injection (Wyeth) (also contains procaine penicillin G)

Bicillin Long-Acting Suspension (Wyeth) (manu-factured for human use)

Dosage form: 300,000 and 600,000 units/ml suspension for IM administration

Bicillin L-A Injection (Wyeth)

Dosage form: Suspension for IM administration

Dual-Pen (Med-Tech) (also contains procaine penicillin G, 150,000 units/ml)

Dosage form: 150,000 units/ml suspension for IM administration

Depo penicillin (Upjohn) (also contains procaine penicillin G, 150,000 units/ml)

Dosage form: 150,000 units/ml suspension for IM or SC administration

Flo-Cillin (Bristol) (also contains procaine penicil-lin G, 150,000 units/ml)

Dosage form: 150,000 units/ml solution for IM or SC administration

Longicil Fortified (Fort Dodge) (also contains pro-caine penicillin G, 150,000 units/ml)

Dosage form: 150,000 units/ml suspension for IM or SC administration

Permapen (Pfizer) (manufactured for human use)

Dosage form: 600,000 units/ml suspension for IM administration

P/M Pen B and G (Pitman-Moore) (also contains procaine penicillin G, 150,000 units/ml)

Dosage form: 150,000 units/ml suspension for IM administration

Benzyl benzoate USP

Benzyl-Hex (Evsco) (also contains rotenone, 0.5%; lindane, 0.25%; and dichlorophen, 0.5%)

Dosage form: 20% solution for topical use

Demodek (Fort Dodge) (also contains terpineol, 1%)

Dosage form: 40% solution for topical use

Demsardex (Burns-Biotec) (also contains lindane)

Dosage form: Solution for topical use

Mange Lotion (Bio-Ceutic) (also contains rote-none, 0.12%; lindane, 0.1%; and dichlorophen, 0.5%)

Dosage form: 30% lotion for topical use

Mitone (Affiliated) (also contains benzocaine, 2%, and rotenone, 0.3%)

Dosage form: 20% solution for topical use

Paramite (Hart-Delta) (also contains rotenone and lindane)

Dosage form: Solution for topical use

Betamethasone

Betasone (Schering)

Dosage form: 7 mg/ml aqueous suspension for IM administration

Betavet (Schering)

Dosage form: 15.9 mg/ml aqueous suspension for intraarticular administration

Celestone (Schering) (manufactured for human use)

Dosage form: 0.6 mg tablets and 0.6 mg/5 ml syrup for po administration; 6 mg/ml inject-able solution for IM or intraarticular admin-istration

Gentocin Otic (Schering) (also contains gentami-cin, 3 mg/ml)

Dosage form: 1 mg/ml otic solution for topical use

Gentocin with Betamethasone (Schering) (also contains gentamicin, 3 mg/ml)

Dosage form: 1 mg/ml ophthalmic solution for topical use

Bile salts (acids)

Bilron (Lilly) (manufactured for human use)

Dosage form: 150 and 300 mg tablets for po administration

Biotin (*see* multiple vitamins; multiple vitamins with minerals)

Bismuth subnitrate

Balmex (Macsil) (manufactured for human use; also contains Peru balsam, zinc oxide, and vi-tamins A and D)

Dosage form: Ointment for topical use

Pellitol (Pitman-Moore) (also contains resorcinol, bismuth subgallate, zinc oxide, calamine, and juniper tar)

Dosage form: Ointment for topical use

Bithionol sulfoxide

Actamer (Monsanto) (not available for use in Unit-ed States)

Boldenone undecylenate

Equipoise (Squibb)

Dosage form: 25 and 50 mg/ml oil solution for IM administration

Bunamidide

Scolaban (Wellcome)

Dosage form: 100, 200, and 400 mg tablets for po administration

Burow's solution USP

Domeboro (Dome) (manufactured for human use)

Dosage form: Soluble tablets and powder to dissolve in water for topical use

Butacaine

Butyn Sulfate Solution (Abbott) (manufactured for human use)

Dosage form: 2% solution for topical use

Butonate

T-113 (Vet-Kem)

Dosage form: 13% solution for administration by stomach tube

Calamine lotion

Calamine Lotion (various) (manufactured for human use)

Dosage form: Suspension for topical use

Calcium borogluconate

C.B.G. (Jen-Sal)

Dosage form: Solution for IV administration

Calcium borogluconate and magnesium

Calcium-D (Diamond) (contains calcium borogluconate, 16.8%; magnesium, 0.055%; and dextrose, 20%)

Dosage form: Solution

Calmadex (Diamond) (contains calcium borogluconate, 22.6%; magnesium 0.055%; and dextrose, 20%)

Dosage form: Solution

DCM Special with Phosphorus (Jen-Sal) (also contains dextrose)

Dosage form: Solution for IV administration

Forcal (Bio-Ceutic) (contains calcium borogluconate, 23%; magnesium chloride, 4.5%; dextrose, 25%; and sodium hypophosphite, 3.43%)

Dosage form: Solution for IV or intraperitoneal administration

Forcal-K (Bio-Ceutic) (contains calcium borogluconate, 23%; magnesium chloride, 4.5%; sodium hypophosphite, 3.43%; dextrose, 25%; and potassium chloride, 0.2%)

Dosage form: Solution for IV or intraperitoneal administration

Norcalcopnos (Norden) (contains calcium borogluconate, 26%; magnesium borogluconate, 6%; dextrose, 15%; and phosphorus 0.5%)

Dosage form: Solution for IV administration

Calcium carbonate

Calcium carbonate (various) (manufactured for human use)

Dosage form: 650 mg tablets and powder for po administration

Calcium gluconate

Calcium 23% Solution (Med-Tech)

Dosage form: 23% solution for IV, IM, or SC administration

Calcium gluconate (various) (manufactured for human use)

Dosage form: 10% solution for IV administration

Calpho Pet Solution (Haver-Lockhart) (also contains calcium hypophosphite, 2.3%)

Dosage form: 6.6% solution for IV or intraperitoneal administration

Calcium gluconate and magnesium

Cal-Phos No. 2 (Med-Tech) (contains calcium gluconate, 28.24%; magnesium chloride; calcium hyophosphite; and dextrose)

Dosage form: Solution for IV or intraperitoneal administration

CGP Solution (Haver-Lockhart) (also contains dextrose, 25%)

Dosage form: 13% calcium, 3% magnesium solution for IV administration

CGP with KCL (Haver-Lockhart) (also contains potassium chloride, 0.1%, and dextrose, 16.6%)

Dosage form: 20% calcium, 0.38% magnesium solution for IV administration

Calcium lactate

Calcium Lactate (various) (manufactured for human use)

Dosage form: 325 and 650 mg tablets and powder for po administration

Calcium phosphate, dibasic

D.C.P. 340 Powder (Parke, Davis) (manufactured for human use)

Dosage form: Powder for po administration

Calcium phosphorus

Fortified Natural Calcium (Med-Tech) (also contains vitamin D)

Dosage form: 32% calcium, 14.5% phosphorus powder for po administration in food, water, or as drench

Natural Calcium Powder (Hart-Delta) (also contains vitamin D_2)

Dosage form: 25% calcium, 12% phosphorus powder for po administration

Pet-Cal (Beecham) (also contains vitamin D_3)

Dosage form: 1500 mg calcium phosphate, 550 mg calcium carbonate tablets for po administration

Vita-Glo Plus (Hart-Delta)

Dosage form: 10% calcium, 5% phosphorus powder for po administration

Calcium–vitamin D
Vet-Cal (Vet-A-Mix)
 Dosage form: Tablets for po administration
California Mastitis Test solution
California Mastitis Test Solution (Haver-Lockhart)
 Dosage form: Aqueous solution
Cambendazole
Camvet (Merck)
 Dosage form: 0.9 gm/ml suspension for admin-
 istration by stomach tube or as drench; as a
 paste for po administration
Camphorated opium tincture (paregoric)
Paregoric (various) (manufactured for human use)
 Dosage form: 2 mg morphine equivalent/5 ml
 liquid for po administration
Cantharidin
Cantharidin (various) (manufactured for human
 use)
 Dosage form: Powder for topical use
Captan
Casteen (Burns-Biotec) (also contains salicylic
 acid and sulfur)
 Dosage form: Shampoo for topical use
E-Z-Dip (Evsco) (also contains carbaryl, 60%)
 Dosage form: 1% powder for topical use
Para Dip (Haver-Lockhart) (also contains carbaryl
 and lindane)
 Dosage form: Dip for topical use
Carbachol (carbamylcholine)
Caride (Haver-Lockhart)
 Dosage form: 0.1% solution for SC adminis-
 tration
Carbaryl (Sevin) (*l*-naphyl *N*-methylcarbamate)
Diryl (Pitman-Moore) (also contains pyrethrins
 and piperonyl butoxide)
 Dosage form: Powder for topical use
E-Z-Dip (Evsco) (also contains captan, 1%)
 Dosage form: 60% powder for topical use
Flair (Jen-Sal) (also contains pyrethrins, piperonyl
 butoxide, malathion, and petroleum distillates)
 Dosage form: Solution for topical use
Flea and Tick Dust (Med-Tech) (also contains
 dichlorophen, 0.5%, and aluminum chlorohy-
 droxy allantoinate, 0.2%)
 Dosage form: 5% powder for topical use
Flea and Tick Powder (Vet-Kem)
 Dosage form: 5% powder for topical use
F.L.T. Bomb (Bio-Ceutic) (also contains dichloro-
 phen, 0.1%; pyrethrins, 0.06%; and piperonyl
 butoxide, 0.6%)
 Dosage form: 1% aerosol for topical use
F-L-T Powder (Bio-Ceutic) (also contains pyre-
 thrins, 0.1%, and piperonyl butoxide, 1%)
 Dosage form: 5% powder for topical use

Mitox (Norden) (also contains neomycin sulfate,
 0.5%; sulfacetamide, 9%; and tetracaine, 0.5%)
 Dosage form: 1% solution for topical use
Mycodex with Carbaryl (Beecham)
 Dosage form: 0.5% shampoo for topical use
Norsect (Norden) (also contains pyrethrins,
 0.075%; piperonyl butoxide, 0.15%; N-octyl
 bicycloheptane dicarboxamide, 0.25%; and
 methoxychlor, 0.5%)
 Dosage form: 0.5% aerosol for topical use
Para Dip (Haver-Lockhart) (also contains lindane
 and captan)
 Dosage form: Dip for topical use
Para-Dust (Hart-Delta) (also contains chlorhy-
 droxy-aluminum allantoinate)
 Dosage form: Powder for topical use
Para Powder (Haver-Lockhart)
 Dosage form: Powder for topical use
Para S-1 (Haver-Lockhart) (also contains pyre-
 thins, 0.06%; piperonyl butoxide, 0.48%; and
 methoxychlor, 0.5%)
 Dosage form: 0.5% aerosol for topical use
Pet Dust (Diamond) (also contains dichlorophen
 and aluminum chlorohydroxy allantoinate)
 Dosage form: Powder for topical use
Pet Spray (Diamond) (also contains pyrethrins
 and rotenone)
 Dosage form: For topical use
Sect-a-spray (Evsco) (also contains pyrethrins,
 0.05%, and piperonyl butoxide, 0.5%)
 Dosage form: 0.5% aerosol for topical use
Sprecto (Pitman-Moore) (also contains pyrethrins,
 piperonyl butoxide, tetrahydrofuraldehyde, and
 dicarboxamide)
 Dosage form: Spray for topical use
Vet-Kem Flea and Tick Powder (Thuron)
 Dosage form: 5% powder for topical use
Carbenicillin
Geocillin (Roerig) (manufactured for human use)
 Dosage form: 382 mg tablets for po adminis-
 tration
Geopen (Roerig) (manufactured for human use)
 Dosage form: 2 gm/vial sterile powder for re-
 constitution to solution for IV or IM adminis-
 tration
Pyopen (Beecham) (manufactured for human use)
 Dosage form: 1, 2, and 5 gm/vial sterile pow-
 der for reconstitution to solution for IV or IM
 administration
Carbon disulfide (*see* carbon disulfide and pipera-
 zine)
Carbon disulfide and piperazine
Parvex (Upjohn)
 Dosage form: Liquid for administration by
 stomach tube

Carotene (*see* multiple vitamins; multiple vitamins with minerals; vitamins A and D; vitamins A, D, and E)

Cascara sagrada
Cas-Evac (Parke, Davis)
Dosage form: Liquid for po administration

Castor oil
Castor Oil (various) (manufactured for human use)
Dosage form: 10 min capsules and liquid for po administration

Cephalexin
Keflex (Lilly) (manufactured for human use)
Dosage form: 250 and 500 mg capsules, 125 and 250 mg/5 ml oral suspension, and 100 mg/10 ml pediatric drops for po administration

Cephaloglycin
Kafocin (Lilly) (manufactured for human use)
Dosage form: 250 mg capsules for po administration

Cephaloridine
Loridine (Lilly) (manufactured for human use)
Dosage form: Powder for reconstitution to 250 and 500 mg/5 ml; 50 and 100 mg/ml solution for IM or IV administration
Loridine Injectable (Elanco)
Dosage form: 100 mg/ml suspension for IM or SC administration

Cephalothin
Keflin (Lilly) (manufactured for human use)
Dosage form: Powder for reconstitution to solution for IV or IM administration

Cephapirin sodium
Cefadyl (Bristol) (manufactured for human use)
Dosage form: Powder for reconstitution to solution for IV or IM administration
Cefa-Lak (Bristol)
Dosage form: 20 mg/ml gel in 10 ml syringe for intramammary administration

Chloramphenicol
Bemacol (Beecham)
Dosage form: Solution for po administration; 1% ophthalmic ointment for topical use
Chloramphenicol (Med-Tech)
Dosage form: 100 and 500 mg capsules for po administration
Chloramphenicol (North American Pharm.)
Dosage form: 100 and 250 mg capsules for po administration
Chlorasol (Evsco)
Dosage form: 5 mg/ml ophthalmic solution for topical use
Chlorasone (Evsco) (also contains prednisolone, 2 mg/gm)

Dosage form: 10 mg/gm ophthalmic ointment for topical use
Chlora-Tabs 100 (Evsco)
Dosage form: 100 mg tablets for po administration
Chloricol (Evsco)
Dosage form: 10 mg/gm ophthalmic ointment for topical use
Chloromycetin (Parke, Davis) (manufactured for human use)
Dosage form: 50, 100, and 250 mg capsules and 150 mg/5 ml palmitate oral suspension for po administration; solution for IV administration; sodium succinate powder for reconstitution to solution for IV administration; 10 mg/gm ophthalmic ointment and 5 mg/ml ophthalmic solution for topical use
Chloromycetin (Parke, Davis)
Dosage form: 1% ophthalmic ointment for topical use
Chloromycetin Otic (Parke, Davis)
Dosage form: Suspension for topical administration
Medichol (Med-Tech)
Dosage form: 100 mg/ml solution for po administration
P/M Chloramphenicol (Pitman-Moore)
Dosage form: 100 mg/ml solution for IM or IV administration; 100 mg/ml oral solution and 50, 100, and 500 mg capsules for po administration

Chlorothiazide
Diuril (Merck Sharp & Dohme)
Dosage form: 2 gm bolus and 0.25 mg tablets for po administration
Diuril (Merck Sharp & Dohme) (manufactured for human use)
Dosage form: 250 and 500 mg tablets and 250 mg/5 ml suspension for po administration; powder for reconstitution to solution for IV administration

Chlorpromazine
Thorazine (Pitman-Moore)
Dosage form: 25 mg/ml solution for IM or IV administration; 10 and 25 mg tablets for po administration
Thorazine (Smith Kline & French) (manufactured for human use)
Dosage form: 10 and 25 mg tablets for po administration; 2.5% solution for IM or IV administration

Chlortetracycline
Aureomycin (Lederle) (manufactured for human use)

Dosage form: Solution for IV administration

Chlorachel (Rachelle)

Dosage form: 10, 50, and 100 gm/pound powder for po administration

Choline (*see* multiple vitamins; multiple vitamins with minerals; vitamin premix)

Chorionic gonadotropin, human (HCG)

Chorionic Gonadotropin Solution (Haver-Lockhart)

Dosage form: 2500 and 10,000 USP units for reconstitution to suspension for IM administration

Chorisol (Burns-Biotec)

Dosage form: 5000 and 10,000 units/vial powder for reconstitution to solution for IM, intrafollicular, or IV administration

Follutein (Squibb) (manufactured for human use)

Dosage form: Lyophilized powder for reconstitution to 1000 IU/ml suspension for IM administration

Gonamone (Fort Dodge)

Dosage form: Powder for reconstitution to solution for IM or intrafollicular administration

Clioxanide (not available in United States)

Cloxacillin

Tegopen (Bristol) (manufactured for human use)

Dosage form: 250 and 500 mg capsules and powder for reconstitution to 125 mg/5 ml suspension for po administration

Cobalt (*see* minerals; multiple vitamins with minerals)

Copper naphthenate

Koppertox (Ayerst)

Dosage form: 37.5% solution for topical use

Copper sulfate

Caustic Dressing Powder (Haver-Lockhart)

Dosage form: Powder for topical use

Coumaphos

Baymix (Cutter)

Dosage form: 11.2% crumbles and feed premix for po administration

Co-ral (Cutter)

Dosage form: 1% dust, emulsifiable liquid, 5% livestock duster, 4% liquid pour-on, 3% spray foam, and 25% wettable powder for topical use

Creosote

Guaiacol Compound (Med-Tech) (also contains guaiacol, 9.7%; cresylic acid, 4.3%; oil of eucalyptus, 0.5%; and camphor, 0.25%)

Dosage form: 0.52% solution for po administration

Cuprimyxin

Unitop (Roche)

Dosage form: 0.5% cream for topical use

Cyanocobalamin (vitamin B_{12}) (*see also* multiple vitamins; multiple vitamins with minerals)

Cyanocobalamin Injection (Med-Tech)

Dosage form: 1 mg/ml solution for IV administration

Cyanocobalamin, Vitamin B_{12} (various) (manufactured for human use)

Dosage form: 500 mg tablets for po administration; 30, 50, 100, and 1000 mg/ml solution for IM administration

Hydrobiomin (Burns-Biotec)

Dosage form: 1 mg/ml solution for IM administration

Hydrox-12 (Med-Tech)

Dosage form: 1 mg/ml solution for IM administration

Ruby B (Parlam)

Dosage form: 5000 μg/15 ml solution for parenteral administration

Vitamin B_{12} (Hart-Delta)

Dosage form: 1000 μg/ml solution for parenteral administration

Vitamin B-12

Dosage form: 1000 μg/ml solution for parenteral administration

Cycloserine

Seromycin (Lilly) (manufactured for human use)

Dosage form: 250 mg capsules for po administration

Demecarium

Humorsol Ophthalmic Solution (Merck Sharp & Dohme) (manufactured for human use)

Dosage form: 0.125% and 0.25% ophthalmic solution for topical use

Deslanoside NF

Cedilanid-D (Sandoz) (manufactured for human use)

Dosage form: 0.2 mg/ml solution for IM or IV administration

Desoxycorticosterone acetate USP

Desoxycorticosterone Acetate Injection (various) (manufactured for human use)

Dosage form: 5 mg/ml solution for IM administration

Doca Acetate (Organon) (manufactured for human use)

Dosage form: 5 mg/ml oil solution for IM administration

Percorten Acetate (Ciba) (manufactured for human use)

Dosage form: 5 mg/ml oil solution for IM administration; pellets for SC implantation

Desoxycorticosterone pivalate

Percorten Pivalate (Ciba) (manufactured for human use)

Dosage form: 25 mg/ml solution for IM administration

Dexamethasone

Azium (Schering)

Dosage form: 2 mg/ml aqueous suspension for IM administration; 2 mg/ml solution for IV administration; 1 and 2 mg/ml solutions, 0.25 mg tablets, 10 mg bolus, and 5 and 10 mg powder packets for po administration

Decadron (Merck Sharp & Dohme) (manufactured for human use)

Dosage form: 0.25, 0.5, 0.75, and 1.5 mg tablets and 0.5 mg/5 ml elixir for po administration; 4 mg/ml phosphate solution for IM or IV administration; 8 mg/ml LA acetate solution for IM administration

Deronil (Schering) (manufactured for human use)

Dosage form: 0.75 mg tablets for po administration

Dexameth (USV) (manufactured for human use)

Dosage form: 0.75 mg tablets for po administration

Dexamethasone (Pfizer)

Dosage form: 2 mg/ml solution for IM or IV administration

Dexamethasone Sodium Phosphate (Maurry)

Dosage form: 0.1% ophthalmic, otic solution for topical use

Dexamethasone Sodium Phosphate Injection USP (Med-Tech)

Dosage form: 4 mg/ml solution for IM or IV administration

Dexasone (Med-Tech)

Dosage form: 2 mg/ml solution for IM or IV administration; 0.25 mg tablets for po administration

Fulvidex (Schering) (also contains nitrofurathiazide, griseofulvin, undecylenic acid, and tetracaine)

Dosage form: Otic suspension for topical use

Gammacorten (Ciba) (manufactured for human use)

Dosage form: 0.75 mg tablets for po administration

Hexadrol (Organon) (manufactured for human use)

Dosage form: 0.5, 0.75, 1.5, and 4 mg tablets and 0.5 mg/5 ml elixir for po administration; 4 mg/ml phosphate solution for IM or IV administration

P/M Dexamethasone (Pitman-Moore)

Dosage form: 2 mg/ml solution for IM or IV administration

Dextrose

DCM Special with Phosphorus (Jen-Sal) (also contains calcium borogluconate and magnesium hypophosphate)

Dosage form: Solution for IV administration

Dextrose (various) (manufactured for human use)

Dosage form: Solution for IV administration

Dextrose 2.5% in Half Strength Lactated Ringer's (Abbott) (contains dextrose, 2.5 gm/100 ml; sodium chloride, 30 mg/100 ml; sodium lactate 155 mg/100 ml; potassium chloride, 15 mg/100 ml; and calcium chloride, 10 mg/100 ml)

Dosage form: 2.5% solution for IV administration

Dextrose 2.5% in Half Strength Lactated Ringer's (Diamond)

Dosage form: Solution for IV administration

Dextrose 2.5% and 5% in Half Strength Saline (Abbott) (contains dextrose, 2.5 or 5 gm/100 ml, and sodium chloride, 450 mg/100 ml)

Dosage form: 2.5% and 5% solution for IV or intraperitoneal administration

Dextrose 2.5% and 5% in Half Strength Saline (Diamond)

Dextrose 5% in Lactated Ringer's (Abbott) (contains dextrose, 5 gm/100 ml; sodium chloride, 600 mg/100 ml; sodium lactate, 310 mg/100 ml; potassium chloride, 30 mg/100 ml; and calcium chloride, 20 mg/100 ml)

Dosage form: 5% solution for IV administration

Dextrose 5% in Saline 0.9% (Abbott) (contains dextrose, 5 gm/100 ml, and sodium chloride, 900 gm/100 ml)

Dosage form: 5% solution for IV administration

5% Dextrose and 0.9% Sodium Chloride (Jen-Sal)

Dosage form: 5% solution for IV administration

Dextrose 5% in Water (Abbott)

Dosage form: 5% solution for IV administration

Dextrose Injection 50% (Abbott)

Dosage form: 50% solution for IV administration

Dextrose Solution 50% (Bio-Ceutic)

Dosage form: 50% solution for IV or intraperitoneal administration

Dextrose Solution 50% (Diamond)

Dosage form: 50% solution for IV administration

Dextrose 50% (Hart-Delta)

Dosage form: 50% solution for IV administration

Dextrose Solution 50% (Jen-Sal)
Dosage form: Solution for IV administration
Dextrose 50% (Med-Tech)
Dosage form: 50% solution for IV administration
Forcal (Bio-Ceutic) (also contains calcium borogluconate, 23%; magnesium chloride, 4.5%; and sodium hypophosphite, 3.43%)
Dosage form: 25% solution for IV or intraperitoneal administration
Forcal-K (Bio-Ceutic) (also contains calcium borogluconate, 23%; magnesium chloride, 4.5%; sodium hypophosphite, 3.43%; and potassium chloride, 1 gm/500 ml)
Dosage form: 25% solution for IV or intraperitoneal administration
Glucose Solution 50% (Fort Dodge)
Dosage form: 50% solution for IV, SC, or intraperitoneal administration
Glucose Solution 50% (Haver-Lockhart)
Dosage form: 50% solution for intraperitoneal, IV, or SC administration
Kaflec (Med-Tech) (also contains potassium chloride, 1.07%, and sodium bicarbonate, 50%)
Dosage form: 48.33% solution for po administration
N.R.G. (Haver-Lockhart) (also contains sorbitol)
Dosage form: Solution for IV or intraperitoneal administration

Diazepam sodium
Valium (Roche) (manufactured for human use)
Dosage form: 2, 5, and 10 mg tablets for po administration; 5 mg/ml solution for IM or IV administration

Dibucaine
Nupercainal (Ciba) (manufactured for human use)
Dosage form: 1% ointment, 1% cream, and 0.25% spray for topical use
Nupercaine (Ciba) (manufactured for human use)
Dosage form: 0.5% solution for spinal anesthesia

Dichlorophen (*see also* dichlorophen and toluene)
Benzyl-Hex (Evsco) (also contains benzyl benzoate, 20%; rotenone C.P.O., 50%; and lindane, 0.25%)
Dosage form: 0.5% solution for topical use
Flea and Tick Dust (Med-Tech) (also contains carbaryl, 5%, and aluminum chlorohydroxy allantoinate, 0.2%)
Dosage form: 0.5% powder for topical use
F.L.T. Bomb (Bio-Ceutic) (also contains carbaryl, 1%; pyrethrins, 0.06%, and piperonyl butoxide, 0.6%)
Dosage form: 0.1% aerosol for topical use

F.L.T. Powder (Bio-Ceutic) (also contains carbaryl, 5%; piperonyl butoxide, 1%; and pyrethrins, 0.1%)
Dosage form: 0.5% powder for topical use
Fungidex (Norden) (also contains zinc undecylenate, 12%; undecylenic acid, 5%; and copper undecylenate, 3%)
Dosage form: 2% creme for topical use
Mange Lotion (Bio-Ceutic (also contains cotenone, 0.12%; lindane, 0.1%; and benzyl benzoate, 30%)
Dosage form: 0.5% lotion for topical use
Pet Dust (Diamond) (also contains aluminum chlorohydroxy allantoinate)
Dosage form: Powder for topical use

Dichlorophen and toluene
Anaplex (Bio-Ceutic)
Dosage form: Capsules for po administration
Difolin (Fort Dodge)
Dosage form: Capsules for po administration
Paracide (Norden)
Dosage form: Capsules for po administration
Vermiplex (Pitman-Moore)
Dosage form: Capsules for po administration

Dichlorphenamide
Daranide (Merck Sharp & Dohme) (manufactured for human use)
Dosage form: 50 mg tablets for po administration
Oratrol (Alcon) (manufactured for human use)
Dosage form: 50 mg tablets for po administration

Dichlorvos (DDVP, Vapona)
Equigard (Shell)
Dosage form: Powder for po administration
Equigel (Shell)
Dosage form: Gel for po administration
Flea Collar for Cats (Shell)
Dosage form: 4.8% in collar for topical use
Flea Collar for Dogs/Cats (Vet-Kem)
Dosage form: 9.6% in collar for topical use
Flea Collar for Dogs/Cats (Vet-Kem)
Dosage form: 4.7% and 9% in collar for topical use
Flea Medallion for Dogs (Vet-Kem)
Dosage form: 18.6% in a medallion (tag) for topical use
Kem-Dip (Vet-Kem) (also contains dioxathion, 3.5%; related compounds, 1.5%; dichloroethane, 9.5%; pine oil, 25%; and petroleum distillate 49%)
Dosage form: 0.93% solution for topical use
Kem-Tox (Vet-Kem) (also contains dioxathion, 10.50%, and tetrachloroethylene, 6%)

Dosage form: 0.93% solution in spray for topical use

Task (Shell)
Dosage form: 136, 204, and 544 mg resin pellets for po administration; 27, 41, 68, 136, and 204 mg capsules and 10 and 25 mg tablets for po administration

Vet-Kem Flea Collar for Cats (Thuron)
Dosage form: 4.37% in collar for topical use

Vet-Kem Flea Collar for Dogs (Thuron)
Dosage form: 8.37% in collar for topical use

Dicloxacillin
Dicloxin (Bristol)
Dosage form: 100 and 500 mg capsules for po administration

Dynapen (Bristol) (manufactured for human use)
Dosage form: 125 and 250 mg capsules and powder for reconstitution to 62.5 mg/5 ml oral suspension for po administration

Pathocil (Wyeth) (manufactured for human use)
Dosage form: 250 mg capsules and powder for reconstitution to 62.5 mg/5 ml suspension for po administration

Veracillin (Ayerst)
Dosage form: 250 and 500 mg capsules for po administration

Dicumarol
Dicumarol (various) (manufactured for human use)
Dosage form: 25, 50, and 100 mg tablets and 25, 50, and 100 mg capsules for po administration

Diethylcarbamazine
Caricide (American Cyanamid)
Dosage form: 60 mg/ml liquid, 50 and 200 mg tablets, and 30 gm/pound powder for po administration

Dec Tabs (Bio-Ceutic)
Dosage form: 50, 200, and 400 mg tablets for po administration

D.E.C. Solution (Hart-Delta)
Dosage form: 60 mg/ml syrup for po administration

Diethylcarbamazine Citrate (Beecham)
Dosage form: 30, 90, and 300 mg tablets for po administration

Difil (Evsco)
Dosage form: 50, 200, and 400 mg tablets and 60 mg/ml syrup for po administration

Dirocide (Squibb)
Dosage form: 60 mg/ml syrup and 100, 200, and 300 mg tablets for po administration

Hetrazan (Lederle) (manufactured for human use)
Dosage form: 50 mg tablets for po administration

Nemacide (Med-Tech)
Dosage form: 60 mg/ml syrup and 50, 100, 200, and 400 mg tablets for po administration

Diethylstilbestrol (DES)
Diethylstibestrol (various) (manufactured for human use)
Dosage form: 5 and 25 mg/ml solutions for IM administration

Stilpel (Fort Dodge)
Dosage form: 15 mg pellet for implantation

Digitalis USP
Digifortis (Parke, Davis) (manufactured for human use)
Dosage form: 100 mg tablets and 100 mg capsules for po administration

Digitalis (various) (manufactured for human use)
Dosage form: 100 mg tablets for po administration

Digitoxin
Cardio-Tabs 5X (Diamond)
Dosage form: 0.5 mg tablets for po administration

Crystodigin (Lilly) (manufactured for human use)
Dosage form: 0.05, 0.1, 0.15, and 0.2 mg tablets for po administration; 0.2 mg/ml solution for IV or IM administration

Digitaline Nativelle (Savage) (manufactured for human use)
Dosage form: 0.1 and 0.2 mg tablets and 0.02 mg/drop oral solution for po administration; 0.2 mg/ml solution for IV or IM administration

Digitox (Med-Tech)
Dosage form: 0.1 mg/ml elixir for po administration

Digitoxin (Haver-Lockhart)
Dosage form: 0.1 mg tablets for po administration; 0.2 mg/ml solution for IM, IV, or SC administration

Digitoxin (Parke, Davis)
Dosage form: 0.1 mg tablets for po administration

Purodigin (Wyeth) (manufactured for human use)
Dosage form: 0.05, 0.1, 0.15, and 0.2 mg tablets for po administration

Digoxin USP
Cardoxin (Evsco)
Dosage form: 0.15 and 0.05 mg/ml elixirs for po administration

Digitone (Med-Tech)
Dosage form: 0.15 mg/ml elixir for po administration

Lanoxin (Burroughs Wellcome)
  Dosage form: 0.05 mg/ml elixir and 0.25 and 0.125 mg tablets for po administration
Lanoxin (Burroughs Wellcome) (manufactured for human use)
  Dosage form: 0.125, 0.25, and 0.5 mg tablets and 0.05 mg/ml elixir for po administration; 0.1 and 0.25 mg/ml solution for IM or IV administration

Dihydrostreptomycin
Bovamycin III (Pitman-Moore) (also contains procaine penicillin G, 100,000 units/25 ml; hydrocortisone, 20 mg/25 ml; and sulfamethazine, 1000 mg/25 ml)
  Dosage form: 5 mg/ml ointment in 25 ml syringe for intramammary administration
Dihydrostreptomycin (Burns-Biotec)
  Dosage form: Solution for intrasinus or IM administration
Dihydrostreptomycin Sulfate (Med-Tech)
  Dosage form: 500 mg/ml for intrasinus or IM administration
HPX-12 Mastitis Syringes (Hamilton Pharm.) (also contains procaine penicillin G, 100,000 units/10 ml; sulfamerazine, 300 mg/10 ml; hydrocortisone acetate, 20 mg/10 ml; and povidone, 200 mg/10 ml)
  Dosage form: 10 mg/ml solution in 10 ml syringe for intramammary administration

Dimethyl sulfoxide (DMSO)
Domoso (Diamond)
  Dosage form: 90% solution and 90% gel for topical use

Dimetridazole (not available in United States)
Dioctyl sodium sulfosuccinate (DSS)
Aurimite (Burns-Biotec) (also contains benzocaine tyrothricin, technical piperonyl butoxide, pyrethrins, petroleum distillate, and hydrocortisone)
  Dosage form: Suspension for topical use
Cerusol (Burns-Biotec)
  Dosage form: Solution for administration as enema or for po, intraruminal, or topical administration
Dioctyl Sodium Sulfosuccinate (various) (manufactured for human use)
  Dosage form: 100 and 250 mg capsules, 100 mg tablets, and 20 mg/5 ml and 50 mg/15 ml syrup for po administration
Disposaject (Pitman-Moore)
  Dosage form: Solution for administration as enema

Premeatrate (Haver-Lockhart)
  Dosage form: Solution for administration by stomach tube, as enema, or for topical use
Diphenoxylate
Lomotil (Searle) (manufactured for human use; also contains atropine sulfate, 0.025 mg)
  Dosage form: 2.5 mg tablet for po administration
Diphenylhydantoin
Dilantin (Parke, Davis)
  Dosage form: 100 mg capsules for po administration
Dilantin (Parke, Davis) (manufactured for human use)
  Dosage form: 100 mg capsules, 125 and 30 mg/5 ml oral suspensions, and 50 mg tablets for po administration
EKKO (Fleming) (manufactured for human use)
  Dosage form: 50, 100, and 250 mg timed-release pellets for po administration
Dipyrone (Hart-Delta)
  Dosage form: 50% solution for IV, IM, or SC administration
Dipyrone (Med-Tech)
  Dosage form: 50% solution for SC, IV, or IM administration
Dipyrone (various) (manufactured for human use)
  Dosage form: 50% solution for IM administration
Myovin (Burns-Biotec)
  Dosage form: 500 mg/ml solution for SC, IM, or IV administration
Narone (Ulmer)
  Dosage form: 650 mg tablets for po administration; 500 mg/ml solution for IM administration
Novin (Haver-Lockhart)
  Dosage form: 5 gr tablets for po administration; 50% solution for IM, IV, or SC administration
Diosphenol
D.N.P. Parenteral (American Cyanamid)
  Dosage form: 4.5% solution for IV administration
Distilled water (sterile)
Distilled Water (Hart-Delta)
Distilled Water (Haver-Lockhart)
Distilled Water (various) (manufactured for human use)
Dithiazanine iodide
Dizan (Elanco)
  Dosage form: 10, 50, 100, and 200 mg tablets and powder for po administration

Doxycycline
Vibramycin (Pfizer) (manufactured for human use)
  Dosage form: 100 and 200 mg/vial powder for reconstitution to solution for IV administration; 50 and 100 mg capsules and powder for reconstitution to 25 mg/5 ml suspension for po administration

Droperidol
Inapsine (McNeil) (manufactured for human use)
  Dosage form: 2.5 mg/ml solution for IM or IV administration

Echothiophate
Phospholine (Ayerst) (manufactured for human use)
  Dosage form: 0.03%, 0.06%, 0.125%, and 0.25% ophthalmic solution for topical use

Electrolyte replacement
Ion-Aid (Diamond Laboratories) (contains sodium chloride, 11.64%; calcium gluconate, 2.2%; magnesium sulfate, 0.61%; monopotassium phosphate, 8.68%; glycine, 21.2%; and dextrose, 55.67%)
  Dosage form: Powder for po administration
Pedialyte (Ross) (manufactured for human use and contains sodium, 30 mEq/liter; potassium, 20 mEq/liter; calcium, 4 mEq/liter; magnesium, 4 mEq/liter; chloride, 30 mEq/liter; citrate, 31 mEq/liter; and dextrose, 50 gm/liter)
  Dosage form: Solution for po administration

Epinephrine
Adrenalin (Parke, Davis)
  Dosage form: 1:1000 solution for IV administration
Adrenalin (Parke, Davis) (manufactured for human use)
  Dosage form: 1 mg/ml solution for IM, IV, intracardial, or SC administration
Epinephrine (Hart-Delta)
  Dosage form: 1:1000 solution for IV administration
Epinephrine (various) (manufactured for human use)
  Dosage form: 1:1000 aqueous solution for IM, intracardial, IV, or SC administration
Epinephrine Hydrochloride (Med-Tech)
  Dosage form: 1:1000 solution for IM, intracardial, IV, or SC administration
Epinephrine Injection (Burns-Biotec)
  Dosage form: 1:1000 solution for IM, intracardial, IM, SC, or topical administration
Epinephrine Injection (Haver-Lockhart)
  Dosage form: 1:1000 solution for IV or SC administration

Epsom salt (magnesium sulfate)
Epsom Salt (Baker)
  Dosage form: Crystals for po administration in water

EQ 335 (lindane 3%/pine oil 35%)
Myzin Smear (Fort Dodge)
  Dosage form: Suspension for topical use

Ergosterol (*see* vitamin D; multiple vitamins; multiple vitamins with minerals)

Erythromycin
Erythro-36 (Abbott)
  Dosage form: Solution for intramammary administration
Erythro-100,-200 (Abbott)
  Dosage form: 100 and 200 mg/ml solution for IM administration
Erythromast "36" (Diamond)
  Dosage form: Solution for intramammary administration
Erythromycin (Diamond)
  Dosage form: 100 mg/ml solution for IM administration
Erythromycin (various) (manufactured for human use)
  Dosage form: 250 mg tablets for po administration; 50 mg/ml ethyl succinate salt solution for IM administration

Erythromycin stearate
Erypar (Parke, Davis) (manufactured for human use)
  Dosage form: 250 and 500 mg tablets for po administration
Erythromycin Stearate (various) (manufactured for human use)
  Dosage form: 250 and 500 mg tablets for po administration

Estradiol
ECP (Upjohn)
  Dosage form: 1 mg/ml sterile solution for IM administration
Estra (Burns-Biotec)
  Dosage form: 2 mg/ml oil solution for IM administration
Estradiol Cypionate Injection (Med-Tech)
  Dosage form: 1, 2, 4, 5 mg/ml solution for IM administration
Estra-Vet (North American Pharm.)
  Dosage form: 2 mg/ml solution for parenteral administration
Progynon (Schering) (manufactured for human use)
  Dosage form: 25 mg pellets for SC implantation
Utonex (Schering) (also contains nitrofurathiazide)

Dosage form: 0.1 mg/ml suspension and suppository for intrauterine administration

Estrogens (*see* diethylstibestrol (DDS); estradiol; estrone)

Estrone

Theelin Aqueous (Parke, Davis) (manufactured for human use)

Dosage form: 1 mg/ml aqueous suspension for IM administration

V-Estrovarin (Affiliate)

Dosage form: 5 mg/ml (50,000 IU/ml) solution for IM administration

Ethozolamide

Cardrase (Upjohn) (manufactured for human use)

Dosage form: 125 mg tablets for po administration

Ethamide (Allergan) (manufactured for human use)

Dosage form: 125 mg tablets for po administration

Ethylenediamine dihydroiodide

Chlor-Ethamine (Pitman-Moore)

Dosage form: 100 and 325 mg tablets for po administration

Ethyodide (Vet-A-Mix)

Dosage form: 45.36 gm/pound powder for po administration in water, feed, or salt

Expectorant Compound (Bio-Ceutic) (also contains ammonium chloride, 226.8 gm/pound, and glyceryl guaiacolate, 36.29 gm/pound)

Dosage form: 36.29 gm/lb powder for po administration

Glycon (Bio-Ceutic) (also contains ammonium chloride, 226.8 gm/pound, and glyceryl guaiacolate, 36.29 gm/pound)

Dosage form: 16.6 gm/pound powder for po administration in drinking water

Guaiamol with Hi-Amine (Pitman-Moore) (also contains guaiacol and ammonium chloride)

Dosage form: Powder for po administration

Hi-Amine Compound (Pitman-Moore)

Dosage form: 1.3 gm/30 gm powder for po administration

Hi-O-Dide (Bio-Ceutic)

Dosage form: Powder for po administration

Hydrodine, Medicated-Double Strength (Affiliated)

Dosage form: 9.2% powder for po administration in feed

Iodal (Haver-Lockhart)

Dosage form: 6 gm bolus for po administration

Orgadine (Fort Dodge)

Dosage form: 4.6% solution for po administration

Fenbendazole

Panacur (National Laboratories)

Dosage form: 10% suspension for po administration

Fentanyl

Sublimaze (McNeil) (manufactured for human use)

Dosage form: 0.05 mg/ml solution for IM or IV administration

Fentanyl-droperidol

Innovar (McNeil) (manufactured for human use)

Dosage form: 0.05 mg fentanyl and 2.5 mg droperidol per milliliter solution for IM or IV administration

Innovar-Vet (Pitman-Moore)

Dosage form: Solution for IM or IV administration

Flumethasone

Flucort (Diamond)

Dosage form: 0.5 mg/ml solution for IM, IV, SC, or intraarticular administration; 0.0625 mg tablets for po administration

Locorten (Ciba) (manufactured for human use)

Dosage form: Cream for topical use

Methagon Injection (Elanco)

Dosage form: 0.5 mg/ml solution for IM, IV, SC, intraarticular or intralesional administration

Flunixin meglumine

Banamine (Schering)

Dosage form: 50 mg/ml solution for IM or IV administration

9-Fluprednisolone acetate

Alphadrol (Upjohn) (manufactured for human use)

Dosage form: 0.75 and 1.5 mg tablets for po administration

Folic acid (*see also* multiple vitamins; multiple vitamins with minerals)

Folic Acid (various) (manufactured for human use)

Dosage form: 0.1 and 1 mg tablets for po administration

Folvite (Lederle) (manufactured for human use)

Dosage form: 0.25 and 1 mg tablets for po administration; 5 mg/ml solution for IM, IV, or SC administration

Follicle-stimulating hormone (FSH)

F.S.H.-P (Burns-Biotec)

Dosage form: 50 mg powder for reconstitution in 10 ml vial for IM, IV, or SC administration

Fospirate (not available in United States)

Furazolidone

Furoxone (Eaton) (manufactured for human use)

Dosage form: 100 mg tablets and 3.33 mg/ml liquid for po administration

Furoxone (Norden)
  Dosage form: 100 mg/ml suspension for po administration
Topazone (Norden)
  Dosage form: Aerosol for topical administration
Furosemide
Lasix (Hoechst-Roussel) (manufactured for human use)
  Dosage form: 20 and 40 mg tablets for po administration; 10 mg/ml solution for IM or IV administration
Lasix (National)
  Dosage form: 12.5 and 50 mg and 2 gm tablets for po administration; 5% solution for injection; 1% syrup for po administration
Gentamicin
Garamycin (Schering) (manufactured for human use)
  Dosage form: 10 and 40 mg/ml solution for IM or IV administration
Gentocin (Schering)
  Dosage form: 50 mg/ml solution for IM or SC administration; 3 mg/ml ophthalmic solution and 3 mg/gm ophthalmic ointment for topical use
Gentocin Otic (Schering) (also contains betamethasone, 1 mg/ml)
  Dosage form: 3 mg/ml otic solution for topical use
Gentocin with Betamethasone (Schering) (also contains betamethasone acetate, 1 mg/ml)
  Dosage form: 3 mg/ml ophthalmic solution for topical use
Gentian and crystal violet
Jayne's P-W Vermifuge (Glenbrook) (manufactured for human use)
  Dosage form: 25 and 9.6 mg tablets for po administration
Pink Eye Spray (Haver-Lockhart) (also contains urea, 0.5%; furfural, 0.2%; tetrahydrofurfural alcohol, 0.025%; and polyvinylpyrrolidone, 2%)
  Dosage form: 1% spray for topical use
Pytenol Lotion (Haver-Lockhart) (also contains isopropyl alcohol, acetone, phenol, clove oil, and tannic acid)
  Dosage form: Lotion for topical use
Ginger root, powdered
Terkaps (Haver-Lockhart) (also contains oil of eucalyptus, oil of cassia, camphor, menthol, salicylic acid, capsicum)
  Dosage form: Solution for po administration, drench, or by stomach tube
Glucagon
Glucagon (Lilly) (manufactured for human use)
  Dosage form: 1 mg powder for reconstitution to 1 mg/ml solution for IM, IV, or SC administration
Glucose (*see* dextrose)
Glycerol
Glycerin (Fort Dodge)
  Dosage form: 95% solution for po administration
Glyceryl guaiacolate
Anti-Tuss with Antihistamine (Med-Tech) (also contains: ammonium chloride, 8 gr/30 ml; sodium citrate, 8 gr/30 ml; pyrilamine maleate, 50 mg/30 ml; phenylephrine HCl, 50 mg/30 ml)
  Dosage form: Solution for po administration
Expectorant Compound (Bio-Ceutic) (also contains ammonium chloride, 226.8 gm/pound, and ethylenediamine dihydroiodide, 16.6 gm/pound)
  Dosage form: 36.29 gm/pound powder for po administration
Glycon (Bio-Ceutic) (also contains ammonium chloride, 226.8 gm/pound, and ethylenediamine dihydroiodide, 16.6 gm/pound)
  Dosage form: 36.29 gm/pound powder for po administration in drinking water
Glytab (Affiliated) (also contains pyrilamine maleate, phenylephrine, and dextromethorphan)
  Dosage form: Tablets for po administration
Glytussin with Iodides (Affiliated) (also contains ammonium chloride, 75%, and potassium iodide, 2%)
  Dosage form: 7% powder for po administration in drinking water
Respacell (Albion) (also contains ammonium chloride, vitamin A, vitamin D₃; potassium iodide, sodium chloride, phosphorus, zinc, and magnesium)
  Dosage form: Bolus for po administration
Respacell "P" (Albion) (also contains ammonium chloride, potassium iodide, sodium chloride, magnesium chloride, and zinc chloride)
  Dosage form: Powder for po administration in water
Vetussin (Parlam) (also contains ascorbic acid, methapyrilene fumarate, ephedrine HCl, sodium citrate, ammonium chloride, and citric acid)
  Dosage form: Solution for po administration
Gonadotropin-releasing hormones (GNRH)
Gonadorelin Acetate (Abbott) (available for investigational use)
Gonadorelin Hydrochloride (Ayerst) (available for investigational use)
  Dosage form: 100, 200, and 500 µg ampules

Gonadotropic hormones (LH + FSH)

A-P Godin-5 (Haver-Lockhart)

Dosage form: Solution for IM administration

A.P. Tropin (Tutag)

Dosage form: 125 Fevold-Hisaw units/5 ml solution for parenteral administration

Gonadovet (Jen-Sal)

Dosage form: 5 mg dessicated hormone for reconstitution to solution for IV administration

Griseofulvin

Fulvicin U/F (Schering)

Dosage form: 2.5 gm bolus, 250 and 500 mg tablets, and 2.5 gm/15 gm powder for po administration

Fulvidex (Schering) (also contains dexamethasone, nitrofurathiazide, undecylenic acid, and tetracaine)

Dosage form: Otic suspension for topical use

Fulvicin-U/F (Schering) (manufactured for human use)

Dosage form: 125, 250, and 500 mg tablets for po administration

Grifulvin V (McNeil) (manufactured for human use)

Dosage form: 125, 250, and 500 mg tablets and 125 mg/5 ml suspension for po administration

Grisactin (Ayerst) (manufactured for human use)

Dosage form: 125 and 250 mg capsules and 500 mg tablets for po administration

Guaiacol

Beucocol (Burns-Biotec) (also contains gomenol, eucalyptol, iodoform, and camphor)

Dosage form: Solution for IM administration

Camphorated Ethereal Oil with Guaiacol (Med-Tech) (also contains ether, 10%, and gum camphor, 22.5%)

Dosage form: 8% solution for IM administration

Guaiacol Compound (Med-Tech) (also contains creosote, 0.52%; cresylic acid, 4.3%; oil of eucalyptus, 0.5%, and camphor, 0.25%)

Dosage form: 9.7% solution for po administration

Guaimol with Hi-Amine (Pitman-Moore) (also contains ethylenediamine dihydroiodide and ammonium chloride)

Dosage form: Powder for po administration

Haloxon

Halox (Wellcome)

Dosage form: Bolus for po administration and powder for reconstitution to suspension for administration as drench

Heparin

Heparin (Burns-Biotec)

Dosage form: 1000 units/ml solution for IM or IV administration

Heparin (various) (manufactured for human use)

Dosage form: 1000, 5000, 10,000, 20,000, and 40,000 units/ml solution for IM, IV, and SC administration

Sodium Heparin Injection (Tutag)

Dosage form: Solution for parenteral administration

Hetacillin

Hetacin-K (Bristol)

Dosage form: 50, 100, and 200 mg tablets and 50 mg/ml liquid for po administration

Versapen (Bristol) (manufactured for human use)

Dosage form: Powder for reconstitution to 112.5 mg ampicillin-equivalent/5 ml suspension for po administration

Versapen-K (Bristol) (manufactured for human use)

Dosage form: 225 and 450 mg ampicillin-equivalent capsules for po administration

Hexachloroethane

Hexadrench (Burns-Biotec)

Dosage form: Solution for po administration as a drench

Hex Drench (Med-Tech)

Dosage form: 10 gm/30 ml solution for po administration as a drench

Hydrochlorothiazide

Esidrix (Ciba) (manufactured for human use)

Dosage form: 25 and 50 mg tablets for po administration

Hydrochlorothiazide (various) (manufactured for human use)

Dosage form: 25 and 50 mg tablets for po administration

HydroDiuril (Merck Sharp & Dohme) (manufactured for human use)

Dosage form: 25, 50, and 100 mg tablets for po administration

Hydrozide Injection (Merck)

Dosage form: 25 mg/ml solution for IM or IV administration

Hydrocortisone

Adrenal Cortex Injection (Med-Tech)

Dosage form: Sterile solution for parenteral administration

Adrenal Cortex Injection NF (North American Pharm.)

Dosage form: 0.5% solution for parenteral administration

Adrenal Cortex Injection (Tutag)

Dosage form: Sterile solution for parenteral administration

Aurimite (Burns-Biotec) (also contains dioctyl sodium sulfosuccinate, benzocaine, tyrothricin, technical piperonyl butoxide, pyrethrins, and petroleum distillate)

Dosage form: Suspension for topical use

Cortef (Upjohn) (manufactured for human use)

Dosage form: 5, 10, and 20 mg tablets and 10 mg/5 ml oral suspension for po administration; 50 mg/ml solution for IM administration

Forte-Topical (Upjohn) (also contains procaine penicillin G, neomycin sulfate, and polymyxin B)

Dosage form: Suspension and otic suspension for topical use

Furacort (Norden) (also contains nitrofurazone, 0.2%)

Dosage form: 1% cream for topical use

Hydrocortisone (various) (manufactured for human use)

Dosage form: 10 and 20 mg tablets for po administration; 25 and 50 mg/ml solutions for IM administration

Kymar Ointment (Burns-Biotec) (also contains neomycin, 3.5 mg/gm, and trypsin-chymotrypsin, 10,000 Armour units/gm)

Dosage form: 2.5 mg/gm ointment for topical use

Neo-Cortef with Tetracaine (also contains neomycin and tetracaine)

Dosage form: Otic ointment for topical use

Neocorticin (Burns-Biotec) (also contains neomycin and sodium sulfacetamide)

Dosage form: Ophthalmic ointment for topical use

Neo-Mast-H (Bio-Ceutic) (also contains procaine penicillin G, 100,000 units/100 ml; neomycin base 1 gm/100 ml; and sulfamethazine 10gm/100 ml)

Dosage form: 200 mg/100 ml solution for intramammary administration

Nolvapent (Fort Dodge) (also contains neomycin, 3.5 mg/ml, and chlorhexidine dihydrochloride, 6.7 mg/ml)

Dosage form: 10 mg/ml ointment for topical use

Hydroxyprogesterone

Delalutin (Squibb) (manufactured for human use)

Dosage form: 125 and 250 mg/ml oil solutions for IM administration

Hygromycin B

Hygromix-8 (Elanco)

Idoxuridine

Dendrid (Alcon) (manufactured for human use)

Dosage form: 0.1% ophthalmic solution for topical use

Herplex (Allergan) (manufactured for human use)

Dosage form: 0.1% ophthalmic solution and 0.5% ophthalmic ointment for topical use

Stoxil (Smith Kline & French) (manufactured for human use)

Dosage form: 0.1% ophthalmic solution and 0.5% ophthalmic solution for topical administration

Interstitial cell–stimulating hormone (ICSH) (*see* luteinizing hormone)

Insulin, intermediate-acting

Globin Zinc Insulin (Burroughs Wellcome) (manufactured for human use)

Dosage form: 40 and 80 units/ml solutions for SC administration

Globin Zinc Insulin (Squibb) (manufactured for human use)

Dosage form: 40 and 80 units/ml solution for SC administration

Lente Iletin (Lilly) (manufactured for human use; 70% insulin zinc suspension, extended, and 30% insulin zinc suspension, prompt)

Dosage form: 40, 80, and 100 units/ml suspensions for SC administration

NPH Iletin (Lilly) (manufactured for human use; NPH insulin)

Dosage form: 40, 80, and 100 units/ml suspensions for SC administration

Insulin, long-acting

Protamine, Zinc and Iletin (Lilly) (manufactured for human use; protamine zinc insulin)

Dosage form: 40, 80, and 100 units/ml suspension for SC administration

Ultralente Iletin (Lilly) (manufactured for human use; insulin zinc suspension, extended)

Dosage form: 40, 80, and 100 units/ml suspension for SC administration

Insulin, NPH (*see* insulin, intermediate-acting)

Insulin, protamine zinc (*see* insulin, long-acting)

Insulin, regular (*see* insulin, short-acting)

Insulin, short-acting

Regular Iletin (Lilly) (manufactured for human use; regular insulin)

Dosage form: 40, 80, and 100 units/ml solution for IV and SC administration

Semilente Iletin (Lilly) (manufactured for human use; insulin zinc suspension, prompt)

Dosage form: 40, 80, and 100 units/ml suspension for SC administration

Insulin, zinc (*see* insulin, intermediate-acting; insulin, long-acting; insulin, short-acting)

Iodides, organic

Weladol (Pitman-Moore)

Dosage form: 1% available iodine in shampoo

base and 2% available iodine in cream for topical administration

Iodine (*see also* iodide, organic; iodine tincture USP; iodine tincture NF, strong)

Hypodermin (Haver-Lockhart)
Dosage form: 1.9% oil solution for SC administration

Hypodermin (Strong) (Haver-Lockhart)
Dosage form: 4% oil solution for SC administration

Iodine Wound Spray (Med-Tech) (contains polyvinyl pyrrolidone-iodine, 3%; sopropyl myristate, 0.3%; and isopropanol, 56.7%)
Dosage form: Aerosol for topical use

Tighten-Up (North American Pharm.) (also contains phenol, tannic acid and camphor)
Dosage form: Liquid for topical administration

Iodine tincture NF, strong

Iodine Strong (Hart-Delta)
Dosage form: Solution for topical administration

Iodine Strong Tincture (various) (manufactured for human use) (contains iodine, 7%, and sodium iodide, 5%)
Dosage form: Solution for topical use

Iodine, Tincture of (Strong) (Fort Dodge)
Dosage form: Solution for topical use

Iodine Tincture, Stronger (Med-Tech) (also contains potassium iodide, 5%)
Dosage form: 7% solution for topical use

Stronger Tincture of Iodine (Bio-Ceutic) (also contains potassium iodide, 5%)
Dosage form: 7% solution for topical use

Tincture of Iodine NF XI Strong (Burns-Biotec)
Dosage form: Solution for topical use

Iodine tincture USP

Iodine Tincture (various) (manufactured for human use) (contains iodine, 2%, and sodium iodide, 2.4%)
Dosage form: Solution for topical use

Iodophor (*see* iodides, organic; iodine; povidone iodine)

Ipecac

Ipecac (various) (manufactured for human use)
Dosage form: Syrup for po administration

Ipronidazole

Ipropran (Roche)
Dosage form: Soluble powder for po administration in drinking water

Iron (*see also* minerals; multiple vitamins with minerals)

Canine Iron (Albion) (also contains copper sulfate, 0.05 mg, and vitamin B_{12}, 5 μg)
Dosage form: 5 mg tablets for po administration

Dexiron-100 (Norden)
Dosage form: 100 mg/ml solution for IM administration

Fenatal Oral Piglet Iron (Albion) (also contains zinc sulfate and vitamin B_{12})
Dosage form: 37.5 mg/ml solution for po administration

Feraplex (Diamond)
Dosage form: 100 mg/ml solution for IM administration

Ferrisol (Fort Dodge) (also contains copper acetate and copper sulfate)
Dosage form: Solution for po administration

Iron-dextran

Ferrextran 100 (Fort Dodge)
Dosage form: 100 mg iron/ml for IM administration

Imferon (Merrell-National) (manufactured for human use)
Dosage form: 50 mg iron/ml solution for IM or IV administration

Iron Dextran Injection (Med-Tech)
Dosage form: 100 mg iron/ml solution for IM administration

Nonemic (Burns-Biotec)
Dosage form: 100 mg iron/ml solution for IM administration

P/M Iron Dextran Complex (Pitman-Moore)
Dosage form: 100 mg iron/ml solution for IM administration

Isoflurophate

Floropryl (Merck Sharp & Dohme) (manufactured for human use)
Dosage form: 0.1% ophthalmic solution and 0.025% ophthalmic ointment for topical use

Isopropamide

Darbazine Injection (Norden) (also contains prochlorperazine)
Dosage form: Solution for SC administration

Darbazine Spansule (Norden) (also contains prochlorperazine)
Dosage form: Timed-release capsules for po administration

Neo-Darbazine Spansule (Norden) (also contains neomycin and prochlorperazine)
Dosage form: Capsules for po administration

Isotonic saline (isotonic sodium chloride) (*see* normal saline)

Kanamycin

Kantrex (Bristol) (manufactured for human use)
Dosage form: 37.5 and 250 mg/ml and 1 gm/3 ml aqueous solutions for IM administration

Kantrim (Bristol)

Dosage form: 50 and 200 mg/ml solutions for IM or SC administration

Kaolin (*see* kaolin and pectin)

Kaolin and pectin

Atropectate (Burns-Biotec) (also contains bismuth subcarbonate and atropine methylnitrate)

Dosage form: Suspension for po administration

Kao-Forte (Vet-A-Mix)

Dosage form: Suspension for po administration

Kaopect (Med-Tech)

Dosage form: Suspension for po administration

Kaopectate (Upjohn)

Dosage form: Suspension for po administration

Kaopectate (Upjohn) (manufactured for human use)

Dosage form: Suspension for po administration

Pektin (Hart-Delta)

Dosage form: Solution for po administration

V-Pektamalt (Affiliated)

Dosage form: Solution for po administration

Lactated Ringer's

Lactated Ringer's (Abbott) (contains sodium chloride, 600 mg/100 ml; sodium lactate, 310 mg/100 ml; potassium chloride, 30 mg/100 ml; and calcium chloride, 20 mg/100 ml)

Dosage form: Solution for IV or SC administration

Lactated Ringer's (Diamond) (contains sodium, 65 mEq/500 ml; potassium, 2 mEq/500 ml; calcium, 1.5 mEq/500 ml; chloride, 54.5 mEq/500 ml; and lactate, 14 mEq/500 ml)

Dosage form: Solution for IV or SC administration

Lactated Ringer's Solution Concentrate (Diamond)

Dosage form: Solution for dilution for IV or SC administration

Lanatoside C NF

Cedilanid (Sandoz) (manufactured for human use)

Dosage form: 0.5 mg tablets for po administration

Lanolin

Flea Soap-L (Burns-Biotec) (also contains rotenone)

Dosage form: For topical use

Levamisole

Levasole Cattle Wormer (Pitman-Moore)

Dosage form: 4.8 gm soluble powder to be mixed with water for administration as a drench; 2.19 gm bolus for po administration

Levasole Sheep Wormer (Pitman-Moore)

Dosage form: 11.7 gm soluble powder to be mixed with water for administration as a drench; 0.184 gm bolus for po administration

Levasole Soluble Pig Wormer (Pitman-Moore)

Dosage form: 18.15 gm soluble powder for po administration in drinking water

Levasole Injectable (Pitman-Moore)

Dosage form: 18.2% solution for SC administration

Ripercol-L (American Cyanamid)

Dosage form: 0.184 and 2.19 gm boluses for po administration; 52 gm soluble powder to be mixed with water for administration as drench; 20.17 gm soluble powder for po administration in water; 18.2% solution for SC administration

Ripercol L-Piperazine (American Cyanamid) (also contains piperazine)

Dosage form: Liquid suspension to be administered by stomach tube or as drench

Lidocaine (*see also* Lidocaine with epinephrine)

Deltacaine (Hart-Delta)

Dosage form: 2% solution for epidural block

Duracaine -E (Burns-Biotec)

Dosage form: Solution for epidural block

Lidocaine (various) (manufactured for human use)

Dosage form: 0.5%, 1%, and 2% solutions for infiltration or nerve, epidural, or caudal block

Lidocaine Hydrochloride (Med-Tech)

Dosage form: 2% solution for epidural block

Lidocaine with epinephrine

Deltacaine Plus (Hart-Delta)

Dosage form: 2% solution with 0.1% epinephrine for infiltration

Lidocaine Hydrochloride with Epinephrine (Med-Tech)

Dosage form: 2% solution with 1:100,000 epinephrine for epidural block

Lidocaine with Epinephrine (various) (manufactured for human use)

Dosage form: 1% and 2% solution for infiltration or nerve, epidural, or caudal block

Lime sulfur

Orthorix Spray (Ortho Chemical)

Dosage form: 26% solution for topical use

Vlem-Dome (Dome) (manufactured for human use)

Dosage form: Powder to be added to water for topical use

Lincomycin

Lincocin (Upjohn)

Dosage form: 100, 200, and 500 mg tablets for po administration; 50 and 100 mg/ml solutions for IM or IV administration

Lincocin (Upjohn)

Dosage form: 250 and 500 mg capsules and 250 mg/5 ml syrup for po administration; 300 mg/

ml solution for IM, IV, or subconjunctival administration

Lindane (gamma benzene hexachloride)

Benzyl-Hex (Evsco) (also contains benzyl benzoate, 20%; rotenone C.P., 0.5%; and dichlorophen, 0.5%)

Dosage form: 0.25% solution for topical administration

Demolene (Hart-Delta) (also contains rotenone)

Dosage form: Solution for topical use

Demsardex (Burns-Biotec) (also contains benzyl benzoate)

Dosage form: Solution for topical use

Fenatox (Burroughs Wellcome) (also contains toxaphene, 45%; kerosene, 34.94%; and petroleum distillates, 5.12%)

Dosage form: 1.96% emulsifiable concentration for topical use

Gammex (Jen-Sal) (also contains xylene)

Dosage form: Suspension for topical use

Kwell (Reed & Carnrick) (Manufactured for human use)

Dosage form: 1% cream, 1% lotion, and 1% shampoo for topical use

Linspray (Norden)

Dosage form: 12% solution for spraying for topical use

Mange Lotion (Bio-Ceutic) (also contains rotenone, 0.12%; dichlorophene, 0.5%; and benzyl benzoate, 30%)

Dosage form: 0.1% lotion for topical use

Mycodex with Lindane (Beecham)

Dosage form: 0.3% shampoo for topical use

Para Dip (Haver-Lockhart) (also contains carbaryl and captan)

Dosage form: Solution for use as dip for topical use

Paramite (Hart-Delta) (also contains rotenone and benzyl benzoate)

Dosage form: Solution for topical use

Screw Worm Medication (Affiliated) (also contains mineral oil, 52.22%)

Dosage form: 1.94% aerosol for topical use

Sectilin (Bio-Ceutic)

Dosage form: 0.097% shampoo for topical use

Thionium with Lindane (Jen-Sal)

Dosage form: Shampoo for topical use

Liniments

Absorbine Veterinary Liniment (W. F. Young)

Dosage form: Solution for topical use

Leg Tone (Haver-Lockhart) (contains iodine tincture strong, camphor, propylene glycol; methyl salicylate, turpentine, ammonium iodide, oil of origanum red, and oil of pennyroyal)

Dosage from: Solution for topical use

Liniment, White (Fort Dodge) (contains ammonium chloride, strong ammonium solutions, gum camphor, turpentine, and oleic acid)

Dosage form: Emulsion for topical use

White Liniment (Med-Tech) (contains gum camphor, ammonium chloride, ammonia water, and turpentine)

Dosage form: Emulsion for topical use

Luteinizing hormone (LH)

P.L.H. (Burns-Biotec)

Dosage form: Lyophilized powder, 25 mg Armour standard/vial, to be reconstituted to solution for IV administration

Magnesium hydroxide

Carmilax (Norden) (also contains nux vomica powdered extract, ginger, and capsicum)

Dosage form: Bolus for po administration

Carmilax Powder (Norden) (also contains nux vomica extract, capsicum, and ginger)

Dosage form: Powder for po administration

Emblo Powder (Haver-Lockhart) (also contains sodium phosphate dibasic and magnesium citrate)

Dosage form: 33% suspendable powder for administration as drench or by stomach tube

Laxalin Bolus (Diamond) (also contains nux vomica, tartar emetic, ginger, and capsicum)

Dosage form: Bolus for po administration

Laxalin Powder (Diamond) (also contains sodium phosphate, sodium thiosulfate, tartar emetic, and strychnine)

Dosage form: Powder for po administration

Lax-A-Mag (Med-Tech) (also contains nux vomica, 10 gr; tartar emetic, 10 gr; ginger, 3 gr; capsicum, 3 gr; and cobalt sulfate, 100 gr)

Dosage form: 400 gr bolus for po administration

Milk of Magnesia (various) (manufactured for human use)

Dosage form: Suspension for po administration

Rumade-C (Burns-Biotec) (also contains tartar emetic, nux vomica extract, capsicum, ginger, dioctyl sodium sulfosuccinate, and cobalt sulfate)

Dosage form: Powder to be mixed with water for administration as a drench

Rumen Compound (Med-Tech) (also contains nux vomica powder, tartar emetic, ginger, capsicum, sodium thiosulfate, and cobalt sulfate)

Dosage form: Powder to be mixed with water for administration as drench

Rumilax (Haver-Lockhart) (also contains nux vomica, antimony potassium tartrate, ginger, capsicum, cobalt sulfate, and dioctyl sodium sulfisuccinate)

Dosage form: Bolus for po administration

Magnesium sulfate (*see* epsom salt)

Malathion

Flair (Jen-Sal) (also contains pyrethrins, piperony butoxide, carbaryl, and petroleum distillates)
Dosage form: Solution for topical use

Kemal (Vet-Kem) (also contains toxaphene, 43%)
Dosage form: 4.3% solution for topical use

Para Bomb-M-1 (Haver-Lockhart) (also contains pyrethrins, 0.06%, and piperonyl butoxide, 0.48%)
Dosage form: 0.5% pressurized spray for topical use

Pet Pest Spray (Affiliated) (also contains pyrethrins, 0.075%; piperonyl butoxide, 0.15%; *N*-octyl bicycloheptane dicarboxamide, 0.25%; methoxychlor, 0.5%; and 2,3:4,5-bis [2-butylene] tetrahydro-2-furaldehyde, 0.2%)
Dosage form: 0.25% aerosol for topical use

Mannitol

Mannitol (Hart-Delta)
Dosage form: 20% solution for IV administration

Mannitol (various) (manufactured for human use)
Dosage form: 25% solution for IV administration

Mannitol IV (Abbott)
Dosage form: 20% solution for IV administration

Osmitrol (Travenol) (manufactured for human use)
Dosage form: 5%, 10%, 15%, and 20% solution for IV administration

Mebendazole

Telmin (Pitman-Moore)
Dosage form: Powder, 166.7 mg/gm, and 200 mg/gm paste for po administration in feed

Telmintic (Pitman-Moore)
Dosage form: Powder for po administration

Vermox Chewable Tablets (Ortho Chemical) (manufactured for human use)
Dosage form: 100 mg tablets for po administration

Meclofenamic acid

Arquel (Parke, Davis)
Dosage form: 5% (500 mg/10 gm) granulation for po administration

Medroxyprogesterone (MAP)

Depo-Provera (Upjohn) (manufactured for human use)
Dosage form: 100 and 400 mg/ml solution for IM administration

Provera (Upjohn) (manufactured for human use)
Dosage form: 2.5 and 10 mg tablets for po administration

Megestrol acetate

Megace (Mead-Johnson) (manufactured for human use)
Dosage form: 20 mg tablets for po administration

Ovaban (Schering)
Dosage form: 5 and 20 mg tablets for po administration

Menichlophalan (experimental drug, not cleared for use in United States)

Meperidine

Demerol Hydrochloride (Winthrop) (manufactured for human use)
Dosage form: 25, 50, 75, and 100 mg/ml solutions for IM, IV or SC administration; 50 and 100 mg tablets and 50 mg/5 ml elixir for po administration

Meralluride (mercurial-theophylline)

Mersalyl and Theophylline (various) (manufactured for human use)
Dosage form: Solution for IM or IV administration

Salyrgan-Theophylline (Winthrop) (manufactured for human use)
Dosage form: Solution for IM or IV administration

Mercuric iodide

Merc-Red Blister (Jen-Sal)

Methenamine

Kidnitone (Parlam)
Dosage form: 60 gr/30 ml solution for po administration

Methenamine (Lilly) (manufactured for human use)
Dosage form: 325 and 500 mg tablets for po administration

Methenamine Tablets (Haver-Lockhart)
Dosage form: 60 gr tablets for po administration

Methenamine Tablets (Med-Tech)
Dosage form: 60 gr tablets to be mixed with water for administration as drench

Methicillin

Azapen (Pfizer) (manufactured for human use)
Dosage form: Powder for reconstitution to solution for IM or IV administration

Celbenin (Beecham) (manufactured for human use)
Dosage form: Powder for reconstitution to solution for IM or IV administration

Staphcillin (Bristol) (manufactured for human use)
Dosage form: Powder for reconstitution to solution for IM or IV administration

Methionine

Alberta (Albion)

Dosage form: 200 mg tablets for po administration

Methigel (Evsco)

Dosage form: 400 mg/5 gm paste for po administration

Methiodol (Med-Tech)

Dosage form: 0.2 and 0.5 gm tablets for po administration

Methio-Form (Vet-A-Mix)

Dosage form: 500 mg tablets for po administration

Methionine (various) (manufactured for human use)

Dosage form: 200 and 500 mg tablets for po administration

Odor-Trol (Haver-Lockhart)

Dosage form: 200 mg tablets for po administration

Uranap (North American Pharm.)

Dosage form: 0.2 gm capsules for po administration

Methocarbamol (glyceryl guaiacol ether carbamate)

Robaxin (Robins) (manufactured for human use)

Dosage form: 500 and 750 mg tablets for po administration

Robaxin-V (Robins)

Dosage form: 100 mg/ml sterile solution for IV administration; 500 mg tablets for po administration

Methoxychlor

Mitecide (Elanco) (also contains mineral oil, 90.05%; piperonyl butoxide, 1%; pyrethrins, 0.1%; and hexachlorophene, 0.5%)

Dosage form: 1% solution for topical use

Norsect (Norden) (also contains carbaryl, 0.5%; pyrethrins, 0.075%; piperonyl butoxide, 0.15%; and N-octyl bicycloheptane dicarboxamide 0.25%)

Dosage form: 0.5% aerosol for topical use

Para S-1 (Haver-Lockhart) (also contains pyrethrins, 0.06%; piperonyl butoxide 0.48%; and carbaryl, 0.5%)

Dosage form: 0.5% aerosol for topical use

Pet Pest Spray (Affiliated) (also contains pyrethrins, 0.075%; piperonyl butoxide; 0.15%; N-octyl bicycloheptane dicarboxamide, 0.25%; malathion, 0.25%; and 2,3:4,5-bis[2-burylene] tetrahydro-2-furaldehyde, 0.2%)

Dosage form: 0.5% aerosol for topical use

Methylcarbamate

Mycodex Flea and Tick Spray (Beecham)

Dosage form: 0.25% spray for topical use

Methylcellulose

Visculose Ophthalmic Solution (Softcon) (manufactured for human use)

Dosage form: 0.5% and 1% ophthalmic solution for topical use

Methylene blue

Decton Blue (Jen-Sal) (also contains dequalinium chloride)

Dosage form: Powder for topical use

Keraplex (Med-Tech) (also contains neomycin, 29.6 mg/30 ml)

Dosage form: 71 mg/30 ml spray for topical use

M-B (Beach)

Dosage form: 65 mg tablets for po administration

Methoform Dressing Powder (Haver-Lockhart) (also contains alum, tannic acid, camphor, cresylic acid, and iodoform)

Dosage form: Powder for topical use

Urolene Blue (Star) (manufactured for human use)

Dosage form: 65 mg tablets for po administration

Methylprednisolone

Depo-Medrol (Upjohn)

Dosage form: 20 and 40 mg/ml aqueous suspensions for IM and intrasynovial administration

Medrol (Upjohn)

Dosage form: 1 mg tablets for po administration

Medrol (Upjohn) (manufactured for human use)

Dosage form: 2, 4, and 16 mg tablets and 2 and 4 mg sustained-action capsules for po administration

Methylscopolamine (methscopolamine)

Pamine Bromide (Upjohn)

Dosage form: 2.5 mg tablets for po administration; 1 mg/ml solution for IM or SC administration

Methyltestosterone

Methyltestosterone (various) (manufactured for human use)

Dosage form: 10 and 25 mg tablets for po administration

Methyl violet

Blulu (Burns-Biotec) (also contains phenol and technical tannic)

Ker-O-Jet (Bio-Ceutic) (also contains furfuryl alcohol, 0.6%; tetrahydrofurfuryl alcohol, 0.03%; urea, 0.6%; and isopropanol, 18%)

Dosage form: 0.06% aerosol for topical use

Pyotannic Blue (Fort Dodge) (also contains aniline, tannic acid, glycerin, oil cloves, and acetone)

Dosage from: Solution for topical use

Pytenol Aero (Haver-Lockhart) (also contains isopropyl alcohol and tannic acid)

Dosage form: Spray for topical use

Tan-O-Blu (Med-Tech) (also contains phenol, 3%, and tannic acid, 2%)

Dosage form: 2.5% solution for topical use

Wound SPRA (Bio-Ceutic) (also contains furfuryl alcohol, 0.6%; urea 0.6%; and isopropanol, 18%)

Dosage form: 0.06% aerosol for topical use

Miconazole

Conofite (Pitman-Moore)

Dosage form: 2% cream for topical use

Micatin (Johnson & Johnson) (manufactured for human use)

Dosage form: 2% cream for topical use

Monistat (Ortho) (manufactured for human use)

Dosage form: 2% cream for topical use

Milk of Magnesia (*see* magnesium hydroxide)

Mineral oil

Laxatone (Evsco) (also contains white petrolatum and linoleic acid)

Dosage form: Ointment for po administration

Mineral Oil (various) (manufactured for human use)

Dosage form: Suspension for po administration; oil solution for topical use

Mitecide (Elanco) (also contains methoxychlor, 1%; piperonyl butoxide, 1%; pyrethrins, 0.1%; and hexachlorophene, 0.5%)

Dosage form: 90.05% solution for topical use

Minerals

Ferro-Coppergen (Norden) (also contains iron and ammonium citrate, 1.3 gm/30 ml; manganese citrate, 65 mg/30 ml; sodium molybdate, 49 mg/30 ml; copper gluconate, 33 mg/30 ml; and cobalt sulfate, 16 mg/30 ml)

Dosage form: Solution for po administration

I.A.T. Cap-Tabs (Fort Dodge) (also contains copper sulfate, 3.89 gm; quebracho extract, 3.89 gm; iron sulfate, 3.89 gm; and calcium carbonate, 3.89 gm)

Dosage form: Tablet for po administration

Medo-Lyle-8X (Med-Tech) (contains calcium lactate, 1.28%; magnesium sulfate, 0.65%; potassium chloride, 1.27%; sodium chloride, 9.68%; sodium citrate, 7.36%; and dextrose, 79.76%)

Dosage form: Soluble powder for reconstitution to solution for IV or intraperitoneal administration

Phos-Aid (Vet-A-Mix) (contains phosphorus, 18%; calcium, 19.8%; sodium chloride, 2.5%; vitamin D_3, 60,000 IU/pound; manganese, 0.25%; zinc, 0.2083%; iron, 0.2083%; copper, 0.0261%; cobalt, 0.0052%; and iodine, 0.0050%)

Dosage form: Powder for po administration

pHOS-pHAID (Fort Dodge) (contains ammonium biphosphate, sodium biphosphate, and sodium acid pyrophosphate)

Dosage form: 250 and 500 mg tablets for po administration

Minocycline

Minocin (Lederle) (manufactured for human use)

Dosage form: 50 and 100 mg capsules and 50 mg/5 ml syrup for po administration; powder for reconstitution to 20 mg/ml solution for IV administration

Vectrin (Parke, Davis) (manufactured for human use)

Dosage form: 50 and 100 mg capsules and 50 mg/5 ml syrup for po administration; 100 mg solution for IV administration

Mitotane (*o,p*-**DDD**)

Lysodren (Calbio) (manufactured for human use)

Dosage form: 500 mg tablets for po administration

Monensin

Coban (Elanco)

Dosage form: Premix for po administration

Morphine

Morphine Sulfate (various) (manufactured for human use)

Dosage form: 8, 10, and 15 mg/ml solution for IV or SC administration

Multiple vitamins

ABCDE Drops (Hart-Delta) (contains vitamins A, B, C, D, E)

Dosage form: Solution for po administration

Abdec (Parke, Davis)

Dosage form: Drops (solution) and capsules for po administration

Aqua B (Upjohn) (contains vitamins B_1, B_2, and B_6; *d*-pantothenyl alcohol; and niacinamide)

Dosage form: Sterile solution for IM, IV, or SC administration

Combex (Parke, Davis) (contains vitamins B_1, B_2, and B_{12})

Dosage form: Capsule for po administration

Hipo B12 (Burns-Biotec) (contains vitamins B_1 and B_2, pantothenyl alcohol, nicotinamide, and vitamins B_6 and B_{12})

Dosage form: Solution for IM or IV administration

Hi-Vite Drops (Evsco) (contains vitamins A, D_2,

E, B_1, B_2, and B_6; nicotinamide; d-panthenol; liver fraction; ferric ammonium citrate; sorbitol; and peptone)

Dosage form: Solution for po administration

Injacom 100+ B Complex (Roche) (contains vitamins A and D_3, niacinamide, vitamins B_1 and B_6, pantothenic acid, vitamin B_2, d-biotin, and vitamin E)

Dosage form: Aqueous emulsion for IM administration

Kit-Vite (Haver-Lockhart) (contains vitamins A, D_2, E, and B_{12}; riboflavin; thiamine; pyridoxine; niacin; and d-calcium pantothenate)

Dosage form: Paste for po administration

Lipo-Aqueous Vitamin Complex (Med-Tech) (contains vitamins A, D_2, B_3, B_6, and B_1; d-panthenol; and vitamin B_2)

Dosage form: Solution for IM or IV administration

Lipo-Form (Vet-A-Mix) (contains choline, methionine, inositol, vitamin E, vitamin B_{12}, niacin, vitamins B_1 and B_2, pantothenic acid, folic acid, and dessicated liver)

Dosage form: Tablets for po administration

Nora-Plex Injection (North American Pharm.) (contains vitamins B_{12}, B_1, B_2, and B_6; choline; niacinamide; inositol; panthenol; and ascorbic acid)

Dosage form: Solution for parenteral administration

Petdrops (Upjohn) (contains vitamins A, D, B_1, and B_2; ascorbic acid, niacinamide; vitamin B_6, dl-α-tocopherol; d-pantothenyl alcohol; and cyanocobalamin (vitamin B_{12})

Dosage form: Solution for po administration

Plex-Sol (Vet-A-Mix) (contains vitamins A, D_3, and E; niacin; calcium d-pantothenate; riboflavin; vitamins B_1 and B_6; folic acid; and vitamin C)

Dosage form: Powder for po administration in drinking water

Puppyatric (Med-Tech) (contains vitamins A, D_2, B_1, B_2, B_6, and B_{12}; panthenol; niacinamide; and liver fraction)

Dosage form: Syrup for po administration

Vitol (Vet-A-Mix) (contains vitamins A, D, E, B_1, and B_2; nicotinic acid; d-panthenol; vitamin B_6; lecithin; vitamin B_{12}; and unsaturated fatty acids)

Dosage form: Solution for po administration

Vita-Plex (Vet-A-Mix) (contains vitamins A, D_3, and B_{12})

Dosage form: Powder for po administration

Vita-Plex Forte (Hart-Delta) (contains amino acids, vitamin B-complex, and vitamin B_{12})

Dosage form: Solution for IM, IV, or SC administration

Vitadrops (Burns-Biotec) (contains vitamins A, D_2, B_1, B_2, and B_6; niacinamide; and pantothenyl alcohol)

Vitec-Sol (Vet-A-Mix) (contains vitamins A, D_3, and B_2; calcium d-pantothenate; vitamins B_6, K, and E; nicotinic acid; and vitamins B_1 and B_{12})

Dosage form: Powder for po administration in water

Vitamin A-D-B_{12} (Med-Tech) (contains vitamins B_{12}, A, and D_3)

Dosage form: Emulsifiable solution for IM or SC administration

Vitamin ADB12 (Bio-Ceutic) (contains vitamins B_{12}, A, and D)

Dosage form: Emulsifiable solution for IM or SC administration

Multiple vitamins with minerals

AA Bolus (Beecham) (contains amino acids; B vitamins; vitamins A, D, and E; minerals; and trace minerals)

Dosage form: 30.8 gm bolus for po administration

Anapram (Tutag) (contains ferrous fumarate; folic acid; bone meal; cobalt; calcium; phosphorus; vitamins A, D_2, E, B_{12}, B_1, and B_2; pyridoxine; niacinamide; ascorbic acid; iodine; calcium; and phosphorus)

Dosage form: Tablets for po administration

Anavites (Tutag) (contains vitamins A, D, B_1, B_2, B_6, and B_{12}; niacinamide; calcium pantothenate; dessicated liver; bone meal; calcium; phosphorus; and vitamin E)

Dosage form: Tablets for po administration

Brytin (Upjohn) (contains vitamins A, D, B_1, and B_2; niacin; vitamin B_6; calcium pantothenate; cyanocobalamin; vitamin E; folic acid; choline; ferrous gluconate; calcium iodate [iodine]; copper oxide; manganese oxide; zinc oxide; cobalt carbonate; and dibasic calcium phosphate)

Dosage form: Pellets for po administration

BVMO (Burns-Biotec) (contains vitamins A, D_2, B_1, B_2, B_6, and B_{12}; liver; niacinamide; pantothenyl alcohol; potassium iodide; iron ammonium citrate; and phosphoric acid)

Dosage form: Tablets and liquid for po administration

BVMO-G (Burns-Biotec) (contains vitamins A, D_2, B_1, B_2, B_6, and B_{12}; liver; niacinamide; pantothenyl alcohol; potassium iodide; iron ammonium citrate; phosphoric acid; copper sulfate; copper acetate; iron peptonate; magnesium stearate; and manganese citrate)

Dosage form: Tablets and liquid for po administration

Calcipet (Burns-Biotec) (contains dicalcium phosphate, calcium carbonate, calcium lactate, vitamin D_3 and calcium gluconate)

Dosage form: Tablet for po administration

Clovite (Fort Dodge) (contains vitamins A, D, and B_{12}; dicalcium phosphate; choline chloride; vitamin E; calcium pantothenate; niacin; pyridoxine; thiamine; riboflavin; and biotin)

Dosage form: Powder for po administration

Dia Glo S.A. (Diamond) (contains vitamins A, B_6 and E; d-pantothenic acid; zinc; and polyunsaturated fatty acids)

Dosage form: Powder for po administration

Equ-Aid, New Formula (Vet-A-Mix) (contains vitamins A, D_3, E, and B_2; nicotinic acid; vitamin B_1; d-pantothenic acid; vitamin B_6 and B_{12}; iodine; iron; copper; cobalt; magnesium; manganese; zinc; phosphorus; calcium; sodium chloride; L-lysine; and unsaturated fatty acids)

Dosage form: Powder for po administration

Equi-Honey-Vite (Med-Tech) (contains cyanocobalamin; pyridoxine; vitamin B_2, niacinamide, thiamine, folic acid, d-panthenol, ferrous sulfate, citric acid, cobalt sulfate, and sorbitol)

Dosage form: Solution for po administration

Equine Atom (North American Pharm.) (contains vitamins B_1, B_2, B_6, B_{12}, and E; niacinamide; folic acid; inositol; panthenol; choline; and iron ammonium citrate)

Dosage form: Liquid form for po administration

Equine Organic Iron Supplement (Albion) (contains iron sulfate, copper sulfate, magnesium sulfate, zinc sulfate, phosphorus, potassium, iodine, vitamin E, thiamine, niacin, pantothenic acid, choline chloride, vitamin B_{12}, folic acid, and vitamin B_2)

Dosage form: Granules for po administration or dissolved in water as a drench

Everglo Portion Paks (Evsco) (contains unsaturated fatty acids, protein, vitamin A, vitamins D_2 and E, thiamine, vitamin B_2, niacinamide, pantothenic acid, biotin, inositol, folic acid, calcium, phosphorus, potassium, sodium, magnesium, manganese, iron, and copper)

Dosage form: Powder for po administration

Felobits (Norden) (contains vitamins A, D_2 and E; thiamine, riboflavin, niacinamide, calcium pantothenate, pyridoxine, inositol, zinc, manganese, magnesium, linoleic acid, choline, calcium, phosphorus, iron, cobalt, and iodine)

Dosage form: Tablets for po administration

Felovite (Evsco) (contains vitamins A, D, E, B_1, B_2 and B_6; calcium pantothenate; nicotinamide; vitamin B_{12}; folic acid; iron; manganese; magnesium; and iodine)

Dosage form: Paste for po administration

Forte-Plex (Vet-A-Mix) (contains vitamins A and D_3, di-calcium pantothenate, vitamin B_2, niacin, and vitamin B_{12})

Dosage form: Powder concentrate po administration

Geribits (Norden) (contains vitamin A, vitamins D_3 and E, thiamine, vitamin B_2, pyridoxine, folic acid, calcium pantothenate, niacinamide, choline, inositol, vitamins B_{12} and B_{15}, linoleic acid, D-sorbitol, iron, copper, cobalt, calcium, phosphorus, zinc, manganese, magnesium, and iodine)

Dosage form: Tablets for po administration

Hemogen Plus (Haver-Lockhart) (contains sorbitol, niacinamide, thiamine, ascorbic acid, riboflavin, folic acid, vitamin B_{12}, pyridoxine, calcium pantothenate, vitamins D_2 and E, ferrous sulfate, cobalt sulfate and copper sulfate)

Dosage form: Tablets for po administration

L-IV-ER (North America Pharm.) (contains ferric ammonium citrate, liver injection, vitamin B_{12}, niacinamide, vitamin B_2 and vitamin B_6)

Dosage form: Solution for parenteral administration

Liver Iron B Complex with Vitamin B12 (Maurry) (contains vitamin B_{12}; iron peptonate; vitamins B_1, B_2, and B_6; calcium pantothenate; niacinamide; and liver)

Dosage form: Solution for IM administration

Liver Iron-B12 Forte (Harte-Delta) (contains liver, iron, B_{12}, folic acid and cobalt)

Dosage form: Solution for IM administration

Liver, Iron, Vitamin with B12 (North American Pharm.) (contains vitamin B_{12}, niacinamide, vitamins B_2 and B_6 and green ferric ammonium citrate)

Dosage form: Solution for parenteral administration

Lixotonic (Beecham) (contains niacinamide; vitamins B_1, B_6, B_{12}, and B_2; peptonized iron; copper, and liver fraction)

Dosage form: Solution for po administration

Mineravite (Med-Tech) (contains vitamins A, D, B_1, and B_2; niacin; pantothenic acid; choline; folic acid; vitamin B_{12}; calcium; phosphorus; sodium chloride; iodine; manganese; copper; cobalt and iron)

Dosage form: Powder for po administration

Multi-Prime (Jen-Sal) (contains ferrous sulfate, choline, inositol, niacinamide, vitamin B_1, *d*-panthenol, and vitamins B_2, B_6, and B_{12})
Dosage form: Syrup for po administration

Nutrimalt Triple Crown (Parlam) (contains vitamins A, D, E, B_1, and B_2; niacin; vitamins B_6, B_{12}, and K; calcium glycerophosphate; sodium iodide; potassium chloride; iron citrate; nickel acetate; magnesium sulfate; manganese citrate; copper sulfate; zinc sulfate; cobalt sulfate; and sodium citrate)
Dosage form: Solution for po administration

Nutri-Mix (Norden) (contains vitamins A, D_2, D_3, B_{12}, B_1 and B_2; calcium pantothenate; niacin; choline; vitamins B_6, K_3, and E; calcium gluconate; dicalcium phosphate; manganese oxide; iron oxide; calcium iodate; cupric oxide; cobalt carbonate; and zinc oxide)
Dosage form: Powder for po administration

Pet-A-Vite (North American Pharm.) (contains liver protein; iron; iodine; vitamins A, D, B_1, B_2, and B_6; niacinamide; vitamins B_{12} and E; and dicalcium phosphate)
Dosage form: Powder for po administration

Pet-A-Vite Mini (North American Pharm.) (contains liver protein; iron; iodine; vitamins A, D, B_1, B_2, and B_6; niacinamide; vitamins B_{12} and E; and dicalcium-calcium phosphate)
Dosage form: Tablets for po administration

Pet-Form (Vet-A-Mix) (contains vitamins A, D_3, E, B_1, and B_2; niacin; vitamins B_6 and B_{12}; pantothenic acid; folic acid; choline; calcium; phosphorus; iron; copper; and cobalt)
Dosage form: Tablets for po administration

Pet-Tabs (Beecham) (contains vitamins A and D_2; niacinamide; vitamins B_1, B_2, B_6, B_{12}, and E; iron peptonized; cobalt sulfate; potassium iodide; cupric acetate; magnesium stearate; manganese sulfate; linoleic acid; calcium phosphate dibasic)
Dosage form: Tablets and granules for po administration

Osteoform 181 (Vet-A-Mix) (contains calcium, phosphorus, vitamins A and D, and ascorbic acid)
Dosage form: Tablets for po administration

Osteoform Improved (Vet-A-Mix) (contains calcium, phosphorus, and vitamins A, D_3, and vitamin C)
Dosage form: Powder for po administration

Super-Plex (Fort Dodge) (contains vitamins A, D (ergosterol), B_1, and B_2; niacinamide; vitamin B_6; calcium pantothenic; vitamin B_{12}; vitamins C and E)
Dosage form: Capsules for po administration

Vi-Sorbits (Norden) (contains elemental iron, vitamin B_{12} and B_6, folic acid, thiamine, vitamin B_2, niacinamide, calcium pantothenate, phosphorus, magnesium, and linoleic acid)
Dosage form: Tablets for po administration

Vita-Bons (Evsco) (contains vitamins A and D; nicotinamide; vitamins B_1, B_2, B_6, B_{12}, and E; methionine; folic acid; fatty acids; iron peptonized; iodine; calcium; manganese; magnesium; phosphorus; copper; and protein)
Dosage form: Tablets for po administration

Vita-Glos (Bio-Ceutic) (contains vitamins A, D_3, B_1, B_2, B_{12}, and B_6; *d*-pantothenic acid; niacin; folic acid; choline; vitamins E and K; polyunsaturated fatty acids; phosphorus; calcium; sodium chloride; iodine; iron; cobalt; magnesium; manganese; zinc; and copper)
Dosage form: Powder for po administration

Vita-Lic (Parlam) (contains vitamins A and D; ergocalciferol; vitamins E, B_1, B_2, and B_6; calcium pantothenate; niacinamide; vitamin B_{12}; manganese; magnesium; and iodine)
Dosage form: Paste for po administration

Vitamycin (Pitman-Moore) (contains cyanocobalamin; niacin; *dl*-calcium pantothenate; vitamins B_1, B_2, and A; cholecalciferol; choline; ferrous sulfate; dibasic calcium phosphate; cupric sulfate; cobalt sulfate; wheat germ oil; menadione; soy lecithin, and zinc sulfate)
Dosage form: Powder for po administration

Vita-Plex Se E (Vet-A-Mix) (contains selenium; vitamins E, A, D_3, and B_2; calcium *di*-pantothenate; niacin; and vitamins B_1 and B_{12})
Dosage form: Powder for po administration

Nafcillin
Nafcil (Bristol) (manufactured for human use)
Dosage form: Powder for reconstitution to 250 mg/ml solution for IM or IV administration
Unipen (Wyeth) (manufactured for human use)
Dosage form: 250 mg capsules, 500 mg tablets, and powder for reconstitution to 250 mg/5 ml oral suspension for po administration

Nalorphine HCL
Nalline (Merck)
Dosage form: 5 mg/ml solution for IV, IM, or SC administration
Nalline (Merck Sharp & Dohme) (manufactured for human use)
Dosage form: 0.2 mg/ml and 5 mg/ml solution for IV or SC administration

Naloxone
Narcan (Endo) (manufactured for human use)
Dosage form: 0.4 and 0.02 mg/ml solution for IM, IV, or SC administration

Nandrolone decanoate

Deca-Durabolin (Organon) (manufactured for human use)

Dosage form: 50 and 100 mg/ml solution for IM administration

Nandrolone phenpropionate

Durabolin (Organon) (manufactured for human use)

Dosage form: 25 and 50 mg/ml solution for IM administration

Naproxen

Equiproxen (Diamond Labs)

Dosage form: Powder for oral administration

Naprosyn (Syntex Puerto Rico) (manufactured for human use)

Dosage form: 250 mg tablets for po administration

N-Butyl chloride

N-Butyl Chloride (Hart-Delta)

Dosage form: 0.25, 0.5, 1, 2, 5 ml capsules for po administration

Neomycin (*see also* neomycin-bacitracin-polymyxin B)

Biosol (Upjohn)

Dosage form: 200 mg/ml liquid, 325 gm/pound soluble powder, and 500 mg bolus for po administration; 50 mg/ml solution for IM administration

Biotef II (Upjohn) (also contains procaine penicillin G)

Dosage form: Ointment for intramammary administration

Hi-po-dri (Burns-Biotec) (also contains procaine penicillin G, 100,000 units/10 ml)

Dosage form: 50 mg/ml suspension in 10 ml syringe for intramammary administration

Hydeltrone (Merck) (also contains prednisolone, 2.5 mg/gm)

Dosage form: 5 mg/gm ophthalmic ointment for topical use

Keraplex (Med-Tech) (also contains methyl violet, 71 mg/30 ml)

Dosage form: 29.6 mg/30 ml for topical use

Kerocin (Bio-Ceutic)

Dosage form: 56.8 mg spray for topical use

Kymar Ointment (Burns-Biotec) (also contains hydrocortisone, 2.5 mg/gm, and trypsin-chymotrypsin, 10,000 Armour units/gm)

Dosage form: 3.5 mg/gm ointment for topical use

Mastimycin (Pitman-Moore) (also contains procaine penicillin G, 100,000 units/syringe)

Dosage form: 500 mg/syringe ointment for intramammary administration

Meti-Derm with Neomycin (Schering) (also contains prednisone, 33.3%)

Dosage form: 33.3% aerosol spray for topical use

Mitox (Norden) (also contains sulfacet, 9%; sevin [carbaryl], 1%; and tetracaine, 0.5%)

Dosage form: 0.5% solution for topical use

Mycifradin Sulfate (Upjohn)

Dosage form: 0.5 gm sterile powder for reconstitution to solution for IM administration

Neo-Aristovet (American Cyanamid) (also contains triamcinolone acetonide, 1 mg/gm)

Dosage form: 5 mg/gm ointment for topical use

Neoblu (Affiliated) (also contains benzocaine, 1%)

Dosage form: 0.1% aerosol for topical use

Neo-Cortef with Tetracaine (Upjohn) (also contains hydrocortisone and tetracaine)

Dosage form: Otic ointment for topical use

Neocorticin (Burns-Biotec) (also contains hydrocortisone and sodium sulfacetamide)

Dosage form: Ophthalmic ointment for topical use

Neo-Darbazine Spansule (Norden) (also contains prochlorperazine and isopropamide)

Dosage form: 25 and 75 mg capsules for po administration

Neo-Delta-Cortef (Upjohn) (also contains prednisolone)

Dosage form: 3.5 mg/ml otic, ophthalmic suspension for topical use

Neo-Delta-Cortef with Tetracaine (Upjohn) (also contains prednisolone and tetracaine)

Dosage form: 3.5 mg/ml otic suspension for topical use

Neo-Mast-H (Bio-Ceutic) (also contains procaine penicillin G, 100,000 units/10 ml hydrocortisone, 200 mg/100 ml; and sulfamethazine, 10 gm/100 ml)

Dosage form: 1 gm/100 ml solution for intramammary administration

Neomycin Sulfate (various) (manufactured for human use)

Dosage form: 0.5 gm sterile powder for reconstitution to suspension for IM administration

Neovet (Med-Tech)

Dosage form: 200 mg/ml solution for po administration or topical use

Nolvapent (Fort Dodge) (also contains chlorhexidine dihydrochloride, 6.7 mg/ml, and hydrocortisone acetate, 10 mg/ml)

Dosage form: 3.5 mg/ml ointment for topical use

Optiprime Opthakote (Diamond) (also contains polymyxin B sulfate, 10,000 units/ml)

Dosage form: 5 mg/ml ophthalmic solution for topical use

Optisone (Evsco) (also contains prednisolone, 2 mg/gm)

Dosage form: 5 mg/gm ophthalmic ointment for topical use

Panalog (Squibb) (also contains nystatin, 100,000 units/ml; thiostreptin, 2500 units/ml; and triamcinolone acetonide, 1 mg/ml)

Dosage form: 2.5 mg/ml ointment for topical use

Topacin (Burns-Biotec) (also contains sulfathiazole, sulfanilamide, and phenacaine)

Dosage form: Powder for topical use

Tylan plus Neomycin (Elanco) (also contains tylosin, 2%)

Dosage form: 0.25% ointment for topical use

Neomycin-bacitracin-polymyxin B

Mycitracin (Upjohn)

Dosage form: Ophthalmic ointment for topical use

Neobacimyx (Burns-Biotec)

Dosage form: Ophthalmic ointment for topical use

Neobacimyx-H (Burns-Biotec) (also contains hydrocortisone)

Dosage form: Ophthalmic ointment for topical use

Neo-Polycin (Dow) (manufactured for human use)

Dosage form: Ointment for topical use

TriOptic-P (Beecham)

Dosage form: Ophthalmic ointment for topical use

TriOptic-S (Beecham) (also contains hydrocortisone acetate)

Dosage form: Ophthalmic ointment for topical use

Vetropolycin (Pitman-Moore)

Dosage form: Ophthalmic ointment for topical use

Vetropolycin HC (Pitman-Moore) (also contains hydrocortisone acetate USP 1%)

Dosage form: Ophthalmic ointment for topical use

Neomycin-polymyxin B

Forte-Topical (Upjohn) (also contains procaine penicillin G and hydrocortisone)

Dosage form: Suspension for topical use and otic administration

Neostigmine

Prostigmin Bromide (Roche) (manufactured for human use)

Dosage form: 15 mg tablets for po administration

Stiglyn 1:500 Injection (Pitman-Moore)

Dosage form: 2 mg/ml solution for SC or IM administration

Niacin (*see also* vitamin B–complex; multivitamins; multivitamins with minerals)

Niacin (various) (manufactured for human use)

Dosage form: 20, 25, 50, 100, and 500 mg tablets for po administration; 10, 50, and 100 mg/ml solution for IM, IV, and SC administration

Niclosamide

Yomesan (Haver-Lockhart)

Dosage form: 357 mg, 500 mg, and 1.428 gm tablets for po administration

Nitrofurantoin

Dantafur (Norden)

Dosage form: 15 mg/ml oral suspension, 10 mg tablets, and 50 mg bolus for po administration

Furadantin (Eaton) (manufactured for human use)

Dosage form: 50 and 100 mg tablets and 25 mg/ml oral suspension for po administration; 9 mg/ml solution for IM or IV administration

Macrodantin (Eaton)

Dosage form: 25, 50, and 100 mg capsules for po administration

Nitrofurantoin (Med-Tech)

Dosage form: 10 and 50 mg tablets for po administration

Nitrofurathiazide

Fulvidex (Schering) (also contains dexamethasone, griseofulvin, undecylenic acid, and tetracaine)

Dosage form: Otic suspension for topical use

Nitrofurazone

Furacin (Eaton) (manufactured for human use)

Dosage form: 0.2% soluble dressing, 0.2% cream, 0.2% solution, and 0.2% soluble powder for topical use

Furacin Micofur (Norden) (also contains nifuroxime, 0.375%, and perodon, 2%)

Dosage form: 0.2% otic solution for topical use

Furacort (Norden) (also contains hydrocortisone acetate, 1%)

Dosage form: 0.2% cream for topical use

Furadex (Norden)

Dosage form: 50 mg bolus and 10 mg tablet for po administration

Nitrofurazone (Med-Tech)

Dosage form: 0.2% dressing, 0.2% dressing with 0.5% butacaine, and 0.2% powder for topical use; 10 and 50 mg tablets, 4.6% soluble powder, and 120 mg bolus (with 12.42 gm urea) for po administration

Nitrosol (Burns-Biotec)

Dosage form: Aerosol powder for topical use

Nitrosol (Med-Tech)
Dosage form: 3.6% aerosol for topical use

Nitrozone-V (Dow B. Hickam)
Dosage form: Spray for topical use

Norepinephrine

Levophed (Winthrop) (manufactured for human use)
Dosage form: 1 mg/ml solution for IV administration

Normal saline

Normal Saline (Abbott; Diamond; Fromm)
Dosage form: 0.9% solution

Physiological Saline Solution (Haver-Lockhart; Med-Tech)
Dosage form: 0.9% solution for IV or SC administration

Saline, Normal (Jen-Sal)
Dosage form: 0.9% solution for IV administration

Salisol (Burns-Biotec)
Dosage form: 0.9% solution

Sodium Chloride (Fort Dodge)
Dosage form: 0.9% sterile solution for IV administration

Sodium Chloride Irrigation (Abbott)
Dosage form: 0.9% solution for topical use

Sodium Chloride Solution 0.9% (Jen-Sal)

Novobiocin

Albamycin (Upjohn) (manufactured for human use)
Dosage form: 250 mg capsules and 125 mg/ml syrup for po administration; 500 mg powder for reconstitution to 100 mg/ml solution for IM or IV administration

Nux vomica (*see* strychnine)

Nystatin

Mycostatin (Upjohn)
Dosage form: 100,000 units/gm ointment and 100,000 units/gm cream for topical use

Nilstat (Lederle) (manufactured for human use)
Dosage form: 100,000 units/gm ointment and 100,000 units/gm cream for topical use

Panalog (Squibb) (also contains neomycin sulfate, 2.5 mg/ml; thiostreptin, 2500 units/ml; and triamcinolone acetonide, 1 mg/ml)
Dosage form: 100,000 units/ml ointment for topical use

Special Formula 17900-Forte (Upjohn) (also contains procaine penicillin G, 100,000 units/10 ml)
Dosage form: 15 mg/ml suspension in 10 ml syringe for intramammary administration

Oil of turpentine

Capsaline (Med-Tech) (also contains camphor, 20 gr/30 ml; salicylic acid, 15 gr/30 ml; oleoresin ginger, 1 min/30 ml; oleoresin capsicum, 1 min/ 30 ml; and methyl salicylate, 2 min/30 ml)
Dosage form: 120 min/30 ml solution for po administration and as drench

Turcapsol (Pitman-Moore) (also contains salicylic acid, methyl salicylate, and camphor)
Dosage form: Solution for po administration and as drench

Oleate, sodium

Osteum (Schering)
Dosage form: 50 mg/ml solution for subperiosteal injection

o,p-DDD (*see* mitotane)

Orgotein

Palosein (Diagnostic Data)
Dosage form: 5 mg/dose lyophilized powder for IM administration

Ouabain USP (strophanthin-G)

Ouabain (Lilly) (manufactured for human use)
Dosage form: 250 mg/ml solution for IV administration

Oxacillin

Bactocill (Beecham) (manufactured for human use)
Dosage form: 500 mg and 1, 2, and 4 gm powders for reconstitution for IM and IV administration

Prostaphlin (Bristol) (manufactured for human use)
Dosage form: 250 and 500 mg capsules and powder for reconstitution to 250 mg/5 ml oral suspension for po administration; 250 and 500 mg and 1, 2, and 4 gm powders for reconstitution to solution for IM or IV administration

Oxyclozanide

Zanil (American Cyanamid)
Dosage form: 3.4% suspension for po administration

Oxytetracycline

Aquachel (Rachelle)
Dosage form: 50 mg/ml solution for IM or IV administration

Biocycline (Upjohn)
Dosage form: 50 mg/ml solution for IM, IV, or SC administration

Bio-Mycin (Bio-Ceutic)
Dosage form: 50 and 100 mg/ml solutions for IM or IV administration

Liquamast (Pfizer)
Dosage form: 30 mg/gm solution for intramammary administration

Liquamycin (Pfizer)
Dosage form: 100 and 50 mg/ml solution for IM, IV, or SC administration

Liquamycin Intramuscular (Pfizer)
  Dosage form: 50 mg/ml solution for IM administration

Medamycin (Med-Tech)
  Dosage form: Solution for IM administration

Natamycin-102 (Professional Vet. Labs)
  Dosage form: 102.4 gm/pound soluble powder for po administration in drinking water

Oxy 500, 1000, 5000 (Med-Tech)
  Dosage form: 0.5, 1, and 5 gm boluses for po administration

Oxy 500, 1000, 5000 Bolus (Professional Vet. Labs)
  Dosage form: 500 mg, 1 gm, and 5 gm boluses for po administration

Oxy 50, 100, 250 Tablets (Professional Vet. Labs)
  Dosage form: 50, 100, and 250 mg tablets for po administration

Terramycin (Pfizer)
  Dosage form: 250 mg capsules for po administration

Terramycin (Pfizer) (manufactured for human use)
  Dosage form: 125 and 250 mg capsules and 125 mg/5 ml syrup for po administration; 50 and 125 mg/ml solution with 2% lidocaine for IM administration

Terramycin Ophthalmic (Pfizer) (also contains polymyxin B, 10,000 units/gm)
  Dosage form: 5 mg/gm ophthalmic ointment for topical use

Oxytocin USP

Butocin (Burns-Biotec)
  Dosage form: Solution for IM, IV, or SC administration

Oxytocin (Diamond)
  Dosage form: 20 USP units/ml solution for IM, IV, or SC administration

Oxytocin Injection (Jen-Sal)
  Dosage form: Sterile solution for parenteral administration

Oxytocin Injection (Fort Dodge; Norden)
  Dosage form: 20 USP units/ml solution for IM, IV, or SC administration

Oxytocin (Synthetic) (Haver-Lockhart)
  Dosage form: 20 USP units/ml solution for IV, IM, or SC administration

Oxytocin Injection (Med-Tech)
  Dosage form: Sterile solution for parenteral administration

Oxytocin Injection (Norden)
  Dosage form: Sterile solution for parenteral administration

Pitocin Injection (Parke, Davis) (manufactured for human use)

  Dosage form: 5 units/0.5 ml vial and 10 units/ml vial solution for IM or IV administration

P.O.P. (Burns-Biotec)
  Dosage form: 20 USP units/ml solution for IV, IM, or SC administration

Syntocin (Affiliated)
  Dosage form: 20 USP units/ml solution for IM or IV administration

Syntocinon Injection (Sandoz) (manufactured for human use)
  Dosage form: 5 USP units/0.5 ml and 10 USP units/ml solution for IM or IV administration

Pancreatic enzymes

Dornavac (Merck Sharp & Dohme)
  Dosage form: Dessicated pancreatic dornase for reconstitution for topical or local application

Digenzymes (Maurry) (contains ox bile extract NF and pancreatin NF)
  Dosage form: Tablets for po administration

Di-Gest (Evsco) (contains pepsin, 100 mg; pancreatin NF, 200 mg; diatase, 25 mg; bile salts, 100 mg; and dimethyl polysiloxane, 40 mg)
  Dosage form: Tablets for po administration

Enzymin (Haver-Lockhart) (contains pepsin, pancreatin, diastase of male, and papain)
  Dosage form: Tablets for po administration

Gastrizyme (Burns-Biotec) (contains pancreatin, pepsin, papain, diastase, and bile constituents [lipase, amylase, prolease])
  Dosage form: Tablets for po administration

Viokase (Viobin) (manufactured for human use; contains lipase, protease, and amylase)
  Dosage form: Powder and tablets for po administration

Viokase-V (Robins) (Contains lipase, protease, and amylase)
  Dosage form: Powder and tablets for po administration

Pantothenic acid (*see* vitamin B–complex; multivitamins; multivitamins with minerals)

Parabendazole (experimental drug, not available for commercial use)

Paramethadione

Paradione (Abbott) (manufactured for human use)
  Dosage form: 300 mg/ml oral solution for po administration

Parathyroid hormone (PTH)

Parathyroid Injection (Lilly) (manufactured for human use)
  Dosage form: 100 units/ml solution for IM, IV, or SC administration

Paregoric (*see* camphorated opium tincture)

Pectin (*see* kaolin and pectin)

Penicillin, phenoxyethyl (phenethicillin)

Maxipen (Pfizer) (manufactured for human use)
Dosage form: 250 mg tablets for po administration

Syncillin (Bristol) (manufactured for human use)
Dosage form: 250 mg tablets for po administration

Penicillin G, potassium

Penicillin G, Potassium (Lilly) (manufactured for human use)
Dosage form: 200,000 and 500,000 units/5 ml, 1 million units/10 ml, and 5 million units/20 ml solution for IM or IV administration

Potassium Penicillin G USP (Squibb)
Dosage form: Powder to be reconstituted to solution for IM or IV administration

Penicillin G, procaine

Biotef II (Upjohn) (also contains neomycin)
Dosage form: Ointment for intramammary administration

Bovamycin III (Pitman-Moore) (also contains dihydrostreptomycin, 125 mg/25 ml; hydrocortisone, 20 mg/25 ml; and sulfamethazine, 1000 mg/25 ml)
Dosage form: 4,000 units/ml ointment in 25 ml syringe for intramammary administration

Forte-Topical (Upjohn) (also contains neomycin sulfate, polymyxin B, and hydrocortisone)
Dosage form: Otic suspension for topical use

Ho-po-dri (Burns-Biotec) (also contains neomycin sulfate 500 mg/10 ml)
Dosage form: 10,000 units/ml suspension in 10 ml syringe for intramammary administration

HPX-12 Mastitis Syringe (Hamilton Pharm.) (also contains dihydrostreptomycin base, 100 mg/10 ml; sulfamerazine, 300 mg/10 ml; hydrocortisone acetate, 20 mg/10 ml; and povidone, 200 mg/10 ml)
Dosage form: 1000 units/ml solution in 10 ml syringe for intramammary administration

Mastimycin (Pitman-Moore) (also contains neomycin, 500 mg/syringe)
Dosage form: 100,000 units ointment in syringe for intramammary administration

Neo-Mast-H (Bio-Ceutic) (also contains neomycin base, 1 gm/100 ml; sulfamethazine, 10 gm/100 ml; hydrocortisone acetate, 200 mg/100 ml)
Dosage form: 10,000 units/ml in 10 ml syringe for intramammary administration

Procaine Penicillin G (Pfizer)
Dosage form: 300,000 units/ml aqueous suspension for IM administration

Procaine Penicillin G USP (Med-Tech)
Dosage form: 300,000 units/ml aqueous suspension for IM administration

Special Formula 17900-Forte (Upjohn) (also contains novobiocin 150 mg/10 ml)
Dosage form: 10,000 units/ml suspension in 10 ml syringe for intramammary administration

TymPen (Vet-A-Mix)
Dosage form: 20,000 units/pound powder for po administration

Wycillin (Wyeth) (manufactured for human use)
Dosage form: Aqueous suspension for IM administration

Penicillin G, procaine-dihydrostreptomycin (penstrep)

Bovamycin II (Pitman-Moore)
Dosage form: Ointment for intramammary administration

Combiotic (Pfizer)
Dosage form: Aqueous suspension for IM administration

Durbiotic (Burns-Biotec)
Dosage form: Suspension for IM administration

Instilin IOX (Jen-Sal)
Dosage form: Oil solution in 10 ml syringe for intramammary administration

Pro-Penstrep (Merck)
Dosage form: Suspension for IM administration

Quartermaster (Hamilton Pharm.)
Dosage form: Oil suspension for intramammary administration

Penicillin V (phenoxymethyl penicillin)

Penicillin V (various) (manufactured for human use)
Dosage form: 125, 250, and 500 tablets for po administration

Pentazocine

Talwin Hydrochloride (Winthrop) (manufactured for human use)
Dosage form: 50 mg tablets for po administration; 30 mg/ml solution for IM, IV, or SC administration

Talwin-V (Winthrop)
Dosage form: 30 mg/ml solution for IV or IM administration

Pentobarbital

Nembutal (Abbott)
Dosage form: 60 mg/ml solution for IV administration

Nembutal (Abbott) (manufactured for human use)
Dosage form: 50 mg/ml solution for IM or IV administration

Peritoneal dialysis solution

Peritoneal Dialysis Solution Concentrate (Diamond) (contains sodium chloride, 5.844 gm; potassium chloride, 0.2609 gm; sodium lactate, 4.5945 gm; magnesium chloride, 0.1525 gm; and calcium lactate, 0.5394 gm)

Perphenazine

Trilafon (Schering) (manufactured for human use)
Dosage form: 2, 4, 8, and 16 mg tablets, 8 mg sustained-action tablets, and 16 mg/5 ml concentration for po administration; 5 mg/ml solution for IV administration

Petrolatum (*see* white petrolatum)

Phenobarbitol

Phenobarbital (Parke, Davis)

Phenobarbital (various) (manufactured for human use)
Dosage form: 8, 16, 32, 65, and 100 mg tablets for po administration

Phenothiazine

Phenothiazine (various)
Dosage form: Powder, bolus, or drench for po administration

Phenothiazine (TBZ Products)
Dosage form: Powder, bolus, or drench for po administration

Phenylbutazone

Azolid (USV) (manufactured for human use)
Dosage form: 100 mg tablets for po administration

Bizolin-100 (Bio-Ceutic)
Dosage form: 100 mg tablets for po administration

Butazolidin (Geigy) (manufactured for human use)
Dosage form: 100 mg tablets for po administration

Butazolidin (Jen-Sal)
Dosage form: 100 mg and 1 and 2 gm tablets for po administration; 20% solution for IV administration

Dinz (North American Pharm.)
Dosage form: 1 gm and 100 mg tablets for po administration; 200 mg/ml solution for parenteral administration

EquiBute (Fort Dodge)
Dosage form: 100 mg tablets for po administration

Phenylbutazone (Beecham; Norden; Haver-Lockhart)
Dosage form: 1 gm and 100 mg tablets for po administration

Phenylbutazone Injection (Haver-Lockhart; Maurry; Med-Tech; Norden; Beecham)
Dosage form: 200 mg/ml solution for parenteral administration

P/M Sterile Phenylbutazone for Injection (Pitman-Moore)
Dosage form: 200 mg/ml (20%) solution for IV administration

Phenylephrine

Phenylephrine HCl (various) (manufactured for human use)
Dosage form: 10% ophthalmic solution for topical use

Steroplex (Evsco) (also contains sulfacetamide sodium, 10%, and prednisolone, 0.2%)
Dosage form: 0.12% ophthalmic solution for topical use

Tri-Ophtho (Maurry) (also contains sodium sulfacetamide, 100 mg/ml, and prednisolone, 5 mg/ml)
Dosage form: 0.12% ophthalmic solution for topical use

Phthalofyne

Whipcide (Pitman-Moore)
Dosage form: 250 mg/ml solution for IV administration; 456, 912, and 2.28 gm tablets for po administration

Physostigmine salicylate

Antilirium (O'Neal, Jones & Feldman) (manufactured for human use)
Dosage form: 1 mg/ml solution for IM or IV administration

Pilocarpine

Pilocarpine HCl (Maurry)
Dosage form: Ophthalmic solution for topical use

Pilocarpine (various) (manufactured for human use)
Dosage form: 0.5%, 1%, 2%, 3%, 4%, and 6% ophthalmic solution for topical use

Piperacetazine

Psymod (Pitman-Moore)
Dosage form: 1 mg tablets for po administration; 0.2% solution for parenteral administration

Quide (Dow) (manufactured for human use)
Dosage form: 10 and 25 mg tablets for po administration

Piperazine

Antepar (Burroughs Wellcome) (manufactured for human use)
Dosage form: 500 mg/5 ml syrup for po administration

Candizine (Norden)
Dosage form: 250 mg tablets for po administration

Parlamate (Parlam)
Dosage form: 250 and 500 mg tablets for po administration; 250 mg/5 ml liquid for administration as drench or by stomach tube

Pipcide (Haver-Lockhart)
Dosage form: 7.5 gr tablets and 1.9 gr toytabs for po administration

Piperate (Fort Dodge)

Dosage form: 10 gm/30 ml solution, 100 mg tablets, and powder for po administration

Piperazine (Vet-A-Mix)

Dosage form: 250 mg tablets for po administration

Piperazine (Double Strength) (Bio-Ceutic)

Dosage form: 34% solution for po administration

Pipersol (Burns-Biotec)

Dosage form: 110 mg solution for po administration

Pipertab 2 (Burns-Biotec)

Dosage form: 100 mg tablets for po administration

Pip-Pop 320 (Vet-A-Mix)

Dosage form: 320 gm powder for po administration

Pipzine (Affiliated)

Dosage form: 34 gm/100 ml (34%) solution and 3.1 gr tablets for po administration

Ripercol L-Piperazine (American Cyanamid) (also contains levamisol)

Dosage form: Liquid suspension for administration by stomach tube or as drench

Syrazine 100 (Vet-A-Mix)

Dosage form: 500 mg/ml solution for po administration

Piperazine–carbon disulfide

Parvex (Upjohn)

Dosage form: 20 gm complex bolus and 7.5 gm complex suspension for po administration

Piperazine–carbon disulfide–phenothiazine

Parvex Plus (Upjohn)

Dosage form: Aqueous suspension for oral administration

Piperocaine

Metycaine Hydrochloride (Lilly) (manufactured for human use)

Dosage form: Powder for reconstitution to solution for topical use

Piperonyl butoxide (*see* pyrethrins–piperonyl butoxide)

Plantago seed

Konsyl (Burton, Parsons) (manufactured for human use)

Dosage form: Powder for po administration

Poloxalene

Therabloat (Norden)

Dosage form: 25 gm/30 ml concentrated solution for administration as drench or by stomach tube

Polymyxin B (*see also* neomycin-bacitracin-polymyxin B)

Optoprime Opthakote (Diamond) (also contains neomycin sulfate)

Dosage form: Ophthalmic solution for topical use

Polymyxin B Sulfate (Pfizer) (manufactured for human use)

Dosage form: 500,000 units for reconstitution to solution for IV or intrathecal administration

Terramycin Ophthalmic (Pfizer) (also contains oxytetracycline, 5 mg/gm)

Dosage form: 10,000 units/gm ophthalmic ointment for topical use

Polymyxin E (colistin)

Coly-Mycin S Oral Suspension (Warner-Chilcott) (manufactured for human use)

Dosage form: Powder for reconstitution to 25 mg/5 ml oral suspension for po administration

Posterior pituitary USP

Pituitrin (Parke, Davis) (manufactured for human use)

Dosage form: 10 units/ml solution for IM or SC administration

Posterior Pituitary Injection (various) (manufactured for human use)

Dosage form: 10 and 20 units/ml solution for IM or SC administration

Potassium chloride

Potassium Chloride (various) (manufactured for human use)

Dosage form: 1, 2, 2.4, and 3.2 mEq/ml solution for IV administration

Potassium Chloride 20 mEq (Abbott)

Dosage form: 2 mEq/ml concentrated solution for IV administration

Potassium Chloride Solution Concentrate (Diamond)

Dosage form: Solution for IV administration

Potassium iodide

Glytussin with Iodides (Affiliated) (also contains glyceryl guaiacolate, 7%, and ammonium chloride, 75%)

Dosage form: 2% powder for po administration in drinking water

Pima (Fleming)

Dosage form: 5 gr/5 ml syrup for po administration

Potassium Iodide (various) (manufactured for human use)

Dosage form: Powder for po administration

Povidone iodine

Betadine (Purdue-Frederick)

Dosage form: Aerosol spray, 10% ointment, solution, and surgical scrub for topical use

Betadine (Purdue-Frederick) (manufactured for human use)
Dosage form: Ointment, solution, shampoo, and surgical scrub for topical use
Metadine (Med-Tech)
Dosage form: Solution for topical use
Pralidoxime chloride
Protopam (Ayerst)
Dosage form: Sterile powder for reconstitution to 1 gm/20 ml solution for IM, intraperitoneal, IV, or SC administration
Protopam Chloride (Ayerst) (manufactured for human use)
Dosage form: 1 gm sterile powder for reconstitution to solution for IM, IV, or SC administration
Prednisolone
Chlorasone (Evsco) (also contains chloramphenicol, 10 mg/gm)
Dosage form: 2 mg/gm ophthalmic ointment for topical use
Cortisate (Burns-Biotec)
Dosage form: 20 mg/ml solution for IV administration
Cortitab (Burns-Biotec)
Dosage form: 5 mg tablet for po administration
Hydeltrone (Merck) (also contains neomycin, 5 mg/gm)
Dosage form: 2.5 mg/gm ophthalmic ointment for topical use
Hydeltrone-T.B.A. (Merck)
Dosage form: 20 mg/ml suspension for IM or intrasynovial administration
Meti-Derm with Neomycin (Schering) (also contains neomycin sulfate, 33.3%)
Dosage form: 33.3% aerosol spray for topical use
Neo-Delta-Cortef (Upjohn) (also contains neomycin, 3.5 mg/ml)
Dosage form: 2.5 mg/ml otic and ophthalmic suspensions for topical use
Neo-Delta-Cortef with Tetracaine (Upjohn) (also contains neomycin, 3.5 mg/ml, and tetracaine, 5 mg/ml)
Dosage form: 2.5 mg/ml otic suspension for topical use
Optisone (Evsco) (also contains neomycin sulfate, 5 mg/gm)
Dosage form: 2 mg/gm ophthalmic ointment for topical use
P/M Prednisolone (Pitman-Moore)
Dosage form: 100 mg/ml suspension for IM or intraarticular administration

Prednisolone (Maurry)
Dosage form: 10 mg/ml and 25 mg/ml suspension for IM or intraarticular administration
Prednisolone (Med-Tech)
Dosage form: 5 mg tablets for po administration
Prednisolone (various) (manufactured for human use)
Dosage form: 1, 2.5, and 5 mg tablets for po administration; 25 and 50 mg/ml acetate solutions for parenteral administration
Solu-Delta-Cortef (Upjohn)
Dosage form: Soluble powder for reconstitution to 10 mg/ml solution for IM or IV administration
Steroplex (Evsco) (also contains sodium sulfacetamide, 10%, and phenylephrine, 0.12%)
Dosage form: 0.2% sterile ophthalmic suspension for topical use
Sterosone A.S. (Med-Tech)
Dosage form: 10 mg/ml sterile suspension for IM, intraarticular, or intrasynovial administration
Tri-Ophtho (Maurry) (also contains sodium sulfacetamide, 100 mg/ml, and phenylephrine hydrochloride, 0.12%)
Dosage form: 5 mg/ml ophthalmic solution for topical use
Prednisolone sodium succinate
Meticortelone (Schering) (manufactured for human use)
Dosage form: 50 mg soluble sterile powder for reconstitution to solution for parenteral administration
Prednisone
Meticorten (Schering)
Dosage form: 10 and 40 mg/ml suspensions for IM administration
Prednisone (Haver-Lockhart)
Dosage form: 5 mg tablets for po administration
Prednisone (Med-Tech)
Dosage form: 5 mg tablets for po administration
Prednisone (various) (manufactured for human use)
Dosage form: 1, 2.5, 5, 20, and 25 mg tablets for po administration
Sterocort (Med-Tech)
Dosage form: 40 mg/ml sterile suspension for IM administration
Zenadrid (Diamond)
Dosage form: 10 and 40 mg/ml suspensions for IM administration
Primidone
Mylepsin (Fort Dodge)
Dosage form: 250 mg tablets for po administration

Mysoline (Ayerst) (manufactured for human use)
  Dosage form: 50 and 250 mg tablets for po administration
Neurosyn (Med-Tech)
  Dosage form: 250 mg tablets for po administration
Primidone Medi-Pets (Ayerst)
  Dosage form: 250 mg chewable tablets for po administration
Primidone Veterinary (Ayerst)
  Dosage form: 250 mg tablets for po administration
Procainamide
Pronestyl (Squibb) (manufactured for human use)
  Dosage form: 250, 375, and 500 mg tablets for po administration; 100 and 500 mg/ml solutions for IM or IV administration
Procaine hydrochloride
Novocain (Winthrop) (manufactured for human use)
  Dosage form: 1%, 2%, and 10% solutions for infiltration anesthesia; nerve, caudal, or other epidural block; and spinal anesthesia
Prochlorperazine
Darbazine Injection (Norden) (also contains isopropamide iodide)
  Dosage form: Solution for SC administration
Darbazine Spansule (Norden) (also contains isopropamide)
  Dosage form: Timed-release capsules for po administration
Neo-Darbarine Spansule (Norden) (also contains neomycin and isopropamide)
  Dosage form: 3.33 and 10 mg capsule for po administration
Progesterone
Progesterone Injection (Med-Tech)
  Dosage form: 50 mg/ml aqueous solution for IM administration
Progesterone Repository Solution (Haver-Lockhart)
  Dosage form: 2.5% solution for IM administration
Progesterone Repository Suspension (Med-Tech)
  Dosage form: 50 mg/ml suspension for IM administration
Repogest (Burns-Biotec)
  Dosage form: 50 mg/ml solution for IM administration
Repositol Progesterone
  Dosage form: 25 and 50 mg/ml solutions for IM administration
Promazine
Promazine (Fort Dodge)
  Dosage form: 50 mg/ml solution for IM or IV

administration; 8 gm/10.25 ounce granules for po administration
Sparine (Wyeth) (manufactured for human use)
  Dosage form: 10, 25, 50, 100, and 200 mg tablets for po administration; 25 and 50 mg/ml solutions for IM or IV administration
Proparacaine
Ophthaine Ophthalmic Solution (Squibb) (manufactured for human use)
  Dosage form: 0.5% sterile ophthalmic solution for topical use
Propiopromazine
Tranvet (Diamond)
  Dosage form: 5 and 10 mg/ml injectable solution for IM or IV administration; 10 and 20 mg tablets for po administration
Propylene glycol
Propylene Glycol USP (Med-Tech)
  Dosage form: Liquid for po administration
Sirlene (Pitman-Moore)
  Dosage form: Solution for po administration
Prostaglandin $F_{2\alpha}$ ($PGF_{2\alpha}$)
Prostin F2 Alpha (Upjohn)
  Dosage form: 5 mg/ml solution for IM administration
Prostalene
Synchrocept (Diamond)
  Dosage form: Sterile solution for parenteral administration
Pyrantel pamoate
Antiminth (Roerig) (manufactured for human use)
  Dosage form: 50 mg/ml oral suspension for po administration
Nemex (Pfizer)
  Dosage form: Suspension for po administration
Strongid T (Pfizer)
  Dosage form: 50 mg/ml suspension for po administration or by stomach tube
Pyrantel tartrate
Strongid (Pfizer)
  Dosage form: Powder for po administration or by stomach tube
Pyrethrins (*see also* Pyrethrins–piperonyl butoxide)
Pet Spray (Diamond) (also contains rotenone and carbaryl)
  Dosage form: Spray for topical use
Pyrethrins–piperonyl butoxide
Aurimite (Burns-Biotec) (also contains diotyl sodium sulfosuccinate, Benzocaine, tyrothricin, petroleum distillate, and hydrocortisone)
  Dosage form: Suspension for topical administration

Cerumite (Evsco) (also contains cerumene [squalene] 25%)
Dosage form: Otic solution for topical use
D-Flea (Evsco)
Dosage form: Shampoo for topical use
Diryl (Pitman-Moore) (also contains carbaryl [sevin])
Dosage form: Powder for topical use
Flair (Jen-Sal) (also contains malathion, carbaryl, and petroleum distillates)
Dosage form: Solution for topical use
Fleatol Shampoo (Haver-Lockhart)
Dosage form: Shampoo for topical use
Fleavol Shampoo (Norden)
Dosage form: Shampoo for topical use
Flick (Affiliated)
Dosage form: Shampoo for topical use
F.L.T. Bomb (Bio-Ceutic) (also contains carbaryl, 1%, and dichlorophen, 0.1%)
Dosage form: Aerosol for topical use
F-L-T Powder (Bio-Ceutic) (also contains carbaryl, 5%, and dichlorophen, 0.5%)
Dosage form: Powder for topical use
Havo-Cide (Haver-Lockhart) (also contains squalene, 25%)
Dosage form: Liquid for topical use
K.F.L. (Pitman-Moore)
Dosage form: Shampoo for topical use
Liqua-Sect (Evsco) (also contains N-octyl bicycloheptane dicarboxamide, 0.333%)
Dosage form: Solution for spraying for topical use
Mange Lotion (Bio-Ceutic) (contains rotenone, 0.12%; lindane, 0.1%; dichlorophen, 0.5%; and benzyl benzoate 30%)
Dosage form: Lotion for topical use
Mitecide (Elanco) (also contains mineral oil, 90.05%; methoxychlor, 1%; and hexachlorophene, 0.5%)
Dosage form: Solution for topical use
Mycodex (Beecham) (also contains hexachlorophene, 2%)
Dosage form: Shampoo for topical use
Norsect (Norden) (also contains carbaryl, 0.5%; N-octyl bicycloheptane dicarboxamide, 0.25%; and methoxychlor 0.5%)
Dosage form: Aerosol for topical use
ParaBomb-M-1 (Haver-Lockhart) (also contains malathion, 0.5%; and 2,3:4,5-bis [2-butylene] tetrahydro-2-furaldehyde, 0.24%)
Dosage form: Pressurized spray for topical use
Para S-1 (Haver-Lockhart) (also contains methoxychlor, 0.5%, and carbaryl, 0.5%)
Dosage form: Aerosol for topical use

Pet Pest Spray (Affiliated) (also contains N-octyl bicycloheptane dicarboxamide, 0.25%; methoxychlor, 0.5%; and 2,3:4,5-bis [2-butylene] tetrahydro-2-furaldehyde, 0.2%)
Dosage form: Aerosol form for topical use
Sebbatix (Winthrop) (also contains N-octyl bicycloheptane dicarboxamide, 0.2%)
Dosage form: Shampoo for topical use
Sect-a-Spray (Evsco) (also contains carbaryl, 0.5%)
Dosage form: Aerosol for topical use
Sprecto (Pitman-Moore) (also contains carbaryl, tetrahydrofuraldehyde, and dicarboxamide)
Dosage form: Spray for topical use
Theradex (Evsco) (also contains hexachlorophene, 2%)
Dosage form: Shampoo for topical use
Pyridoxine (vitamin B_6) (*see* vitamin B complex; multiple vitamins; multiple vitamins with minerals)
Quinidine gluconate
Quinaglute Dura-Tabs (Cooper) (manufactured for human use)
Dosage form: 330 mg tablets for po administration
Quinidine Gluconate (Lilly) (manufactured for human use)
Dosage form: 80 mg/ml solution for IV or IM administration
Quinidine polygalacturonate
Cardioquin Tablets (Purdue Frederick) (manufactured for human use)
Dosage form: 275 mg tablets for po administration
Quinidine sulfate
Quinidine Sulfate (various) (manufactured for human use)
Dosage form: 200 mg tablets for po administration; 200 mg/ml solution for IM or IV administration
Quinine
Quinine Sulfate (various) (manufactured for human use)
Dosage form: 3 and 5 gr capsules for po administration
Rafoxanide
Ranide (Merck Sharp & Dohme)
Dosage form: Not yet available in the United States
Riboflavin (vitamin B_2) (*see* vitamin B complex; multiple vitamins; multiple vitamins with minerals)
Red iodide of mercury (*see* mercuric iodide)
Ringer's solution
Ringer's Injection (Abbott) (contains sodium chlo-

ride, 800 mg/100 ml; potassium chloride, 30 mg/100 ml; and calcium chloride, 33 mg/100 ml)

Dosage form: Solution for IV administration

Ringer's Solution (Concentrate) (Diamond) (contains 8 gm/1000 ml sodium chloride; potassium chloride, 0.3 gm/1000 ml; and calcium chloride, 0.33 gm/1000 ml)

Dosage form: Solution for dilution for IV or SC administration

Ronidazole (not available in United States)

Ronnel

Catron (Bio-Ceutic) (also contains xylene, 0.5%)

Dosage form: 2.5% aerosol spray for topical use

Ectoral (Pitman-Moore)

Dosage form: 250 and 500 mg and 1 gm tablets for po administration; 33.33% emulsifiable concentrate for topical use

Screw Worm Spray with Ronnel (Med-Tech) (also contains xylene, 2.5%)

Dosage form: 2.5% spray for topical use

Rotenone

Benzyl-Hex (Evsco) (also contains benzyl benzoate, 20%; lindane, 0.25%; and dichlorophen, 0.5%)

Dosage form: 0.5% solution for topical administration

Flea-Soap-L (Burns-Biotec) (also contains lanolin)

Dosage form: Soap for topical use

Mange Lotion (Bio-Ceutic) (also contains lindane, 0.1%; dichlorophen, 0.5%; and benzyl benzoate, 30%)

Dosage form: 0.12% lotion for topical use

Mitone (Affiliated) (also contains benzyl benzoate, 20%, and benzocaine, 2%)

Dosage form: 0.3% solution for topical use

Paramite (Hart-Delta) (contains lindane and benzyl benzoate)

Dosage form: Solution for topical use

Pet Spray (Diamond) (also contains pyrethrins and carbaryl)

Dosage form: Spray for topical use

Ruelene

Ruelene 350 Insecticide (Dow)

Dosage form: Liquid for topical administration

Ruelene 25E Insecticide (Dow)

Dosage form: Liquid for topical administration

Ruelene R Insecticide (Dow)

Dosage form: Liquid for topical administration

Ruelene Wormer Drench (Dow)

Dosage form: Liquid for po administration

Salicylazosulfapyridine

Azulfidine (Pharmacia) (manufactured for human use)

Dosage form: 500 mg tablets for po administration

Sulcolon (Lederle) (manufactured for human use)

Dosage form: 500 mg tablets for po administration

Salicylic acid

Cerbinol (Pitman-Moore) (also contains neutral and benzoic acids of propylene glycol, acid ester calculated as propylene glycol monomalic ester, malic acid, and benzoic acid)

Dosage form: Solution and cream for topical use

Keralyte Gel (Westwood) (manufactured for human use)

Dosage form: 6% gel for topical use

Pragmatar (Norden) (also contains colorless crude coal tar, 0.35%, and sulfur, 3%)

Dosage form: 3% shampoo and ointment for topical use

Turcapsol (Pitman-Moore) (also contains methyl salicylate, camphor, and oil of turpentine)

Dosage form: Solution and cream for topical use

Scarlet oil

Scarlet Oil (Fort Dodge) (contains Biebrich scarlet, carbolic acid, thymol, menthol, eucalyptol, camphor, balsam of Peru, oil of cade, castor oil, acetone, and alcohol)

Dosage form: Solution for topical use

Scarlet Oil (Med-Tech) (contains oil of eucalyptus, methyl salicylate, carbolic acid, Biebrich scarlet, and hydrocarbon oil)

Dosage form: Solution for topical use

Scarlet Oil Improved (Med-Tech) (contains menthol, oil of eucalyptus, carbolic acid, pine tar oil, Biebrich scarlet, oil of thyme, and Peru balsam)

Dosage form: Solution for topical use

Scarlet Oil Aerosol Spray (Bio-Ceutic) (contains Biebrich scarlet red, thyme oil, menthol, eucalyptus oil, camphor oil, phenol, cade oil, and mineral oil)

Dosage form: Aerosol for topical use

Scarletol (Haver-Lockhart) (contains balsam peruvian, oil of camphor, thyme oil red, eucalyptus oil, scarlet red, cottonseed oil, menthol, pine tar, and castor oil)

Dosage form: Aerosol spray for topical use

Selenium

Exsel (Herbert Laboratories) (manufactured for human use)

Dosage form: 2.5% lotion for topical use

Seleen (Abbott)

Dosage form: Suspension for topical use

Selsun (Abbott) (manufactured for human use)

Dosage form: 2.5% lotion for topical use

Simethicone

Mylicon (Stuart) (manufactured for human use)
    Dosage form: 40 and 80 mg chewable tablets
    and 40 mg/0.6 ml drops for po administration

Sodium bicarbonate

Alkisol (Burns-Biotec)
    Dosage form: Solution for IV or SC adminis-
    tration

Sodium Bicarbonate (Abbott)
    Dosage form: 5% and 8.4% solution for IV ad-
    ministration

Sodium Bicarbonate (Hart-Delta)
    Dosage form: 8.4% solution for IV adminis-
    tration

Sodium Bicarbonate (Med-Tech)
    Dosage form: 7.5% solution for IV adminis-
    tration

Sodium chloride (*see* normal saline)

Sodium hydroxide and calcium hydroxide

Franklin Dehorning Paste (Franklin)
    Dosage form: Paste for topical administration

Sodium iodide

Sodium Iodide (Bio-Ceutic; Med-Tech; Jen-Sal)
    Dosage form: 20% solution for IV administration

Sodium Iodide (various) (manufactured for human
    use)
    Dosage form: 100 mg/ml solution for IV admin-
    istration

Sodium Iodide Solution (Haver-Lockhart)
    Dosage form: Sterile solution for parenteral
    administration

Sodium lactate (*see* peritoneal dialysis solution)

Sodium phosphate

Fleet Veterinary Enema (Pitman-Moore) (also
    contains sodium biphosphate)
    Dosage form: solution for administration as
    enema

Sodium phosphate dibasic

Neutra-Phos (Willen) (manufactured for human
    use; also contains potassium phosphate dibasic
    and sodium and potassium phosphate mono-
    basic)
    Dosage form: 250 mg phosphorus-equivalent
    capsules for po administration

Sodium selenite (*see* sodium selenite and vita-
    min E)

Sodium selenite and vitamin E

Bo-Se (Burns-Biotec)
    Dosage form: 2.19 mg sodium selenite and 50
    mg vitamin E per milliliter emulsion for IM
    or SC administration

E-SE (Burns-Biotec)
    Dosage form: 5.48 mg sodium selenite and 50
    mg vitamin E per milliliter solution for IM
    or IV administration

L-SE (Burns-Biotec)
    Dosage form: 0.55 mg sodium selenite and 50
    mg vitamin E per milliliter solution for IM
    or SC administration

Mu-SE (Burns-Biotec)
    Dosage form: Emulsion for IM or SC admin-
    istration

Seletoc (Burns-Biotec)
    Dosage form: Solution for IM or SC adminis-
    tration; capsules and minicaps for po admin-
    istration

Spectinomycin

Spectam Scour-Halt (Abbott)
    Dosage form: 50 mg/ml solution for po admin-
    istration

Spectinomycin (Diamond)
    Dosage form: Injectable solution for IM admin-
    istration; 100 mg tablets and oral liquid for
    po administration

Trobicin (Upjohn) (manufactured for human use)
    Dosage form: Sterile powder for reconstitution
    to 400 mg/ml solution for IM administration

Spironolactone

Aldactone (Searle) (manufactured for human use)
    Dosage form: 25 mg tablets for po adminis-
    tration

Spironolactone-hydrochlorothiazide

Aldactazide (Searle) (manufactured for human use)
    Dosage form: Tablets for po administration

Stanozolol

Winstrol (Winthrop) (manufactured for human
    use)
    Dosage form: 2 mg tablets for po administration

Winstrol-V (Winthrop)
    Dosage form: 2 mg tablets for po administration;
    50 mg/ml suspension for IM administration

Streptomycin (*see also* Penicillin G, procaine di-
    hydrostreptomycin)

Streptomycin Sulfate (various) (manufactured for
    human use)
    Dosage form: 1 and 5 gm powders for recon-
    stitution to solution for IM administration

Strychnine

Strychnine Sulfate (Haver-Lockhart)
    Dosage form: 1 gr tablets for SC administra-
    tion

Sulfabromomethazine

Sulfabrom (Merck) (also contains sodium)
    Dosage form: 2.5 and 15 gm boluses for po ad-
    ministration

Sulfacetamide

Mitox (Norden) (also contains neomycin sulfate
    0.5%; sevin (carbaryl) 1%; and tetracaine, 0.5%)
    Dosage form: 9% solution for topical use

Neocorticin (Burns-Biotec) (also contains hydro-cortisone and neomycin)

Dosage form: Ophthalmic ointment for topical use

Steroplex (Evsco) (contains prednisolone, 0.2%, and phenylephrine, 0.12%)

Dosage form: 10% sterile ophthalmic suspension for topical use

Sulf-10 (Maurry)

Dosage form: 10% ophthalmic solution for topical use

Sulfacetamide (various) (manufactured for human use)

Dosage form: 10% and 30% ophthalmic solution for topical use

Tri-Optho (Maurry) (also contains prednisolone, 5 mg/ml, and phenylephrine hydrochloride, 0.12%)

Dosage form: 100 mg/ml ophthalmic solution for topical use

Sulfadiazine

Sulfadiazine (various) (manufactured for human use)

Dosage form: 325 and 500 mg tablets for po administration

Sulfadimethoxine

Agribon (Roche)

Dosage form: 12.5% concentrated solution for po administration in drinking water

Albon (Roche)

Dosage form: 94.6 gm powder, 12.5% concentrated solution, and 2.5, 5, and 15 gm boluses and 12.5 gm sustained-release bolus for po administration in water; 40% solution for parenteral administration

Bactrovet (Pitman-Moore)

Dosage form: 10% solution for IM, IV, or SC administration; 125 and 250 mg tablets and 12.5% oral suspension for po administration

Medacide-SDM Injection (Med-Tech)

Dosage form: 10% solution for IV administration

Sudine (Affiliated)

Dosage form: 125, 250, and 1000 mg tablets for po administration

Symbio (Affiliated)

Dosage form: 100 mg/ml solution for IM or IV administration

Sulfaguanidine

Guantanate (Med-Tech)

Dosage form: 240 gr bolus for po administration

Sulfaguanidine (Med-Tech)

Dosage form: 7.7 gr tablets and bolus for po administration

Sulfamerazine

HPX-12 Mastitis Syringe (Hamilton Pharm.) (also contains procaine penicillin G, 100,000 units/10 ml; dihydrostreptomycin base, 100 mg/10 ml; hydrocortisone acetate, 20 mg/10 ml; and povidone, 200 mg/10 ml)

Dosage form: 30 mg/ml solution in 10 ml syringe for intramammary administration

Sulfamerazine (various) (manufactured for human use)

Dosage form: Powder for po administration

Sulfamethazine

Bovamycin III (Pitman-Moore) (also contains procaine penicillin G, 100,000 units/25 ml; dihydrostreptomycin, 125 mg/25 ml; and hydrocortisone, 20 mg/5 ml)

Dosage form: 40 mg/ml ointment in 25 ml syringe for intramammary administration

Durameth (Burns-Biotec)

Dosage form: 15 gm bolus for po administration

Hava-Span (Haver-Lockhart)

Dosage form: 22.5 gm prolonged-release bolus for po administration

Neo-Mast-H (Bio-Ceutic) (also contains procaine penicillin G, 100,000 units/100 ml; neomycin base, 1 gm/100 ml; and hydrocortisone acetate, 200 mg/100 ml)

Dosage form: 10 gm/100 ml solution for intramammary administration

SM (Med-Tech)

Dosage form: 15 and 30 gm bolus for po administration

Sodium Sulfamethazine (American Cyanamid)

Dosage form: 12.5% solution and soluble powder for reconstitution to 12.5% solution for administration as drench or for po administration in drinking water; 25% solution for parenteral administration

Sodium Sulfamethazine (Med-Tech)

Dosage form: 12.5% solution for po administration

Sulfachel-M (Rachelle)

Dosage form: 35, 100, and 454 gm/pound soluble powders, 15 gm bolus, and 12.5% oral solution for po administration; 25% injectable solution for parenteral administration

Sulfamethazine (American Cyanamid)

Dosage form: 15 and 2.5 gm bolus for po administration

Sulfamethazine (Med-Tech)

Dosage form: 0.5 gm tablets, 12.5% and 25% sorbitol solution, and 25% plain solution for po administration

Sulfamethazine (Professional Vet. Labs)
Dosage form: Bolus for po administration
Sulfamethazine Spanbole II (Norden)
Dosage form: 27 gm sustained-release tablet for po administration
Veta-Meth (Vet-A-Mix)
Dosage form: 12.5% solution for parenteral administration; 5, 15, and 25 gm tablets for po administration

Sulfamethizole
Thiosulfil (Ayerst) (manufactured for human use)
Dosage form: 250 and 500 mg tablets and 250 mg/5 ml oral suspension for po administration

Sulfanilamide
Spad Eye Ointment (Haver-Lockhart) (also contains sulfathiazole, phenacaine, and vitamins A and D)
Dosage form: Ophthalmic ointment for topical use
Topacin (Burns-Biotec) (also contains neomycin, sulfathiazole, and phenacaine)
Dosage form: Powder for topical use

Sulfathiazole
Sodium Sulfathiazole (Med-Tech)
Dosage form: Soluble powder for po administration in water
Spad Eye Ointment (Haver-Lockhart) (also contains sulfanilamide, phenacaine, and vitamins A and D)
Dosage form: Ointment for topical use
Sulfathiazole (Med-Tech)
Dosage form: 240 gr bolus for po administration
Sul-Thi-Zol (Merck)
Dosage form: Soluble powder for po administration
Topacin (Burns-Biotec) (also contains neomycin, sulfanilamide, and phenacaine)
Dosage form: Powder for topical use

Sulfa-urea
Sulfarea (Haver-Lockhart) (contains sulfanilamide and urea)
Dosage form: Solution for topical use
Sulfa-Urea (Norden) (contains sulfathiazole, 5%, and urea, 10%)
Dosage form: Creme for topical use

Sulfisoxazole
Gantrisin (Roche) (manufactured for human use)
Dosage form: 500 mg tablets, 500 mg/5 ml syrup, and 500 mg/5 ml suspension for po administration; 400 mg/ml solution for IV administration
Soxisol (Fort Dodge)
Dosage form: 260 mg (4 gr) tablets for po administration

Sulfisoxizole (various) (manufactured for human use)
Dosage form: 500 mg tablets for po administration

Sulfur
Orthorix Spray (Ortho Chemical) (contains calcium polysulfide)
Dosage form: 25% suspension for topical use
Pragmatar (Norden) (also contains colorless crude coal tar, 0.35%, and salicylic acid, 3%)
Dosage form: 3% shampoo and ointment for topical use
Redux (Burns-Biotec) (contains cupric sulfate and flowers of sulfur)
Dosage form: Ointment for topical use

Tars
Coal Tar Solution (various) (manufactured for human use)
Dosage form: 20% solution for topical use
L.C.D. (Almay) (manufactured for human use)
Dosage form: 20% solution for topical use

Temephos (not yet available in United States)

Testosterone
Repotest (Burns-Biotec)
Dosage form: 25 mg/ml solution for IM administration
Testosterone (various) (manufactured for human use)
Dosage form: 25, 50, and 100 mg/ml aqueous suspension for IM administration
Testosterone Enanthate Injection USP (Med-Tech)
Dosage form: 1000 mg/ml aqueous solution for IM administration
Testosterone Repository Solution (Haver-Lockhart)
Dosage form: 25 mg/ml solution for IM administration

Tetracaine
Pontocaine Hydrochloride (Winthrop) (manufactured for human use)
Dosage form: 1% solution for spinal anesthesia

Tetrachlorethylene USP
Nema (Parke, Davis)
Dosage form: 0.2, 0.5, 2.5, and 5 ml capsules for po administration

Tetracycline
Panmycin (Upjohn)
Dosage form: 100 mg/ml suspension and 500 mg bolus for po administration
Panmycin (Upjohn) (manufactured for human use)
Dosage form: 100 mg powder for reconstitution to aqueous suspension for IM administration; 250 mg in solution for IV administration; 250 and 500 mg tablets for po administration

P/M Tetracycline Hydrochloride (Pitman-Moore)
Dosage form: 100 and 250 mg tablets for po administration

Polyotic (American Cyanamid)
Dosage form: 500 mg tablets and soluble powder for po administration

Tetrachel-Vet-25, -102, -324 (Rachelle)
Dosage form: 25, 102.4, and 324 gm/pound powder for po administration

Tetracycline (Tutag)
Dosage form: Capsules for po administration

Tetracycline Hydrochloride USP (Squibb)
Dosage form: Capsules for po administration

Tetravite (Burns-Biotec)
Dosage form: Soluble powder for po administration

Thiabendazole *(see also* thiabendazole and piperazine; thiabendazole and trichlofon)

Equizole (Merck)
Dosage form: Powder for administration by stomch tube or as drench and for po administration

Mintezol (Merck Sharp & Dohme) (manufactured for human use)
Dosage form: 500 mg tablets and 500 mg/5 ml oral suspension for po administration

Omnizole (Merck)
Dosage form: 2 and 15 gm boluses; 30 gm/pound (6.6%) granules, and 43% paste for po administration; 6 gm/30 ml suspension for po administration or as drench

Thibenzole (Merck)
Dosage form: 15 gm bolus, drench, pellets, and paste for po administration

Thiabendazole and piperazine
Equizole A (Merck)
Dosage form: Liquid for administration by stomach tube or as drench; powder for po administration

Thiabendazole and trichlorfon
Equizole B (Merck)
Dosage form: Soluble powder to be mixed with water for administration as drench or by stomach tube and for po administration

Thiacetarsamide
Arsenamide Sodium (Haver-Lockhart)
Dosage form: 10 mg/ml solution for IV administration

Caparsolate Sodium (Abbott)
Dosage form: 1% solution for IV administration

Caparsolate (Diamond)
Dosage form: 1% solution for IV administration

Filaramide (Fort Dodge)
Dosage form: Solution for IV administration

Thiamin (vitamin B1) *(see also* vitamin B complex; multiple vitamins; multiple vitamins with minerals)

Thiaject (Burns-Biotec)
Dosage form: Sterile solution for parenteral administration

Thiamine Hydrochloride (Med-Tech)
Dosage form: 250 mg/ml solution for IM or IV administration

Thiamylal
Bio-Tal (Bio-Ceutic)
Dosage form: Solution for IV administration

Surital (Parke, Davis) (manufactured for human use)
Dosage form: Powder for reconstition to solution for IV administration

Thyroid hormone
S-P-T "Liquid" (Fleming)
Dosage form: 1, 2, 3, and 5 gr capsules for po administration

Thyroid USP (various) (manufactured for human use)
Dosage form: 5, 6.5, 8, 16, 32, 65, 98, 130, 195, 260, and 325 mg capsules for po administration

Thyroid-stimulating hormone (TSH)
Dermathycin (Jen-Sal)
Dosage form: Sterile solution for parenteral administration

Thytropar (Armour) (manufactured for human use)
Dosage form: 10 IU lyophilized powder for reconstition to suspension for IM or SC administration

Thyroxine
Letter (Armour) (manufactured for human use)
Dosage form: 0.025, 0.05, 0.1, 0.2, 0.3, and 0.5 mg tablets for po administration

Synthroid (Flint) (manufactured for human use)
Dosage form: 0.025, 0.05, 0.1, 0.15, 0.2, 0.3, and 0.5 mg tablets for po administration; 0.5 mg powder for reconstition to 0.1 mg/ml solution for IV administration

Tincture opium *(see* camphorated opium tincture)

Tobramycin
Nebcin (Lilly) (manufactured for human use)
Dosage form: 40 mg/ml solution for IM or IV administration

Tolnaftate USP
Tinactin (Schering) (manufactured for human use)
Dosage form: 10 mg/gm cream, 10 mg/gm powder, 10 mg/ml solution, and powder aerosol for topical use

Tinavet (Schering)
Dosage form: 1% cream for topical use

Toluene (*see also* dichlorophen and toluene)
Methacide (Affiliated)
  Dosage form: 0.1, 0.25, 0.5, 1, and 3 gm capsules for po administration
Toluene and dichlorophen (*see* dichlorophen and toluene)
Toxaphene
Fenatox (Burroughs Wellcome) (also contains lindane, 1.96%; kerosene, 34.94%; and petroleum distillates, 5.12%)
  Dosage form: 45% emulsifiable concentrate for topical use
Kemal (Vet-Kem) (also contains malathion, 4.3%)
  Dosage form: 43% solution for topical use
Triamcinolone acetonide
Aristocort (Lederle) (manufactured for human use)
  Dosage form: 0.1% and 0.5% ointments and 0.025%, 0.1%, and 0.5% cream for topical use
Aristovet (American Cyanamid)
  Dosage form: 0.5 mg tablets for po administration
Kenalog (Squibb) (manufactured for human use)
  Dosage form: 10 mg/ml and 40 mg/ml suspensions for IM, intraarticular, or intradermal administration; 0.025%, 0.1%, and 0.5% ointments and 0.025%, 0.1%, and 0.5% creams for topical use
Neo-Aristovet (American Cyanamid) (also contains neomycin sulfate 5 mg/gm)
  Dosage form: 1 mg/gm ointment for topical use
Panalog (Squibb) (also contains nystatin, 100,000 units/ml; neomycin sulfate, 2.5 mg/ml; and thiostreptin, 2500 units/ml)
  Dosage form: 1 mg/ml ointment for topical use
Vetalog (Squibb)
  Dosage form: 0.1% cream for topical use; 2 and 6 mg/ml sterile suspension for IM or SC administration; 0.5 and 1.5 mg tablets for po administration
Trichlorfon (*see also* trichlorfon-piperazine-phenothiazine)
Casect (Bio-Ceutic)
  Dosage form: 8% solution for topical use
ComBot (Haver-Lockhart)
  Dosage form: Liquid for administration by stomach tube
Dyrex (Fort Dodge)
  Dosage form: Granules and bolus for po administration
Freed (Fort Dodge) (also contains atropine)
  Dosage form: Tablets for po administration
Grub and Louse Pour-On (Vet-Kem)
  Dosage form: 8% solution for topical use

Vet-Kem Grub and Louse Pour-On Cattle Insecticide (Thuron)
  Dosage form: 8% solution for topical use
Trichlorfon-piperazine-phenothiazine
Dyrex T.F. (Fort Dodge)
  Dosage form: Powder for administration by stomach tube
Trimeprazine
Temaril (Smith Kline & French) (manufactured for human use)
  Dosage form: 2.5 mg tablets, 5 mg sustained-action capsules, and 2.5 mg/5 ml syrup for po administration
Temaril-P (Norden)
  Dosage form: 4.7 mg sustained-release capsules with 1 mg prednisolone, 9.4. mg sustained-action capsules with 2 mg prednisolone, and 5 mg tablets with 2 mg prednisolone for po administration
Triple sulfas
Orsol (Bio-Ceutic) (contains sulfamethazine sodium, 3%; sulfathiazole sodium, 7.2%; and sulfapyridine sodium, 2%)
  Dosage form: Solution for po administration in water or as drench
Soxifour (Fort Dodge) (contains sulfamethazine, 5.63%; sulfathiazole, 5.75%; and sulfamerazine, 1.12%)
  Dosage form: 12.5% solution for po administration
Sulfa (Haver-Lockhart) (contains sulfamerazine, sulfathiazole, and sulfadiazine)
  Dosage form: Tablets for po administration
Sulfa-24-Tri-Sulfa (Bio-Ceutic) (contains sodium sulfamethazine, 8%; sodium sulfapyridine, 8%; and sodium sulfathiazole, 8%)
  Dosage form: Solution for IV administration
Thipyrimeth (Burns-Biotec) (contains sulfathiazole, sulfapyridine, and sulfamethazine)
Triple Sulfa (various) (manufactured for human use; contains sulfadiazine, sulfamerazine, and sulfamethazine)
  Dosage form: Tablets for po administration
Tri-Vet-Sul (Haver-Lockhart) (contains sulfathiazole, 51 mg/ml; sulfamethazine, 41 mg/ml; and sulfamerazine, 10 mg/ml)
  Dosage form: Solution for po administration
Tri-Sulfa-G (Norden) (contains sulfamethazine, 45 mg; sulfathiazole, 45 mg; and sulfapyridine, 20 mg)
  Dosage form: Solution for po administration
Trisul (Burns-Biotec) (contains sulfathiazole, sulfapyridine, and sulfamethazine)
Triple Sulfa (Med-Tech) (contains sulfamethazine,

2.5 gr; sulfathiazole, 2.5 gr; and sulfanilamide, 2.5 gr)

Dosage form: 7.5 gr tablets for po administration

Triple Sulfa (Med-Tech) (contains sulfamethazine, 8%; sulfamerazine, 8%; and sulfathiazole, 8%)

Dosage form: 24% oral solution for po administration in water

Triple Sulfa (Med-Tech) (contains sulfanilamide, 90 gr; sulfamethazine, 60 gr; and sulfathiazole, 90 gr)

Dosage form: Bolus for po administration

Triple Sulfa Injectable (Med-Tech) (contains sulfamethazine, 8% or 4%; sulfapyridine, 8% or 4%; and sulfathiazole, 8% or 4%)

Dosage form: 24% and 12% solution for intraperitoneal, IV, IM, or SC administration

Tropicamide

Mydriacyl Ophthalmic Solution (Alcon) (manufactured for human use)

Dosage form: 0.5% and 1% ophthalmic solution for topical use

Tylosin

Tylan Injection (Elanco)

Dosage form: 50 and 200 mg/ml solution for IM administration

Tylan plus Neomycin (Elanco) (also contains neomycin, 0.25%)

Dosage form: 2% eye powder for topical use

Tylocine (Elanco)

Dosage form: 50 mg/ml solution for parenteral administration; 200 mg tablets for po administration

Undecylenic acid

Desenex (Pharmacraft Consumer Prods.) (manufactured for human use)

Dosage form: 5% ointment, 2% powder, 10% solution and powder spray-on for topical use

Fulvidex (Schering) (also contains dexamethasone, nitrofurathiazide, griseofulvin; and tetracaine)

Dosage form: Otic suspension for topical use

Fungidex (Norden) (also contains zinc undecylenate, 12%; copper undecylenate, 3%, and dichlorophen, 2%)

Dosage form: 5% creme for topical use

Unsaturated fatty acids (linoleic, linolenic, and oleic acids)

Diet-Derm (Vet-A-Mix) (also contains lecithin, 54 mg/5 ml; vitamin A, 1250 IU/5 ml; vitamin D_3, 250 IU/5 ml; and vitamin E, 10 IU/5 ml)

Dosage form: 3827.5 mg/5 ml liquid for po administration

Linoplex (Evsco) (also contains lecithin, vitamin A, vitamin D_2, and vitamin E)

Dosage form: Solution for po administration

Urea

Ureaphil (Abbott) (manufactured for human use)

Dosage form: 40 gm/150 ml sterile solution for IV administration

Uredofos

Sansalid (Beecham)

Dosage form: Tablets for po administration

Vasopressin (antidiuretic hormone, ADH) USP

Pitressin (Parke, Davis) (manufactured for human use)

Dosage form: 20 pressor units/ml solution for IM or SC administration

Vegetable oil

Bloat-Pac (Vet-A-Mix) (also contains polyglycerol oleate, polyethylene glycol monoleate, butylated hydroxyanisole, butylated hydroxytoluene, citric acid, ethoxyquin, propylene glycol, and propyl gallate)

Dosage form: Solution for intraruminal administration or as drench or by stomach tube

Vitamins A and D

A-D Special (Burns-Biotec)

Dosage form: Sterile solution for parenteral administration

Cod Liver Oil (Parke, Davis)

Dosage form: Liquid for po administration

Injacom-100 (Roche)

Dosage form: 200,000 units/ml aqueous emulsion for IM administration

P/M Vitamin A and D (Pitman-Moore)

Dosage form: Emulsifiable solution for IM or intraruminal administration

Vitamin A and D (Pfizer)

Dosage form: Emulsion for IM or SC administration

Vitamin A-D3 (Med-Tech)

Dosage form: Emulsifiable solution for IM, SC, or intraruminal administration

Vitamin A-D 500 (Bio-Ceutic)

Dosage form: Emulsifiable solution for IM administration

Vitamin A-D3 Forte (Med-Tech)

Dosage form: Emulsifiable solution for IM, SC, or intraruminal administration

Vitamin AD-M (Bio-Ceutic)

Dosage form: Emulsifiable solution for IM administration

Vitamins A, D, and E (*see also* multiple vitamins; multiple vitamins with minerals)

Ade Powder (Affiliated)

Dosage form: Powder for po administration in drinking water

ADE-Sol (Vet-A-Mix)

Dosage form: Powder for po administration in drinking water

Ade Vet (North American Pharm.)

Dosage form: Solution for parenteral administration

Emulsade Injection (Haver-Lockhart)

Dosage form: Emulsifiable solution for IM or SC administration

Injacom (Roche)

Dosage form: Solution for IM administration

Rocavit (Roche)

Dosage form: Solution for IM administration

Vitamin B complex

Albee (Robins) (contains vitamins B_1 and B_2, niacin, pantothenic acid, and vitamin B_6)

Dosage form: Capsules for po administration

B-Sol (Fort Dodge) (contains thiamine, 10 mg/ml; riboflavin 2 mg/ml; panthenol, 50 mg/ml; nicotinamide, 100 mg/ml; and pyridoxine, 2 mg/ml)

Dosage form: Solution for IM, SC, or intraperitoneal administration

Buco-B (Burns-Biotec) (contains vitamins B_1, B_2, and B_6; niacinamide; pantothenyl alcohol; and vitamin B_{12})

Dosage form: Solution for po administration

Combiplex-B (Med-Tech) (contains thiamin, 12.5 mg/ml; riboflavin, 2 mg/ml; niacinamide, 100 mg/ml; d-panthenol, 10 mg/ml; pyridoxine, 5 mg/ml; and cyanocobalamin, 5 mEq/ml)

Dosage form: Solution for IM or IV administration

Multi-B Super (Med-Tech) (also contains vitamins B_1 and B_2, niacinamide, d-panthenol, and vitamins B_6 and B_{12})

Dosage form: Solution for IM or IV administration

Vitamin "B" Complex (Norden) (contains vitamins B_1 and B_2, calcium pantothenate, niacinamide, vitamins B_6 and B_{12})

Dosage form: Solution for IM, IV, or SC administration

Vitamin B_{12} (*see* cyanocobalamin)

Vitamin C (ascorbic acid)

Ascorbic Acid (various) (manufactured for human use)

Dosage form: 50, 100, 250, 500, and 1000 mg tablets, 250 and 500 mg capsules, and 100 mg wafers for po administration

Hydro-C (Hart-Delta)

Dosage form: 500 mg capsules and 250 mg/ml solution for po administration

Vitac-V (Dow B. Hickman)

Dosage form: 500 mg timed disintegration capsules for po administration; 300 mg/ml solu-

tion and 300 mg/ml gel injection for parenteral administration

Vitamin D (*see also* Calcium–Vitamin D)

Vitamin D (Parke, Davis)

Dosage form: Capsules for po administration

Vitamin D (various) (manufactured for human use)

Dosage form: 25,000 and 50,000 IU capsules for po administration

Vitamin E (*see also* sodium selenite and vitamin E; multiple vitamins; multiple vitamins with minerals)

Vitamin E (Hart-Delta)

Dosage form: 125,000 IU/pound powder for po administration

Vitamin E (various) (manufactured for human use)

Dosage form: 30, 50, 100, 200, 400, 600, 800, and 1000 IU capsules for po administration; 100 and 200 mg/ml solution for parenteral administration

Vitamin E Injectable (Med-Tech)

Dosage form: 200 IU/ml solution for IM administration

Vitamin K

K-5,-50 (Burns-Biotec)

Dosage form: 5 and 50 ml/ml solution for IV administration

K-Sol (Vet-A-Mix)

Dosage form: 17.6 mg/gm powder for po administration

K-Vite (North American Pharm.)

Dosage form: 5.2 mg/ml solution for parenteral administration

Mephyton (Merck Sharp & Dohme) (manufactured for human use)

Dosage form: 5 mg tablets for po administration

Vitamin K Injection (Med-Tech)

Dosage form: 50 mg/ml solution for IM or SC administration

Vitamin K3 (Haver-Lockhart)

Dosage form: 10 and 48 mg/ml solution for IM administration

Vitamin K3 Injection (Haver-Lockhart)

Dosage form: Solution for IM administration

Vitamin K3 Injection (Haver-Lockhart)

Dosage form: 48 mg/ml solution for IM administration

Vitamin premix

ADD-Plex (Vet-A-Mix) (contains vitamins A, D, D_3, B_{12}, and E; thiamine; vitamin K; cobalt; sulfate monohydrate; dicalcium phosphate; riboflavin; pantothenic acid; and niacin)

Dosage form: Food premix for po administration

Complete Custom Premix No. 1 (Vet-A-Mix) (contains calcium, phosphorus, vitamins A and D_3, dicalcium pantothenate, riboflavin, niacin, vitamin B_{12}, iodine, manganese, iron, copper, cobalt, and zinc)

Dosage form: Food premix for po administration

Complete Custom Premix No. 2 (Vet-A-Mix) (contains arsanilic acid, calcium, phosphorus, salt, vitamins A and D_3, *dl*-calcium pantothenate, riboflavin, niacin, vitamin B_{12}, iodine, manganese, iron, copper, cobalt, and zinc)

Dosage form: Food premix for po administration

White liniment (*see* liniments)

White petrolatum

Cat-A-Lax (Parlam-Ormont) (also contains vitamin A, 100 units/30 ml. vitamin D, 33 units/30 ml; vitamin E, 33 units/30 ml; and vitamin B_1, 2 mg/30 ml)

Dosage form: Ointment for po administration

Kat-A-Lax (Pitman-Moore) (also contains cod liver oil)

Dosage form: Paste for po administration

Kit-Tonne (Haver-Lockhart) (also contains vitamins A, D, and E and thiamine)

Dosage form: Paste for po administration

Laxatone (Evsco) (also contains liquid petrolatum [mineral oil] and linoleic acid)

Dosage form: Ointment for po administration

Lax-O-Cat (North American Pharm.) (contains vitamins A, D_2, E, and B_1 and linoleic acid)

Dosage form: Ointment for po administration

Ophthalmic Base Ointment (Haver-Lockhart) (also contains petrolatum liquid)

Dosage form: Ophthalmic ointment for topical use

White Petrolatum (various) (manufactured for human use)

Dosage form: Ointment for topical use

Xylazine

Rompun (Haver-Lockhart)

Dosage form: 100 mg/ml solution for IM or IV administration

Zinc

Orazinc (Mericon) (manufactured for human use)

Dosage form: 220 mg capsules for po administration

Zinc Sulfate (Mericon) (manufactured for human use)

Dosage form: 66 mg tablets for po administration

Glossary

Because students may use this text prior to learning the meaning of medical terms and because many students may be unfamiliar with the jargon used in veterinary practice, we have attempted to define such words and expressions used in the text. Many of the explanations in the following list vary from standard definitions. However, all are defined in accordance with their use in the text.

acidosis A condition in which the body fluids are at a lower pH than normal. (See also *metabolic acidosis* or *respiratory acidosis.*)

acidotic Distinguished by acidosis.

acid rebound The process by which the stomach produces an excess of acid in response to the use of certain alkaline drugs.

active immunity The process by which an animal produces antibodies and develops an immune status as a result of exposure to an antigen.

acute Having a brief but harsh duration.

adjuvant Substances that when added to an antigen increase the immune response. Generally, adjuvants delay the absorption of biologicals from the site of administration.

adrenalin Trademark name for epinephrine.

adsorb To attract and keep substances on the surface of an object.

adsorbent A material that adsorbs substances.

afferent nerve A nerve that carries an impulse toward the brain or spinal cord.

agent A word commonly used synonymously with the terms "drug" or "microorganism." (See also *necrotizing agent* and *preanesthetic agent.*)

aldosterone One of the mineralocorticoids given off by the outer layer of the adrenal gland. Aldosterone causes the kidney to retain body sodium and secrete potassium.

alkaloid One of a group of bitter basic substances contained in plants. Alkaloids have a variety of biological effects.

alkalosis A condition distinguished by the loss of acid from the body or an excess of base.

anabolic effect An effect that promotes construction processes. In this process, elementary substances are changed by living cells into proteins, fats, and complex carbohydrates. This results in the retention of nitrogen and an increase in muscle mass.

anabolism The building-up process in which elementary substances are changed by living cells into proteins, fats, and complex carbohydrates.

analgesic A drug that relieves pain.

analog A chemical compound that is structurally related to another compound.

anamnestic reaction Swift recurrence of an antibody in the blood after the employment of an antigen to which the animal had earlier developed an active immune response. Often the second response results in higher levels of antibodies than that of the first.

anaphylatoxin The chemical substance that causes anaphylaxis.

anaphylaxis An extreme allergic reaction to a substance to which an animal had previously been sensitized.

androgen The male sex hormones.

anemia Decrease in the number of red blood cells to fewer than normal. (See also *aplastic anemia.*)

anesthesia A loss of sensation. (See also *general anesthesia* and *local anesthesia.*)

anestrus Without estrus. A failure of a female animal to come into estrus or heat.

aneurysm A sac caused by the irreversible abnormal dilation of an artery.

angioedema Edema that is caused by functional disturbance in the peripheral nervous system.

anterior segment The iris and ciliary body of the eye (the anterior segment of the uvea).

anterior synechiae Adhesions between the iris and cornea.

anterior uveitis Inflammation of the iris and ciliary body.

anthelmintic A drug used for the treatment of parasitism by worms.

antibiotic A chemical manufactured by living microorganisms that has an inhibiting or lethal effect on other microorganisms.

antibody A large complex protein manufactured by the body in response to an antigen. The antibody may react with the antigen in a variety of ways.

anticholinergic Blocking the effects of the parasympathetic nervous system generally by blocking the muscarinic effects of acetylcholine.

anticholinesterase drugs Drugs that block the action of the enzyme cholinesterase. The result is a greater response than normal to both the muscarinic and nicotinic effects of acetylcholine.

anticonvulsant An anticonvulsive drug.

anticonvulsive A drug that reduces or eliminates the frequency or severity of convulsions.

antiemetic A substance that stops or reduces vomiting and nausea.

antiflatulent A substance relieving gastrointestinal gas.

antigen A substance that triggers the production of antibodies.

antigenic mass The amount of antigen present.

antihistamine Drug used to prevent the effects of histamine.

anti-infective A drug that inhibits or kills microorganisms responsible for disease. Anti-infectives include sulfonamides, nitrofurans, antibiotics, and others.

anti-inflammatory A substance that reduces inflammation.

antipruritic A substance that stops or relieves itching or itching sensations.

antipyretic A substance that reduces or relieves fever.

antiserum A watery fluid that includes antibodies.

antispasmodic A substance alleviating spasm of smooth muscle, usually of the gastrointestinal tract.

antitoxin An antibody that the body forms in response to the introduction of a toxin or toxinlike substance. This antibody is able to neutralize the toxin that triggered the antibody's appearance.

antitussive A substance that stops or reduces coughing.

antivagal A substance that reduces or eliminates the effects of stimulation of the vagus nerve. Antivagal drugs speed the heart rate and reduce gastrointestinal secretions and motility.

aplastic anemia A form of anemia resulting from a reduction in the production of red blood cells.

aqueous humor The fluid that fills the anterior and posterior chambers of the eye.

arachnid A member of the class Arthropoda. This class includes such creatures as spiders, ticks, mites, and scorpions.

arrhythmia Unusual cardiac rate and/or rhythm.

arteriole A tiny branch of an artery, larger than a capillary.

arteritis Inflammation of an artery.

articular Relating to a joint.

aseptic The state in which pathogenic microorganisms are found lacking, prevented, or excluded.

atonic A condition in which muscular contractions lack normal strength.

attenuate A process by which living organisms are modified so that their virulence is reduced or lost.

attenuated vaccine A vaccine that is made from microorganisms which have been made less virulent.

autogenous Produced within or from material taken from the patient's body or from the bodies of a specific group of patients.

autoimmune disease Disease characterized by the body's production of antibodies against its own tissue(s).

avirulent Not able to resist or destroy the protective mechanism of the host; lacking the ability to cause disease.

AVMA The American Veterinary Medical Association.

bactericidal A substance that kills bacteria.

bacterin A vaccine containing killed bacteria.

bacteriostatic Drug preventing multiplication of bacteria, thus enabling the body's defense mechanisms to fight infection.

barbiturate A derivative of barbituric acid and used in animals as either an anticonvulsant or general anesthetic.

benzimidazoles A group of anthelmintic drugs that include cambendazole, fenbendazole, mebendazole, and thibendazole.

biological A product such as a vaccine, toxoid, serum, antigen, or antitoxin. These tend to be identified by the source and/or purpose for which they are used (e.g., feline panleukopenia vaccine).

bitch A female member of the canine family.

bivalent vaccine A vaccine that contains two distinct antigens.

blister A class of drugs used on the skin of horses that causes a chemical burn and blister formation.

bloat The accumulation of excessive gas in the rumen. (See also *primary bloat* and *secondary bloat*.)

blood dyscrasia Abnormality in the cellular content of the blood.

bolus A large tablet dosage form for administration to livestock.

bound drug A drug that has an affinity for or collects in certain body tissues or substances such as proteins. The bound drug is usually inactive.

brain stem The stemlike section of the brain that unites the cerebral hemispheres with the spinal cord.

broad spectrum Effective against a wide range. Thus broad-spectrum antibiotics are effective against a wide variety of organisms.

brucellosis A bacterial infectious disease caused by *Brucella* species. It is called "undulant fever" in humans.

bursa (pl. *bursae*) A fluid-filled sac placed at strategic sites in the tissues to prevent friction.

calving The act of a cow giving birth to a calf.

capillary permeability The degree of penetration that a capillary wall allows.

cartilage The elastic tissue that forms certain parts of the skeletal system. Cartilage is attached to the articular bone surfaces.

carbamate A pesticide that is an ester of carbamic acid. The pesticide functions by blocking the action of cholinesterase.

cardia The area of the stomach adjacent to the terminal end of the esophagus.

cardiac output The amount of blood pumped out by ventricles of the heart in a given period of time.

catabolism The tearing down process in which compounds are reduced by living cells to simpler substances.

cathartic A drug that promotes evacuation of the bowels.

cerebral cortex The part of the brain that rules behavior, thought, and their interrelation.

cerebral spinal fluid The fluid contained in the spaces in the brain and spinal cord and in the space between the arachnoid and pia mater.

cervical Relating to the neck.

cesticidal Able to kill cestodes.

cestode Generally a platyhelminth or flatworm parasite. Specifically the cestodes are tapeworms.

chelated Having undergone chelation.

chelation The binding of metals in soluble chemical complexes.

chemotherapy The use of chemicals to treat infectious diseases or cancer.

cholinergic A drug that mimics the muscarinic effects of acetylcholine.

cholinergic blocking drug A substance that blocks the action of acetylcholine. As generally used, the term refers to blocking the muscarinic effects of acetylcholine. Therefore atropine and related compounds are cholinergic blocking drugs.

chronic Prevailing over a lengthy duration of time; appearing for a lengthy period.

clinical pathology A part of pathology that uses laboratory techniques to aid in the diagnosis of disease.

colibacillosis A condition resulting from infection with *Escherichia coli*.

colic Severe abdominal pain, specifically recurrent visceral pain resulting from spasm, distention, or obstruction. (See also *spasmodic colic*.)

colostrum The fluid secreted by a female mammal a few days prior, during, or after birth. It has up to 20% protein, more minerals, and less fat than does milk.

complement A substance triggering certain antibody-antigen reactions.

conjunctivitis An inflammation of the conjunctiva of the eye, usually distinguished by tearing and engorgement of the blood vessels of the affected area.

contraindicated Improper or undesirable.

convulsion A syndrome resulting from a central nervous system disturbance that is manifested by one or more of the following: a severe involuntary contraction or a number of contractions of muscles, abnormal body movements, a loss or disturbance of consciousness, abnormal behavior, or involuntary urination and defecation.

coumarin Colorless crystals made from tonka beans, sweet clover, and other plants, which act on the blood to reduce its ability to coagulate.

crystalluria A condition in which crystals are excreted in the urine. The excretion may cause irritation or blockage of the urethra.

cycloplegic drug A drug that paralyzes the ciliary muscle of the eye.

DEA The Drug Enforcement Administration, a branch of the U.S. Department of Justice.

demineralization The condition in which minerals are reduced in body structures. For example, demineralization of bone occurs when calcium and/or phosphate contents of bone are reduced.

denuded Stripped or bared, usually of the outer covering of hair or skin.

dermatitis Inflammation of the skin.

dermatomycotic Relating to a fungal infection of the skin.

dermatosis (pl. *dermatoses*) A skin disease.

detoxify To remove the poisonous abilities of a substance; Also commonly used to describe the process by which drugs are chemically changed to facilitate their removal from the body.

diaphragm A muscular sheet that separates the thorax from the abdomen, which by contraction causes air to enter the lungs.

diastole A dilation of the heart during which the heart fills with blood; the opposite of systole.

dorsal Relating to the surface of an animal located adjacent to the spine. When an animal stands on four legs, the upper surface of the animal is the dorsal surface.

downer-cow A bovine that is unable to rise and stand on all four feet.

drug A chemical or biological substance used to aid in the treatment, prevention, or diagnosis of a disease process. A drug is usually described by a generic name. (See also *bound drug, cholinergic blocking drug, cycloplegic drug, generic drug, keratolytic drug, legend drug,* and *over-the-counter drug.*)

drug residue Small amounts of drugs remaining in feeds or animal products.

edema Swelling caused by the abnormal collection of fluid in spaces between the body's cells.

efferent nerve A nerve that carries impulses away from the brain or spinal cord.

efficacious Possessing the ability to give an intended effect.

efficacy The ability to generate effects; effectiveness.

electrolyte A substance that in solution forms ions and so becomes able to conduct electricity.

embolus (pl. *emboli*) A particle present in blood vessels that travels in the blood until it plugs a vessel.

emetic A substance that triggers vomiting.

empirically Depending solely on experience as opposed to depending on the results of scientific investigation.

emulsify To produce an emulsion.

emulsion A mixture of mutually insoluble liquids in which minute particles of one liquid are suspended in the volume of the other liquid.

endocarditis A condition in which the membrane lining the heart's cavities becomes inflamed.

endometrial cystic hyperplasia Abnormal proliferation of the lining of the uterine cavity, which may also contain numerous small cysts.

endometrium The mucous membrane lining the interior of the uterus.

endotoxins Chemicals present in the cell wall of certain bacteria that when released in the body result in fever and increased capillary permeability, causing inflammation, hemorrhage, and shock.

enterococci Any streptococcus living in the intestines.

enzootic A disease found in an animal population. It is synonymous with the word "endemic" used to describe human disease.

enzyme A member of a group of complex organic materials that speed up certain chemical changes within animals' bodies.

epilepsy A disease state in animals characterized by periodic convulsions.

episcleritis Inflammation of the tissues covering the sclera (the white covering of the eye).

epithelium The material forming the cover of the exterior of the body, internal surfaces, and lining small cavities.

epizootic A disease occasionally present in an animal population that attacks many animals in a region simultaneously. It is synonymous with the word "epidemic" used to describe human disease.

equine A member of the horse family.

eructation Belching; the process of bringing air or gases from the stomach or rumen to the mouth and expelling them.

esophagus The tubelike structure that connects the pharynx to the stomach.

estrus The cyclic limited period during which female animals are sexually receptive to the male; in heat.

etiology The cause of disease.

exogenous Due to external causes.

exotoxin Harmful chemicals produced by bacteria, the effect of which is often seen in tissues distant from the site of infection. Exotoxins stimulate the production of antibodies.

expectorant A drug that promotes an increased secretion or mobilization of upper respiratory fluids or mucus.

extracellular Outside of cells.

exudate Debris made of fluid and cells that are deposited in tissues in reaction to inflammation.

farrow The process of a sow giving birth to a litter of pigs.

FDA The Food and Drug Administration.

feed conversion The rate of gain compared with pounds consumed.

fermentation The process of chemically changing organic materials by the action of microorganisms.

fibrillation Rapid contractions of muscle fibers that lack functional rate or rhythm.

fibrosis The formation of fibrous connective tissue.

field strain Strains of microorganisms found in naturally occurring outbreaks of disease.

fit See *convulsion*.

flaccid Limp, soft, not giving resistance.

flora Referring to a population of bacteria and fungi (e.g., the flora of the gastrointestinal tract refers to the bacterial and fungal population of the intestinal tract).

foal (1) A newly born animal of the horse family. (2) The process of a mare giving birth.

gamma globulin Globulin found in plasma, which contains antibodies that attack foreign substances.

general anesthesia An anesthesia producing muscle relaxation, unconsciousness, and a loss of sensation throughout the body.

generic drug A nontrademarked drug with a name usually referring to its composition.

globulin A class of proteins that are involved in the makeup of antibodies. (See also *gamma globulin*.)

glomerular filtrate The substance that passes from the blood to the kidney tubules at the glomerulus.

glucocorticoid A corticosteroid that causes some degree of gluconeogenesis in the body.

gluconeogenesis The body process of manufacturing carbohydrates from molecules that are not carbohydrates but are primarily proteins.

glucose precursors Chemicals such as glycerol that the body can readily convert to glucose.

glycogen A starch produced in an animal's body and stored in muscle or liver tissue.

glycosuria The presence of sugar in the urine.

gonad A general term to describe the sexual glands, ovary, or testicle.

gonadotropin A hormone substance that stimulates the gonads. The gonadotropins are follicle-stimulating hormone and luteinizing hormone.

gram-negative bacteria Bacteria that, when stained with Gram's stain, lose the violet stain while retaining the counterstain.

gram-positive bacteria Bacteria that, when stained with Gram's stain, retain the characteristic violet stain.

half-life The amount of time it takes for half of a given dose to be either changed to an inactive form or eliminated from the body.

heat The period when a female animal is receptive to being bred; estrus.

hematoma Blood assembled extravascularly in a space, tissue, or organ.

hemoconcentration An increase in the blood's cellular and protein concentration caused by a decrease in the liquid content.

hemolytic toxin A toxin that causes the red blood cells to rupture.

hepatic Relating to, affecting, or resembling the liver.

hepatic portal vein The vein that extends from the intestinal tract to the liver.

hepatotoxic Injurious to the liver.

hepatotoxicity The ability to destroy or poison the liver or cells of the liver.

hormone A substance carried in the body that has an effect on other cell activities far from its source.

host A plant or animal nurturing another organism. The organism so nurtured is called a "parasite." (See also *intermediate host*.)

hydrolyze To fracture a compound by the addition of water.

hyperacidity An unusually great amount of acid.

hyperglycemia An unusually high level of glucose in the blood.

hyperglycemic Having increased levels of glucose in the blood.

hyperkalemia Elevated blood potassium levels.

hypermotility An abnormal degree of motility (spontaneous movement). This term is often used to refer to increased activity in the gastrointestinal tract.

hyperplasia A condition in which the number of normal cells in a tissue increase to an unusually large quantity.

hypersalivation Excessive salivation.

hypersensitivity A condition in which an animal's body responds more strongly than usual to an antigen. The reaction is harmful ranging from slight edema to anaphylaxis.

hyperthyroidism A condition in which an animal secretes excessive thyroid hormones.

hypertonic Having greater osmotic pressure than body fluids.

hypnotic A drug that encourages sleep.

hypoglycemia An unusually low level of glucose in the blood.

hypokalemia Decreased level of potassium in the blood.

hypotension Blood pressure lower than normal.

IBR See *infectious bovine rhinotracheitis*.

icterus The condition known as "jaundice." Jaundice is distinguished by the yellow color of the affected animal due to increased blood levels of bilirubin.

ileocecal valve The opening between the terminal ileum (the small intestine) and the cecum of the horse.

immunity Resistance to disease through appropriate antibodies that provide partial or total resistance to the harmful effects of specific infecting microorganisms. (See also *active immunity* and *passive immunity*.)

inactivated Refers to the type of microorganism contained in a vaccine; synonymous with the word "killed."

inactivated vaccine A vaccine containing killed organisms.

infectious bovine rhinotracheitis A viral upper respiratory disease of cattle.

infective larvae Immature parasite forms which are at a stage of development that renders them capable of infecting a host.

ingesta Substances taken into the stomach or rumen.

ingestion The process of taking in food.

innervation The number and types of nerves in a section.

instar An insect of the phylum Arthropoda that is between molts. After the last molt, the insect is an adult.

interference phenomenon Theory stating that a cell can only be infected by one virus at a time. Thus the presence of one virus type in a cell precludes the infection of the cell by another virus type.

intermediate host The animal or other organism, in which a parasite passes a mandatory larval stage. The adult parasite resides in a species other than the intermediate host.

interstitial fluid The liquid between cells.

interstitial space The space between cells.

intraarticular Being found or contained in a joint.

intracellular Within cells.

intracellular space The space within cells.

intussusception A telescoping of the intestines; the collapse of the intestines into themselves.

ionized Divided into a group of ions; atoms with an electrical charge.

irreversible shock Shock that cannot be remedied by treatment, resulting in death.

isotonic Having the same osmotic pressure as body fluids.

keratinization Formation of a simple protein that forms structures such as hair, nails, and horny tissue.

keratitis Inflammation of the cornea of the eye.

keratoconjunctivitis Inflammation of the conjunctiva and cornea of the eye.

keratoconjunctivitis sicca The inflammation and drying of the cornea and conjunctiva. This condition often hinders vision.

keratolytic drug A drug that makes the outer layer of skin peel or soften.

ketone bodies Chemical compounds containing the carbonyl group ($C=O$) that result from the metabolic breakdown of fats. Specifically the ketone bodies are acetoacetic acid, acetone, and β-hydroxybutyric acid.

ketosis An abnormally high level of ketone bodies in the blood.

kinetics That part of dynamics that deals with the rate of change of specific factors.

lacrimation The production of tears.

laminae Thin intermeshing sheetlike structures that line both the inner surface of the hoof and lie over the periosteum of the third phalanx bone. Laminae on the inner surface of the hoof are nonsensitive laminae, and those that lay over the third phalanx are sensitive laminae. Sensitive laminae contain blood vessels and nerves and supply nutrition to the hoof by way of the nonsensitive laminae.

laminitis Inflammation of the sensitive laminae of the hoof.

lapinized The process of weakening a microorganism by infecting rabbits in succession to modify its characteristics.

larva (pl. *larvae*) The immature form of an insect after hatching and before its maturation into adult form.

latent Hidden, unapparent potential.

LD$_{50}$ The dose that when given to a group of animals will cause death in 50% of the population.

legend drug A drug that must either be dispensed or prescribed by a veterinarian; the opposite of an over-the-counter drug.

legume A group of plants generally rich in proteins with broad leaves. Examples are alfalfa and peas.

lesion Recognizable abnormal tissue.

leukotoxin A substance toxic to white blood cells.

ligament Fibrous tissue that supports a joint by connecting bones.

lipid Referring to fat (e.g., "lipid-soluble," or soluble in fat or oil).

local anesthesia The loss of sensation in a limited area.

lumen The inside space of a tubular organ.

mange A disease distinguished by skin irritation caused by mites.

metabolic acidosis Acidosis resulting from increased production and retention of acid compounds or from abnormal losses of alkaline ions.

metabolism The chemical and energy transformations that occur in the body.

metabolize The process of making chemical and energy transformations. For example, metabolizing drugs refers to the process in which drugs are changed chemically.

MIC See *minimum inhibitory concentration.*

microflora Microorganisms.

micronize To pulverize a substance into very small particles that are measured in microns.

microorganism An extremely small living organism. This group includes fungi, bacteria, and viruses.

milk let-down The process of contraction of small muscles surrounding the saclike structures that produce milk in the mammary gland, forcing the milk into the milk cistern and teat cistern.

Millipore filter A product designed to filter solutions, removing very small particles often including bacteria.

mineralocorticoid A steroid manufactured by the outer layer of the adrenal gland (adrenal cortex) that causes sodium retention and potassium loss by way of the kidney.

minimum inhibitory concentration The concentration of an anti-infective drug required to inhibit growth of a particular organism.

miotic A drug that causes the pupil of the eye to constrict.

MLV See *modified live virus.*

modified live virus A living virus that has been changed so that when given in a vaccine it does not cause disease but results in the production of antibodies.

molt The process by which immature arthropods form a new second body covering under the first covering and subsequently shed the outside first covering.

monovalent vaccine A vaccine that contains only one type of antigen.

mucosa A mucous membrane.

muscarinic effect A reaction in which the parasympathetic nervous system is stimulated.

musculoskeletal Pertaining to or made up of the skeleton and muscles.

mycotic Referring to a fungus.

mydriasis A condition in which the pupils of the eye are dilated.

mydriatic A drug that causes the pupil of the eye to dilate.

myocardium The heart muscle.

myositis Inflammation of a muscle.

narrow spectrum Active against a narrow range of organisms. Thus narrow-spectrum antibiotics are active against relatively few bacterial strains.

necrosis Death of body tissues, especially in small areas.

necrotizing agent A substance causing necrosis.

nematode Any worm of the class Nematoda. Many nematodes are parasites and are commonly called "roundworms."

nephrotoxic Poisonous to kidney cells.

nerve See *afferent nerve, efferent nerve, parasympathetic nerve, peripheral nerve,* and *sympathetic nerve.*

neuromuscular blocking drug A drug that prevents the normal reaction at the area where nerves stimulate the release of acetylcholine and muscular contraction.

neurotoxic Damaging to nerve tissue.

neurotoxicity The ability of being neurotoxic.

neurotoxin A substance toxic to nerve tissue, often destroying the peripheral nerve sheaths.

neutropenia A condition in which the neutrophilic white blood cells are decreased in number.

nicotinic effect The effect of acetylcholine on the skeletal muscles.

nonionized Atoms or molecules without electrical charge.

normograph A chart that plots a given result against a known stimulus (e.g., a chart that predicts when puppies will lose material antibodies based on the serum levels of antibodies in the mother).

nymphomania A condition in which an animal shows continuous signs of heat.

nystagmus Rapid, involuntary movement of the eyeball.

organophosphate One of a class of external and internal pesticides that work by inhibiting the action of cholinesterase (an enzyme that breaks down acetylcholine to an inactive form).

osmosis The travel of water through a membrane that separates two solutions, tending to equalize the osmotic pressure of the solutions on both sides of the membrane.

OTC Over the counter, an expression referring to a nonprescription drug.

over-the-counter drug A drug that can be sold directly without a prescription; the opposite of a legend drug.

ovine Relating to sheep; sheeplike.

ovulation The process by which the ovum is released from the ovary.

oxygenation Supplying or combining with oxygen.

pacemaker The structure that sets the pace of or controls the rate at which the heart beats.

pannus The infiltration of the cornea of the eye with blood vessels.

panophthalmitis Disease or inflammation of the entire eye.

paradoxical Varying from the normal expected reaction, often reacting contrary to the expected reaction.

parasympathetic nerve The involuntary nerves that are responsible for the maintenance of the animal in a state of rest. Parasympathetic nerves tend to stimulate digestive processes, slow heart rate, and constrict the pupil of the eye.

parasympatholytic A substance that interrupts the effects of impulses carried by the parasympatholytic nerves. Such drugs counter the muscarinic effects of acetylcholine. Parasympatholytics typically slow intestinal movement, increase heart rate, and cause the pupil to dilate.

parasympathomimetic A substance that generates effects like those produced by stimulation of the parasympathetic nerves. They mimic the muscarinic effects of acetylcholine.

parenteral Commonly used to describe the administration of drugs by injection.

parturition Delivery or the process of giving birth.

passive immunity A means of providing antibodies by transferring them from one animal to another.

pathogen An organism that causes disease.

pathogenic Capable of causing disease.

pathology A field of medicine that studies the effects of disease on the structure and function of tissues.

penicillinase An enzyme produced by some bacteria that destroys certain penicillins.

perfusion Liquid poured over or through an organ or tissue.

pericardium The saclike membrane that contains the heart.

periosteum The connective tissue covering bones.

peripheral nerve Nerves other than those in the brain or spinal cord.

permeability The degree of penetration possible; the ability to be crossed.

pH Symbol used to indicate acidity or alkalinity. pH values are numbered from 0 to 14, 7 being neutral, 7 to 14 expressing alkalinity, and 0 to 7 expressing acidity. It is the negative log of the hydrogen ion concentration of a system.

pharyngitis Inflammation of the pharynx.

phlebitis Inflammation of a vein.

photophobia Intolerance to light.

phylogenetic Relating to the entire evolution of a group of animals.

placebo A substance with no biologic activity given to an animal as if it is an active drug.

plasma Blood's liquid fraction, containing separate suspended particles. It is the blood minus the blood cells.

polymerized The combining of simpler molecules of the same type into a more complex compound.

posterior segment The choroid of the eye (the posterior section of the uvea).

posterior synechiae Adhesions between the iris and lens.

potentiate To increase the activity.

potentiation The action of increasing the degree of a predicted response.

preanesthetic agent A drug that is given before an anesthetic to make the induction of the anesthetic safer and smoother.

primary bloat The accumulation of gas in the rumen due to the presence of foam.

proglottid One of the sections in the body of the mature tapeworm. The proglottids make up most of the mature tapeworm's body.

prophylactic Relating to prevention of disease.

proprietary compound A drug or formulation that is kept from free competition by a patent, copyright, trademark, or other means.

protozoan A one-celled organism of the phylum Protozoa.

pruritic Related to itching.

pruritus Itching.

pseudopregnancy A condition in which females exhibit a prolonged diestrus that resembles pregnancy; a false pregnancy.

pulmonary Relating to the lungs.

pylorus The opening from the stomach to the intestine.

pyoderma A primary or secondary infection of the skin by pus-forming bacteria.

pyometra The collecting of pus in the uterus.

pyrogen A substance that causes fever.

queen (1) A female cat. (2) The process of a female cat giving birth.

rate of gain The amount of weight gained by an animal over a defined period of time.

recumbent Lying down; not standing.

renal Pertaining to the kidney.

reservoir (1) An animal or group of animals that are infected with pathogenic microorganisms and that serve as a potential source of infection for a population. (2) A chemical or tissue in the body that tends to attract and hold specific drugs.

residue See *drug residue.*

respiratory acidosis Acidosis due to the retention of carbon dioxide from too little exchange of oxygen and carbon dioxide in the lungs.

retractor peni muscle The muscle that is used to pull the penis into the prepuce.

rhinitis Inflammation of the mucous membranes of the nose.

rubifacient A class of drugs that irritate the skin.

ruminant An animal that has a stomach divided into four digestive cavities. These animals constitute a separate order, including cattle, sheep, goats, and deer.

ruminatoric A drug that stimulates the movement of the rumen.

saline laxative A laxative consisting of nonabsorbable electrolytes that draw water into the intestinal tract and thereby increase intestinal movement.

scolex The head of a tapeworm that attaches to a host.

scours Diarrhea. This term is used often for diarrhea of infant animals or calves.

secondary bloat The accumulation of gas in the rumen due to obstruction in the esophagus.

sedation The process of calming animals.

sedative A drug that calms animals.

seizure See *convulsion.*

serotype The definition of microorganisms by the kinds of antigens present in their cells.

serum The clear fluid that separates from blood on clotting. It is blood minus the cells and clotting factors.

shock A condition of severe decrease in the effective circulatory blood volume caused by disturbance of circulatory control or loss of fluid. (See also *irreversible shock*).

shunt To shift or turn fluid from one place to another.

skeletal muscle Striated muscles attached to bones and that are under voluntary control.

slough To shed diseased tissue from the body, separating it from healthy tissue.

smooth muscle Nonstriated involuntary muscle.

spasmodic colic Abdominal pain resulting from hyperactivity of the equine gastrointestinal tract.

specific gravity The weight of a substance compared to the weight of an equal volume of another substance, usually water.

spectrum Range of activity, which is usually measurable. Thus narrow-spectrum antibiotics have activity against relatively few bacterial strains, whereas broad-spectrum antibiotics have activity against a wide range of bacterial strains.

sprain To wrench a joint, rupturing some fibers of a ligament but leaving most of the ligament intact; the condition resulting from overstraining a ligament.

stasis A lack of movement.

status epilepticus A continuous state of convulsions due to brain malfunction.

sternal recumbency To lie down in a position in which the body is in a normal dorsal ventral position relative to the ground; lying on the breast bone.

stomach tube Commonly used to describe a nasogastric tube that is placed in the nose of a horse and passed down the esophagus to the stomach. Liquid medication can be given to horses through a stomach tube.

subacute The stage between acute and chronic.

subconjunctival Under the conjunctiva (the membrane lining the eyelid and a portion of the sclera of the eye).

subcutaneous Under the skin; usually used to describe a route of injection.

suprainfection Infection by resistant bacteria, yeast, or fungi as a result of anti-infective therapy; especially used to describe the colonization of such organisms of the intestinal tract.

surfactants A compound that reduces the surface tension of a liquid.

sympathetic nerve Involuntary nerves that tend to prepare the animal for "flight or fighting." Sympathetic nerves cause the eye to dilate and the heart to beat faster and decrease activity of the gastrointestinal tract.

sympathomimetic A drug whose effects are like those of impulses given by sympathetic nervous system fibers.

syndrome A certain set of signs that appear together.

synechia The abnormal adhesion or sticking together of separate parts. (See also *anterior synechiae* and *posterior synechiae.*)

synergistic An action of two or more substances that is greater than the sum of the components.

synovial Relating to synovia, a fluid found in joint cavities.

synovial fluid The viscous fluid in joint cavities.

systole A contraction of the heart during which blood is forced into the arteries; the opposite of diastole.

tendon Dense connective tissues that connect muscle to another part such as a bone.

tetany A syndrome recognized by sharp spasms, convulsions, and muscle twitching.

therapeutician A person involved in the selection, use, or administration of therapy.

therapeutics Treatment and prevention of disease.

thrombocyte A platelet; a blood cell involved in the clotting process.

thrombophlebitis Inflammation of a vein associated with a vascular obstruction.

thromboplastic A substance that starts or encourages clotting.

thrombus Blood clot in and attached to a blood vessel at its site of origin.

tissue culture The growing of animal or plant cells in artificial environments.

titer Levels of antibodies as measured in the serum.

titrate To raise and lower a dose of a drug until the clinically effective level is obtained.

tocopherol Any alcohol having the properties of vitamin E.

topical Local application; external use.

torsion The action of twisting; especially used to describe the twisting of intestinal loops.

toxemia The presence of toxins or poisons in the blood.

toxic Relating to, resulting from, or similar to a poison; poisonous.

toxicosis A condition caused by poisons.

toxin A poisonous substance. (See also *hemolytic toxin.*)

toxoids Nonharmful chemicals, closely related to toxins, that are used to produce an active immunity against specific toxins.

trachea A tubular organ bringing air to the lungs (windpipe).

tranquilizer A drug that at clinical doses calms or quiets the animal without causing unconsciousness or depression of cardiac or respiratory function.

transient Passing, temporary.

tropic hormones Those hormones which stimulate the production and release of other hormones: adrenocorticotropic hormone (ACTH); the gonadotropic, follicle-stimulating, and luteinizing hormones; and thyroid-stimulating hormone.

tube worming The administration of an anthelmintic to horses through a nasogastric (stomach) tube.

turbinate bones Thin, fragile bones located in the nasal cavity.

unit A measure of biological activity accepted as a standard.

unthriftiness Referring to livestock that are underweight and generally in poor condition.

uremia A condition in which the body retains large amounts of waste products usually excreted in the urine.

urinary incontinence An inability to retain a normal amount of urine in the bladder resulting in involuntary passing of urine.

urolithiasis The obstruction of the urethra with a stone that formed in the urinary tract.

USP United States Pharmacopoeia, an organization that has determined standards of strength, quality, and purity for drugs.

uterine involution The return of the uterus after delivery to its normal nonpregnant condition.

uvea The vascular coat of the eye, which consists of the anterior segment (the iris and ciliary body) and posterior segment (the choroid).

vaccine A suspension of killed or attenuated bacteria or viruses that is inoculated to produce partial or complete immunity to a specific disease. (See also *attenuated vaccine, bivalent vaccine, inactivated vaccine,* and *monovalent vaccine.*)

vacuolization Referring to spaces or cavities.

vascular Relating to blood vessels.

vascularization The process of invasion with blood vessels.

vasoconstriction The constriction or narrowing of blood vessels.

vasodilation The expansion of a blood vessel lumen; usually the expansion of arterioles.

vasodilator A substance triggering dilation of arterioles.

vasopressor A substance triggering contraction of the muscular tissue of blood vessels, narrowing their lumen.

vehicle A substance in which a drug is dissolved, suspended, or mixed.

ventral Relating to the underside, belly, or abdomen; the opposite of dorsal.

venule Any small vessel that joins others to form veins. Venules receive blood from the capillary network and carry it to the veins.

virulence The degree to which an infectious substance can resist or destroy the protective mechanism of the host; the degree to which a substance can cause disease.

virus A substance belonging to a group of infectious organisms. Viruses lack the ability to metabolize independently of living cells, and living host cells are necessary for virus reproduction.

visceral pain Pain arising from a body organ, especially from the abdominal organs.

vitamins Organic substances that must be present in the body in small amounts for normal metabolism to take place.

volatile Tending to evaporate rapidly.

withdrawal time The interval between the last administration of a drug and the earliest time that either an animal can be slaughtered for food or milk or eggs from the animal can be used for food.

zoonotic infections Those infectious diseases transmitted from animals to humans.

Index

☐Page references to illustrations appear in italics; page numbers followed by t indicate tables.